Ear Diseases: Diagnostic Imaging and Therapeutics

Ear Diseases: Diagnostic Imaging and Therapeutics

Editor: Norma Hendricks

AMERICAN
MEDICAL PUBLISHERS
www.americanmedicalpublishers.com

AMERICAN
MEDICAL PUBLISHERS
www.americanmedicalpublishers.com

Cataloging-in-Publication Data

Ear diseases : diagnostic imaging and therapeutics / edited by Norma Hendricks.
p. cm.
Includes bibliographical references and index.
ISBN 979-8-88740-081-5
1. Ear--diseases. 2. Ear--diseases--Imaging. 3. Ear--diseases--Treatment. 4. Diagnostic imaging.
5. Ear--diseases--Diagnosis. I. Hendricks, Norma.
RF123.5.I4 E27 2023
617.807 54--dc23

American Medical Publishers,
41 Flatbush Avenue,
1st Floor, New York,
NY 11217, USA

ISBN 979-8-88740-081-5 (Hardback)

Contents

Preface

Over the recent decade, advancements and applications have progressed exponentially. This has led to the increased interest in this field and projects are being conducted to enhance knowledge. The main objective of this book is to present some of the critical challenges and provide insights into possible solutions. This book will answer the varied questions that arise in the field and also provide an increased scope for furthering studies.

The ear is a sensory system consisting of organs which help in hearing sounds. The main ear diseases include otosclerosis, Ménière's disease, tinnitus, barotrauma and presbycusis. Tinnitus is an ear disease which results in perception of sound in absence of any external sound. Otosclerosis is a disease caused due to the development of small bones in the ear. Ménière's disease is a condition affecting the inner parts of the ear resulting in hearing loss and pressure in the ear. The diagnosis of ear diseases generally involves a physical exam, assessment of medical and health history, and undertaking a hearing test. The requirement for imaging studies arises in case of suspicion of complications and when treatment does not work effectively. Computed tomography and magnetic resonance imaging are utilized to diagnose inner ear pathology. The drugs that are utilized to tackle the inner ear diseases include neurotrophins, corticosteroids, antioxidants, anesthetics and aminoglycoside antibiotics. This book provides comprehensive insights on ear diseases. It includes some of the vital pieces of work being conducted across the world, on various topics related to diagnostic imaging and therapeutics for diseases related to the ear. Medical professionals and students actively engaged in the study and management of these diseases will find this book full of crucial and unexplored concepts.

I hope that this book, with its visionary approach, will be a valuable addition and will promote interest among readers. Each of the authors has provided their extraordinary competence in their specific fields by providing different perspectives as they come from diverse nations and regions. I thank them for their contributions.

Editor

1

The Neural Mechanisms of Tinnitus: A Perspective from Functional Magnetic Resonance Imaging

Jinghua Hu[1†], Jinluan Cui[2†], Jin-Jing Xu[1], Xindao Yin[2], Yuanqing Wu[1] and Jianwei Qi[1*]*

[1] *Department of Otolaryngology, Nanjing First Hospital, Nanjing Medical University, Nanjing, China,* [2] *Department of Radiology, Nanjing First Hospital, Nanjing Medical University, Nanjing, China*

***Correspondence:**
Yuanqing Wu
cnnxdd@163.com
Jianwei Qi
qjw70818@163.com*

† These authors have contributed equally to this work

Tinnitus refers to sound perception in the absence of external sound stimulus. It has become a worldwide problem affecting all age groups especially the elderly. Tinnitus often accompanies hearing loss and some mood disorders like depression and anxiety. The comprehensive adverse effects of tinnitus on people determine the severity of tinnitus. Understanding the mechanisms of tinnitus and related discomfort may be beneficial to the prevention and treatment, and then getting patients out of tinnitus distress. Functional magnetic resonance imaging (fMRI) is a powerful technique for characterizing the intrinsic brain activity and making us better understand the tinnitus neural mechanism. In this article, we review fMRI studies published in recent years on the neuroimaging mechanisms of tinnitus. The results have revealed various neural network alterations in tinnitus patients, including the auditory system, limbic system, default mode network, attention system, and some other areas involved in memory, emotion, attention, and control. Moreover, changes in functional connectivity and neural activity in these networks are related to the perception, persistence, and severity of tinnitus. In summary, the neural mechanism of tinnitus is a complex regulatory mechanism involving multiple networks. Future research is needed to study these neural networks more accurately to refine the tinnitus models.

Keywords: tinnitus, neural mechanism, MRI, fMRI, functional connectivity

INTRODUCTION

Tinnitus

Tinnitus is defined as a phantom auditory perception without external sound stimulation. Tinnitus is common in otolaryngology, with a prevalence rate of 10–15% in adults (Henry et al., 2020) and about 32.0% in an elderly population (Chang et al., 2019). Bothersome tinnitus can cause mood disorders like depression, anxiety, and also leads to sleep disorders. In turn, these disorders can further exacerbate tinnitus (Bhatt et al., 2017). There could be a common neurobiological pathway involved in the development of both depression and tinnitus so that tinnitus sufferers may be particularly susceptible to the stress of the phantom sound (Pinto et al., 2014).

A universally agreed classification system for tinnitus has not been realized yet. Tinnitus can be classified by different methods based on clinical and etiological factors such as pulsatile or non-pulsatile (persistent), subjective or objective, conductive or sensorineural paralleling the way hearing loss is classified (Coelho et al., 2020). Pulsatile tinnitus (PT) is less frequent than non-pulsatile tinnitus (NPT) (Weissman and Hirsch, 2000). PT may be subjective or objective, while

NPT is subjective only (Weissman and Hirsch, 2000). The mechanisms of PT and NPT are different. The cause of PT can be vascular or myogenic, which can be diagnosed by imaging methods like CT and MRI (Pegge et al., 2017), but the cause of NPT is not entirely clear. Moreover, studies have found that patients with PT have abnormal functional connectivity (FC) in specific areas of the brain. Similar to NPT, long-term PT patients experience changes in auditory cortex and limbic system, which may be related to negative emotions like anxiety and depression (Zheng et al., 2019). There is an fMRI study that found a changed baseline brain activity in some limbic, frontal, and occipital areas. However, because of the relatively clear pathogenesis of PT, the changes in the brain were considered as results following the long-term sound stimulation but not the origin of tinnitus (Lv et al., 2016).

Since NPT is more common than PT clinically, when we use the term "tinnitus," it habitually refers to NPT. Early research on tinnitus focused on auditory pathways. It has been assumed for some time that cochlear dysfunction caused by environmental noise overexposure or cochlear trauma is the trigger of tinnitus (Shore and Wu, 2019). However, a small number of studies indicated that many patients still experience tinnitus after the cochlear lesions' complete recovery (Pulec, 1995). Although cochlear dysfunction is strongly associated with tinnitus, CNS must play a main contributory role (Bauer et al., 2008). As a result, an increasing number of researchers have investigated the CNS of a tinnitus brain.

There are several hypotheses about the central mechanism of tinnitus generation. It was found that normal auditory stimuli trigger gamma activity at the thalamus level (Metherate and Cruikshank, 1999), which is enhanced in tinnitus patients (Lorenz et al., 2009). So it was supposed that tinnitus may arise from ongoing inhibitory auditory alpha activity and enhanced gamma activity synchronization (Lorenz et al., 2009). In addition, another important hypothesis advocated that tinnitus originates from central neuroplasticity changes (Jinsheng, 2013; Kapolowicz and Thompson, 2020). It is assumed that the imbalance of excitatory and inhibitory inputs to auditory neurons leads to the plasticity change in the central auditory system (CAS). Sometimes this kind of plasticity adjustment goes beyond the CAS, eventually triggering abnormal activation of multiple systems including increased neuron spontaneous discharges and neural synchrony (Kaltenbach, 2011), so that the non-auditory systems associated with tinnitus deserves comprehensive studies too. The current tinnitus studies increasingly focus on the view that tinnitus is a multisystem problem, which involves memory, emotion, attention, and control networks. They together contribute to the generation and development of tinnitus sound perception and related characteristics (Laureano et al., 2014; Pattyn et al., 2016; Maudoux et al., 2017). Jastreboff (1990) proposed a neuropsychological model that demonstrates that whether tinnitus triggers anxiety or depression depends on whether the limbic systems are involved (Jastreboff and Hazell, 1993). Although there are many studies on the neural mechanism of tinnitus over the years, the exact mode of action and its associated pathophysiology remains an enigma.

Functional Magnetic Resonance Imaging

During the past several years, the rapid development of neuroimaging techniques has contributed greatly in the non-invasive imaging studies of tinnitus. Increasing numbers of studies on tinnitus have focused on cerebral FC. Previous electrophysiological studies using magnetoencephalography (MEG) or electroencephalography (EEG) have shown alterative neural activities and connectivity in the brain of tinnitus (Nathan et al., 2005; Vanneste and De Ridder, 2012). EEG and MEG techniques have a better temporal resolution but poor anatomical resolution, while functional brain imaging techniques have better structural resolution to make better interpretation on the exact location of the source of the signal (e.g., fMRI) (Han et al., 2016).

The fMRI in a narrow sense only refers to blood oxygen level-dependent fMRI (BOLD-fMRI), which uses blood contrast to observe changes in blood oxygenation in the progress of neural activity. Two main research methods are task-based fMRI and rest-state fMRI (rs-fMRI). In studies of tinnitus mechanism and treatment, task-based fMRI design generally utilizes sound stimulus to induce the blood oxygen changes in some related areas (James et al., 2017; Zimmerman B. et al., 2019), while rs-fMRI is usually used to analyze the FC between different seeds in regions of interest (ROI). Compared to task-based fMRI, the rs-fMRI technique does not require complex task design and cooperation of patients with the task (Sair et al., 2016), so that it can directly and comprehensively reflects the spontaneous nerve activity and functional connection networks. Since tinnitus is characterized by highly subjective sound hallucinations, and there is no task-based modulation of the tinnitus signal, rs-fMRI has been proven to be a powerful technique for characterizing the intrinsic brain activity in patients with tinnitus (Husain and Schmidt, 2014; Zhou et al., 2019). The amplitude of low frequency fluctuations (ALFF) and regional homogeneity (ReHo) are methods commonly used in rs-fMRI data analysis to reflect different aspects of regional neural activity, while FC density analysis, seed-based FC analysis, independent component analysis (ICA), and graph analysis are used to analyze the FC of different brain regions (Lv et al., 2018).

In a broader sense, fMRI also includes diffusion weighted imaging (DWI), perfusion weighted imaging (PWI), susceptibility weighted imaging (SWI), and magnetic resonance spectroscopy (MRS). Diffusion tensor imaging (DTI) is a special form of DWI. It can evaluate the anisotropy of white matter (WM), so that WM fiber bundles can be observed and tracked effectively. DTI was widely used in some neurological disorders, such as Alzheimer's disease (Bigham et al., 2020) and schizophrenia (Ochi et al., 2020). Chen Q. et al. (2020) conducted a tinnitus study by using DTI. The results showed that tinnitus is related to changes in WM integrity in some brain regions including corpus callosum and cingulum. ASL is one kind of PWI technique to quantify cerebral blood flow (CBF) using the labeling arterial blood as an endogenous tracer (Ferré et al., 2013). One of the latest ASL study of tinnitus found decreased CBF in the auditory and prefrontal cortex. Interestingly, the degree of headache of tinnitus patients is related to the CBF decrease (Chen Y. C. et al., 2020). SWI shows intrinsic differences in magnetic sensitivity between tissues, such as bleeding and abnormal deposition of iron ions, thus reflecting pathological changes (Guo et al., 2020). At present, it is rarely used in the study of subjective tinnitus. In view of an ASL study on CBF changes in a tinnitus patient, it may be valuable for tinnitus research in the future. MRS is an emerging MRI technology. Taking ^{1}H or ^{31}P as the object of spectrum examination, the concentration of metabolite markers can be calculated, such as N-acetyl aspartate (NAA), lactic acid (Lac), choline (Cho), and so on (He et al., 2020). It is usually used in the differential diagnosis of tumors (Hekmatnia et al., 2019) and neurological disease study, such as epilepsy (Abedi-Firouzjah et al., 2020), Alzheimer's disease, and cognitive impairment (Chandra et al., 2019). Studies have explored the connection between chronic tinnitus and mild cognitive impairment. Maybe the MRS technique will be of help in the further related study. Combining two or more fMRI tools can help with a comprehensive analysis of neuropathological changes from multiple perspectives (Yeo et al., 2018). That is called multimodal fMRI analysis technique. A number of researches have combined functional and structural measurements on tinnitus studies (Luan et al., 2019). This technique has a great application foreground for its comprehensiveness.

Thanks to the rapid development of fMRI technology, we have found a range of abnormal changes in both central auditory system (CAS) and some non-auditory system of people with tinnitus (Kim et al., 2012; Maudoux et al., 2017; Minami et al., 2018). In addition, the DMN, the attention system, and some other areas responsible for memory, emotion, attention, and control are involved in tinnitus, as well as the distress associated with these persistent phantom (more on that below). To better understand the neural network of tinnitus, this review provides a critical review of fMRI studies published in recent years on the neuroimaging mechanisms of tinnitus. **Figure 1** gives an overview of the tinnitus-related brain areas based on fMRI.

Central Auditory System

Important structures in the auditory pathway of tinnitus patients, such as the cochlear nucleus, lateral colliculus, inferior colliculus nucleus, medial geniculate body, and cerebral auditory cortex, are likely to play a role in the occurrence of the phantom sound of tinnitus (Kris et al., 2014), suggesting that the initial tinnitus signal is produced by hyperactivity in the central auditory pathway (Rauschecker et al., 2010). Structural and functional anomalies of the CAS have been found in tinnitus (Cai et al., 2019). Studies have found gray matter and white matter alert in the auditory cortex of tinnitus patients (Boyen et al., 2013; Schmidt et al., 2018). A recent fMRI study found decreased ReHo in the primary auditory cortex and increased ReHo in some secondary auditory regions like supramarginal and angular gyri (Anthony et al., 2019). Emmert et al. combined ASL, task-based, and rest-state fMRI to study how tinnitus patients regulate their own brain activity by continuous and intermittent feedback. It was found that secondary auditory areas might be more susceptible to intermittent feedback modulation (Emmert et al., 2017). This may be related to a compensation mechanism in these secondary auditory areas of tinnitus.

However, a contradicting result was obtained that shows that there are no significant differences in the auditory cortical FC between chronic subjective tinnitus and the control group after correcting for multiple statistical comparisons (Davies et al., 2014). This result indicated that auditory network connectivity was not modified by the experience of tinnitus. They also found altered FC in brain regions related to attention and emotional

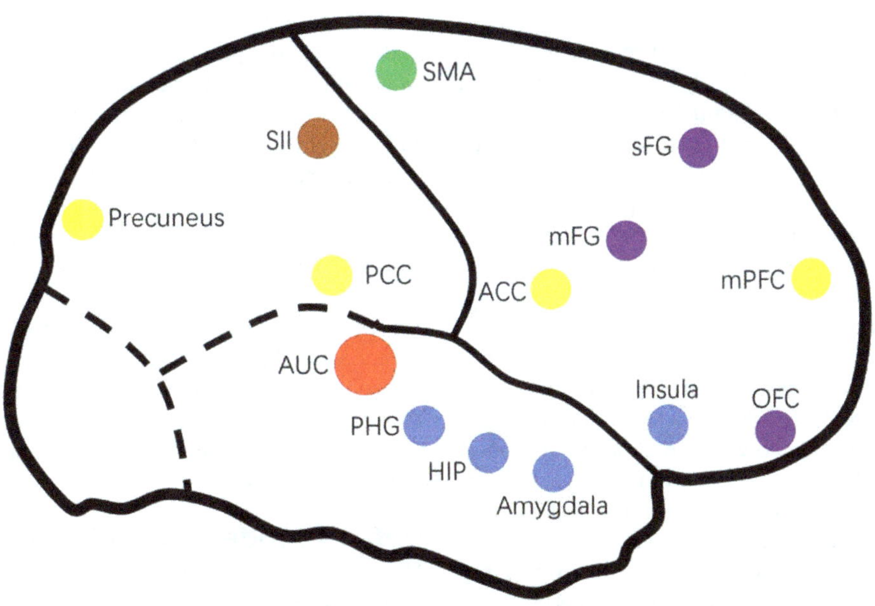

FIGURE 1 | Overview of the tinnitus-related brain areas based on fMRI. AUC, auditory cortex; ACC, anterior cingulate cortex; HIP, hippocampus; mFG, medial frontal cortex; mPFC, medial prefrontal cortex; OFC, orbitofrontal cortex; PCC, posterior cingulate cortex; PHG, parahippocampus; sFG, superior frontal gyrus.

processing only in bothersome tinnitus. The different result may be caused by many factors such as the tinnitus laterality, the hearing threshold, the severity of the distress, and annoyance. So more studies need to be conducted to compare subgroups with different levels of the abovementioned tinnitus-related features in order to confirm the mechanism of CAS in tinnitus.

Tinnitus is often accompanied by hearing loss but not vice versa (Ovidiu et al., 2006). Some studies attempted to dissociate the effect of tinnitus from hearing loss. It was found that hearing loss causes greater gray and white matter alterations than tinnitus (Husain et al., 2011a), especially in the primary auditory cortex and limbic area of the frontal lobe (Boyen et al., 2013). Hearing loss patients with or without tinnitus have different neural activities and functional changes in the CNS (Kris et al., 2014). Increased connectivity was found between the limbic and auditory regions of hearing loss with tinnitus (Schmidt et al., 2013). To tinnitus patients, hearing loss seems to drive the communication between these two areas and enhance memory-related activity of the hippocampus (Vanneste and De Ridder, 2016). The association of tinnitus and hearing loss makes patients suffer more severe discomfort (Savastano, 2008). Therefore, in the study of the tinnitus neural network, hearing loss should be taken into consideration as an especially important factor.

Limbic System

The limbic system is termed as the "feeling and reacting brain," which can respond to emotional stimulation. It is also implicated in memory, especially the emotional-related part (Rajmohan and Mohandas, 2007). The composition of the limbic system is controversial, but it includes the parahippocampus, amygdala, hippocampus, anterior cingulate cortex (ACC), and partial basal ganglia (Rajmohan and Mohandas, 2007).

Jastreboff (1990) regarded the limbic system as the main source of psychological responses related to tinnitus for its important role in behavior and emotional expression (Jastreboff and Hazell, 1993). The indispensable role of the limbic system in tinnitus is well established. The initial tinnitus signal may generate from parts of the auditory system, which can be blocked by the limbic system. However, in patients with chronic tinnitus, limbic system damage and resulting inefficiency of auditory–limbic interactions lead to the failure of this inhibition (Rauschecker et al., 2010; Leaver et al., 2016). There were also researchers suggesting that abnormal activation of the limbic structures may occur at an early stage of tinnitus and maintaining this condition throughout the tinnitus period (Kapolowicz and Thompson, 2020). The exact relationship between the limbic system and auditory system has become a hot topic in recent years. Numerous brain imaging studies and conceptual models of tinnitus has demonstrated increased functional and anatomical connectivity between the auditory and limbic regions (Maudoux et al., 2012; Seydell-Greenwald et al., 2014; Chen et al., 2017b).

It is thought that sustained increase in the activity of the parahippocampus leads to adaptive dysfunction, which inhibits adaptation to tinnitus and mis-transmits auditory memory stored in the hippocampus (Sven et al., 2011). The hippocampus and amygdala could also have a role in the persistence of tinnitus by updating auditory memory for tinnitus (Elham and Ghassem, 2018). Gunbey et al. (2017) conducted a DTI study finding a negative relation between the hippocampus–amygdala fractional anisotropy values and tinnitus severity. A recent study applied cyclicity analysis to fMRI data, revealing that the pairs of brain regions connected to the amygdala contributed most to the differences between tinnitus and controls (Zimmerman B. J. et al., 2019). Another fMRI study examined how amygdala acted on emotional sound processing in tinnitus subjects. It suggested enhanced amygdala activation in bothersome tinnitus. To those who successfully adapted to the emotionally negative sound, the emotional response of the amygdala decreased (Davies et al., 2017). These evidences reveal that some of tinnitus brain generators share common resources with brain memory and emotion generators, which may contribute to the persistence of the phantom bothersome sound.

In patients with tinnitus, spontaneous nerve activity and FC are enhanced in the insula (Carpenter-Thompson et al., 2014). The increased response in the insula, mainly the anterior part, may reflect adaption to the tinnitus perception by focusing attention on non-auditory events (van der Loo et al., 2011; Harold et al., 2012). Furthermore, the insula is one of the key nodes in the common brain circuit of both chronic tinnitus and pain (Dirk et al., 2011; Rauschecker et al., 2015). Areas including insula, ventromedial prefrontal cortex (vmPFC), and nucleus accumbens (NAc) act as a central gating system for sensory perception, which determines the sentimental value of sensory stimuli and modulates information transmission in the brain (Rauschecker et al., 2015). Dirk et al. (2011) thought this gating system is a non-specific distress network through the involvement of learning mechanisms and memory mechanisms, and then proposed a working model for the origin of phantom pain and phantom sound. Tinnitus and chronic pain occur when this system is compromised (Chen et al., 2017a). It suggested that tinnitus and neuropathic pain share an overlapping brain network with common activation and connectivity patterns and are differentiated by a specific mechanism (Vanneste et al., 2019). Furthermore, NAc, vmPFC, and subgenual ACC (sgACC) form a frontostriatal top–down gating system, which related to top–down noise cancelation and perceptual learning (Hullfish et al., 2019). A study (Xu et al., 2019) that combined MRI with granger causality analysis (GCA) found directional connectivity were enhanced between the NAc and PFC in the chronic tinnitus group compared to the control group, and this enhancement was positively correlated with tinnitus duration and distress. It is confirmed that the frontostriatal gating control system is important in tinnitus and pain perception. These hypotheses can help us better understand the mechanism of the distress associated with tinnitus and may extend to other similar phantoms.

Default Mode Network (DMN)

The DMN is a brain system in which the activity increases in the resting state and decreases in the task state (Shulman et al., 1997). DMN is generally considered to be composed of the posterior cingulate cortex (PCC)/precuneus, ACC, medial prefrontal cortex(mPFC), and angular gyrus (Mantini et al., 2007).

Some studies proposed that the generation of tinnitus may be associated with the abnormalities in the DMN. Lanting et al. (2016) conducted an fMRI study combined with independent component analysis (ICA). The data of the two kinds of state (fixed-state and resting state) were obtained for both tinnitus and control group. They found in the tinnitus patients that the DMN was less extensive and showed significantly less connectivity in both states. At the same time, the activity of DMN was not stronger during the resting-state than during the fixed-state. They attribute this pattern to the unremitting engaging effect of the tinnitus perception.

Chronic tinnitus patients show significantly enhanced FC between the ACC and left precuneus, which was correlated with the tinnitus duration (Chen et al., 2018b). In addition, enhanced FC between the PCC and mPFC was positively correlated with the tinnitus distress (Chen et al., 2018a,c). Among them, lack of cognitive control function caused by alterations in PFC may play a pivotal role in tinnitus generation and persistence (Seydell-Greenwald et al., 2012; Rodrigo et al., 2018). This result is similar to a previous study of Schmidt et al., which examined two sources of variability in the subgroups: tinnitus severity and duration. They observed decreased correlations between DMN and the precuneus, which were consistent across individuals with long-term tinnitus. More bothersome tinnitus demonstrated stronger decrease. So the connectivity of the precuneus could serve as a marker for long duration tinnitus and index tinnitus severity (Schmidt et al., 2017). They hypothesize that the enhancement of DMN-precuneus connectivity could reduce the severity of tinnitus. The role of DMN in tinnitus was verified from another aspect that the neurofeedback training of the PCC can relieve tinnitus-related distress (Sven et al., 2018). Moreover, there are studies that revealed that DMN was related to the severity of mood symptoms and cognitive dysfunction in some mental illnesses like Alzheimer's disease, schizophrenia, and infantile autism (Binnewijzend et al., 2012; Olivito et al., 2017; Lee et al., 2019). Perhaps DMN plays a similar role in tinnitus, so a neural model of these similar mental illness can be a reference.

Attention and Control System

There is a lot of evidence indicating that some cortical area of the brain, particularly those networks responsible for attention, focus, and cognitive control also have abnormal activity and FC in tinnitus (Harold et al., 2012).

Attentional network can be divided into the dorsal attention network (DAN) and ventral attention network (VAN). The DAN comprises the intraparietal sulcus (IPS) and the frontal eye fields (FEF), while the the VAN comprises the temporoparietal junction (TPJ) and the ventral frontal cortex (VFC) (Vossel et al., 2014). Many fMRI studies have focused on these brain regions. Husain et al. (2011b) found a decreased activation in the DAN areas, which may be involved in auditory attention and short-term memory network, and a pivotal difference between tinnitus and hearing loss in neural bases. Schmidt et al. (2013, 2017) found an increased FC in tinnitus patients between the DAN and parahippocampus as well as the precuneus, and that was associated with tinnitus severity. Besides, it was found in bothersome tinnitus that the FC for primary visual cortex involved significant negative correlations in CAS, VAN, and some executive control network components. It indicated a dissociation activity between visual, auditory, attention, and control networks in tinnitus. That might reflect a mechanism of adaptation to chronic bothersome tinnitus that reduces the salience of phantom noises and directing attention to non-auditory events (Burton et al., 2012). These studies suggested that improving the function of attention system and mitigating the connectivity between limbic regions, attention, and auditory system could be an effective therapy to reduce tinnitus and related distress.

The cognitive control network (CCN), which directs attentional focus may have a basic role in tinnitus maintenance (Trevis et al., 2016). Decreased activation of the CCN (right middle frontal gyrus is the core node), decreased connectivity between the CCN and salience network (SN), and increased connectivity between the CCN and autobiographical memory networks (AMN) were found in tinnitus (Trevis et al., 2017). The dysfunction and ineffective connection of CCN leading to failure of switching attention away from the noisy environment to a task that requires cognition, contributes to persistent awareness of the phantom sound (Trevis et al., 2017).

CONCLUSION

Combined with prior fMRI research literatures on tinnitus neural network, it is believed that both auditory and non-auditory systems play an important role in tinnitus. The damaged structure and function of the auditory system leads to the origin of tinnitus, but the non-auditory system is indispensable in the continuous perception of tinnitus and is related to some tinnitus characteristics such as duration, severity, loudness, and tinnitus-related distress. Future research should confirm whether the neural network changes found in non-auditory areas of the brain of tinnitus patients are a cause of tinnitus or the result of tinnitus signals being continuously transmitted in these networks. fMRI is certainly a useful tool for exploring neural networks of the tinnitus and similar mental disorders. Research combined with multiple MRI tools would be more helpful. A relatively explicit mechanism can contribute to therapeutical intervention of tinnitus.

AUTHOR CONTRIBUTIONS

JH and JC checked the references and wrote the manuscript. J-JX and XY helped review and revise the manuscript. YW and JQ contributed to the discussion and manuscript revision. All authors contributed to the article and approved the submitted version.

REFERENCES

Abedi-Firouzjah, R., Rostamzadeh, A., Banaei, A., Shafiee, M., Moghaddam, Z. M., and Vafapour, H. (2020). Exploring changes in thalamus metabolites as diagnostic biomarkers in idiopathic generalised epilepsy patients using magnetic resonance spectroscopy. *Malays. J. Med. Sci. MJMS* 27, 78–86. doi: 10.21315/mjms2020.27.1.8

Anthony, G., Jeremy, D., Nicolas, M. D. C., Jean-Luc, P., Emmanuelle, L. B., and Frédéric, V. (2019). Alterations in regional homogeneity in patients with unilateral chronic tinnitus. *Trends Hear.* 23, 1–12.

Bauer, C. A., Turner, J. G., Caspary, D. M., Myers, K. S., and Brozoski, T. J. (2008). Tinnitus and inferior colliculus activity in chinchillas related to three distinct patterns of cochlear trauma. *J. Neurosci. Res.* 86, 2564–2578. doi: 10.1002/jnr.21699

Bhatt, J. M., Bhattacharyya, N., and Lin, H. W. (2017). Relationships between tinnitus and the prevalence of anxiety and depression. *Laryngoscope* 127, 466–469. doi: 10.1002/lary.26107

Bigham, B., Zamanpour, S. A., Zemorshidi, F., Boroumand, F., Zare, H., and Initiative, A. S. D. N. (2020). Identification of superficial white matter abnormalities in alzheimer's disease and mild cognitive impairment using diffusion tensor imaging. *J. Alzheimer's Dis. Rep.* 4, 49–59. doi: 10.3233/adr-190149

Binnewijzend, M. A., Schoonheim, M. M., Sanz-Arigita, E., Wink, A. M., van der Flier, W. M., Tolboom, N., et al. (2012). Resting-state fMRI changes in Alzheimer's disease and mild cognitive impairment. *Neurobiol. Aging* 33, 2018–2028.

Boyen, K., Langers, D. R., De Kleine, E., and Van Dijk, P. (2013). Gray matter in the brain: differences associated with tinnitus and hearing loss. *Hear. Res.* 295, 67–78. doi: 10.1016/j.heares.2012.02.010

Burton, H., Wineland, A., Bhattacharya, M., Nicklaus, J., Garcia, K. S., and Piccirillo, J. F. (2012). Altered networks in bothersome tinnitus: a functional connectivity study. *BMC Neurosci.* 13:3.

Cai, W. W., Li, Z. C., Yang, Q. T., and Zhang, T. (2019). Abnormal spontaneous neural activity of the central auditory system changes the functional connectivity in the tinnitus brain: a resting-state functional MRI study. *Front. Neurosci.* 13:1314. doi: 10.3389/fnins.2019.01314

Carpenter-Thompson, J. R., Akrofi, K., Schmidt, S. A., Dolcos, F., and Husain, F. T. (2014). Alterations of the emotional processing system may underlie preserved rapid reaction time in tinnitus. *Brain Res.* 1567, 28–41. doi: 10.1016/j.brainres.2014.04.024

Chandra, A., Dervenoulas, G., Politis, M., and Initiative, A. S. D. N. (2019). Magnetic resonance imaging in Alzheimer's disease and mild cognitive impairment. *J. Neurol.* 266, 1293–1302.

Chang, N. C., Dai, C. Y., Lin, W. Y., Yang, H. L., Wang, H. M., Chien, C. Y., et al. (2019). Prevalence of persistent tinnitus and dizziness in an elderly population in Southern Taiwan. *J. Int. Adv. Otol.* 15, 99–105. doi: 10.5152/iao.2019.6257

Chen, Q., Wang, Z., Lv, H., Zhao, P., Yang, Z., Gong, S., et al. (2020). Reorganization of brain white matter in persistent idiopathic tinnitus patients without hearing loss: evidence from baseline data. *Front. Neurosci.* 14:591. doi: 10.3389/fnins.2020.00591

Chen, Y. C., Chen, H., Bo, F., Xu, J. J., Deng, Y., Lv, H., et al. (2018a). Tinnitus distress is associated with enhanced resting-state functional connectivity within the default mode network. *Neuropsychiatr. Dis. Treat.* 14, 1919–1927. doi: 10.2147/ndt.s164619

Chen, Y. C., Hu, J. H., Cui, J. L., Shang, S. A., Yong, W., Xu, J. J., et al. (2020). Headache is associated with aberrant cerebral blood flow in chronic tinnitus revealed by perfusion functional MRI. *Res. Square* [Epub ahead of print].

Chen, Y. C., Liu, S., Lv, H., Bo, F., Feng, Y., Chen, H., et al. (2018b). Abnormal resting-state functional connectivity of the anterior cingulate cortex in unilateral chronic tinnitus patients. *Front. Neurosci.* 12:9. doi: 10.3389/fnins.2018.00009

Chen, Y. C., Wang, F., Wang, J., Bo, F., Xia, W., Gu, J. P., et al. (2017a). Resting-state brain abnormalities in chronic subjective tinnitus: a meta-analysis. *Front. Hum. Neurosci.* 11:22. doi: 10.3389/fnhum.2017.00022

Chen, Y. C., Xia, W., Chen, H., Feng, Y., Xu, J. J., Gu, J. P., et al. (2017b). Tinnitus distress is linked to enhanced resting-state functional connectivity from the limbic system to the auditory cortex. *Hum. Brain Mapp.* 38, 2384–2397. doi: 10.1002/hbm.23525

Chen, Y. C., Zhang, H., Kong, Y., Lv, H., Cai, Y., Chen, H., et al. (2018c). Alterations of the default mode network and cognitive impairment in patients with unilateral chronic tinnitus. *Quant. Imaging Med. Surg.* 8, 1020–1029. doi: 10.21037/qims.2018.11.04

Coelho, C. B., Santos, R., Campara, K. F., and Tyler, R. (2020). Classification of tinnitus: multiple causes with the same name. *Otolaryngol. Clin. North Am.* 53, 515–529.

Davies, J., Gander, P. E., Andrews, M., and Hall, D. A. (2014). Auditory network connectivity in tinnitus patients: a resting-state fMRI study. *Int. J. Audiol.* 53, 192–198. doi: 10.3109/14992027.2013.846482

Davies, J. E., Gander, P. E., and Hall, D. A. (2017). Does chronic tinnitus alter the emotional response function of the amygdala?: a sound-evoked fMRI study. *Front. Aging Neurosci.* 9:31. doi: 10.3389/fnagi.2017.00031

Dirk, D. R., Belen, E. A., Ranulfo, R., and Berthold, L. (2011). Phantom percepts: tinnitus and pain as persisting aversive memory networks. *Proc. Natl. Acad. Sci. U.S.A.* 108, 8075–8080. doi: 10.1073/pnas.1018466108

Elham, T., and Ghassem, M. (2018). A different view on the link between tinnitus and cognition; is there a reciprocal link? *Int. J. Neurosci.* 128, 1188–1198. doi: 10.1080/00207454.2018.1503185

Emmert, K., Kopel, R., Koush, Y., Maire, R., Senn, P., Van De Ville, D., et al. (2017). Continuous vs. intermittent neurofeedback to regulate auditory cortex activity of tinnitus patients using real-time fMRI - A pilot study. *NeuroImage Clin.* 14, 97–104. doi: 10.1016/j.nicl.2016.12.023

Ferré, J. C., Bannier, E., Raoult, H., Mineur, G., Carsin-Nicol, B., and Gauvrit, J. Y. (2013). Arterial spin labeling (ASL) perfusion: techniques and clinical use. *Diagn. Intervent. Imaging* 94, 1211–1223. doi: 10.1016/j.diii.2013.06.010

Gunbey, H. P., Gunbey, E., Aslan, K., Bulut, T., Unal, A., and Incesu, L. (2017). Limbic-auditory interactions of tinnitus: an evaluation using diffusion tensor imaging. *Clin. Neuroradiol.* 27, 221–230. doi: 10.1007/s00062-015-0473-0

Guo, X., Ma, L., Li, H., Qi, X., Wei, Y., Duan, Z., et al. (2020). Brainstem iron overload and injury in a rat model of brainstem hemorrhage. *J. Stroke Cerebrovas. Dis.* 29:104956. doi: 10.1016/j.jstrokecerebrovasdis.2020.104956

Han, Y., Lei, D., Min, Z., Vadim, Z., Raquel, P., and Jerzy, B. (2016). Reconstructing large-scale brain resting-state networks from high-resolution EEG: spatial and temporal comparisons with fMRI. *Brain Connect.* 6, 122–135. doi: 10.1089/brain.2014.0336

Harold, B., Andre, W., Mousumi, B., Joyce, N., Keith, S. G., and Jay, F. P. (2012). Altered networks in bothersome tinnitus: a functional connectivity study. *BMC Neurosci.* 13:3. doi: 10.1186/1471-2202-13-3

He, Y. N., Meng, Y., Gao, N.-N., Zhang, B.-J., Li, H., and Ji, S.-S. (2020). Effect of injecting mouse nerve growth factor in different ways on motor development, cerebral hemodynamics and biochemical metabolism in children with cerebral palsy. *Chinese Acupuncture Moxibustion* 40, 839–844.

Hekmatnia, A., Sabouri, M., Ghazavi, A. H., Far, P. S., Hekmatnia, F., Sofi, G. J., et al. (2019). Diagnostic value of magnetic resonance spectroscopy (MRS) for detection of brain tumors in patients. *Med. Sci.* 23, 939–945.

Henry, J. A., Reavis, K. M., Griest, S. E., Thielman, E. J., Theodoroff, S. M., Grush, L. D., et al. (2020). Tinnitus: an epidemiologic perspective. *Otolaryngol. Clin. North Am.* 53, 481–499.

Hullfish, J., Abenes, I., Yoo, H. B., De Ridder, D., and Vanneste, S. (2019). Frontostriatal network dysfunction as a domain—general mechanism underlying phantom perception. *Hum. Brain Mapp.* 40, 2241–2251. doi: 10.1002/hbm.24521

Husain, F. T., Medina, R. E., Davis, C. W., Szymko-Bennett, Y., Simonyan, K., Pajor, N. M., et al. (2011a). Neuroanatomical changes due to hearing loss and chronic tinnitus: a combined VBM and DTI study. *Brain Res.* 1369, 74–88. doi: 10.1016/j.brainres.2010.10.095

Husain, F. T., Pajor, N. M., Smith, J. F., Kim, H. J., Rudy, S., Zalewski, C., et al. (2011b). Discrimination task reveals differences in neural bases of tinnitus and hearing impairment. *PLoS One* 6:e26639. doi: 10.1371/journal.pone.0026639

Husain, F. T., and Schmidt, S. A. (2014). Using resting state functional connectivity to unravel networks of tinnitus. *Hear. Res.* 307, 153–162. doi: 10.1016/j.heares.2013.07.010

James, G. A., Thostenson, J. D., Brown, G., Carter, G., Hayes, H., Tripathi, S. P., et al. (2017). Neural activity during attentional conflict predicts reduction in tinnitus perception following rTMS. *Brain Stimul.* 10, 934–943. doi: 10.1016/j.brs.2017.05.009

Jastreboff, P. J. (1990). Phantom auditory perception (tinnitus): mechanisms of generation and perception. *Neurosci. Res.* 8, 221–254. doi: 10.1016/0168-0102(90)90031-9

Jastreboff, P. J., and Hazell, J. W. (1993). A neurophysiological approach to tinnitus: clinical implications. *Br. J. Audiol.* 27, 7–17. doi: 10.3109/03005369309077884

Jinsheng, Z. (2013). Auditory cortex stimulation to suppress tinnitus: mechanisms and strategies. *Hear. Res.* 295, 38–57. doi: 10.1016/j.heares.2012.05.007

Kaltenbach, J. A. (2011). Tinnitus: models and mechanisms. *Hear. Res.* 276, 52–60. doi: 10.1016/j.heares.2010.12.003

Kapolowicz, M. R., and Thompson, L. T. (2020). Plasticity in limbic regions at early time points in experimental models of tinnitus. *Front. Syst. Neurosci.* 13:88. doi: 10.3389/fnsys.2019.00088

Kim, J. Y., Kim, Y. H., Lee, S. H., Seo, J. H., Song, H. J., Cho, J. H., et al. (2012). Alteration of functional connectivity in tinnitus brain revealed by resting-state fMRI?: a pilot study. *Int. J. Audiol.* 51, 413–417. doi: 10.3109/14992027.2011.652677

Kris, B., Emile, D. K., Pim, V. D., and Langers, D. R. M. (2014). Tinnitus-related dissociation between cortical and subcortical neural activity in humans with mild to moderate sensorineural hearing loss. *Hear. Res.* 312, 48–59. doi: 10.1016/j.heares.2014.03.001

Lanting, C., Wozaniak, A., Van Dijk, P., and Langers, D. R. M. (2016). Tinnitus- and task-related differences in resting-state networks. *Adv. Exp. Med. Biol.* 894, 175–187. doi: 10.1007/978-3-319-25474-6_19

Laureano, M. R., Onishi, E. T., Bressan, R. A., Castiglioni, M. L. V., Batista, I. R., Reis, M. A., et al. (2014). Memory networks in tinnitus: a functional brain image study. *PLoS One* 9:e87839. doi: 10.1371/journal.pone.0087839

Leaver, A. M., Seydell-Greenwald, A., and Rauschecker, J. P. (2016). Auditory–limbic interactions in chronic tinnitus: challenges for neuroimaging research. *Hear. Res.* 334, 49–57. doi: 10.1016/j.heares.2015.08.005

Lee, H., Lee, D. K., Park, K., Kim, C. E., and Ryu, S. (2019). Default mode network connectivity is associated with long-term clinical outcome in patients with schizophrenia. *NeuroImage Clinical* 22:101805. doi: 10.1016/j.nicl.2019.101805

Lorenz, I., Müller, N., Schlee, W., Hartmann, T., and Weisz, N. (2009). Loss of alpha power is related to increased gamma synchronization—A marker of reduced inhibition in tinnitus? *Neurosci. Lett.* 453, 225–228. doi: 10.1016/j.neulet.2009.02.028

Luan, Y., Wang, C., Jiao, Y., Tang, T., Zhang, J., and Teng, G.-J. (2019). Prefrontal-temporal pathway mediates the cross-modal and cognitive reorganization in sensorineural hearing loss with or without tinnitus: a multimodal MRI study. *Front. Neurosci.* 13:222. doi: 10.3389/fnins.2019.00222

Lv, H., Wang, Z., Tong, E., Williams, L. M., Zaharchuk, G., Zeineh, M., et al. (2018). Resting-state functional MRI: everything that nonexperts have always wanted to know. *AJNR Am. J. Neuroradiol.* 39, 1390–1399.

Lv, H., Zhao, P., Liu, Z., Wang, G., Zeng, R., Yan, F., et al. (2016). Frequency-dependent neural activity in patients with unilateral vascular pulsatile tinnitus. *Neural Plast.* 2016:4918186.

Mantini, D., Perrucci, M. G., Del Gratta, C., Romani, G. L., and Corbetta, M. (2007). Electrophysiological signatures of resting state networks in the human brain. *Proc. Natl. Acad. Sci. U.S.A.* 104, 13170–13175. doi: 10.1073/pnas.0700668104

Maudoux, A., Lefebvre, P., Cabay, J. E., Demertzi, A., Vanhaudenhuyse, A., Laureys, S., et al. (2012). Connectivity graph analysis of the auditory resting state network in tinnitus. *Brain Res.* 1485, 10–21. doi: 10.1016/j.brainres.2012.05.006

Maudoux, A., Lefebvre, P., Cabay, J.-E., Demertzi, A., Vanhaudenhuyse, A., Laureys, S., et al. (2017). Auditory resting-state network connectivity in tinnitus: a functional MRI study. *PLoS One* 7:e36222. doi: 10.1371/journal.pone.0036222

Metherate, R., and Cruikshank, S. J. (1999). Thalamocortical inputs trigger a propagating envelope of gamma-band activity in auditory cortex in vitro. *Exp. Brain Res.* 126, 160–174. doi: 10.1007/s002210050726

Minami, S. B., Oishi, N., Watabe, T., Uno, K., and Ogawa, K. (2018). Auditory related resting state fMRI functional connectivity in tinnitus patients: tinnitus diagnosis performance. *Otol. Neurotol.* 39, 1–5. doi: 10.1097/mao.0000000000001626

Nathan, W., Stephan, M., Marcus, M., Katalin, D., and Thomas, E. (2005). Tinnitus perception and distress is related to abnormal spontaneous brain activity as measured by magnetoencephalography. *PLoS Med.* 2:e153. doi: 10.1371/journal.pmed.0020153

Ochi, R., Noda, Y., Tsuchimoto, S., Tarumi, R., Honda, S., Matsushita, K., et al. (2020). White matter microstructural organizations in patients with severe treatment-resistant schizophrenia: a diffusion tensor imaging study. *Prog. Neuro Psychopharmacol. Biol. Psychiatry* 100:109871. doi: 10.1016/j.pnpbp.2020.109871

Olivito, G., Clausi, S., Laghi, F., Tedesco, A. M., Baiocco, R., Mastropasqua, C., et al. (2017). Resting-state functional connectivity changes between dentate nucleus and cortical social brain regions in autism spectrum disorders. *Cerebellum* 16, 283–292. doi: 10.1007/s12311-016-0795-8

Ovidiu, K., Roland, S., Richard, K., and Manfred, G. (2006). Course of hearing loss and occurrence of tinnitus. *Hear. Res.* 221, 59–64. doi: 10.1016/j.heares.2006.07.007

Pattyn, T., Van Den Eede, F., Vanneste, S., Cassiers, L., Veltman, D., Van De Heyning, P., et al. (2016). Tinnitus and anxiety disorders: a review. *Hear. Res.* 333, 255–265. doi: 10.1016/j.heares.2015.08.014

Pegge, S. A., Steens, S. C., Kunst, H. P., and Meijer, F. J. (2017). Pulsatile tinnitus: differential diagnosis and radiological work-up. *Curr. Radiol. Rep.* 5:5.

Pinto, P. C. L., Marcelos, C. M., Mezzasalma, M. A., Osterne, F. J. V., De Melo Tavares De Lima, M. A., and Nardi, A. E. (2014). Tinnitus and its association with psychiatric disorders: systematic review. *J. Laryngol. Otol.* 128, 660–664. doi: 10.1017/s0022215114001030

Pulec, J. L. (1995). Cochlear nerve section for intractable tinnitus. *Ear Nose Throat J.* 74, 468–476. doi: 10.1177/014556139507400708

Rajmohan, V., and Mohandas, E. (2007). The limbic system. *Indian J. Psychiatry* 49, 132–139.

Rauschecker, J. P., Leaver, A. M., and Muhlau, M. (2010). Tuning out the noise: limbic-auditory interactions in tinnitus. *Neuron* 66, 819–826. doi: 10.1016/j.neuron.2010.04.032

Rauschecker, J. P., May, E. S., Maudoux, A., and Ploner, M. (2015). Frontostriatal gating of tinnitus and chronic pain. *Trends Cogn. Sci.* 19, 567–578. doi: 10.1016/j.tics.2015.08.002

Rodrigo, A., Laurent, R., Laurence, D., Monique, D., Daniela, E.-K., Naïma, D., et al. (2018). A key role of the prefrontal cortex in the maintenance of chronic tinnitus: an fMRI study using a Stroop task. *NeuroImage Clin.* 17, 325–334. doi: 10.1016/j.nicl.2017.10.029

Sair, H. I., Yahyavi-Firouz-Abadi, N., Calhoun, V. D., Airan, R. D., Agarwal, S., Intrapiromkul, J., et al. (2016). Presurgical brain mapping of the language network in patients with brain tumors using resting-state fMRI: comparison with task fMRI. *Hum. Brain Mapp.* 37, 913–923. doi: 10.1002/hbm.23075

Savastano, M. (2008). Tinnitus with or without hearing loss: are its characteristics different? *Eur. Arch. Oto Rhino Laryngol.* 265, 1295–1300. doi: 10.1007/s00405-008-0630-z

Schmidt, S. A., Akrofi, K., Carpenter-Thompson, J. R., and Husain, F. T. (2013). Default mode, dorsal attention and auditory resting state networks exhibit differential functional connectivity in tinnitus and hearing loss. *PLoS One* 8:e76488. doi: 10.1371/journal.pone.0076488

Schmidt, S. A., Carpenter-Thompson, J., and Husain, F. T. (2017). Connectivity of precuneus to the default mode and dorsal attention networks: a possible invariant marker of long-term tinnitus. *Neuroimage Clin.* 16, 196–204. doi: 10.1016/j.nicl.2017.07.015

Schmidt, S. A., Zimmerman, B., Bido Medina, R. O., Carpenter-Thompson, J. R., and Husain, F. T. (2018). Changes in gray and white matter in subgroups within the tinnitus population. *Brain Res.* 1679, 64–74. doi: 10.1016/j.brainres.2017.11.012

Seydell-Greenwald, A., Leaver, A. M., Turesky, T. K., Morgan, S., Kim, H. J., and Rauschecker, J. P. (2012). Functional MRI evidence for a role of ventral prefrontal cortex in tinnitus. *Brain Res.* 1485, 22–39. doi: 10.1016/j.brainres.2012.08.052

Seydell-Greenwald, A., Raven, E. P., Leaver, A. M., Turesky, T. K., and Rauschecker, J. P. (2014). Diffusion imaging of auditory and auditory-limbic connectivity in tinnitus: preliminary evidence and methodological challenges. *Neural Plast.* 2014:145943.

Shore, S. E., and Wu, C. (2019). Mechanisms of noise-induced tinnitus: insights from cellular studies. *Neuron* 103, 8–20. doi: 10.1016/j.neuron.2019.05.008

Shulman, G. L., Fiez, J. A., Corbetta, M., Buckner, R. L., Miezin, F. M., Raichle, M. E., et al. (1997). Common blood flow changes across visual tasks: II. Decreases in cerebral cortex. *J. Cogn. Neurosci.* 9, 648–663. doi: 10.1162/jocn.1997.9.5.648

Sven, V., Kathleen, J., Jan, O., and Dirk, D. R. (2018). Influencing connectivity and cross-frequency coupling by real-time source localized neurofeedback of the posterior cingulate cortex reduces tinnitus related distress. *Neurobiol. Stress* 8, 211–224. doi: 10.1016/j.ynstr.2016.11.003

Sven, V., Paul, V. D. H., and Dirk, D. R. (2011). The neural network of phantom sound changes over time: a comparison between recent-onset and chronic tinnitus patients. *Eur. J. Neurosci.* 34, 718–731. doi: 10.1111/j.1460-9568.2011.07793.x

Trevis, K. J., Mclachlan, N. M., and Wilson, S. J. (2016). Cognitive mechanisms in chronic tinnitus: psychological markers of a failure to switch attention. *Front. Psychol.* 7:1262. doi: 10.3389/fpsyg.2016.01262

Trevis, K. J., Tailby, C., Grayden, D. B., Mclachlan, N. M., Jackson, G. D., and Wilson, S. J. (2017). Identification of a neurocognitive mechanism underpinning awareness of chronic tinnitus. *Sci. Rep.* 7, 1–9.

van der Loo, E., Congedo, M., Vanneste, S., Van De Heyning, P., and De Ridder, D. (2011). Insular lateralization in tinnitus distress. *Auton. Neurosci. Basic Clin.* 165, 191–194. doi: 10.1016/j.autneu.2011.06.007

Vanneste, S., and De Ridder, D. (2012). The auditory and non-auditory brain areas involved in tinnitus. An emergent property of multiple parallel overlapping subnetworks. *Front. Syst. Neurosci.* 6:31. doi: 10.3389/fnsys.2012.00031

Vanneste, S., and De Ridder, D. (2016). Deafferentation-based pathophysiological differences in phantom sound: tinnitus with and without hearing loss. *NeuroImage* 129, 80–94. doi: 10.1016/j.neuroimage.2015.12.002

Vanneste, S., To, W. T., and De Ridder, D. (2019). Tinnitus and neuropathic pain share a common neural substrate in the form of specific brain connectivity and microstate profiles. *Prog. Neuro Psychopharmacol. Biol. Psychiatry* 88, 388–400. doi: 10.1016/j.pnpbp.2018.08.015

Vossel, S., Geng, J. J., and Fink, G. R. (2014). Dorsal and ventral attention systems: distinct neural circuits but collaborative roles. *Neuroscientist* 20, 150–159. doi: 10.1177/1073858413494269

Weissman, J. L., and Hirsch, B. E. (2000). Imaging of tinnitus: a review. *Radiology* 216, 342–349.

Xu, J. J., Cui, J. L., Feng, Y., Yong, W., Chen, H. Y., Chen, Y. C., et al. (2019). Chronic tinnitus exhibits bidirectional functional dysconnectivity in frontostriatal circuit. *Front. Neurosci.* 13:1299. doi: 10.3389/fnins.2019.01299

Yeo, C. J. J., Hutton, G. J., and Fung, S. H. (2018). Advanced neuroimaging in Balo's concentric sclerosis: MRI, MRS, DTI, and ASL perfusion imaging over 1 year. *Radiol. Case Rep.* 13, 1030–1035. doi: 10.1016/j.radcr.2018.04.010

Zheng, W., Peng, Z., Pengfei, Z., Jing, L., Heyu, D., Hongxia, Y., et al. (2019). Long−term reactions to pulsatile tinnitus are marked by weakened short−range functional connectivity within a brain network in the right temporal lobe. *J. Magn. Reson. Imaging* 49, 1629–1637. doi: 10.1002/jmri.26545

Zhou, G. P., Shi, X. Y., Wei, H. L., Qu, L. J., Yu, Y. S., Zhou, Q. Q., et al. (2019). Disrupted intraregional brain activity and functional connectivity in unilateral acute tinnitus patients with hearing loss. *Front. Neurosci.* 13:1010. doi: 10.3389/fnins.2019.01010

Zimmerman, B., Finnegan, M., Paul, S., Schmidt, S., Tai, Y., Roth, K., et al. (2019). Functional brain changes during mindfulness-based cognitive therapy associated with tinnitus severity. *Front. Neurosci.* 13:747. doi: 10.3389/fnins.2019.00747

Zimmerman, B. J., Abraham, I., Schmidt, S. A., Baryshnikov, Y., and Husain, F. T. (2019). Dissociating tinnitus patients from healthy controls using resting-state cyclicity analysis and clustering. *Netw. Neurosci.* 3, 67–89. doi: 10.1162/netn_a_00053

2

Cortical Oscillatory Signatures Reveal the Prerequisites for Tinnitus Perception: A Comparison of Subjects with Sudden Sensorineural Hearing Loss with and without Tinnitus

Sang-Yeon Lee[1], *Byung Yoon Choi*[1], *Ja-Won Koo*[1], *Dirk De Ridder*[2] *and Jae-Jin Song*[1*]

[1] *Department of Otorhinolaryngology-Head and Neck Surgery, Seoul National University Bundang Hospital, Seongnam, South Korea,* [2] *Unit of Neurosurgery, Department of Surgical Sciences, Dunedin School of Medicine, University of Otago, Dunedin, New Zealand*

Correspondence:
Jae-Jin Song
jjsong96@snubh.org;
jjsong96@gmail.com

Just as the human brain works in a Bayesian manner to minimize uncertainty regarding external stimuli, a deafferented brain due to hearing loss attempts to obtain or "fill in" the missing auditory information, resulting in auditory phantom percepts (i.e., tinnitus). Among various types of hearing loss, sudden sensorineural hearing loss (SSNHL) has been extensively reported to be associated with tinnitus. However, the reason that tinnitus develops selectively in some patients with SSNHL remains elusive, which led us to hypothesize that patients with SSNHL with tinnitus (SSNHL-T) and those without tinnitus (SSNHL-NT) may exhibit different cortical activity patterns. In the current study, we compared resting-state quantitative electroencephalography findings between 13 SSNHL-T and 13 SSNHL-NT subjects strictly matched for demographic characteristics and hearing thresholds. By performing whole-brain source localization analysis complemented by functional connectivity analysis, we aimed to determine the as-yet-unidentified cortical oscillatory signatures that may reveal potential prerequisites for the perception of tinnitus in patients with SSNHL. Compared with the SSNHL-NT group, the SSNHL-T group showed significantly higher cortical activity in Bayesian inferential network areas such as the frontopolar cortex, orbitofrontal cortex (OFC), and pregenual anterior cingulate cortex (pgACC) for the beta 3 and gamma frequency bands. This suggests that tinnitus develops in a brain with sudden auditory deafferentation only if the Bayesian inferential network updates the missing auditory information and the pgACC-based top-down gatekeeper system is actively involved. Additionally, significantly increased connectivity between the OFC and precuneus for the gamma frequency band was observed in the SSNHL-T group, further suggesting that tinnitus derived from Bayesian inference may be linked to the default mode network so that tinnitus is regarded as normal. Taken together, our preliminary results suggest a possible mechanism for the selective development of tinnitus in patients with SSNHL. Also, these areas could serve as the potential targets of neuromodulatory approaches to preventing the development or prolonged perception of tinnitus in subjects with SSNHL.

Keywords: tinnitus, sudden sensorineural hearing loss, bayes, cingulate gyrus, electroencephalography

INTRODUCTION

Non-pulsatile tinnitus is a common otologic symptom characterized by conscious auditory perception in the absence of an external stimulus. This is often called a "phantom sound" because there is no corresponding genuine physical source of the sound (Vanneste et al., 2018b; Lee et al., 2019; Han et al., 2020). Although the exact mechanism of tinnitus has yet to be elucidated, peripheral auditory deafferentation has been suggested as the most important factor in increased spontaneous neuronal firing in the central auditory system and cortical maladaptive plasticity between auditory and non-auditory brain regions, leading to the development of tinnitus (Eggermont and Roberts, 2012; Elgoyhen et al., 2015). Hearing loss has been strongly implicated in tinnitus, as demonstrated by a relationship between tinnitus pitch and maximum hearing loss frequency, which suggests that tinnitus is a fill-in phenomenon (Schecklmann et al., 2012). Recently, growing evidence has shown that the brain works in a Bayesian manner to minimize perceptual uncertainty regarding external stimuli. If the brain is deprived of auditory input, it attempts to "fill in" the missing auditory information from auditory memory, leading to the perception of auditory phantoms (i.e., tinnitus) (Friston et al., 2014; Eggermont and Kral, 2016; Lee et al., 2017, 2020a). Specifically, according to the theoretical multiphase compensation model, the brain attempts to overcome missing auditory information input, generating predictions via increasing topographically restricted tones, widening receptive fields, rewiring dendrites and axons, and retrieving auditory memories, resulting in brain reorganization (De Ridder et al., 2014b).

Sudden sensorineural hearing loss (SSNHL), a complex and challenging emergency in the otology field, is typically defined as a sensorineural hearing loss of more than 30 dB across three consecutive frequencies in a pure-tone audiogram occurring within a 72-h period. Importantly, tinnitus was reportedly accompanied by SSNHL in 66–93% of cases (Ding et al., 2018). Similar to ordinary progressive sensorineural hearing loss, the Bayesian brain model may explain how sudden auditory deprivation (i.e., SSNHL) elicits auditory phantom percepts, namely by increasing the need to compensate for prediction errors by upregulating neural firing in specific tonotopic regions and retrieving extant memories from the parahippocampal gyrus (Lee et al., 2017), depending on the amount of hearing loss (Vanneste and De Ridder, 2016). However, why not all patients with SSNHL experience tinnitus remains unexplained. That is, although tinnitus persists in some patients with SSNHL even after treatment, other patients do not experience tinnitus, or tinnitus is perceived temporarily but resolves spontaneously afterward. This, in turn, led us to hypothesize that tinnitus may develop in subjects with SSNHL only if the requisite cortical changes occur secondary to SSNHL.

Zhang et al. demonstrated altered white matter integrity in the auditory neural pathway of patients with SSNHL, which may be associated with the severity of tinnitus (Zhang et al., 2020). Furthermore, a recent study by Cai et al. showed more specific inhibition of neural activity and functional connectivity in patients with SSNHL and tinnitus compared with healthy controls (Cai et al., 2019), shedding further light on the putative association between SSNHL and tinnitus from the perspective of brain activity. However, neural substrates for selective development of tinnitus have thus far not been investigated among patients with SSNHL.

To test this hypothesis, we investigated neural substrates accounting for the development of tinnitus exclusively in patients with SSNHL by comparing resting-state quantitative electroencephalography (rs-qEEG) findings between SSNHL patients with and others without tinnitus (SSNHL-T and SSNHL-NT). Using whole-brain source localization analysis complemented by functional connectivity analysis, we aimed to determine the as-yet-unidentified cortical oscillatory signatures that could reveal the prerequisites for tinnitus development and to discuss the possible mechanism of the selective development of tinnitus in patients with SSNHL. Although this study includes a relatively small number of patients, which may have weakened the clinical implications of the results and statistical power, the results presented herein seem a more significant undertaking than we initially envisioned. Indeed, there is currently no consensus on the neurobiological markers for selective development of tinnitus in patients with SSNHL. Overall, our study stands out in this precision medicine era for incorporating neuroimaging in a tinnitus study to establish a future guide for the treatment of tinnitus in patients with SSNHL that incorporates neuroimaging as the "new normal."

MATERIALS AND METHODS

Participants

We performed a retrospective review of the medical records of patients with unilateral idiopathic SSNHL who visited the outpatient clinic at Seoul National University Bundang Hospital (SNUBH) between January 2014 and March 2020. For the SSNHL-NT group, we were able to identify only 18 patients who met the criteria for unilateral SSNHL with no complaint of tinnitus. Two of the 18 were excluded due to an insufficient follow-up period (i.e., <2 months). Of the remaining 16 patients,

3 were disqualified due to delayed emergence of tinnitus or significant hearing improvement during the follow-up period of at least 2 months after the onset of SSNHL. Ultimately, 13 patients were enrolled in the SSNHL-NT group. No patients in this group were diagnosed with Meniere's disease, vestibular schwannoma, or psychiatric/neurological disorders.

As outlined in **Table 1**, 51 SSNHL-T patients whose Tinnitus Handicap Index (THI) score was ≤36 (grades 1 or 2), which was administered to minimize potential bias caused by distress-induced changes in cortical activity, were initially selected from the SNUBH database (1,196 rs-qEEG-available subjects). Subsequently, 13 subjects matched for sex, laterality, and audiogram (i.e., >70 dB HL in the affected ear and <40 dB HL in the unaffected ear) with the SSHL-NT subjects but blinded to rs-qEEG findings were finally enrolled in the SSNHL-T group. None of the subjects in the SSNHL-T group had a history of objective tinnitus or etiologies such as Meniere's disease, head injuries, brain surgery, or neurological disorders. The study was approved by the Institutional Review Board of the Clinical Research Institute at Seoul National University Bundang Hospital and was conducted in accordance with the Declaration of Helsinki (IRB-B-2006-621-105).

TABLE 1 | Demographics and clinical characteristics.

	SSNHL-NT group (*N* = 13)	SSNHL-T group (*N* = 13)	*P*-value
Age			
Median	70	62	0.129
Range	30–81	30–74	
Sex			
Male	6	6	1.000
Female	7	7	
Laterality			
Right	8	8	1.000
Left	5	5	
Duration (months)[a]			
Median	16	11	0.696
Range	3–84	3–106	
Hearing threshold (dB HL)			
250 Hz	71.15 ± 24.93	60.00 ± 29.86	0.597
500 Hz	80.00 ± 22.82	72.31 ± 24.12	0.037
1 kHz	86.15 ± 14.74	77.31 ± 22.04	0.400
2 kHz	85.00 ± 16.20	83.46 ± 26.09	0.024
3 kHz	89.23 ± 15.53	85.38 ± 27.27	0.588
4 kHz	89.62 ± 15.34	90.77 ± 21.30	0.240
8 kHz	90.77 ± 14.56	94.23 ± 18.53	0.101
Average hearing threshold (dB HL)[b]			
Mean (SD)	80.96 ± 20.38	85.19 ± 14.83	0.551
THI score[b]			
Mean (SD)	NA	26.46 ± 8.37	NA
Range		8–36	

SSNHL-NT, sudden sensorineural hearing loss without tinnitus; SSNHL-T, sudden sensorineural hearing loss with tinnitus; SD, standard deviation; HL, hearing loss; THI, tinnitus handicap inventory; NA, not available.

[a] Note that duration refers to the period between SSNHL onset and EEG acquisition.

[b] Note that the mean hearing threshold was calculated using the average of the hearing thresholds at 0.5, 1, 2, and 4 kHz.

Audiological and Psychoacoustic Evaluation

The hearing thresholds for seven different octave frequencies (0.25, 0.5, 1, 2, 3, 4, and 8 kHz) were evaluated using pure-tone audiometry in a soundproof booth. The mean hearing threshold was calculated using the average of the hearing thresholds at 0.5, 1, 2, and 4 kHz (Han et al., 2019; Shim et al., 2019; Bae et al., 2020; Huh et al., 2020; Lee et al., 2020b; Song et al., 2020). At each subject's initial visit, we obtained a structured history of the characteristics of tinnitus including its presence, laterality, and psychoacoustic nature (pure-tone or narrow-band noise).

EEG Recording

We performed qEEG data acquisition and pre-processing procedures according to a previously reported protocol (Kim et al., 2016; Song et al., 2017; Han et al., 2018; Vanneste et al., 2018b; Lee et al., 2019). Prior to EEG recording, we instructed the enrolled patients not to drink alcohol for 24 h and to avoid caffeine on the day of recording to exclude alcohol-induced changes in the EEG signal (Korucuoglu et al., 2016) and caffeine-induced reductions in alpha and beta power (Siepmann and Kirch, 2002). EEGs were recorded with the patient seated upright with the eyes closed for 5 min using a tin-electrode cap (ElectroCap, Eaton, OH, USA), a Mitsar amplifier (EEG-201; Mitsar, St. Petersburg, Russia), and WinEEG software, version 2.84.44 (Mitsar) in a fully lit room insulated from sound and stray electric fields. The EEG data were obtained using WinEEG software (ver. 2.84.44; Mitsar) (available at http://www.mitsar-medical.com). The impedances of all electrodes were maintained below 5 kΩ. Data were obtained at a sampling rate of 1,024 Hz and filtered using a high-pass filter with a cutoff of 0.15 Hz and a low-pass filter with a cutoff of 200 Hz. After initial data acquisition, the raw data were resampled at 128 Hz and band-pass filtered using a fast Fourier transform filter with a Hanning window at 2–44 Hz. After importing the data into Eureka! Software (Sherlin and Congedo, 2005), all episodic artifacts were evaluated manually and removed from the EEG stream. We eliminated additional artifacts using independent component analysis with ICoN software (http://sites.google.com/site/marcocongedo/software/nica) (Koprivova et al., 2011; White et al., 2012). All subjects' vigilance levels, including slowing of alpha rhythm or emergence of sleep spindles, were meticulously monitored. No patients included in this study exhibited any abnormal EEG patterns during the measurements.

Source Localization Analysis

Standardized low-resolution brain electromagnetic tomography (sLORETA) was employed to estimate the scalp-recorded electrical activity in each of the eight frequency bands (i.e., intracerebral sources). The sLORETA software includes a toolbox for the functional localization of standardized current densities based on electrophysiological and neuroanatomical constraints (Pascual-Marqui, 2002). We identified the cortical sources that generated the activities recorded by the scalp electrodes in each of the following eight frequency bands: delta (2–3.5 Hz), theta (4–7.5 Hz), alpha 1 (8–10 Hz), alpha 2 (10–12 Hz), beta 1 (13–18 Hz), beta 2 (18.5–21 Hz), beta 3 (21.5–30 Hz), and gamma (30.5–44 Hz). sLORETA computes neuronal electrical activity as current density (A/m^2) without assuming a predefined number of active sources. The sLORETA solution space consists of 6,239 voxels (voxel size: 5 × 5 × 5 mm) and is restricted to the cortical gray matter and hippocampus, as defined by the digitized Montreal Neurological Institute (MNI) 152 template (Fuchs et al., 2002). Scalp electrode coordinates on the MNI brain are derived from the International 5% System (Jurcak et al., 2007). A total of 5,000 random permutations, with correction for multiple testing (i.e., for tests performed for all electrodes and/or voxels and for all time samples and/or different frequencies) were carried out; thus, further correction for multiple comparisons was unnecessary. The locations of significant clusters were confirmed using a LORETA-KEY toolbox, such as the Anatomy toolbox, and the Talairach and Tournoux atlas (Talairach and Tornoux, 1988).

Functional Connectivity Analysis

As for the functional connectivity analysis, a total of 16 regions of interest, defined by their respective Brodmann areas (BAs) and known to relate to tinnitus according to previously published literature (Vanneste et al., 2018b), were selected as possible nodes. These included the bilateral superior parietal lobule (BA7), the bilateral frontopolar cortices (BA10), the bilateral orbitofrontal cortices (BA11), the bilateral posterior cingulate cortices (BA27), the bilateral pregenual cortices (BA32), the bilateral parahippocampi (BA36), and the bilateral primary auditory cortices (BA41 and BA42).

Statistical Analyses

Statistical non-parametric mapping (SnPM) was adopted for permutation tests for source localization and functional connectivity. To identify between-group differences in resting-state cortical oscillatory activities, sLORETA built-in voxel-wise randomization tests (5,000 permutations) were used to perform nonparametric statistical analyses of functional images with a threshold $P < 0.05$. We also employed a between-groups t-statistic with a threshold of $P < 0.05$. Correction for multiple comparisons in SnPM using random permutations has been shown to yield similar results to those obtained from a statistical parametric mapping approach using a general linear model with multiple-comparison corrections (Nichols and Holmes, 2002). For lagged linear connectivity differences, we assessed between-group differences for each contrast using a paired t-test with a threshold of $P < 0.05$. We also corrected for multiple comparisons using sLORETA's built-in voxel-wise randomization tests for all of the voxels included in the 16 regions of interests for connectivity analysis (5,000 permutations). Although the between-groups t-statistic was used for source localization and the paired t-test was used for connectivity analysis, these are nonparametric analyses based on 5,000 permutations. All analyses were done and illustrated using the R statistical package (version 3.3.2, R Foundation for Statistical Computing, Vienna, Austria). All statistical tests were two-tailed, and $P < 0.05$ was considered significant.

RESULTS

Demographics and Clinical Characteristics: SSNHL-T vs. SSNHL-NT

The demographic and clinical characteristics of the two groups are summarized in **Figure 1**. The laterality of the hearing loss and sex distribution were matched between the SSNHL-NT and SSNHL-T groups. No significant differences in age at onset of SSNHL or duration of hearing loss (from the onset of SSNHL to the timepoint at rs-qEEG measurement) were observed between the two groups. Furthermore, hearing thresholds across all frequencies for the affected- and non-affected ears did not differ between the two groups. The median THI score of the SSNHL-T group was 12 (range, 4–36).

Source-Localization Analysis: SSNHL-T vs. SSNHL-NT

Compared with the SSNHL-NT group, the SSNHL-T group showed significantly increased cortical activity in the frontopolar cortex (FPC, BA10), the orbitofrontal cortex (OFC, BA11), and the pregenual anterior cingulate cortex (pgACC, BA32) for the beta 3 and gamma frequency bands ($P < 0.05$) (**Figure 2**). No significant effects were observed for the delta, theta, alpha 1, alpha 3, beta 1, and beta 2 frequency bands.

Connectivity Analyses: SSNHL-T vs. SSNHL-T

Compared with the SSNHL-NT group, the SSNHL-T group showed significantly increased functional connectivity between the left OFC and the right precuneus (BA7) for the gamma frequency band ($P < 0.05$) (**Figure 3**). For the other seven frequency bands, there were no significant between-group differences in functional connectivity among ROIs.

DISCUSSION

This is the first study to explore cortical activity and connectivity differences between SSNHL subjects with and those without tinnitus and to attempt to reveal the cortical oscillatory signatures for selective development of tinnitus among patients with SSNHL. In this study, the SSNHL-T group had abnormally increased activity in the FPC, OFC, and pgACC for the beta 3 and gamma frequency bands compared with the SSNHL-NT group. These findings suggest that auditory phantom percepts may develop when the brain experiences sudden decreased peripheral auditory input as the Bayesian inferential network updates the missing auditory information with the involvement of the pgACC-based top-down gatekeeper system. Furthermore, the lagged linear connectivity between the left OFC and the right precuneus was significantly increased for the gamma frequency band in the SSNHL-T group compared with the SSNHL-NT group, indicating that tinnitus deriving from Bayesian updating seems to involve the default mode network (DMN); thus, tinnitus seemed to be perceived as normal by the SSNHL-T group.

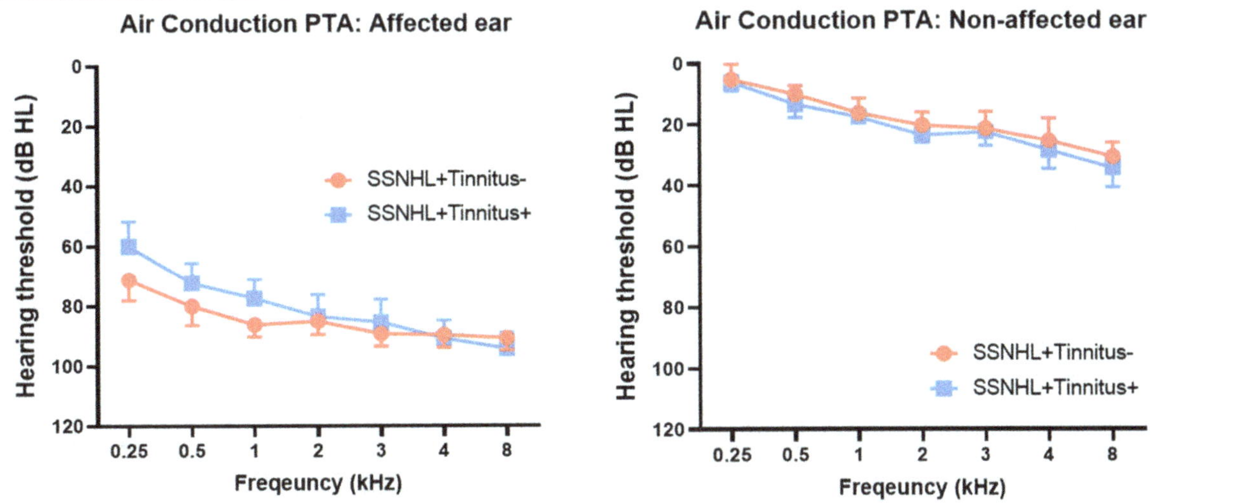

FIGURE 1 | Comparison of hearing thresholds across all frequencies between patients with sudden sensorineural hearing loss with and without tinnitus (SSNHL-T and SSNHL-NT, respectively). Air conduction pure-tone audiometry (PTA) revealed nearly matched hearing thresholds across all frequencies between the two groups in both the affected and the non-affected ear.

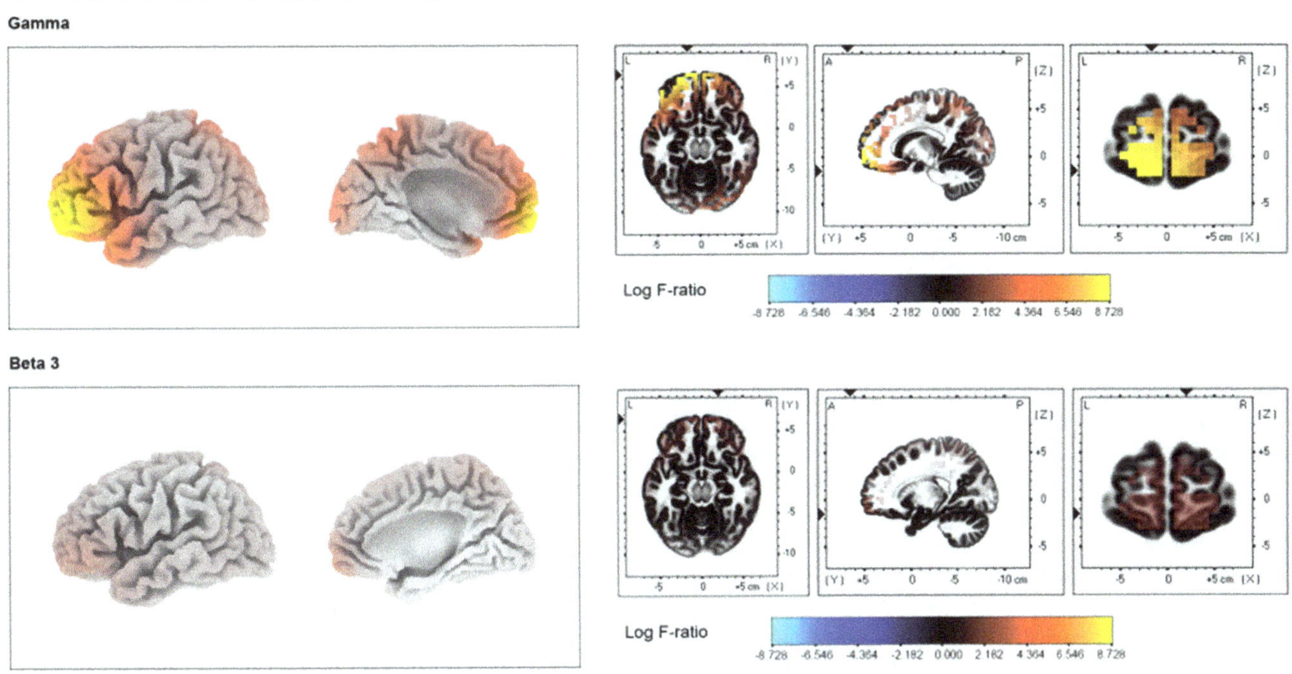

FIGURE 2 | Source-localized cortical power comparison in sudden sensorineural hearing loss with and without tinnitus (SSNHL-T and SSNHL-NT, respectively) groups using resting-state quantitative electroencephalography data. The SSNHL-T group showed increased activity in the frontopolar cortex, orbitofrontal cortex, and pregenual anterior cingulate cortex for the gamma and beta 3 frequency bands compared with the SSNHL-NT group.

The Bayesian Inferential Network Updates Missing Auditory Information via Bottom-Up Deafferentation

The Bayesian brain model, an extension of a predictive brain model, has been suggested as an explanation for the development of tinnitus. According to this model, tinnitus is a response to peripheral auditory deafferentation that aims to reduce perceptual uncertainty (Morcom and Friston, 2012; De Ridder et al., 2014b). In other words, deafferentation-induced auditory phantom percepts, namely tinnitus, are preceded by peripheral auditory input-based memory, and tinnitus develops when prediction error occurs due to peripheral

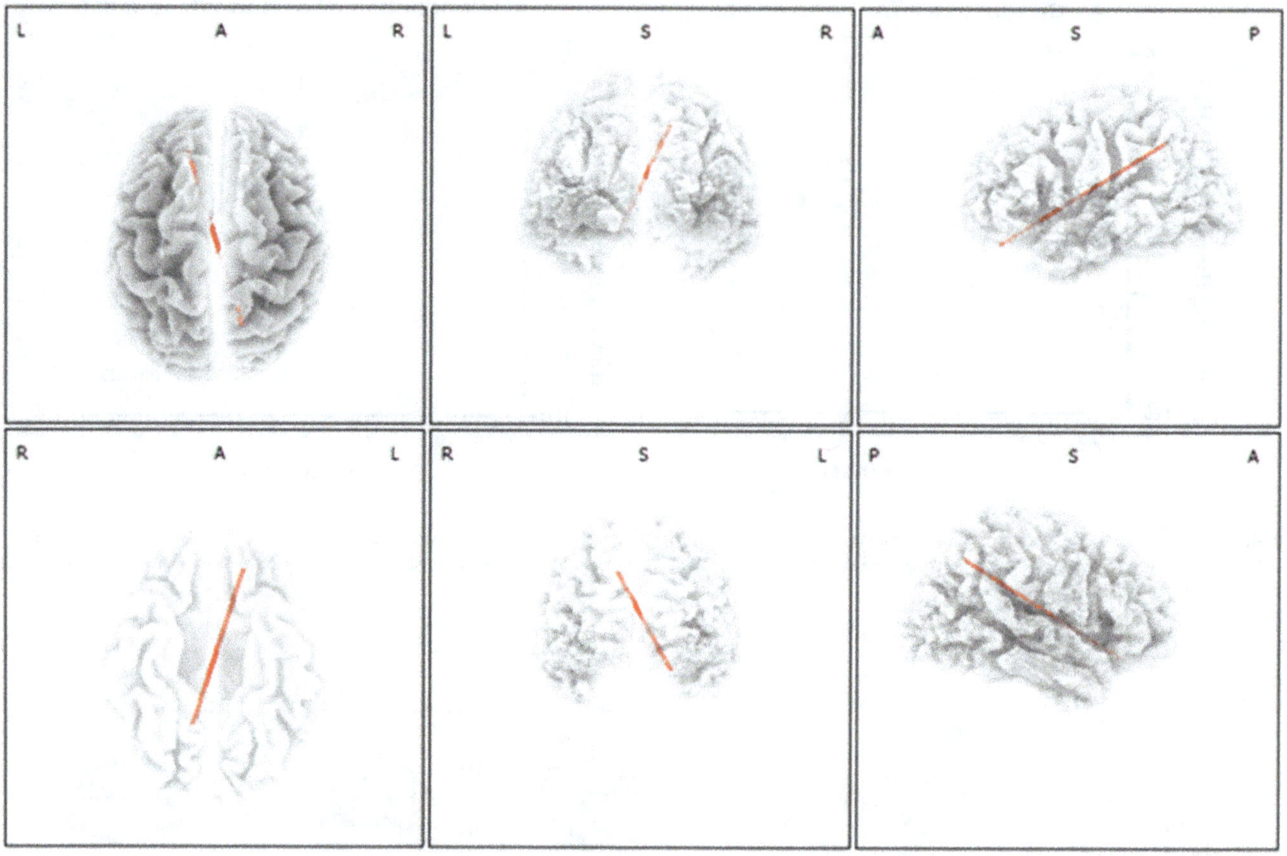

FIGURE 3 | Functional connectivity analysis with regard to selective development of tinnitus in subjects with sudden sensorineural hearing loss (SSNHL). Increased functional connectivity between the left orbitofrontal cortex and the right precuneus for the gamma frequency band was significant in the SSNHL with tinnitus (SSNHL-T) compared with the SSNHL without tinnitus (SSNHL-NT) group.

hearing loss (De Ridder et al., 2014a; Lee et al., 2017). In the same context, we have recently reported that approximately 70% of patients with unilateral SSNHL experience ipsilesional tinnitus (Lee et al., 2017), indicating that missing auditory information (i.e., prediction error) may stimulate neural circuit interactions between lower-order (peripheral auditory input) and higher-order (prediction-driving process of auditory perception) auditory systems to reduce uncertainty in a bottom-up fashion due to sudden hearing deterioration. In this regard, significantly increased source-localized activity in the OFC and FPC in the SSNHL-T group in the current study may reflect the role of active Bayesian inferential prefrontal cortical processes (Donoso et al., 2014) in tinnitus generation in the context of a sudden decrease in peripheral auditory input. The prefrontal cortices are considered to employ probabilistic inferential processes (i.e., Bayesian inferences), enabling optimizing behavioral adaptations in uncertain situations based on available information (Koechlin, 2016; Parr et al., 2018). In particular, polar to lateral prefrontal cortices such as the OFC and FPC are involved in making probabilistic inferences and exploring new strategies formed from long-term memory in uncertain environments (Donoso et al., 2014). Therefore, increased source-localized activity in the prefrontal cortices (i.e., OFC and FPC) in the SSNHL-T group may reflect the Bayesian inferential processes of updating sensory prediction and thereby adopting new strategies (phantom auditory perception) based on stored auditory memory in the context of suddenly decreased peripheral auditory input. Of note, we have recently revealed significantly increased information inflow in cortical areas associated with Bayesian inference in progressive sensorineural hearing loss patients with tinnitus as compared to those without tinnitus (unpublished data), in accordance with the current findings.

The OFC has also been suggested as responsible for the emotional processing of sounds (Blood et al., 1999), and is connected to other limbic areas involved in emotion processing (Beauregard, 2007; Vanneste and De Ridder, 2012). In an integrative model of tinnitus (De Ridder et al., 2014c), once the aberrant activity that causes tinnitus percepts is deemed salient, the autonomic nervous system, the limbic system, and their interaction could be further involved in distributing tinnitus-related distress signals across the brain. Indeed, the OFC has been reported to play a pivotal role in the top-down modulation of autonomic and peripheral physiological responses accompanying emotional experiences (Ohira et al., 2006), supporting neural activity in the OFC might link to biopsychosocial processes of disease (Hänsel and von Känel, 2008). Furthermore, neural activity in the OFC extending to the FPC in beta 1 and beta 2 has shown to differ between sex during emotional processing and emotional regulation (Vanneste et al., 2012). Additionally, tinnitus perception and tinnitus-related distress are closely associated with these brain areas (Schlee et al., 2009), and correlated with the audiological handicap associated with unilateral SSNHL.

Additionally, tinnitus loudness and distress are correlated with the audiological handicap associated with unilateral SSNHL (Chiossoine-Kerdel et al., 2000). Although we attempted to minimize distress-related cortical changes by recruiting SSNHL-T subjects with only mild distress, distress cannot be completely eliminated in tinnitus. In this regard, the activity changes in the FPC and OFC may also reflect the emotional weight attached to aberrant auditory perception (i.e., tinnitus) in patients with SSNHL.

A Top-Down Gatekeeper System Is Activated to Cancel Internally Generated Auditory Phantoms

Recent studies have suggested that auditory phantom percepts can be associated with bottom-up (ascending) deafferentation as well as with a dysfunctional top-down (descending) noise-canceling mechanism (De Ridder et al., 2014b; Song et al., 2015; Vanneste et al., 2019). This top-down mechanism is a putative central gatekeeper that functions as an "auditory gate," evaluating the relevance and affective meaning of sensory stimuli and modulating information transmission via descending inhibitory pathways to the thalamic reticular nucleus (Hullfish et al., 2019; Vanneste et al., 2019). In previous pain studies, the degree of improvement after spinal cord stimulation depended on activation of the pgACC (Moens et al., 2012), which is a part of the descending pain inhibitory pathway (Fields, 2004; Kong et al., 2010), the somatosensory analog of the noise canceling system. Additionally, Vanneste et al. demonstrated that altered neural activity of the pgACC likely increases tinnitus loudness in patients who are Met carriers (i.e., COMT $Val^{158}Met$ polymorphism), probably due to reduced canceling-out of irrelevant auditory input. Furthermore, increased activity in the parahippocampus and the pgACC for the theta and gamma frequency bands, as well as decreased activity in the auditory cortex, is found exclusively in tinnitus patients with hearing loss compared with those who have hearing loss but without tinnitus (Vanneste et al., 2018a). While the activation of a top-down noise-canceling mechanism works predominantly in the alpha frequency band during the resting state, dysfunctional noise canceling resulting in tinnitus is hypothesized to be linked to the theta and gamma frequency bands (Vanneste et al., 2019). These findings are consistent with our data showing increased source-localized activity in the pgACC for the gamma frequency band in the SSNHL-T group. That is, the pgACC, which normally functions as a central gatekeeper, is activated to abate behaviorally irrelevant phantom auditory signals that stem from Bayesian updating via bottom-up deafferentation.

Overall, our data suggest that auditory phantom percepts may develop in a brain with suddenly decreased peripheral auditory input when the Bayesian inferential network actively updates the missing auditory information. Furthermore, as an attempt to minimize this auditory phantom, the pgACC-based top-down gatekeeper system may be activated in brains with sudden auditory deafferentation.

Tinnitus Percepts May Be Considered the Norm When Bayesian Updating-Based Tinnitus Is Actively Linked to the Default Mode Network

As shown in **Figure 3**, a significant increase in connectivity between the OFC (BA11) and the precuneus (BA7) was observed in the SSNHL-T group compared with the SSNHL-NT group. The posterior cingulate cortex and precuneus are considered critical nodes of the brain's DMN, a specific group of brain regions activated when people are occupied with an internally focused task (i.e., the task-negative mode) (Vanneste and De Ridder, 2012). Therefore, our data may indicate that patients with SSNHL perceive tinnitus when Bayesian updating-based tinnitus is actively linked to the DMN. The DMN may regard the salient but irrelevant auditory information (i.e., tinnitus) arising from the Bayesian updating as normal, ultimately leading to continuous tinnitus perception. We have recently shown that localized activation of brain areas involved in the DMN may act as a negative predictor of improvement in tinnitus after partial auditory reafferentation by the use of hearing aids or cochlear implants, as tinnitus perception may already seem normal due to activation of DMN-related brain areas (Song et al., 2013; Han et al., 2020). Collectively, these findings reinforce the existing notion that the brain regions involved in generating tinnitus may become integrated into the DMN in patients with tinnitus (De Ridder et al., 2011; Vanneste and De Ridder, 2012). Based on the literature as well as the current findings, our results justify the evaluation of localized activity and functional connectivity using functional neuroimaging in patients with SSNHL. The rationale behind such an effort lies in the expectation that altered brain activity and connectivity, including that of the DMN, may predict the prognosis with regard to the chronification of tinnitus or treatment responses in subjects with tinnitus.

Limitations and Future Perspectives

Taken together, the results of the present study merit special attention in that they are grossly in line with the recently proposed Bayesian brain model for the generation of tinnitus and offer a key to unraveling the conundrum of the selective development of tinnitus in patients with SSNHL. Our study also raises an important issue that may stimulate further research incorporating customized neuromodulation approaches based on the status of neural substrates responsible for the perception of tinnitus in patients with SSNHL.

Nevertheless, there are some limitations that should be addressed in future studies. First, the results presented here are limited by the relatively small number of subjects in both groups, mainly due to the difficulty of recruiting SSNHL patients without tinnitus. Future follow-up studies in a larger number of subjects should be performed to replicate the current results. Additionally, the current study was designed as a cross-sectional evaluation, which, along with the retrospective study design, may weaken the clinical implications of our results. These limitations require future prospective and longitudinal follow-up studies to determine the origination of these differences of cortical activity and connectivity between SSNHL subjects with and those without tinnitus. Particularly, recruiting patients showing immediate tinnitus following sudden auditory deprivation but improved thereafter, as negative plasticity compensates for itself, would be important to elicit more significant findings. Second, confounding related to distress-induced cortical activity changes was minimized by including SSNHL subjects with tinnitus who had low THI scores; however, such confounding was not completely eliminated because tinnitus with no distress is almost nonexistent. A future prospective study including SSNHL with "very minimally" distressing tinnitus should be conducted to confirm the reproducibility of the current findings. Third, this study did not consider the possibility of combined hyperacusis in the SSNHL-T group. A recent study using rs-qEEG showed that increased "circuit-breaker" activity was associated with hyperacusis-related neural substrates (Han et al., 2018), which suggests that cortical activity may be biased if tinnitus subjects with combined hyperacusis are included. Future studies recruiting a SSNHL-T group without combined hyperacusis should be performed to address this limitation.

CONCLUSION

Our preliminary study explored cortical activity and connectivity differences between SSNHL subjects with and without tinnitus, shedding light on the cortical oscillatory signatures for selective development of tinnitus among patients with SSNHL. These areas could serve as potential targets of neuromodulatory approaches to prevent the development or prolonged perception of tinnitus in subjects with SSNHL.

ETHICS STATEMENT

The study was approved by the Institutional Review Board of the Clinical Research Institute at Seoul National University Bundang Hospital, and was conducted in accordance with the Declaration of Helsinki (IRB-B-2006-621-105). The patients/participants provided their written informed consent to participate in this study.

AUTHOR CONTRIBUTIONS

S-YL and J-JS led the analysis and interpretation of the results and drafted the first manuscript. BC, J-WK, and DD conceived the investigation and revised the manuscript for important intellectual content. All authors contributed to all aspects of the investigation, including methodological design, data collection and analysis, interpretation of the results, revision of the manuscript for important intellectual content, and approved the final version of the manuscript and agree to be accountable for all aspects of the work.

ACKNOWLEDGMENTS

The English in this document has been checked by at least two professional editors, both native speakers of English. For a certificate, please see: http://www.textcheck.com/certificate/8QiQBI.

REFERENCES

Bae, E. B., Lee, J. H., and Song, J. J. (2020). Single-session of combined tDCS-TMS may increase therapeutic effects in subjects with tinnitus. *Front. Neurol.* 11:160. doi: 10.3389/fneur.2020.00160

Beauregard, M. (2007). Mind does really matter: evidence from neuroimaging studies of emotional self-regulation, psychotherapy, and placebo effect. *Prog. Neurobiol.* 81, 218–236. doi: 10.1016/j.pneurobio.2007.01.005

Blood, A. J., Zatorre, R. J., Bermudez, P., and Evans, A. C. (1999). Emotional responses to pleasant and unpleasant music correlate with activity in paralimbic brain regions. *Nat. Neurosci.* 2, 382–387. doi: 10.1038/7299

Cai, Y., Li, J., Chen, Y., Chen, W., Dang, C., Zhao, F., et al. (2019). Inhibition of brain area and functional connectivity in idiopathic sudden sensorineural hearing loss with tinnitus based on resting-state EEG. *Front. Neurosci.* 13:851. doi: 10.3389/fnins.2019.00851

Chiossoine-Kerdel, J. A., Baguley, D. M., Stoddart, R. L., and Moffat, D. A. (2000). An investigation of the audiologic handicap associated with unilateral sudden sensorineural hearing loss. *Otol. Neurotol.* 21, 645–651.

De Ridder, D., Elgoyhen, A. B., Romo, R., and Langguth, B. (2011). Phantom percepts: tinnitus and pain as persisting aversive memory networks. *Proc. Natl. Acad. Sci.* 108, 8075–8080. doi: 10.1073/pnas.1018466108

De Ridder, D., Joos, K., and Vanneste, S. (2014a). The enigma of the tinnitus-free dream state in a Bayesian world. *Neural Plast.* 2014:612147. doi: 10.1155/2014/612147

De Ridder, D., Vanneste, S., and Freeman, W. (2014b). The Bayesian brain: phantom percepts resolve sensory uncertainty. *Neurosci. Biobehav. Rev.* 44, 4–15. doi: 10.1016/j.neubiorev.2012.04.001

De Ridder, D., Vanneste, S., Weisz, N., Londero, A., Schlee, W., Elgoyhen, A. B., et al. (2014c). An integrative model of auditory phantom perception: tinnitus as a unified percept of interacting separable subnetworks. *Neurosci. Biobehav. Rev.* 44, 16–32. doi: 10.1016/j.neubiorev.2013.03.021

Ding, X., Zhang, X., Huang, Z., and Feng, X. (2018). The characteristic and short-term prognosis of tinnitus associated with sudden sensorineural hearing loss. *Neural Plast.* 2018:6059697. doi: 10.1155/2018/6059697

Donoso, M., Collins, A. G., and Koechlin, E. (2014). Human cognition. Foundations of human reasoning in the prefrontal cortex. *Science* 344, 1481–1486. doi: 10.1126/science.1252254

Eggermont, J. J., and Kral, A. (2016). Somatic memory and gain increase as preconditions for tinnitus: insights from congenital deafness. *Hear. Res.* 333, 37–48. doi: 10.1016/j.heares.2015.12.018

Eggermont, J. J., and Roberts, L. E. (2012). The neuroscience of tinnitus: understanding abnormal and normal auditory perception. *Front. Syst. Neurosci.* 6:53. doi: 10.3389/fnsys.2012.00053

Elgoyhen, A. B., Langguth, B., De Ridder, D., and Vanneste, S. (2015). Tinnitus: perspectives from human neuroimaging. *Nat. Rev. Neurosci.* 16, 632–642. doi: 10.1038/nrn4003

Fields, H. (2004). State-dependent opioid control of pain. *Nat. Rev. Neurosci.* 5, 565–575. doi: 10.1038/nrn1431

Friston, K. J., Stephan, K. E., Montague, R., and Dolan, R. J. (2014). Computational psychiatry: the brain as a phantastic organ. *Lancet Psychiatry* 1, 148–158. doi: 10.1016/S2215-0366(14)70275-5

Fuchs, M., Kastner, J., Wagner, M., Hawes, S., and Ebersole, J. S. (2002). A standardized boundary element method volume conductor model. *Clin. Neurophysiol.* 113, 702–712. doi: 10.1016/S1388-2457(02)00030-5

Han, J. J., Jang, J. H., Ridder, D. D., Vanneste, S., Koo, J.-W., and Song, J.-J. (2018). Increased parietal circuit-breaker activity in delta frequency band and abnormal delta/theta band connectivity in salience network in hyperacusis subjects. *PLoS ONE* 13:e0191858. doi: 10.1371/journal.pone.0191858

Han, J. J., Ridder, D. D., Vanneste, S., Chen, Y.-C., Koo, J.-W., and Song, J.-J. (2020). Pre-treatment ongoing cortical oscillatory activity predicts improvement of tinnitus after partial peripheral reafferentation with hearing aids. *Front. Neurosci.* 14:410. doi: 10.3389/fnins.2020.00410

Han, S. A., Choe, G., Kim, Y., Koo, J. W., Choi, B. Y., and Song, J. J. (2019). Beware of a fragile footplate: lessons from ossiculoplasty in patients with ossicular anomalies related to second pharyngeal arch defects. *J. Clin. Med.* 8:2130. doi: 10.3390/jcm8122130

Hänsel, A., and von Känel, R. (2008). The ventro-medial prefrontal cortex: a major link between the autonomic nervous system, regulation of emotion, and stress reactivity? *Biopsychosoc. Med.* 2:21. doi: 10.1186/1751-0759-2-21

Huh, G., Bae, Y. J., Woo, H. J., Park, J. H., Koo, J. W., and Song, J. J. (2020). Vestibulocochlear symptoms caused by vertebrobasilar dolichoectasia. *Clin. Exp. Otorhinolaryngol.* 13, 123–132. doi: 10.21053/ceo.2019.00780

Hullfish, J., Abenes, I., Yoo, H. B., De Ridder, D., and Vanneste, S. (2019). Frontostriatal network dysfunction as a domain-general mechanism underlying phantom perception. *Hum. Brain Mapp.* 40, 2241–2251. doi: 10.1002/hbm.24521

Jurcak, V., Tsuzuki, D., and Dan, I. (2007). 10/20, 10/10, and 10/5 systems revisited: their validity as relative head-surface-based positioning systems. *Neuroimage* 34, 1600–1611. doi: 10.1016/j.neuroimage.2006.09.024

Kim, S. H., Jang, J. H., Lee, S. Y., Han, J. J., Koo, J. W., Vanneste, S., et al. (2016). Neural substrates predicting short-term improvement of tinnitus loudness and distress after modified tinnitus retraining therapy. *Sci. Rep.* 6:29140. doi: 10.1038/srep29140

Koechlin, E. (2016). Prefrontal executive function and adaptive behavior in complex environments. *Curr. Opin. Neurobiol.* 37, 1–6. doi: 10.1016/j.conb.2015.11.004

Kong, J., Loggia, M. L., Zyloney, C., Tu, P., Laviolette, P., and Gollub, R. L. (2010). Exploring the brain in pain: activations, deactivations and their relation. *Pain* 148, 257–267. doi: 10.1016/j.pain.2009.11.008

Koprivova, J., Congedo, M., Horacek, J., Prasko, J., Raszka, M., Brunovsky, M., et al. (2011). EEG source analysis in obsessive-compulsive disorder. *Clin. Neurophysiol.* 122, 1735–1743. doi: 10.1016/j.clinph.2011.01.051

Korucuoglu, O., Gladwin, T. E., and Wiers, R. W. (2016). The effect of acute alcohol on motor-related EEG asymmetries during preparation of approach or avoid alcohol responses. *Biol. Psychol.* 114, 81–92. doi: 10.1016/j.biopsycho.2015.12.012

Lee, J. M., Kim, Y., Ji, J.-Y., Koo, J.-W., and Song, J.-J. (2020a). "Auditory experience, for a certain duration, is a prerequisite for tinnitus: lessons from subjects with unilateral tinnitus in the better-hearing ear," in *Progress in Brain Research*, eds W. Schlee, B. Langguth, T. Kleinjung, S. Vanneste, and D. De Ridder (Amsterdam: Elsevier).

Lee, S. Y., Kim, M. K., Bae, Y. J., An, G. S., Lee, K., Choi, B. Y., et al. (2020b). Longitudinal analysis of surgical outcome in subjects with pulsatile tinnitus originating from the sigmoid sinus. *Sci. Rep.* 10:18194. doi: 10.1038/s41598-020-75348-3

Lee, S. Y., Nam, D. W., Koo, J. W., De Ridder, D., Vanneste, S., and Song, J. J. (2017). No auditory experience, no tinnitus: lessons from subjects with congenital- and acquired single-sided deafness. *Hear. Res.* 354, 9–15. doi: 10.1016/j.heares.2017.08.002

Lee, S. Y., Rhee, J., Shim, Y. J., Kim, Y., Koo, J. W., De Ridder, D., et al. (2019). Changes in the resting-state cortical oscillatory activity 6 months after modified tinnitus retraining therapy. *Front. Neurosci.* 13:1123. doi: 10.3389/fnins.2019.01123

Moens, M., Sunaert, S., Marien, P., Brouns, R., De Smedt, A., Droogmans, S., et al. (2012). Spinal cord stimulation modulates cerebral function: an fMRI study. *Neuroradiology* 54, 1399–1407. doi: 10.1007/s00234-012-1087-8

Morcom, A. M., and Friston, K. J. (2012). Decoding episodic memory in ageing: a Bayesian analysis of activity patterns predicting memory. *Neuroimage* 59, 1772–1782. doi: 10.1016/j.neuroimage.2011.08.071

Nichols, T. E., and Holmes, A. P. (2002). Nonparametric permutation tests for functional neuroimaging: a primer with examples. *Hum. Brain Mapp.* 15, 1–25. doi: 10.1002/hbm.1058

Ohira, H., Nomura, M., Ichikawa, N., Isowa, T., Iidaka, T., Sato, A., et al. (2006). Association of neural and physiological responses during voluntary emotion suppression. *Neuroimage* 29, 721–733. doi: 10.1016/j.neuroimage.2005.08.047

Parr, T., Rees, G., and Friston, K. J. (2018). Computational neuropsychology and Bayesian inference. *Front. Hum. Neurosci.* 12:61. doi: 10.3389/fnhum.2018.00061

Pascual-Marqui, R. D. (2002). Standardized low-resolution brain electromagnetic tomography (sLORETA): technical details. *Methods Find. Exp. Clin. Pharmacol.* 24 (Suppl. D), 5–12.

Schecklmann, M., Vielsmeier, V., Steffens, T., Landgrebe, M., Langguth, B., and Kleinjung, T. (2012). Relationship between audiometric slope and tinnitus pitch in tinnitus patients: insights into the mechanisms of tinnitus generation. *PLoS ONE* 7:e34878. doi: 10.1371/journal.pone.0034878

Schlee, W., Hartmann, T., Langguth, B., and Weisz, N. (2009). Abnormal resting-state cortical coupling in chronic tinnitus. *BMC Neurosci.* 10:11. doi: 10.1186/1471-2202-10-11

Sherlin, L., and Congedo, M. (2005). Obsessive-compulsive dimension localized using low-resolution brain electromagnetic tomography (LORETA). *Neurosci. Lett.* 387, 72–74. doi: 10.1016/j.neulet.2005.06.069

Shim, Y. J., Bae, Y. J., An, G. S., Lee, K., Kim, Y., Lee, S. Y., et al. (2019). Involvement of the internal auditory canal in subjects with cochlear otosclerosis: a less acknowledged third window that affects surgical outcome. *Otol. Neurotol.* 40, e186–e190. doi: 10.1097/MAO.0000000000002144

Siepmann, M., and Kirch, W. (2002). Effects of caffeine on topographic quantitative EEG. *Neuropsychobiology* 45, 161–166. doi: 10.1159/000054958

Song, J.-J., Punte, A. K., De Ridder, D., Vanneste, S., and Van de Heyning, P. (2013). Neural substrates predicting improvement of tinnitus after cochlear implantation in patients with single-sided deafness. *Hear. Res.* 299, 1–9. doi: 10.1016/j.heares.2013.02.001

Song, J. J., Kim, K., Sunwoo, W., Mertens, G., Van de Heyning, P., De Ridder, D., et al. (2017). A quantitative electroencephalography study on cochlear implant-induced cortical changes in single-sided deafness with tinnitus. *Front. Hum. Neurosci.* 11:210. doi: 10.3389/fnhum.2017.00210

Song, J. J., Ku, E. J., Kim, S., Kim, E., Choi, Y. S., and Jung, H. J. (2020). Increased risk of psychopathological abnormalities in subjects with unilateral hearing loss: a cross-sectional study. *Clin. Exp. Otorhinolaryngol.* doi: 10.21053/ceo.2020.00283. [Epub ahead of print].

Song, J. J., Vanneste, S., and De Ridder, D. (2015). Dysfunctional noise cancelling of the rostral anterior cingulate cortex in tinnitus patients. *PLoS ONE* 10:e0123538. doi: 10.1371/journal.pone.0123538

Talairach, J., and Tornoux, P. (1988). *Co-Planar Stereotaxic Atlas of the Human Brain: 3-Dimensional Proportional System: An Approach to Cerebral Imaging.* Stuttgart: Georg Thieme.

Vanneste, S., Alsalman, O., and De Ridder, D. (2018a). COMT and the neurogenetic architecture of hearing loss induced tinnitus. *Hear. Res.* 365, 1–15. doi: 10.1016/j.heares.2018.05.020

Vanneste, S., Alsalman, O., and De Ridder, D. (2019). Top-down and bottom-up regulated auditory phantom perception. *J. Neurosci.* 39, 364–378. doi: 10.1523/JNEUROSCI.0966-18.2018

Vanneste, S., and De Ridder, D. (2012). The auditory and non-auditory brain areas involved in tinnitus. An emergent property of multiple parallel overlapping subnetworks. *Front. Syst. Neurosci.* 6:31. doi: 10.3389/fnsys.2012.00031

Vanneste, S., and De Ridder, D. (2016). Deafferentation-based pathophysiological differences in phantom sound: tinnitus with and without hearing loss. *Neuroimage* 129, 80–94. doi: 10.1016/j.neuroimage.2015.12.002

Vanneste, S., Joos, K., and De Ridder, D. (2012). Prefrontal cortex based sex differences in tinnitus perception: same tinnitus intensity, same tinnitus distress, different mood. *PLoS ONE* 7:e31182. doi: 10.1371/journal.pone.0031182

Vanneste, S., Song, J. J., and De Ridder, D. (2018b). Thalamocortical dysrhythmia detected by machine learning. *Nat. Commun.* 9:1103. doi: 10.1038/s41467-018-02820-0

White, D. J., Congedo, M., Ciorciari, J., and Silberstein, R. B. (2012). Brain oscillatory activity during spatial navigation: theta and gamma activity link medial temporal and parietal regions. *J. Cogn. Neurosci.* 24, 686–697. doi: 10.1162/jocn_a_00098

Zhang, Z., Jia, X., Guan, X., Zhang, Y., Lyu, Y., Yang, J., et al. (2020). White matter abnormalities of auditory neural pathway in sudden sensorineural hearing loss using diffusion spectrum imaging: different findings from tinnitus. *Front. Neurosci.* 14:200. doi: 10.3389/fnins.2020.00200

3

Pre-Treatment Ongoing Cortical Oscillatory Activity Predicts Improvement of Tinnitus After Partial Peripheral Reafferentation with Hearing Aids

*Jae Joon Han[1], Dirk De Ridder[2], Sven Vanneste[3,4], Yu-Chen Chen[5], Ja-Won Koo[6] and Jae-Jin Song[6]**

[1] Department of Otorhinolaryngology-Head and Neck Surgery, Soonchunhyang University College of Medicine, Seoul Hospital, Seoul, South Korea, [2] Unit of Neurosurgery, Department of Surgical Sciences, Dunedin School of Medicine, University of Otago, Dunedin, New Zealand, [3] Lab for Clinical and Integrative Neuroscience, Trinity College of Neuroscience, Trinity College Dublin, Dublin, Ireland, [4] Lab for Clinical and Integrative Neuroscience, School of Behavioral and Brain Sciences, The University of Texas at Dallas, Dallas, TX, United States, [5] Department of Radiology, Nanjing First Hospital, Nanjing Medical University, Nanjing, China, [6] Department of Otorhinolaryngology-Head and Neck Surgery, Seoul National University Bundang Hospital, Seoul, South Korea

***Correspondence:**
Jae-Jin Song
jjsong96@snubh.org;
jjsong96@gmail.com

Although hearing aids (HAs) are sometimes efficacious in abating tinnitus, the precise mechanism underlying their effect is unclear and predictors of symptom improvement have not been determined. Here, we examined the correlation between the amount of tinnitus improvement and pre-HA quantitative electroencephalography (qEEG) findings to investigate cortical predictors of improvement after wearing HAs. QEEG data of thirty-three patients with debilitating tinnitus were retrospectively correlated with the percentage improvements in tinnitus handicap inventory and the numerical rating scale scores of tinnitus. Activation of brain areas involved in the default mode network (DMN; inferior parietal lobule, parahippocampus, and posterior cingulate cortex) were found to be a negative predictor of improvement in tinnitus-related distress after wearing HAs. In addition, higher pre-HA cortical power at the medial auditory processing system or higher functional connectivity of the lateral/medial auditory pathway to the DMN was found to serve as a positive prognostic indicator with regard to improvement of tinnitus-related distress. In addition, insufficient activity of the pre-treatment noise canceling system tended to be a negative predictor of tinnitus perception improvement after wearing HAs. The current study may serve as a milestone toward a pre-HAs prediction strategy for tinnitus improvements in subjects with hearing loss and severe tinnitus.

Keywords: tinnitus, hearing aids, hearing loss, treatment, electroencephalography, neural plasticity

INTRODUCTION

Tinnitus is an auditory symptom characterized by the perception of sound or noise in the absence of an external sound source. The overall prevalence of tinnitus in the general population is 10–15% (Henry et al., 2005; Bhatt et al., 2016) with about 7.2% of affected individuals reporting their symptom as a major problem and about half having discussed their symptom with a physician

(Bhatt et al., 2016). Various treatment modalities, such as medication, sound therapy, cognitive behavioral therapy, tinnitus retraining therapy, cochlear implants, non-invasive brain stimulation, and hearing aids (HAs), have been suggested for the management of tinnitus (Langguth et al., 2013; Bae et al., 2020), yet no treatment exists that benefits all patients (Langguth et al., 2013).

Since Saltzman and Ersner first reported effectiveness of HAs for controlling tinnitus about 70 years ago (Saltzman and Ersner, 1947), many studies have supported the use of HAs as a treatment option for tinnitus (Kiessling, 1980; Brooks and Bulmer, 1981; Surr et al., 1985; Surr et al., 1999). Even though at a meta-analytic level there is no support for the use of HAs with or without maskers (Sereda et al., 2018), still approximately half of patients using HAs experience an improvement of tinnitus (Surr et al., 1999; Shekhawat et al., 2013). In addition, a recent review indicated that 17 of 18 original research studies showed positive evidence suggesting that using HAs for tinnitus management is beneficial (Shekhawat et al., 2013). Therefore, HAs have been recommended as a useful treatment option for tinnitus patients with hearing loss (Tunkel et al., 2014).

Several hypotheses have been proposed to explain the possible mechanism of tinnitus improvement associated with the use of HAs (Del Bo and Ambrosetti, 2007). For example, HAs have been suggested to be beneficial for tinnitus patients by helping the brain to distinguish between true sounds and tinnitus, decreasing annoyance by partial masking of tinnitus using augmented environmental sounds, and enhancing the ability to cope with tinnitus by reducing communication stress (Del Bo and Ambrosetti, 2007; Shekhawat et al., 2013). In addition, the neurophysiological rationale of HAs usage suggested that sound amplification by HAs may restore the activity of auditory neurons and cortical activity (Gabriel et al., 2006; Norena and Eggermont, 2006), and therefore may lead to neuroplastic changes of the auditory pathway and neural correlates related to the generation of tinnitus.

Previous researchers have suggested several mechanisms of tinnitus generation in subjects with reduced peripheral auditory input. That is, auditory deprivation may result in a compensation mechanism called "homeostatic plasticity," a phenomenon affecting the neuronal activity of the auditory system at several levels along the ascending auditory pathway to compensate for the reduced peripheral input (Norena, 2011; Langguth et al., 2013). At the cortical level, peripheral deafferentation-induced changes such as reduced lateral inhibition in the deafferented cortical areas have been reported (Yang et al., 2011). Also, other researchers have suggested stochastic resonance serves to increase signals above the increased neuronal thresholds after peripheral hearing loss, thereby partly compensating for the hearing loss and possibly leading to the development of tinnitus (Krauss et al., 2016, 2018). Considering that all these models are based on the assumption that the ascending auditory system from the cochlea to the cerebral cortex attempts to maintain a neuronal network similar to the one before the peripheral auditory deprivation occurred, HA-assisted partial restoration of the cochlear input may abate tinnitus if these mechanisms are not totally irreversible. In other words, homeostatic plasticity along with reduced lateral inhibition or the stochastic resonance resulting in phantom auditory perception would become less active because less compensatory mechanisms are needed due to increased peripheral input assisted by HAs.

Hearing aid have long been proposed as one of the most useful treatment options for tinnitus, and most previous studies have reported positive effects of HAs on tinnitus. However, the mechanism underlying tinnitus improvement associated with HA usage remains unclear. In particular, despite previously suggested theories of tinnitus improvement by HAs implying the possible involvement of cortical neuroplastic changes, the neural substrates associated with the improvement of tinnitus by HAs have not been investigated. Based on previous studies of ours showing that pre-treatment cortical activities in the auditory cortex, posterior cingulate cortex, and the parahippocampus are important predictors of tinnitus improvement after hearing restoration by cochlear implantation (Song et al., 2013), and also showing that tinnitus in patients with hearing loss may be related to the parahippocampal mechanism (Vanneste and De Ridder, 2016), we surmised that similar areas might also be important in predicting tinnitus improvement associated with HA usage. The present study was performed to identify pre-treatment neural substrates associated with tinnitus improvement after using HAs in subjects with tinnitus. We also compared the cortical oscillatory activities of patients who showed marked improvement of tinnitus after wearing HAs with those who experienced slight improvement of tinnitus using source localization, complemented by connectivity analysis.

MATERIALS AND METHODS

Participants

A total of 33 non-pulsatile subjective tinnitus subjects with hearing loss who had used HAs for more than 6 months were enrolled in this study. The mean age of the participants was 64.6 ± 14.6 years (range: 26–88 years), and 14 (42.4%) were male. During the initial visit, we obtained a structured medical history regarding the characteristics of tinnitus, such as the affected side, the psychoacoustic nature (pure-tone, narrow-band noise, or warble-tone), matched tinnitus frequency and loudness, and the duration of tinnitus perception. Out of the total of 33 subjects, 14 (42.4%) complained of unilateral tinnitus, while the remaining 19 had bilateral tinnitus. More than half of the participants (19 of 33, 57.6%) reported pure-tone tinnitus, while 11 (33.3%) had narrow-band noise, and one (3.0%) had warble-tone tinnitus. The most frequently matched frequency of tinnitus was 8 kHz (12 subjects, 36.4%), and the others showed variable tinnitus frequencies (4 kHz, five subjects; 3 kHz, one subject; 2 kHz, four subjects, 1 kHz, one subject; 500 Hz, four subjects; 250 Hz, two subjects). The mean duration of tinnitus perception was 8.4 ± 9.8 years (range: 3 months – 40 years). This retrospective study was approved by the Seoul National University Bundang Hospital Institutional Review Board (IRB) and the requirement for informed consent from the subjects was waived (IRB- B-1702/383-104) and the IRB waived the need for informed consent for this study. All methods were performed in accordance with the relevant guidelines and regulations.

The perceived tinnitus handicap was measured using the tinnitus handicap inventory (THI), a self-reported tinnitus handicap measure consisting of 25 items evaluating the extent of tinnitus-related distress (Newman et al., 1996). We evaluated tinnitus loudness (response to the question "How loud is your tinnitus?" on a scale from 0 to 10), tinnitus-related distress (response to the question "How bothered are you by your tinnitus?" on a scale from 0 to 10), and tinnitus perception (response to the question "What is the percentage of the daytime during which you are aware of the tinnitus?" from 0 to 100%) based on numerical rating scale (NRS) scores. The questionnaires were evaluated both before and after 6 months of using HAs. We excluded subjects with Ménière's disease, pulsatile tinnitus, histories of drug or alcohol abuse, psychiatric/neurological disorders, and chronic headache; those using current psychotropic or central nervous system-active medications; those with a history of seizures; and those with any history of head injury resulting in loss of consciousness.

We used the median split method (Schlee et al., 2012; Song et al., 2013), a data-driven *post hoc* stratification approach, to compare the resting-state oscillatory brain activities between the subjects who showed marked improvement (MI group) and slight improvement (SI group) after tinnitus treatment with HAs. The MI and SI groups were assigned according to percentage improvement of NRS tinnitus distress scores. All subjects in the MI group showed >44.4% improvement of NRS tinnitus distress intensity, while all subjects in the SI group showed improvement <37.5%.

Hearing Aids Fitting and Usage

At the initial visit, the hearing level of all participants was evaluated with pure tone audiometry (PTA) and speech audiometry, and all subjects were shown to have mild to severe hearing loss. The average hearing threshold (calculated by averaging the PTA thresholds at 500, 1000, 2000, and 4000 Hz) (Lee et al., 2017; Sunwoo et al., 2017; Song et al., 2018; Bae et al., 2019; Han et al., 2019; Huh et al., 2019; Lee et al., 2019b; Shim et al., 2019) of participants was 53.4±15.0 dB (range: 15.0 – 105.0) and the average speech discrimination score was 62.7 ± 25.7% (range: 12–100%). The selection of HAs was based on patients' preferences and needs among all products available at our institute (Oticon, Resound, Siemens, Starkey, and Widex). The choice of HAs was also determined based on individual needs and choice from entry to advanced level. Therefore, the implemented technology and types of HAs were relatively variable. Fitting of HAs was performed by routine procedures according to each manufacturer's guidelines and programmed via NOAH or NOAH-Link® equipment using the algorithm provided by each manufacturer's software. The presence of tinnitus and its matched frequency were not considered during the fitting process, and additional functions for tinnitus management, such as sound generation implemented in HAs, were not applied in this study so as to evaluate pure contribution of HAs to the improvement of tinnitus. HAs were fitted according to the individual's configuration of hearing loss as well as to participant's comfort and preference. The participants were counseled to increase the usage time of HAs gradually, up to full-time usage. Follow-up and re-fitting were performed 2 – 3 times a month until the patients were satisfied with the amplification of sound and alleviation of discomfort from HAs. After using HAs for over 6 months with proper fitting and full-time usage, aided threshold levels at frequencies of 250, 500, 1000, 2000, 3000, and 4000 Hz were evaluated. The average follow-up duration was 5.3 ± 0.9 months (range, 3 – 7 months). In addition, questionnaires on THI and NRS scores were obtained after 6 months of HA usage.

EEG Recording

To identify the neural correlates related with tinnitus improvement after wearing HAs, we performed EEG recording before applying the HAs. Data acquisition and pre-processing procedures were performed according to the methods described previously (Song et al., 2017; Han et al., 2018; Vanneste et al., 2018; Lee et al., 2019a). Resting-state EEGs were recorded for about 5 min without any sound stimuli at 19 scalp sites using a tin electrode cap (ElectroCap, Eaton, OH, United States) connected to a Mitsar amplifier (Mitsar EEG-201; Mitsar, Saint Petersburg, Russia) in a fully lit room shielded from sound and stray electric fields. The participants sat upright on a comfortable chair during EEG recording. The EEG data were saved using WinEEG software (ver. 2.84.44; Mitsar)[1]. The impedances at all electrodes were maintained below 5 kΩ. Data were obtained at a sampling rate of 1024 Hz and then filtered using a high-pass filter with a cutoff of 0.15 Hz and a low-pass filter with a cutoff of 200 Hz. After initial data acquisition, the raw data were processed with resampling to 128 Hz and then with band-pass filtering using a fast Fourier transform filter and application of a Hanning window at 2 – 44 Hz. The data were then imported into Eureka! Software (Sherlin and Congedo, 2005). All episodic artifacts related to eye blinks, eye movements, teeth clenching, or body movements were inspected manually and removed from the EEG stream with Eureka! software. Further artifact removal was conducted by performing independent component analysis using ICoN software[2] (Koprivova et al., 2011; White et al., 2012).

Caffeinated and alcoholic beverages were prohibited for 24 h prior to EEG recording to avoid caffeine-induced alpha and beta power decreases (Siepmann and Kirch, 2002) or alcohol-induced changes in the EEG stream (Volkow et al., 2000). Participants' vigilance was monitored to prevent abnormal EEG signals, such as slowing of the alpha rhythm or enhancement of theta power (Moazami-Goudarzi et al., 2010). The participants included in the present study did not show drowsiness-related EEG changes.

Source Localization Analysis

The localization of the intracerebral sources from the recorded EEG streams was performed using low-resolution brain electromagnetic tomography (LORETA)-KEY software[3], a toolbox for the functional localization of standardized current

[1] http://www.mitsar-medical.com
[2] http://sites.google.com/site/marcocongedo/software/nica
[3] http://www.uzh.ch/keyinst/NewLORETA/Software/Software.htm

densities based on electrophysiological and neuroanatomical constraints (Pascual-Marqui, 2002). Source localization was performed based on each of the following eight frequency bands: delta (2 – 3.5 Hz), theta (4 – 7.5 Hz), alpha1 (8 – 10 Hz), alpha2 (10 – 12 Hz), beta 1 (13 – 18 Hz), beta 2 (18.5 – 21 Hz), beta 3 (21.5 – 30 Hz), and gamma (30.5 – 44 Hz) bands (Kim et al., 2016; Song et al., 2017; Han et al., 2018; Vanneste et al., 2018). The electrical activity was computed as current density ($\mu A/mm^2$) without assuming a predefined number of active sources. The LORETA-KEY software divides the Montreal Neurological Institute (MNI)-152 volume (Fuchs et al., 2002), including the hippocampus and anterior cingulate cortex, into 6239 voxels with dimensions of 5 mm × 5 mm × 5 mm. Scalp electrode coordinates on the MNI brain are derived from the international 5% system (Jurcak et al., 2007). Performing 5000 random permutations, correction for multiple testing (i.e., for tests performed for all electrodes and/or voxels, and for all time samples and/or different frequencies) was carried out and, thus, no further correction for multiple comparison was needed. LORETA-KEY assumes related orientations and strengths of neighboring neuronal sources and, thus, the inverse problem, which is derived from source reconstruction from electric neuronal activity based on extracranial measurements, is solved by the algorithm. Anatomical labeling of significant clusters was performed automatically by an embedded toolbox within LORETA-KEY, and these labels were reconfirmed by matching the centroids of significant clusters with the Talairach and Tournoux atlas (Talairach and Tornoux, 1988).

Functional Connectivity Analysis

Phase synchronization and the extent of coherence between the MI group and SI group corresponding to different regions of interest (ROIs) were calculated to evaluate the difference of functional connectivity between two groups using the LORETA-KEY connectivity toolbox. This toolbox defines measures of linear and non-linear dependence (i.e., coherence and phase synchronization) between multivariate time series; the measures are expressed as the sums of lagged/instantaneous dependencies. For functional connectivity analysis, a total of 16 ROIs defined by the Brodmann area (BA), known to be related to tinnitus according to the literature, were selected as possible nodes: the bilateral primary auditory cortices (A1, BAs 41 and 42) (Rolls, 2004; Kringelbach, 2005; Smits et al., 2007), the bilateral parahippocampus (PHC, BA 27) (Landgrebe et al., 2009), the bilateral dorsal/pregenual/subgenual anterior cingulate cortices (dACC, BA 24; pgACC, BA 32; sgACC, BA 25) (Damasio, 1996; Vanneste et al., 2010; De Ridder et al., 2011b), the bilateral orbitofrontal cortices (OFC, BA 10) (Song et al., 2015), and the bilateral inferior parietal lobule (IPL, BA 40) (Houdayer et al., 2015; Chen et al., 2018).

Region of Interest (ROI) Analysis

For ROIs that showed a significant correlation with the percentage improvements in NRS tinnitus-related distress or perception, log-transformed electric current density was averaged. Each ROI was defined by a single voxel that was closest to the center of the area where a significant difference was found in the source localization analysis. Then, the correlation between the log-transformed electric current density in each ROI and the percentage improvements in NRS tinnitus-related distress or perception was evaluated by calculating the Pearson correlation coefficient.

Statistical Analysis

To identify the resting-state cortical oscillatory activities related to tinnitus improvement, the LORETA-KEY images were analyzed by the statistical non-parametric mapping (SnPM) method for each contrast using LORETA-KEY's built-in voxel-wise randomization tests (5000 permutations). In this way, we correlated pre-HAs source-localized activities among whole-brain areas and a connectivity of 16 ROIs with the percentage improvement in the THI score, NRS loudness, NRS distress, and NRS perception. Also, to test the reliability of our results, we have split the enrolled subjects into 2 groups according to the order of enrollment (an odd-numbered subject group and an even-numbered subject group) and performed the same analyses to see if the correlations are maintained in these two subgroups. Moreover, we employed a t statistic between MI and SI groups with a threshold of $P < 0.05$. Correction for multiple comparisons in SnPM using random permutations has been shown to yield similar results to those obtained from a statistical parametric mapping approach using a general linear model with multiple comparison corrections (Nichols and Holmes, 2002). For lagged linear connectivity differences, we compared the differences between the MI and SI groups for each contrast using the paired t statistic with a threshold of $P < 0.05$. We also corrected for multiple comparisons using LORETA-KEY's built-in voxel-wise randomization tests on all of the voxels included in the 16 ROIs for connectivity analysis (5000 permutations). All other descriptive statistical analyses were performed using SPSS software (version 20.0, SPSS, Inc., Chicago, IL, United States). In all analyses, $P < 0.05$ was taken to indicate statistical significance.

RESULTS

Functional Gain and Tinnitus Improvement

For 33 tinnitus participants included, the average aided hearing thresholds with HAs were significantly better than unaided air conduction thresholds at all frequencies [250 Hz, 27.0 ± 10.6 vs. 33.9 ± 19.0; 500 Hz, 31.2 ± 11.9 vs. 38.6 ± 17.5; 1 kHz (32.0 ± 12.3 vs. 50.6 ± 18.7; 2 kHz, 37.7 ± 13.1 vs. 56.1 ± 19.2; 3 kHz, 44.7 ± 13.9 vs. 63.3 ± 18.4; 4 kHz, 50.2 ± 13.7 vs. 68.3 ± 19.4; $P < 0.01$ for all frequencies)] (**Supplementary Figure S1**). The average functional gains of HAs were 7.0 ± 14.7 dB at 250 Hz, 7.4 ± 12.6 dB at 500 Hz, 18.6 ± 12.2 dB at 1 kHz, 18.3 ± 14.1 dB at 2 kHz, 18.6 ± 12.8 dB at 3 kHz, and 18.2 ± 12.7 dB at 4 kHz.

All questionnaire scores pertaining to tinnitus severity improved significantly after using HAs (**Table 1**). The mean THI scores after using HAs were significantly lower than pre-HA THI scores (27.9 ± 18.0 vs. 56.8 ± 24.0, respectively, $P < 0.01$). In addition, NRS tinnitus loudness (4.8 ± 2.1 vs. 7.0 ± 2.1,

TABLE 1 | Changes in tinnitus handicap inventory and numeric rating scale scores 6 months after using hearing aids.

	Pre-HAs	Post-HAs	*P*-value
THI score	56.8 ± 24.0	27.9 ± 18.0	<0.01
NRS loudness	7.0 ± 2.1	4.8 ± 2.1	<0.01
NRS distress	6.7 ± 3.0	4.3 ± 2.6	<0.01
NRS perception (%)	79.1 ± 27.5	59.7 ± 36.4	<0.01

THI, tinnitus handicap inventory; NRS, numeric rating scale; HAs, hearing aids.

respectively, $P < 0.01$), tinnitus distress (4.3 ± 2.6 vs. 6.7 ± 3.0, respectively, $P < 0.01$), and tinnitus perception (59.7 ± 36.4 vs. 79.1 ± 27.5, respectively, $P < 0.01$) improved significantly after 6 months of wearing HAs. To evaluate the relationship between the degree of tinnitus improvement and the functional gain with HAs, we performed simple correlation analysis between the functional gains and the tinnitus questionnaire scores. The percentage improvements in the THI scores were not significantly correlated with the average functional gain with use of HAs ($r = 0.02$, $P = 0.92$). The percentage changes of NRS loudness ($r = -0.13$, $P = 0.48$), distress ($r = 0.049$, $P = 0.78$), and perception ($r = -0.01$, $P = 0.94$) were also not significantly correlated with the functional gain in use of HAs.

Source-Localized Correlation Analysis Between Pre-HAs qEEG and Post-HAs Tinnitus Improvement

The percentage improvements in NRS tinnitus-related distress were negatively correlated with the pre-HA source-localized activities at the right IPL (BA 40), right PHC (BA 27), and right posterior cingulate cortex (PCC, BA 23) for the gamma frequency band ($P < 0.01$) (**Figure 1**). The correlation analysis between the log-transformed mean current density for the gamma frequency band at BA 40 and the percentage improvements in NRS tinnitus-related distress showed a significant negative correlation ($r = -0.39$, $P = 0.03$). In subgroup analysis, we have confirmed negative correlations between the percentage improvements in NRS tinnitus-related distress and the right IPL, PHC, and PCC in each subgroup (**Supplementary Figure S2**), in accordance with the results for all subjects (**Figure 1**). For the other seven frequency bands, there were no significant correlations between the percentage improvements of NRS distress and the pre-HA source-localized activities.

The activities of the bilateral sgACC (BA 25) exhibited negative correlations of marginal significance with the percentage improvements in NRS tinnitus perception for the beta 3 frequency band ($P = 0.08$) (**Figure 2**). The log-transformed mean current density for the beta 3 frequency band at the right BA 25 showed a tendency of negative correlation with the percentage improvements in NRS tinnitus-related perception ($P = 0.10$). In subgroup analysis, the tendency of negative correlation between the percentage improvements in NRS tinnitus-related perception and the bilateral sgACC for beta 3 frequency band was also confirmed in each subgroup (**Supplementary Figure S3**), in accordance with the results for all subjects (**Figure 2**). No significant correlations were evident between the percentage improvements of NRS perception and the pre-HA source-localized activities for the other seven frequency bands.

Meanwhile, the percentage improvement of NRS tinnitus loudness did not show significant correlations with pre-HA source-localized activities at any of the eight frequency bands examined.

With regard to the percentage improvement of NRS tinnitus distress, in comparison to the SI group, the MI group showed significantly higher cortical powers in the bilateral dorsolateral prefrontal cortices (DLPFC, BA 9), bilateral dACC (BA 24), and bilateral sgACC (BA 32) for the alpha 1 frequency band ($P < 0.01$) (**Figure 3**). There were no significant differences between the two groups for the other seven frequency bands (delta, theta, alpha 2, beta 1, 2, and 3).

Connectivity Analyses

On correlation analysis between lagged linear functional connectivity of the 16 ROIs and questionnaire scores (THI and NRS scores), no significant correlations were found. However, on lagged linear functional connectivity analysis with regard to tinnitus-related distress, the MI group showed significantly increased functional connectivities in comparison to the SI group between the left A1 and left IPL for the delta frequency band (**Figure 4A**), between the left A1 and right PHC for the theta frequency band (**Figure 4B**), between the left OFC and left IPL for the alpha 1 frequency band (**Figure 4C**), and between the bilateral dACC and right IPL for the alpha 2 frequency band (**Figure 4D**) ($P < 0.05$). For the other four frequency bands (beta 1, 2, 3, and gamma), no significant differences were found between the MI and SI groups with regard to functional connectivity among the 16 ROIs.

DISCUSSION

In the current study, we sought to evaluate the treatment effect of HAs in subjects with debilitating tinnitus and to gain a better understanding of the underlying neural predictors of a beneficial effect related to HAs. We observed significant tinnitus improvement 6 months after wearing HAs and found several positive- and negative pre-treatment cortical indicators that may be important for predicting the amount of improvement with regard to tinnitus-related distress and tinnitus perception during the daytime. In addition to previous observational studies showing improvement of tinnitus after wearing HAs in subjects with tinnitus, the current study is the first to demonstrate treatment outcome may be predictable based on the status of the brain before HAs are applied.

Activation of the Default Mode Network as a Negative Predictor of Tinnitus-Related Distress Improvements Even After Partial Peripheral Reafferentation by HAs

As described above, the percentage improvements in NRS tinnitus-related distress showed statistically significant negative

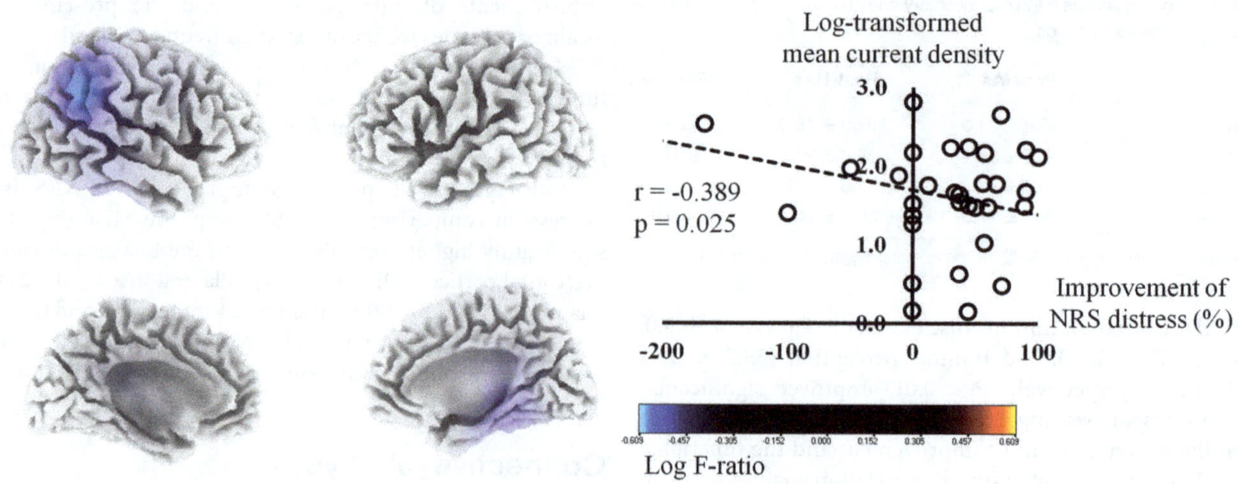

FIGURE 1 | Source-localized correlation analysis between the percentage improvements in the numerical rating scale (NRS) of tinnitus distress and the resting-state quantitative electroencephalography data before wearing hearing aids (HAs). The percentage improvements in NRS tinnitus-related distress correlated negatively with the pre-HA source-localized activities at the right inferior parietal lobule, right parahippocampus, and right posterior cingulate cortex for the gamma frequency band.

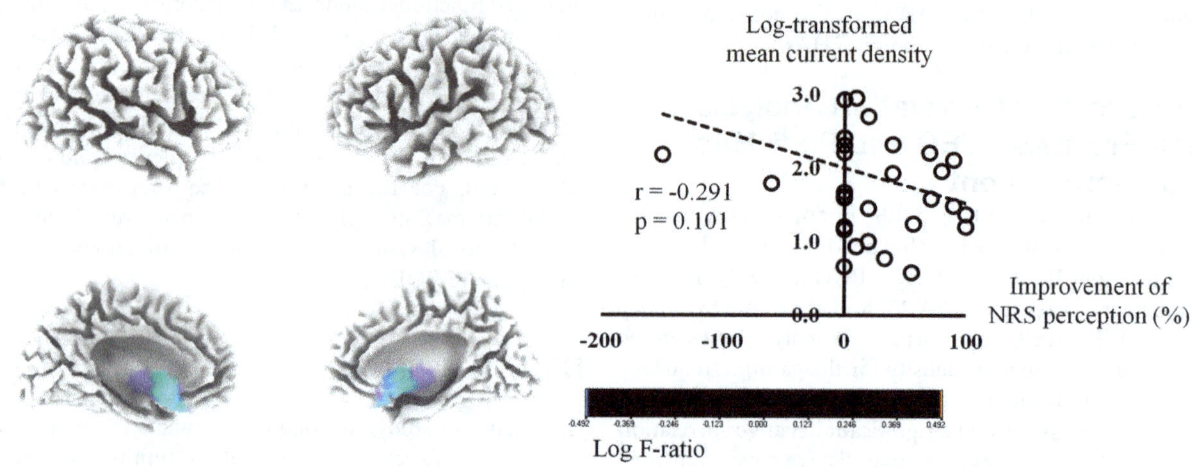

FIGURE 2 | Source-localized correlation analysis between the percentage improvements in the numerical rating scale (NRS) of tinnitus perception and the resting-state quantitative electroencephalography data before wearing hearing aids (HAs). The activities of the bilateral subgenual anterior cingulate cortex exhibited negative correlations of marginal significance with the percentage improvements in NRS tinnitus perception for the beta 3 frequency band (*P* = 0.08).

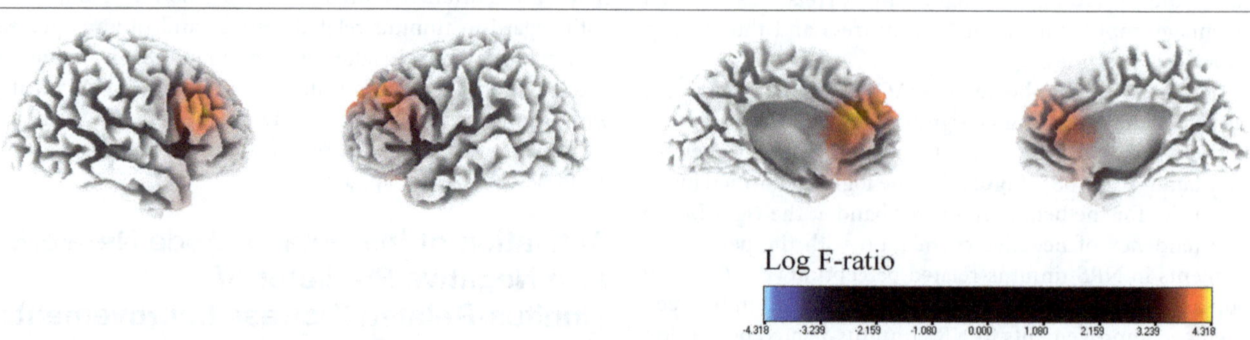

FIGURE 3 | Median-split source-localized comparison between the marked improvement (MI) group and the slight improvement (SI) group with regard to tinnitus-related distress. The MI group showed significantly higher cortical powers in the bilateral dorsolateral prefrontal cortices, bilateral dorsal anterior cingulate cortices, and bilateral subgenual anterior cingulate cortices for the alpha 1 frequency band in comparison with the SI group.

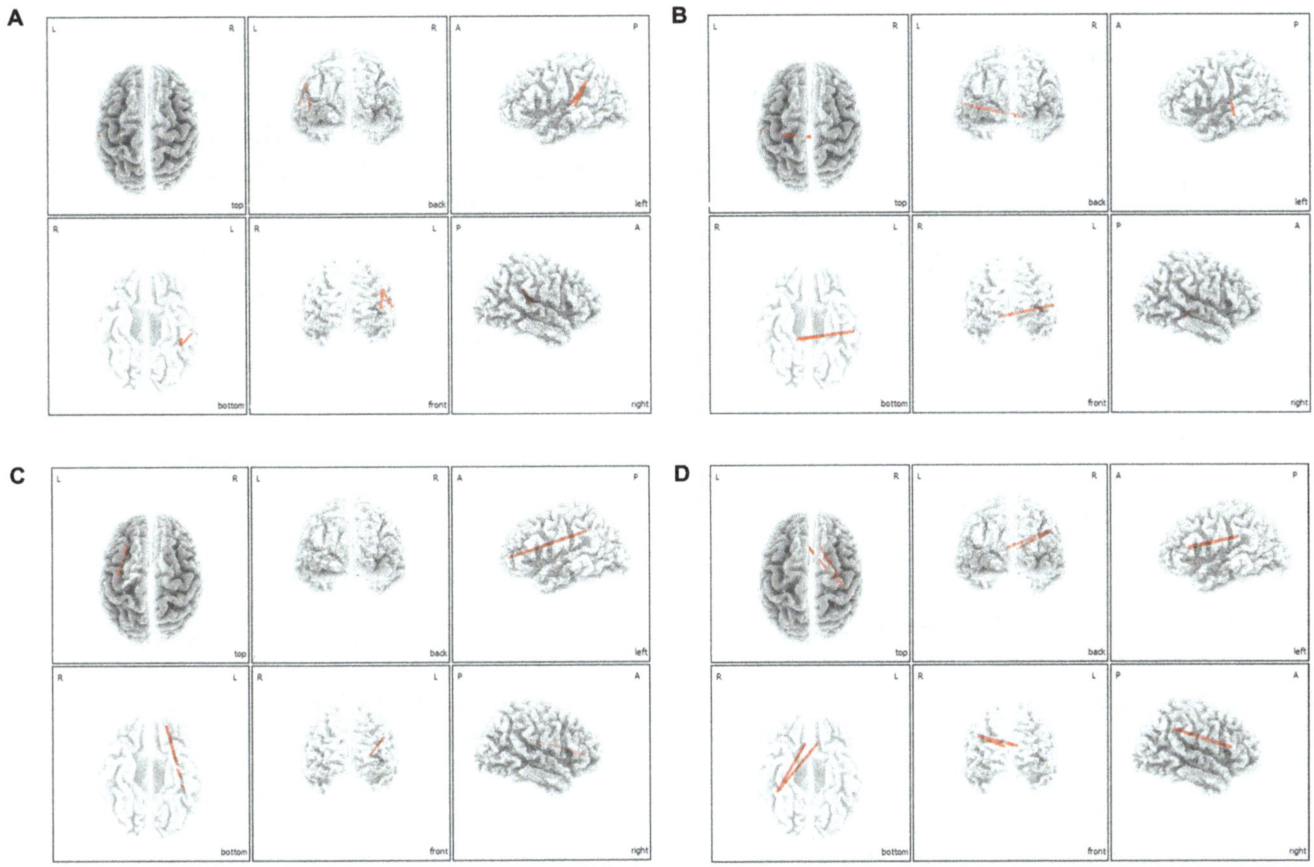

FIGURE 4 | Median-split lagged linear functional connectivity analysis with regard to tinnitus-related distress. The marked improvement (MI) group showed significantly increased functional connectivities in comparison with the slight improvement (SI) group between the left primary auditory cortices and left inferior parietal lobule for the delta frequency band **(A)**, between the left primary auditory cortex and right parahippocampus for the theta frequency band **(B)**, between the left orbitofrontal cortex and left inferior parietal lobule for the alpha 1 frequency band **(C)**, and between the bilateral dorsal anterior cingulate cortex and right inferior parietal lobule for the alpha 2 frequency band **(D)**.

correlations with the pre-HAs source-localized activities at the right IPL, right PHC, and right PCC for the gamma frequency band (**Figure 1**). These three areas have been regarded as the components of the brain's default mode network (DMN) (Raichle et al., 2001; Raichle and Snyder, 2007; Raichle, 2015), a specific group of brain regions activated when people are occupied with internally focused tasks.

Previous studies have suggested that tinnitus generators may become integrated in the DMN in subjects with tinnitus (De Ridder et al., 2011a; Vanneste and De Ridder, 2012). In this regard, an abnormally increased activity in tinnitus patients with hearing loss may be an ominous sign with regard to symptom improvement after wearing HAs. That is, even after partial reafferentation by HAs, tinnitus-related distress may not be successfully improved because tinnitus itself may already have become a norm due to activation of the components of the DMN. This is also consistent with a previous report showing relatively unsatisfactory improvement of tinnitus after cochlear implantation in single-sided deafness subjects who showed relatively high preoperative cortical power at the components of the DMN (Song et al., 2013).

Tinnitus Subjects With Higher Medial Auditory Processing System Activity May Respond More to HA-Assisted Increased Auditory Input

On median split analysis with regard to tinnitus-related distress, the MI group showed significantly higher cortical powers in the bilateral DLPFC, bilateral dACC, and bilateral sgACC for the alpha 1 frequency band in comparison with the SI group (**Figure 3**). Analogous to the medial pain system (Price, 2000; Kulkarni et al., 2005), a medial auditory processing system in charge of affective components of sound processing has recently been proposed (Leaver et al., 2011; De Ridder et al., 2014). As the DLPFC, dACC, and sgACC are components of the medial auditory processing system, we posit that tinnitus subjects with higher medial auditory processing system activity may respond better to HA-assisted increased auditory input. That is, partial peripheral reafferentation by HAs may abate the affective component of tinnitus to a greater extent in subjects with abnormally increased activity in the affective sound processing system.

This is also consistent with a previous electrical stimulation study indicating activation of the DLPFC and the dACC in patients with limb and back pain undergoing burst stimulation of the spinal cord (De Ridder et al., 2013). As the DLPFC and the dACC are also components of the medial pain pathway (De Ridder et al., 2013), the results of the present study showing higher cortical powers in the DLPFC and dACC in the MI group reconfirm previous reports suggesting analogies between chronic pain and tinnitus (Tonndorf, 1987; De Ridder et al., 2011a; Rauschecker et al., 2015). That is, in addition to previously suggested analogies, such as central phantom perception after peripheral injury or hypersensitivity to sensory stimulation, both chronic pain and tinnitus may respond well to peripheral stimulation when the medial pain or auditory pathway is activated.

Functional Connection of the Lateral/Medial Auditory Pathway to the IPL and PHC May Ameliorate the Negative Influence of the DMN With Regard to the Improvement of Tinnitus-Related Distress

Functional connectivity contrast analysis between the MI and SI groups revealed significantly increased functional connectivities between the left A1 and the left IPL in the MI group compared to those in the SI group for the delta frequency band (**Figure 4A**), and between the left A1 and right PHC for the theta frequency band (**Figure 4B**). Together with the findings of source-localized correlation analysis showing higher pre-HA cortical powers at the IPL and the PHC as negative prognostic factors with regard to improvement of tinnitus-related distress after wearing HAs, the median split connectivity analysis results may indicate that tinnitus distress would be abated more if the IPL and PHC, the components of DMN, are functionally connected to A1. That is, if the lateral auditory pathway is activated by HA-assisted partial peripheral reafferentation and if A1 is functionally connected to the IPL or the PHC, this may offset the negative influence of the IPL and the PHC with regard to improvement of tinnitus-related distress after wearing HAs. In this regard, increased functional connectivity between the bilateral dACCs and right IPL for the alpha 2 frequency band in the MI group, as compared to the SI group, could also be interpreted in the same way. That is, if a tinnitus subject's functional connection between the medial auditory pathway and the DMN is relatively increased before wearing HAs, there is a relatively greater chance of tinnitus-related distress improvement after wearing HAs because abnormally increased activity in the DMN may be mitigated by increased activity of the medial auditory pathway after wearing HAs. This is in agreement with direct modulation of the dACC and auditory cortex by implants. If a patient has increased functional connectivity between the auditory cortex and the parahippocampus, the patient is more likely to respond to the implant on the auditory cortex (De Ridder and Vanneste, 2014). Similarly, if a patient has increased functional connectivity from the dACC, an implant is more likely to be effective in improving tinnitus (De Ridder et al., 2016).

Pre-treatment Noise-Canceling System Activity May Determine the Improvement of Tinnitus Perception After Wearing Hearing Aids

The percentage improvements in NRS tinnitus-related perception showed a trend toward a negative correlation ($P = 0.08$) with the pre-HA source-localized activities at the bilateral sgACC (**Figure 2**). Although not statistically significant, these results were consistent with our previous report positing the sgACC as one of the core components of the descending noise-canceling mechanism that counteracts peripheral auditory deafferentation-based phantom sound (i.e., tinnitus) generation (Lee et al., 2019a). That is, our results suggest that if the pre-treatment cortical oscillatory power of the noise canceling system consisting of the rostral ACC as well as the sgACC is not sufficient, the perception of tinnitus may not be improved even after partial restoration of the auditory input by HAs. This is another analogy with chronic pain. That is, when performing spinal cord stimulation, the amount of improvement depends on the activation of the pgACC (Moens et al., 2012), which is part of the descending pain inhibitory pathway (Fields, 2004; Kong et al., 2010), the somatosensory analog of the noise canceling system.

The sgACC itself extends into the ventromedial prefrontal cortex (vmPFC), which was suggested in previous functional MRI studies to form part of the core of tinnitus perception (Leaver et al., 2011, 2012). Other groups have proposed that the vmPFC and the nucleus accumbens are part of a central "gatekeeping" system that evaluates the relevance of sensory stimuli and modulates information flow via descending pathways (Rauschecker et al., 2015). In this regard, it was suggested that tinnitus occurs when the function of the vmPFC is compromised. Considering the anatomical proximity between the sgACC and vmPFC, we conjecture that a dysfunctional sgACC (or vmPFC) may be responsible for the failure of descending noise canceling and, thus, induction of tinnitus perception. Judging from the results of the present study showing a trend-level negative correlation between pre-HA sgACC activities and post-HA improvements in tinnitus perception (**Figure 2**), we surmised that partial reafferentation by HAs may not be effective for tinnitus subjects with dysfunctional sgACCs with regard to the reduction of tinnitus perception.

Strengths and Limitations of This Study

To our knowledge, this is the first study to show the possibility of treatment outcome prediction with regard to the amount of tinnitus improvement using pre-HA cortical oscillatory features.

However, several limitations of the present study should be noted. First, as we evaluated the treatment outcomes of HAs 6 months after the first fitting, the long-term effects of HAs with regard to improvement of tinnitus should be re-evaluated in a follow-up study. That is, future studies correlating pre-treatment rs-qEEG data with long-term outcomes should be conducted to determine the cortical predictors of the final tinnitus treatment outcome after wearing HAs. Second, information on the post-HA status of the included subjects was limited because only questionnaires, such as THI and NRS scales, were used for outcome evaluation of tinnitus improvement. In this regard, future follow-up studies exploring post-HA qEEG changes to determine objective cortical oscillatory activity changes after partial peripheral reafferentation by HAs, and to correlate changes in cortical oscillatory activities with changes in subjective tinnitus and tinnitus-related distress, should be performed. Third, we enrolled tinnitus patients with severe distress (i.e., mean THI score of 56.8, NRS loudness of 7.0, and NRS distress of 6.7). That is, only a few subjects had mild distress in this retrospective cohort. To explore HA-related tinnitus improvement and relevant cortical activity changes, and to minimize the effects of improved distress, further studies are required to explore subjective symptom changes and objective oscillatory power changes in subjects with tinnitus, with minimal distress caused by their symptoms. Fourth, dividing the subjects into groups with- and without meaningful THI improvements, and comparing pre-HAs qEEGs to see the pre-treatment differences between good- and poor responders to HAs would give us further valuable information on the clinical setting. However, there were only 3 of 33 subjects who showed clinically an "improvement," defined as a decrease of more than 20% in the THI score (Khedr et al., 2008), and thus the current study group precluded the possibility of the group comparison between good- and poor responders. Future follow-up studies in a larger number of subjects are warranted to discover pre-HAs predictors of clinically significant improvements in tinnitus after wearing HAs.

CONCLUSION

Taken together, we evaluated the effects of HAs in subjects with severe tinnitus, with reference to pre-treatment cortical oscillatory patterns measured by rs-qEEG. This study underscored activation of the DMN as a negative predictor of tinnitus-related distress improvements even after partial peripheral reafferentation by HAs. In addition, we found that higher pre-HA cortical oscillatory power at the medial auditory processing system or functional connection of the lateral/medial auditory pathway to the DMN may act as positive prognostic indicators with regard to improvement of tinnitus-related distress. Finally, we observed a tendency toward insufficient activity of the pre-treatment noise canceling system as a negative predictor of tinnitus perception improvement after wearing HAs. The present study may facilitate the development of a pre-HA prediction strategy for tinnitus improvements in subjects with hearing loss and severe tinnitus.

ETHICS STATEMENT

The studies involving human participants were reviewed and approved by Seoul National University Bundang Hospital Institutional Review Board. Written informed consent for participation was not required for this study in accordance with the national legislation and the institutional requirements.

AUTHOR CONTRIBUTIONS

J-JS led the analysis and interpretation of the result, and drafted the first manuscript. JH and J-JS conceived the investigation, revised the manuscript for important intellectual content. JH, DR, SV, Y-CC, J-WK, and J-JS contributed to all aspects of the investigation, including methodological design, data collection and analysis, interpretation of the results, and revision of the manuscript for important intellectual content. All authors approved the final version of the manuscript and agreed to be accountable for all aspects of the work.

REFERENCES

Bae, E. B., Lee, J. H., and Song, J.-J. (2020). Single-session of combined tDCS-TMS may increase therapeutic effects in subjects with Tinnitus. *Front. Neurol.* 11:160. doi: 10.3389/fneur.2020.00160

Bae, Y. J., Shim, Y. J., Choi, B. S., Kim, J. H., Koo, J. W., and Song, J. J. (2019). "Third Window" and "Single Window" effects impede surgical success: analysis of Retrofenestral Otosclerosis involving the internal auditory canal or round window. *J. Clin. Med.* 8:1182. doi: 10.3390/jcm8081182

Bhatt, J. M., Lin, H. W., and Bhattacharyya, N. (2016). Prevalence, severity, exposures, and treatment patterns of Tinnitus in the United States. *JAMA Otolaryngol. Head Neck Surg.* 142, 959–965. doi: 10.1001/jamaoto.2016.1700

Brooks, D. N., and Bulmer, D. (1981). Survey of binaural hearing aid users. *Ear Hear.* 2, 220–224.

Chen, Y. C., Liu, S., Lv, H., Bo, F., Feng, Y., Chen, H., et al. (2018). Abnormal Resting-State Functional Connectivity of the Anterior Cingulate Cortex in Unilateral Chronic Tinnitus Patients. *Front. Neurosci.* 12:9. doi: 10.3389/fnins.2018.00009

Damasio, A. R. (1996). The somatic marker hypothesis and the possible functions of the prefrontal cortex. *Philos. Trans. R. Soc. Lond. B Biol. Sci.* 351, 1413–1420. doi: 10.1098/rstb.1996.0125

De Ridder, D., Elgoyhen, A. B., Romo, R., and Langguth, B. (2011a). Phantom percepts: tinnitus and pain as persisting aversive memory networks. *Proc. Natl. Acad. Sci. U.S.A.* 108, 8075–8080. doi: 10.1073/pnas.1018466108

De Ridder, D., Vanneste, S., and Congedo, M. (2011b). The distressed brain: a group blind source separation analysis on tinnitus. *PLoS One* 6:e24273. doi: 10.1371/journal.pone.0024273

De Ridder, D., Joos, K., and Vanneste, S. (2016). Anterior cingulate implants for tinnitus: report of 2 cases. *J. Neurosurg.* 124, 893–901. doi: 10.3171/2015.3.JNS142880

De Ridder, D., Plazier, M., Kamerling, N., Menovsky, T., and Vanneste, S. (2013). Burst spinal cord stimulation for limb and back pain. *World Neurosurg.* 80:642-649.e1. doi: 10.1016/j.wneu.2013.01.040

De Ridder, D., and Vanneste, S. (2014). Targeting the parahippocampal area by auditory cortex stimulation in tinnitus. *Brain Stimul.* 7, 709–717. doi: 10.1016/j.brs.2014.04.004

De Ridder, D., Vanneste, S., and Freeman, W. (2014). The Bayesian brain: phantom percepts resolve sensory uncertainty. *Neurosci. Biobehav. Rev.* 44, 4–15. doi: 10.1016/j.neubiorev.2012.04.001

Del, Bo L., and Ambrosetti, U. (2007). Hearing aids for the treatment of tinnitus. *Prog. Brain Res.* 166, 341–345. doi: 10.1016/s0079-6123(07)66032-4

Fields, H. (2004). State-dependent opioid control of pain. *Nat. Rev. Neurosci.* 5, 565–575. doi: 10.1038/nrn1431

Fuchs, M., Kastner, J., Wagner, M., Hawes, S., and Ebersole, J. S. (2002). A standardized boundary element method volume conductor model. *Clin. Neurophysiol.* 113, 702–712.

Gabriel, D., Veuillet, E., Vesson, J. F., and Collet, L. (2006). Rehabilitation plasticity: influence of hearing aid fitting on frequency discrimination performance near the hearing-loss cut-off. *Hear. Res.* 213, 49–57. doi: 10.1016/j.heares.2005.12.007

Han, J. J., Jang, J. H., Ridder, D., Vanneste, S., Koo, J. W., and Song, J. J. (2018). Increased parietal circuit-breaker activity in delta frequency band and abnormal delta/theta band connectivity in salience network in hyperacusis subjects. *PLoS One* 13:e0191858. doi: 10.1371/journal.pone.0191858

Han, S. A., Choe, G., Kim, Y., Koo, J. W., Choi, B. Y., and Song, J. J. (2019). Beware of a Fragile Footplate: lessons from Ossiculoplasty in patients with ossicular anomalies related to second pharyngeal arch defects. *J. Clin. Med.* 8:2130. doi: 10.3390/jcm8122130

Henry, J. A., Dennis, K. C., and Schechter, M. A. (2005). General review of tinnitus: prevalence, mechanisms, effects, and management. *J. Speech Lang. Hear Res.* 48, 1204–1235. doi: 10.1044/1092-4388(2005/084)

Houdayer, E., Teggi, R., Velikova, S., Gonzalez-Rosa, J. J., Bussi, M., Comi, G., et al. (2015). Involvement of cortico-subcortical circuits in normoacousic chronic tinnitus: a source localization EEG study. *Clin. Neurophysiol.* 126, 2356–2365. doi: 10.1016/j.clinph.2015.01.027

Huh, G., Bae, Y. J., Woo, H. J., Park, J. H., Koo, J. W., and Song, J. J. (2019). Vestibulocochlear symptoms caused by vertebrobasilar dolichoectasia. *Clin. Exp. Otorhinolaryngol.* doi: 10.21053/ceo.2019.00780 [Online ahead of print].

Jurcak, V., Tsuzuki, D., and Dan, I. (2007). 10/20, 10/10, and 10/5 systems revisited: their validity as relative head-surface-based positioning systems. *Neuroimage* 34, 1600–1611. doi: 10.1016/j.neuroimage.2006.09.024

Khedr, E. M., Rothwell, J. C., Ahmed, M. A., and El-Atar, A. (2008). Effect of daily repetitive transcranial magnetic stimulation for treatment of tinnitus: comparison of different stimulus frequencies. *J. Neurol. Neurosurg. Psychiatry* 79, 212–215. doi: 10.1136/jnnp.2007.127712

Kiessling, J. (1980). [Masking of tinnitus aurium by maskers and hearing aids (author's transl)]. *HNO* 28, 383–388.

Kim, S. H., Jang, J. H., Lee, S. Y., Han, J. J., Koo, J. W., Vanneste, S., et al. (2016). Neural substrates predicting short-term improvement of tinnitus loudness and distress after modified tinnitus retraining therapy. *Sci. Rep.* 6:29140. doi: 10.1038/srep29140

Kong, J., Loggia, M. L., Zyloney, C., Tu, P., Laviolette, P., and Gollub, R. L. (2010). Exploring the brain in pain: activations, deactivations and their relation. *Pain* 148, 257–267. doi: 10.1016/j.pain.2009.11.008

Koprivova, J., Congedo, M., Horacek, J., Prasko, J., Raszka, M., Brunovsky, M., et al. (2011). EEG source analysis in obsessive-compulsive disorder. *Clin. Neurophysiol.* 122, 1735–1743. doi: 10.1016/j.clinph.2011.01.051

Krauss, P., Tziridis, K., Metzner, C., Schilling, A., Hoppe, U., and Schulze, H. (2016). Stochastic resonance controlled upregulation of internal noise after hearing loss as a putative cause of tinnitus-related neuronal hyperactivity. *Front. Neurosci.* 10:597. doi: 10.3389/fnins.2016.00597

Krauss, P., Tziridis, K., Schilling, A., and Schulze, H. (2018). Cross-modal stochastic resonance as a universal principle to enhance sensory processing. *Front. Neurosci.* 12:578. doi: 10.3389/fnins.2018.00578

Kringelbach, M. L. (2005). The human orbitofrontal cortex: linking reward to hedonic experience. *Nat. Rev. Neurosci.* 6, 691–702. doi: 10.1038/nrn1747

Kulkarni, B., Bentley, D. E., Elliott, R., Youell, P., Watson, A., Derbyshire, S. W., et al. (2005). Attention to pain localization and unpleasantness discriminates the functions of the medial and lateral pain systems. *Eur. J. Neurosci.* 21, 3133–3142. doi: 10.1111/j.1460-9568.2005.04098.x

Landgrebe, M., Langguth, B., Rosengarth, K., Braun, S., Koch, A., Kleinjung, T., et al. (2009). Structural brain changes in tinnitus: grey matter decrease in auditory and non-auditory brain areas. *Neuroimage* 46, 213–218. doi: 10.1016/j.neuroimage.2009.01.069

Langguth, B., Kreuzer, P. M., Kleinjung, T., and De Ridder, D. (2013). Tinnitus: causes and clinical management. *Lancet Neurol.* 12, 920–930. doi: 10.1016/s1474-4422(13)70160-1

Leaver, A. M., Renier, L., Chevillet, M. A., Morgan, S., Kim, H. J., and Rauschecker, J. P. (2011). Dysregulation of limbic and auditory networks in tinnitus. *Neuron* 69, 33–43. doi: 10.1016/j.neuron.2010.12.002

Leaver, A. M., Seydell-Greenwald, A., Turesky, T. K., Morgan, S., Kim, H. J., and Rauschecker, J. P. (2012). Cortico-limbic morphology separates tinnitus from tinnitus distress. *Front. Syst. Neurosci.* 6:21. doi: 10.3389/fnsys.2012.00021

Lee, S. Y., Nam, D. W., Koo, J. W., De Ridder, D., Vanneste, S., and Song, J. J. (2017). No auditory experience, no tinnitus: lessons from subjects with congenital- and acquired single-sided deafness. *Hear. Res.* 354, 9–15. doi: 10.1016/j.heares.2017.08.002

Lee, S. Y., Rhee, J., Shim, Y. J., Kim, Y., Koo, J. W., De Ridder, D., et al. (2019a). Changes in the resting-state cortical oscillatory activity 6 months after modified tinnitus retraining therapy. *Front. Neurosci.* 13:1123. doi: 10.3389/fnins.2019.01123

Lee, S. Y., Song, S. K., Park, S. J., Park, H. G., Choi, B. Y., Koo, J. W., et al. (2019b). Jugular bulb resurfacing with bone cement for patients with high dehiscent jugular bulb and Ipsilateral Pulsatile Tinnitus. *Otol. Neurotol.* 40, 192–199. doi: 10.1097/MAO.0000000000002093

Moazami-Goudarzi, M., Michels, L., Weisz, N., and Jeanmonod, D. (2010). Temporo-insular enhancement of EEG low and high frequencies in patients with chronic tinnitus. QEEG study of chronic tinnitus patients. *BMC Neurosci.* 11:40. doi: 10.1186/1471-2202-11-40

Moens, M., Sunaert, S., Marien, P., Brouns, R., De Smedt, A., Droogmans, S., et al. (2012). Spinal cord stimulation modulates cerebral function: an fMRI study. *Neuroradiology* 54, 1399–1407. doi: 10.1007/s00234-012-1087-8

Newman, C. W., Jacobson, G. P., and Spitzer, J. B. (1996). Development of the Tinnitus handicap inventory. *Arch. Otolaryngol. Head Neck Surg.* 122, 143–148.

Nichols, T. E., and Holmes, A. P. (2002). Nonparametric permutation tests for functional neuroimaging: a primer with examples. *Hum. Brain Mapp.* 15, 1–25.

Norena, A. J. (2011). An integrative model of tinnitus based on a central gain controlling neural sensitivity. *Neurosci. Biobehav. Rev.* 35, 1089–1109. doi: 10.1016/j.neubiorev.2010.11.003

Norena, A. J., and Eggermont, J. J. (2006). Enriched acoustic environment after noise trauma abolishes neural signs of tinnitus. *Neuroreport* 17, 559–563.

Pascual-Marqui, R. D. (2002). Standardized low-resolution brain electromagnetic tomography (sLORETA): technical details. *Methods Find. Exp. Clin. Pharmacol.* 24(Suppl. D), 5–12.

Price, D. D. (2000). Psychological and neural mechanisms of the affective dimension of pain. *Science* 288, 1769–1772. doi: 10.1126/science.288.5472.1769

Raichle, M. E. (2015). The brain's default mode network. *Annu. Rev. Neurosci.* 38, 433–447. doi: 10.1146/annurev-neuro-071013-014030

Raichle, M. E., MacLeod, A. M., Snyder, A. Z., Powers, W. J., Gusnard, D. A., and Shulman, G. L. (2001). A default mode of brain function. *Proc. Natl. Acad. Sci. U.S.A.* 98, 676–682. doi: 10.1073/pnas.98.2.676

Raichle, M. E., and Snyder, A. Z. (2007). A default mode of brain function: a brief history of an evolving idea. *Neuroimage* 37, 1083–1090. doi: 10.1016/j.neuroimage.2007.02.041

Rauschecker, J. P., May, E. S., Maudoux, A., and Ploner, M. (2015). Frontostriatal gating of Tinnitus and Chronic pain. *Trends Cogn. Sci.* 19, 567–578. doi: 10.1016/j.tics.2015.08.002

Rolls, E. T. (2004). The functions of the orbitofrontal cortex. *Brain Cogn.* 55, 11–29. doi: 10.1016/S0278-2626(03)00277-X

Saltzman, M., and Ersner, M. S. (1947). A hearing aid for the relief of tinnitus aurium. *Laryngoscope* 57, 358–366.

Schlee, W., Leirer, V., Kolassa, I. T., Weisz, N., and Elbert, T. (2012). Age-related changes in neural functional connectivity and its behavioral relevance. *BMC Neurosci.* 13:16. doi: 10.1186/1471-2202-13-16

Sereda, M., Xia, J., El Refaie, A., Hall, D. A., and Hoare, D. J. (2018). Sound therapy (using amplification devices and/or sound generators) for tinnitus. *Cochrane Database. Syst. Rev.* 12, CD013094. doi: 10.1002/14651858.CD013094.pub2

Shekhawat, G. S., Searchfield, G. D., and Stinear, C. M. (2013). Role of hearing AIDS in tinnitus intervention: a scoping review. *J. Am. Acad. Audiol.* 24, 747–762. doi: 10.3766/jaaa.24.8.11

Raichle, M. E., and Snyder, A. Z. (2007). A default mode of brain function: a brief history of an evolving idea. *Neuroimage* 37, 1083–1090. doi: 10.1016/j.neuroimage.2007.02.041

Rauschecker, J. P., May, E. S., Maudoux, A., and Ploner, M. (2015). Frontostriatal gating of Tinnitus and Chronic pain. *Trends Cogn. Sci.* 19, 567–578. doi: 10.1016/j.tics.2015.08.002

Rolls, E. T. (2004). The functions of the orbitofrontal cortex. *Brain Cogn.* 55, 11–29. doi: 10.1016/S0278-2626(03)00277-X

Saltzman, M., and Ersner, M. S. (1947). A hearing aid for the relief of tinnitus aurium. *Laryngoscope* 57, 358–366.

Schlee, W., Leirer, V., Kolassa, I. T., Weisz, N., and Elbert, T. (2012). Age-related changes in neural functional connectivity and its behavioral relevance. *BMC Neurosci.* 13:16. doi: 10.1186/1471-2202-13-16

Sereda, M., Xia, J., El Refaie, A., Hall, D. A., and Hoare, D. J. (2018). Sound therapy (using amplification devices and/or sound generators) for tinnitus. *Cochrane Database. Syst. Rev.* 12, CD013094. doi: 10.1002/14651858.CD013094.pub2

Shekhawat, G. S., Searchfield, G. D., and Stinear, C. M. (2013). Role of hearing AIDS in tinnitus intervention: a scoping review. *J. Am. Acad. Audiol.* 24, 747–762. doi: 10.3766/jaaa.24.8.11

Sherlin, L., and Congedo, M. (2005). Obsessive-compulsive dimension localized using low-resolution brain electromagnetic tomography (LORETA). *Neurosci. Lett.* 387, 72–74. doi: 10.1016/j.neulet.2005.06.069

Shim, Y. J., Bae, Y. J., An, G. S., Lee, K., Kim, Y., Lee, S. Y., et al. (2019). Involvement of the internal auditory canal in subjects with cochlear otosclerosis: a less acknowledged third window that affects surgical outcome. *Otol. Neurotol.* 40, e186–e190. doi: 10.1097/MAO.0000000000002144

Siepmann, M., and Kirch, W. (2002). Effects of caffeine on topographic quantitative EEG. *Neuropsychobiology* 45, 161–166.

Smits, M., Kovacs, S., de Ridder, D., Peeters, R. R., van Hecke, P., and Sunaert, S. (2007). Lateralization of functional magnetic resonance imaging (fMRI) activation in the auditory pathway of patients with lateralized tinnitus. *Neuroradiology* 49, 669–679. doi: 10.1007/s00234-007-0231-3

Song, J. J., Hong, S. K., Lee, S. Y., Park, S. J., Kang, S. I., An, Y. H., et al. (2018). Vestibular manifestations in subjects with enlarged vestibular aqueduct. *Otol. Neurotol.* 39, e461–e467. doi: 10.1097/MAO.0000000000001817

Song, J. J., Kim, K., Sunwoo, W., Mertens, G., Van de Heyning, P., De Ridder, D., et al. (2017). A quantitative electroencephalography study on cochlear implant-induced Cortical changes in single-sided deafness with Tinnitus. *Front. Hum. Neurosci.* 11:210. doi: 10.3389/fnhum.2017.00210

Song, J. J., Punte, A. K., De Ridder, D., Vanneste, S., and Van de Heyning, P. (2013). Neural substrates predicting improvement of tinnitus after cochlear implantation in patients with single-sided deafness. *Hear. Res.* 299, 1–9. doi: 10.1016/j.heares.2013.02.001

Song, J. J., Vanneste, S., Schlee, W., Van de Heyning, P., and De Ridder, D. (2015). Onset-related differences in neural substrates of tinnitus-related distress: the anterior cingulate cortex in late-onset tinnitus, and the frontal cortex in early-onset tinnitus. *Brain Struct. Funct.* 220, 571–584. doi: 10.1007/s00429-013-0648-x

Sunwoo, W., Jeon, Y. J., Bae, Y. J., Jang, J. H., Koo, J. W., and Song, J. J. (2017). Typewriter tinnitus revisited: the typical symptoms and the initial response to carbamazepine are the most reliable diagnostic clues. *Sci. Rep.* 7:10615. doi: 10.1038/s41598-017-10798-w

Surr, R. K., Kolb, J. A., Cord, M. T., and Garrus, N. P. (1999). Tinnitus Handicap Inventory (THI) as a hearing aid outcome measure. *J. Am. Acad. Audiol.* 10, 489–495.

Surr, R. K., Montgomery, A. A., and Mueller, H. G. (1985). Effect of amplification on tinnitus among new hearing aid users. *Ear Hear.* 6, 71–75.

Talairach, J., and Tornoux, P. (1988). *Co-Planar Stereotaxic Atlas of the Human Brain: 3-Dimensional Proportional System: An Approach to Cerebral Imaging.* Stuttgart: Georg Thieme.

Tonndorf, J. (1987). The analogy between tinnitus and pain: a suggestion for a physiological basis of chronic tinnitus. *Hear. Res.* 28, 271–275. doi: 10.1016/0378-5955(87)90054-2

Tunkel, D. E., Bauer, C. A., Sun, G. H., Rosenfeld, R. M., Chandrasekhar, S. S., Cunningham, E. R., et al. (2014). Clinical practice guideline: tinnitus. *Otolaryngol. Head Neck Surg.* 151 (2 Suppl), S1–S40. doi: 10.1177/0194599814545325

Vanneste, S., and De Ridder, D. (2012). The auditory and non-auditory brain areas involved in tinnitus. An emergent property of multiple parallel overlapping subnetworks. *Front. Syst. Neurosci.* 6:31. doi: 10.3389/fnsys.2012.00031

Vanneste, S., and De Ridder, D. (2016). Deafferentation-based pathophysiological differences in phantom sound: Tinnitus with and without hearing loss. *Neuroimage* 129, 80–94. doi: 10.1016/j.neuroimage.2015.12.002

Vanneste, S., Plazier, M., der Loo, E., de Heyning, P. V., Congedo, M., and De Ridder, D. (2010). The neural correlates of tinnitus-related distress. *Neuroimage* 52, 470–480. doi: 10.1016/j.neuroimage.2010.04.029

Vanneste, S., Song, J. J., and De Ridder, D. (2018). Thalamocortical dysrhythmia detected by machine learning. *Nat. Commun.* 9:1103. doi: 10.1038/s41467-018-02820-0

Volkow, N. D., Logan, J., Fowler, J. S., Wang, G. J., Gur, R. C., Wong, C., et al. (2000). Association between age-related decline in brain dopamine activity and impairment in frontal and cingulate metabolism. *Am. J. Psychiatry* 157, 75–80. doi: 10.1176/ajp.157.1.75

White, D. J., Congedo, M., Ciorciari, J., and Silberstein, R. B. (2012). Brain oscillatory activity during spatial navigation: theta and gamma activity link medial temporal and parietal regions. *J. Cogn. Neurosci.* 24, 686–697. doi: 10.1162/jocn_a_00098

Yang, S., Weiner, B. D., Zhang, L. S., Cho, S. J., and Bao, S. (2011). Homeostatic plasticity drives tinnitus perception in an animal model. *Proc. Natl. Acad. Sci. U.S.A.* 108, 14974–14979. doi: 10.1073/pnas.1107998108

Loss of Vision Dominance at the Preresponse Level in Tinnitus Patients: Preliminary Behavioral Evidence

Zhicheng Li[1,2†], Ruolei Gu[3†], Min Qi[1], Jintian Cen[1], Shuqi Zhang[1], Jing Gu[1], Xiangli Zeng[1] and Qi Chen[2*]*

[1] Department of Otolaryngology-Head and Neck Surgery, Third Affiliated Hospital of Sun Yat-sen University, Guangzhou, China, [2] Department of Psychology and Center for Studies of Psychological Application, South China Normal University, Guangzhou, China, [3] Key Laboratory of Behavioral Science, Institute of Psychology, Chinese Academy of Sciences, Beijing, China

***Correspondence:**
Xiangli Zeng
zxiangl@mail.sysu.edu.cn
Qi Chen
qi.chen27@gmail.com

† These authors have contributed equally to this work

At present, the mechanisms underlying changes in visual processing in individuals with tinnitus remain unclear. Therefore, we investigated whether the vision dominance of individuals with tinnitus disappears at the preresponse level through behavioral study. A total of 38 individuals with tinnitus and 31 healthy controls completed a task in which they were asked to attend to either visual or auditory stimuli while ignoring simultaneous stimulus inputs from the other modality. We manipulated three levels of congruency between the simultaneous visual and auditory inputs: congruent (C), incongruent at the preresponse level (PRIC), and incongruent at the response level (RIC). Thus, we differentiated the cross-modal conflict explicitly into the preresponse (PRIC > C) and response (RIC > PRIC) levels. The results revealed no significant difference in the size of the preresponse level conflict between the auditory attention and visual attention conditions in tinnitus group. In brief, the preresponse level of individuals with tinnitus showed a loss in vision dominance. This may be due to the reduced interference of visual information in auditory processing.

Keywords: tinnitus, cross-modal interference, vision dominance, attention, behavioral research

INTRODUCTION

Vision and audition are important functions through which individuals obtain information about the external environment. When individuals attend to information from one sensory modality, they tend to "look without seeing" or "listen without hearing" to the information received by other sensory modalities. However, the information received by the non-attended modality affects the information processing of that received by the attended modality, and this phenomenon is known as cross-modal interference. Previous studies have reported that when the input information of visual and auditory modalities is inconsistent, the processing time is prolonged and the accuracy of responses to attended stimuli decrease (Colavita, 1974; Chen and Zhou, 2013). Moreover, visual distractors cause more interference to auditory processing than auditory distractors do to visual processing (as vision dominance) at the preresponse level, but auditory distractors cause more interference to visual processing than visual distractors do to auditory processing (as audition dominance) at the response level (Repp and Penel, 2004; Kato and Konishi, 2006; Mayer et al., 2009; Koppen et al., 2009; Chen and Zhou, 2013).

Tinnitus, a subjective auditory experience, emerges independent of external stimuli, and its occurrence and maintenance require attentional resources (Roberts et al., 2013). Previous studies have shown that visual processing in individuals with tinnitus is significantly worse than that of healthy controls (Stevens et al., 2007; Heeren et al., 2014; Araneda et al., 2015a,b; Li et al., 2018), and is more susceptible to cross-modal interference of auditory information (Araneda et al., 2015b). Meanwhile, the decrease in signal detection (the early stage of cognitive processing) might underlie the impaired visual processing in individuals with tinnitus (Li et al., 2018). With this in mind, the "visual dominance effect" (i.e., allocating more attentional resources to visual rather than auditory information, which leads to stronger interference of visual distractors on auditory targets) at the preresponse level might function abnormally in individuals with tinnitus. Clarifying this problem will facilitate further understanding of the effect of tinnitus on individuals' cognitive processing (particularly cross-channel information integration), and will provide a reference for improving strategies concerning the evaluation and management of tinnitus. However, the changes and mechanisms of visual processing in individuals with tinnitus are unclear.

The current study aimed to investigate whether the vision dominance of individuals with tinnitus disappears at the preresponse level. To this aim, we used the experimental design of Chen and Zhou (2013), which could help investigate cross-modal conflict at the preresponse and response levels. Participants simultaneously received visual and auditory stimuli (i.e., cross-modal inputs), and were asked to attend to one modality and ignore the other. All experimental stimuli were presented as one of four colors (red/green/blue/yellow), two of which (red and green) were targets, while the other two (blue and yellow) were distractors (**Figure 1A**); only stimuli in the "target" category required press the button. The task included the two following factors: modality (attending to visual/auditory stimuli) and congruency (cross-modal congruency, C; incongruent at preresponse level, PRIC; incongruent at both the preresponse and response levels, RIC). In the C condition, bimodal inputs referred to the same target (e.g., participants saw a red block and heard "red"). In the PRIC condition, the stimulus in the attended channel (visual/auditory) was a target, but the stimulus in the unattended channel was a distractor that did not require a response (e.g., participants saw a red block but heard "blue"); therefore, the cross-modal conflict emerged at the preresponse level but not the response level. In the RIC condition, the stimuli in the attended channel and the unattended channel were two different targets that required different responses (e.g., participants saw a red block but heard "green") (**Figure 1B**); therefore, the cross-modal conflict emerged at both the preresponse and response levels. According to Chen and Zhou (2013), the classical findings in this task are that visual distractors cause larger preresponse-level interference (PRIC > C in reaction time) to auditory processing than vice versa, while auditory distractors cause larger response-level interference (RIC > PRIC in reaction time) to visual processing than vice versa.

Based on these previous studies, we hypothesized that the vision dominance of individuals with tinnitus would disappears at the preresponse level, and there would be no significant difference between the interference of visual information in auditory processing and vice versa. In line with this hypothesis, we found that there was no significant difference in preresponse-level interference between the modalities attended. This study did not have any specific predictions concerning the disappearance of visual dominance.

METHODS

The experimental protocol was reviewed and approved by the Ethics Committee of the Third Affiliated Hospital of Sun Yat-sen University [approval number: (2018) 02-358-01]. All enrolled participants were required to sign an informed consent form.

Participants

Individuals with tinnitus admitted to the Outpatient Department of Otorhinolaryngology, the Third Affiliated Hospital of Sun Yat-sen University due to tinnitus as a major complaint were enrolled (21 men, 17 women, mean age = 28.23 ± 6.20 years). All individuals were diagnosed as having chronic subjective tinnitus, without hyperacusis, and the pure-tone threshold from 125 to 8000 Hz, including the semioctave range, were ≤40 dB HL. Healthy controls, who had no history of hearing loss (both pure-tone threshold ≤25 dB HL), tinnitus, dizziness, or other ear diseases, were recruited from online and poster adverts at the Sun Yat-sen University (16 men, 15 women, mean age = 22.63 ± 2.24 years). All participants were right-handed, had normal or corrected-to-normal vision (5.0 or above in the Logarithmic Visual Acuity Chart), and no color blindness or weakness. No participant had a history of neurological or psychiatric disorders.

Experimental Design and Stimuli

We adopted a 2 (group: tinnitus and control groups) × 2 (modality attended: Attend-Visual and Attend-Auditory) × 3 (congruency: C, PRIC, and RIC) hybrid design.

Visual stimuli (color blocks) were presented on an LED monitor at a viewing distance of 70 cm. Auditory stimuli (verbal pronunciations) were voice recordings of a male speaker and were delivered binaurally via stereo headphones. The volume was adjusted for each participant such that the auditory stimuli could be clearly heard.

The experimental task was to judge whether the attended color block or verbal pronunciation was red or green. Throughout the experiment, all color blocks and verbal pronunciations were potential targets that required responses. Participants used the index and middle fingers of their right hand to respond by pressing one key on the response box for red or another key for green. The mapping between the two response keys and red versus green color was counterbalanced across participants.

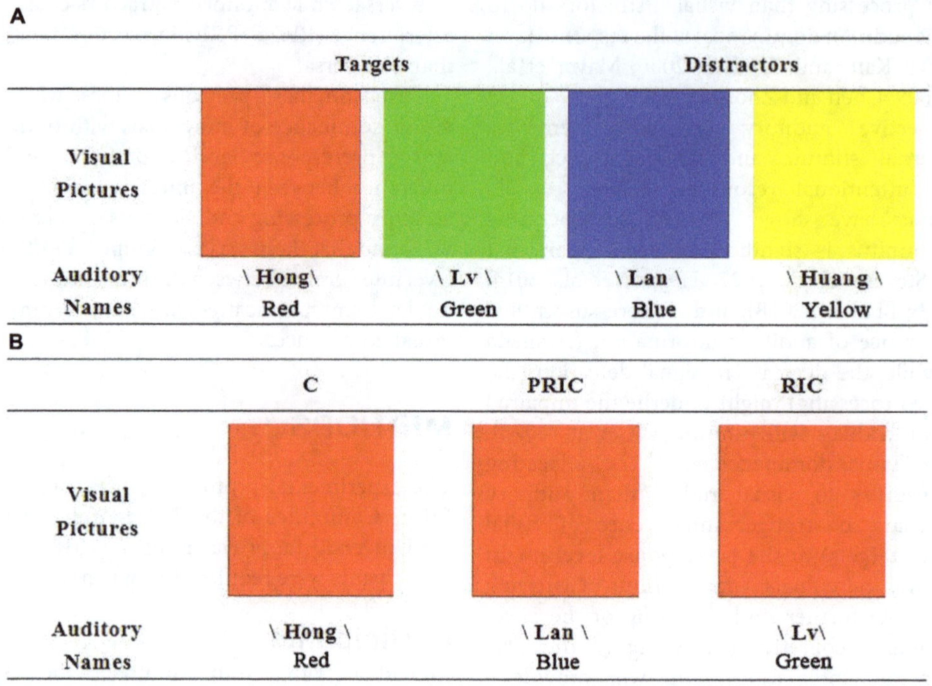

FIGURE 1 | Exemplar stimuli **(A)** and design **(B)** in experiment. **(A)** Two color pictures and their verbal sounds served as targets. Another two color pictures and their verbal sounds served as distractors. **(B)** Examples of the manipulation of the three levels of congruency are provided for the situation in which the visual modality was attended. In the C condition, the auditory name and visual picture refer to the same target. In the PRIC condition, the auditory name refers to the distractors and the visual picture refers to the target. In the RIC condition, the auditory name and visual picture refer to different targets. The auditory names were played in Mandarin, like /Hong/、/Lv/、/Lan/, and /Huang/.

Procedure

The stimuli were presented using a hybrid design in which the attended modality was blocked, and the C, PRIC, and RIC trials were mixed randomly within each block. In each block, participants were asked to focus on either the visual or auditory stimuli while ignoring stimuli from the other modality. They were instructed to fixate on the central cross throughout the experiment without moving their eyes. In each trial, a color block and verbal pronunciation were simultaneously presented for 300 ms. Each of the six experimental conditions had 48 trials, resulting in a total of 384 trials (288 experimental trials and 96 null trials). In a null trial, only the central fixation cross was displayed. For the visual attention condition and auditory attention condition, respectively, null trials and C, PRIC, and RIC trials were randomly mixed and then divided into 24 test blocks. Each block comprised 8 trials and lasted for 20 s. The visual attention condition and auditory attention condition blocks were alternated. Each block started with a 2-s visual instruction about which modality was to be attended.

Statistical Analyses

Within each of the six experimental conditions, omissions, incorrect responses, and trials with reaction times (RTs) three standard deviations away from the mean RT were excluded from further analyses. The mean RTs of the remaining trials were subsequently calculated. Normally distributed data were analyzed using repeated measures analysis of variance (ANOVA) and *t*-tests. Otherwise, median and quartile ranges were presented, and differences were tested using Wilcoxon Signed Ranks Test. $p < 0.05$ was considered statistically significant.

RESULTS

The 2 (group: tinnitus and control groups) × 2 (modality attended: Attend-Visual and Attend-Auditory) × 3 (congruency: C, PRIC, and RIC) repeated measures ANOVA showed a significant main effect of Group [$F(1,67) = 9.15$, $p = 0.004$], whereby the tinnitus group had significantly longer RTs than those of the control group, irrespective of the attended modality or congruency condition ($p < 0.05$; **Figure 2A**).

Moreover, there was a significant main effect of attended modality [$F(1,67) = 76.94$, $p < 0.001$], whereby RTs to the visual targets were significantly shorter than those to the auditory targets. There was also a main effect of congruency [$F(2,134) = 284.53$, $p < 0.001$]; further pairwise comparisons using Bonferroni correction indicated that RTs in the PRIC condition were significantly longer than those in the C condition ($p < 0.001$), and RTs in the RIC condition were significantly longer than those in the PRIC condition ($p = 0.02$). This result indicated significant cross-modal conflicts at both the preresponse and response levels.

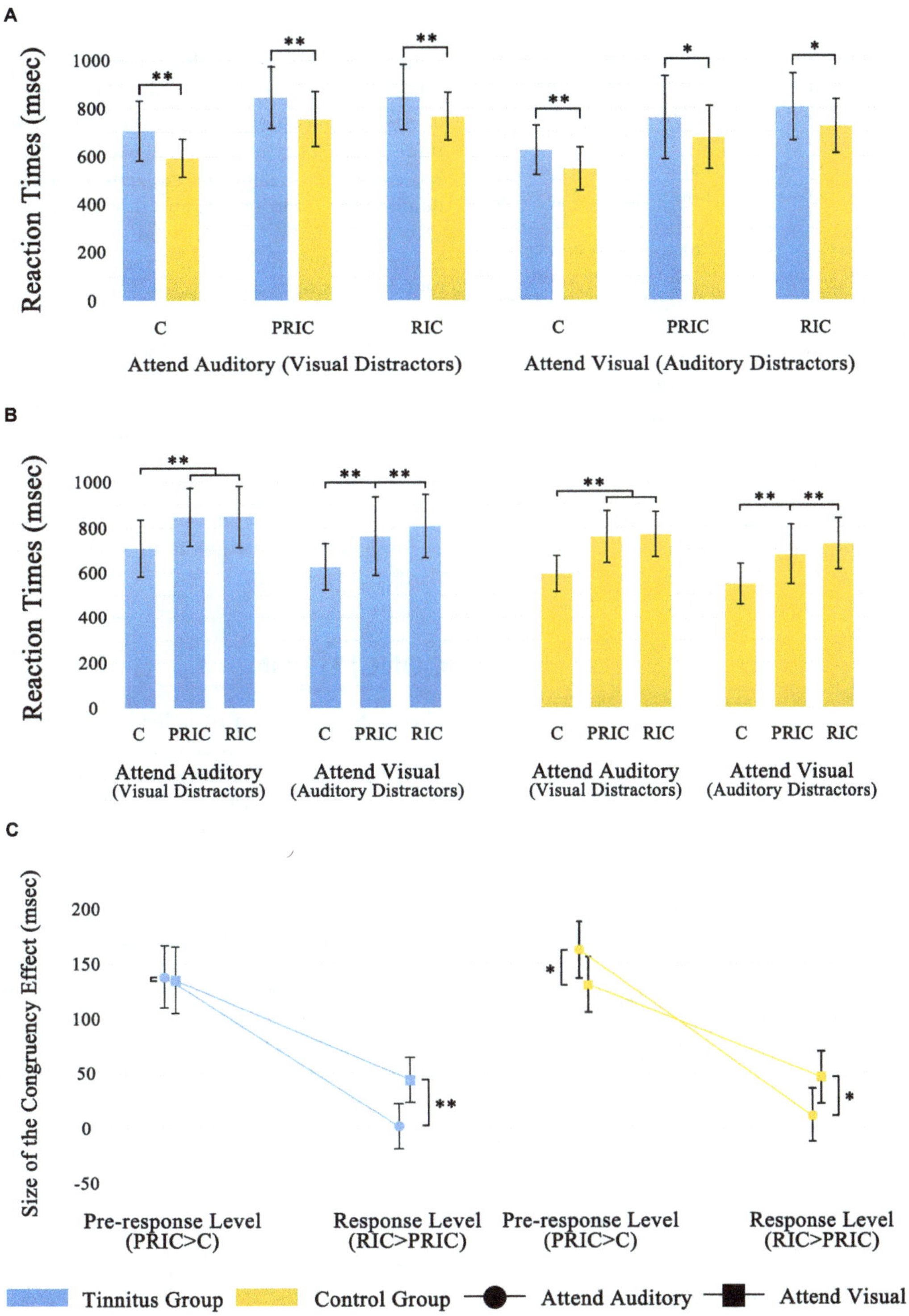

FIGURE 2 | Behavioral results of Experiment. **(A)** Inter-group differences of the six experimental conditions. **(B)** Intra-group differences of the six experimental conditions. **(C)** Inter-group differences of sizes of cross-modal conflict at the preresponse (PRIC > C) and response (RIC > PRIC) levels are shown as a function of the attended modality. $^{*}p < 0.05$; $^{**}p < 0.01$.

There was a significant interaction between the attended modality and congruency [$F(2,134) = 7.44$, $p = 0.001$], and planned t-tests on simple effects indicated that the preresponse level conflict was significant both in the auditory attention condition ($p < 0.001$) and visual attention condition ($p < 0.001$). Conversely, the response level conflict was only significant in the visual attention condition (p = 0.001), and not in the auditory attention condition (p = 0.40). There were no significant interactions between attended modality and group [$F(1,67) = 1.38$, $p = 0.25$], consistency and group [$F(2,134) = 0.50$, $p = 0.61$], attended modality, consistency, and group [$F(2,134) = 1.80$, $p = 0.17$]. This indicated that the pattern between attended modality and consistency were similar between the tinnitus group and control group (**Figure 2B**).

Within the control group, the size of the preresponse level conflict was significantly larger when the auditory modality was attended vs. when the visual modality was attended (p = 0.02), whereas the size of the response level conflict was significantly larger when visual modality was attended vs. when the auditory modality was attended (p = 0.04) (**Figure 2C**, right). Within the tinnitus group, the size of the preresponse level conflict was not significantly different between the auditory attention and visual attention conditions (p = 0.85) (**Figure 2C**, left).

For both the auditory attention and visual attention conditions, further independent samples t-tests did not reveal any significant between-group differences in the size of the congruency effect at the preresponse and response levels groups (p = 0.24, 0.59, 0.82, and 0.91, respectively).

DISCUSSION

The brain can process a limited amount of information per unit time; therefore, the brain needs to allocate limited attention resources to process the most pertinent information in complex situations (Mishra and Gazzaley, 2012). The occurrence and maintenance of tinnitus both require attentional resources, which eventually affects cognitive processing (Roberts et al., 2013). The present study found that the RTs of the tinnitus group in both experimental conditions were significantly longer than those of the control group, thus supporting the reduction of visual and auditory processing in individuals with tinnitus.

More importantly, we found that the vision dominance of individuals with tinnitus disappeared at the preresponse level, as hypothesized. Although the size of the congruency effect at the preresponse level did not show significant differences between the tinnitus and control groups, it reduced from 162 ms in the control group to 138 ms in the tinnitus group in the auditory attention condition, while it maintained a similar effect in the tinnitus (135 ms) and control (130 ms) groups in the visual attention condition. Therefore, we speculate that the disappearance of visual dominance at the preresponse level in individuals with tinnitus is mainly due to the reduced interference of visual information in auditory processing. This finding also indicates that the auditory modality may demand a greater allocation of attention, which consequently weakens the interference of the visual modality.

However, we must also realize that tinnitus may be a product of brain dysfunction (Elgoyhen et al., 2015), and brain dysfunction may also affect other cognitive processes, other than auditory processing. Thus, whether the reduction of visual processing in individuals with tinnitus is due to tinnitus, or, like tinnitus, still needs to be further explored. Moreover, the default mode network is involved in visual dominance at the preresponse level (Chen and Zhou, 2013), and many brain regions and neural connections in the default mode network of individuals with tinnitus have been found to exhibit changes (Elgoyhen et al., 2015). We aim to explore the relationship between the disappearance of visual dominance at the preresponse level and the change in the default mode network in our follow-up EEG and imaging studies. Furthermore, this study only focused on individuals with chronic subjective tinnitus. Therefore, the results of the study cannot be extended to other groups of individuals with tinnitus. Follow-up studies should gradually incorporate different groups of individuals of tinnitus, such as those with acute tinnitus or objective tinnitus, to further clarify this viewpoint.

CONCLUSION

The preresponse level of individuals with tinnitus revealed a loss of vision dominance, which may be due to the reduced interference of visual information in auditory processing. Further studies are warranted to verify our findings and to explore the neural mechanisms underlying behavioral changes using EEG and imaging techniques.

AUTHOR CONTRIBUTIONS

ZL designed and performed the experiments, analyzed the data, and wrote the manuscript. RG analyzed the data and perfected the manuscript. XZ modified the research approach and chose the patients. QC directed and modified the research approach and provided the critical revision. ZL, RG, XZ, and QC discussed the results and implications and commented on the manuscript at all stages. MQ, JC, SZ, and JG in charge of preliminary screening and contacted with subject.

ACKNOWLEDGMENTS

Thanks to Xia Jing, Fang Ying, and Zou Guijing from School of Psychology, South China Normal University for their help in experimental programming and Sun Tienan, Fan Huiyang, Zhuang Jinkun, and Wei Xin from the Zhongshan School of Medicine, Sun Yat-sen University, for their help in data acquisition.

REFERENCES

Araneda, R., De Volder, A., Deggouj, N., Philippot, P., Heeren, A., Lacroix, E., et al. (2015a). Altered top-down cognitive control and auditory processing in tinnitus: evidences from auditory and visual spatial stroop. *Restor. Neurol. Neurosci.* 33, 67–80. doi: 10.3233/RNN-140433

Araneda, R., De Volder, A., Deggouj, N., and Renier, L. (2015b). Altered inhibitory control and increased sensitivity to cross-modal interference in tinnitus during auditory and visual tasks. *PLoS One* 10:e0120387. doi: 10.1371/journal.pone.0120387

Chen, Q., and Zhou, X. (2013). Vision dominates at the preresponse level and audition dominates at the response level in cross-modal interaction: behavioral and neural evidence. *J Neurosci.* 33, 7109–7121. doi: 10.1523/JNEUROSCI.1985-12.2013

Colavita, F. (1974). Human sensory dominance. *Percept. Psychophys.* 16, 409–412. doi: 10.3758/bf03203962

Elgoyhen, A., Langguth, B., De Ridder, D., and Vanneste, S. (2015). Tinnitus: perspectives from human neuroimaging. *Nat. Rev. Neurosci.* 16, 632–642. doi: 10.1038/nrn4003

Heeren, A., Maurage, P., Perrot, H., De Volder, A., Renier, L., Araneda, R., et al. (2014). Tinnitus specifically alters the top-down executive control sub-component of attention: evidence from the attention network task. *Behav. Brain. Res.* 269, 147–154. doi: 10.1016/j.bbr.2014.04.043

Kato, M., and Konishi, Y. (2006). Auditory dominance in the error correction process: a synchronized tapping study. *Brain Res.* 1084, 115–122. doi: 10.1016/j.brainres.2006.02.019

Koppen, C., Levitan, C., and Spence, C. (2009). A signal detection study of the Colavita visual dominance effect. *Exp. Brain Res.* 196, 353–360. doi: 10.1007/s00221-009-1853-y

Li, Z., Gu, R., Zeng, X., Qi, M., Cen, J., Zhang, S., et al. (2018). Eyes and ears: cross-modal interference of tinnitus on visual processing. *Front. Psychol.* 9:1779. doi: 10.3389/fpsyg.2018.01779

Mayer, A., Franco, A., Canive, J., and Harrington, D. L. (2009). The effects of stimulus modality and frequency of stimulus presentation on cross-modal distraction. *Cereb. Cortex* 19, 993–1007. doi: 10.1093/cercor/bhn148

Mishra, J., and Gazzaley, A. (2012). Attention distributed across sensory modalities enhances perceptual performance. *J. Neurosci.* 32, 12294–12302. doi: 10.1523/JNEUROSCI.0867-12.2012

Repp, B., and Penel, A. (2004). Rhythmic movement is attracted more strongly to auditory than to visual rhythms. *Psychol. Res.* 68, 252–270.

Roberts, L., Husain, F., and Eggermont, J. (2013). Role of attention in the generation and modulation of tinnitus. *Neurosci. Biobehav. Rev.* 37, 1754–1773. doi: 10.1016/j.neubiorev.2013.07.007

Stevens, C., Walker, G., Boyer, M., and Gallagher, M. (2007). Severe tinnitus and its effect on selective and divided attention. *Int. J. Audiol.* 46, 208–216. doi: 10.1080/14992020601102329

5

Chronic Tinnitus Exhibits Bidirectional Functional Dysconnectivity in Frontostriatal Circuit

Jin-Jing Xu[1†], Jinluan Cui[2†], Yuan Feng[2], Wei Yong[2], Huiyou Chen[2], Yu-Chen Chen[2], Xindao Yin[2*] and Yuanqing Wu[1*]*

[1] Department of Otolaryngology, Nanjing First Hospital, Nanjing Medical University, Nanjing, China, [2] Department of Radiology, Nanjing First Hospital, Nanjing Medical University, Nanjing, China

***Correspondence:**
Yu-Chen Chen
chenyuchen1989@163.com;
chenyuchen1989@126.com
Xindao Yin
y.163yy@163.com
Yuanqing Wu
15366110097@163.com

[†] These authors have contributed equally to this work

Purpose: The phantom sound of tinnitus is considered to be associated with abnormal functional coupling between the nucleus accumbens (NAc) and the prefrontal cortex, which may form a frontostriatal top-down gating system to evaluate and modulate sensory signals. Resting-state functional magnetic resonance imaging (fMRI) was used to recognize the aberrant directional connectivity of the NAc in chronic tinnitus and to ascertain the relationship between this connectivity and tinnitus characteristics.

Methods: Participants included chronic tinnitus patients (n = 50) and healthy controls (n = 55), matched for age, sex, education, and hearing thresholds. The hearing status of both groups was comparable. On the basis of the NAc as a seed region, a Granger causality analysis (GCA) study was conducted to investigate the directional connectivity and the relationship with tinnitus duration or distress.

Results: Compared with healthy controls, tinnitus patients exhibited abnormal directional connectivity between the NAc and the prefrontal cortex, principally the middle frontal gyrus (MFG), orbitofrontal cortex (OFC), and inferior frontal gyrus (IFG). Additionally, positive correlations between tinnitus handicap questionnaire (THQ) scores and increased directional connectivity from the right NAc to the left MFG ($r = 0.357$, $p = 0.015$) and from the right MFG to the left NAc ($r = 0.626$, $p < 0.001$) were observed. Furthermore, the enhanced directional connectivity from the right NAc to the right OFC was positively associated with the duration of tinnitus ($r = 0.599$, $p < 0.001$).

Conclusion: In concurrence with expectations, tinnitus distress was correlated with enhanced directional connectivity between the NAc and the prefrontal cortex. The current study not only helps illuminate the neural basis of the frontostriatal gating control of tinnitus sensation but also contributes to deciphering the neuropathological features of tinnitus.

Keywords: tinnitus, nucleus accumbens, prefrontal cortex, directional connectivity, resting-state fMRI

INTRODUCTION

Tinnitus is defined as a phantom auditory perception that may bother many patients to the extent that it changes their lives (Baguley et al., 2013; Bauer, 2018). Because of the aging population and unavoidable noise pollution, the incidence of chronic tinnitus has increased sharply over the past 15 years (Shargorodsky et al., 2010; Knipper et al., 2013). Currently, the mechanism of action of chronic and irreversible tinnitus is unknown. Hence, many investigators have applied themselves to unraveling the nature of tinnitus (Galazyuk et al., 2012), notably subjective chronic tinnitus without organic lesions. Abnormal cochlear function has been considered to be the primary cause of tinnitus over the years. However, a small number of studies indicated that many patients failed to experience relief from tinnitus after the complete recovery of cochlear lesions (Rauschecker et al., 2010). The central nervous system is integral when considering the occurrence and development of tinnitus. A series of anomalies in the auditory center were observed in tinnitus cases in prior research studies (Leaver et al., 2011, 2016a; Kim et al., 2012; Song et al., 2012, 2015; Vanneste and De Ridder, 2012; Adjamian et al., 2014; Husain and Schmidt, 2014; Chen et al., 2015, 2016; Hinkley et al., 2015; Gunbey et al., 2017; Schmidt et al., 2017; Hullfish et al., 2019), simultaneously covering synaptic remodeling (Eggermont and Roberts, 2004), neuronal spontaneous hyperactivity or hypoactivity (Chen et al., 2014), increased neuronal synchronicity (Eggermont, 2007; Langers et al., 2012), and changes in tonotopic representation of sound (Langers et al., 2012). Tinnitus activations may also involve the non-auditory center, in which the limbic system and the autonomic nervous system are especially important (Crippaa et al., 2010; Rauschecker et al., 2010; Leaver et al., 2011, 2016a; Kim et al., 2012; Vanneste and De Ridder, 2012; Carpenter-Thompson et al., 2014; Kreuzer et al., 2015; Song et al., 2015; Chen et al., 2016; Gunbey et al., 2017; Schmidt et al., 2017; Hullfish et al., 2019). As a result, an increasing number of researchers have investigated tinnitus from the periphery to the central nervous system. Although many studies have investigated this area over the years, the neuropathological mechanism underlying tinnitus generation remains an enigma.

Comprehensively accumulated evidence from functional neuroimaging studies indicated that the limbic system plays an intermediary role in evaluating and modulating tinnitus perception signals, for instance, identifying and eliminating phantom sounds normally as well as canceling the noise at the level of the limbic system by providing feedback to the thalamic reticular nucleus (TRN) (Muhlau et al., 2006; Rauschecker et al., 2010, 2015; Leaver et al., 2011; Barry et al., 2015; Gunbey et al., 2017). At the level of the thalamus, the inhibition and stimulation of the medial geniculate nucleus (MGN) and TRN are determined by the pathway above (Rauschecker et al., 2010, 2015; Barry et al., 2015). Research has also indicated that one of the reasons for the generation and maintenance of tinnitus is the breakdown of auditory circuitry, especially in the thalamic regions, including the MGN and TRN (Rauschecker et al., 2010; Barry et al., 2015). Moreover, the functional connectivity between the nucleus accumbens (NAc) and MGN single neurons as well as the modulation of auditory neuron activity in the MGN by the NAc may play a part in the development of tinnitus (Barry et al., 2015).

Furthermore, the generation of tinnitus may be ascribed to the reaction of the NAc to dysfunctional sensory gating control (Barry et al., 2015). The study of Rauschecker et al. demonstrated that as part of a central gatekeeping system in tinnitus, the subcallosal area, which is composed of the ventromedial prefrontal cortex (vmPFC) and the NAc, evaluates the relevance and emotional value of sensory stimuli, and controls the flow of information (Rauschecker et al., 2010). Previous studies have suggested that the NAc and vmPFC and subgenual anterior cingulate cortex (sgACC) form a frontostriatal gating circuit in tinnitus patients (Leaver et al., 2011, 2016b; Rauschecker et al., 2015; Hullfish et al., 2019). Therefore, functional magnetic resonance imaging (fMRI) was used to measure the neural activity within frontostriatal network in tinnitus.

The interconnection within cerebral networks, which is structurally segregated and functionally specialized, may be further understood by resting-state low-frequency (0.01–0.1 Hz) fluctuations of blood oxygenation level-dependent (BOLD) fMRI (Biswal et al., 1995; Raichle et al., 2000; Barkhof et al., 2014). Recent MRI studies on tinnitus have raised awareness of altered structural and functional brain alterations in auditory and limbic regions (Leaver et al., 2011, 2016a; Vanneste and De Ridder, 2012; Meyer et al., 2016; Hullfish et al., 2019). The NAc, vmPFC, and sgACC could be the kernel regions of tinnitus dysfunction. The highest degree of hyperactivity, specifically to sounds frequency matched in the NAc area, as well as complementary structural differences in the vmPFC, has been shown in tinnitus patients (Leaver et al., 2016a). Increased gray matter (GM) and decreased white matter (WM) concentrations in the vmPFC within tinnitus patients have been detected (Middleton and Tzounopoulos, 2012), in which the functional changes in the NAc and auditory cortex were closely associated with the degree of structural changes. Moreover, Meyer et al. (2016) demonstrated that the reduced GM in sgACC was correlated with tinnitus duration in a large sample of tinnitus patients, suggesting that ongoing tinnitus may be related to progressive reorganization of the sgACC, which is consistent with the gating model (Rauschecker et al., 2015). Likewise, Hinkley et al. (2015) investigated the presence of increased functional connectivity in the NAc and vmPFC with the auditory cortex of tinnitus patients. While many studies have shown that tinnitus involves changes in the functional connectivity between the whole brain and the NAc as well as the vmPFC (Leaver et al., 2011; Adjamian et al., 2014; Hullfish et al., 2019), the directionality or specificity of the dysfunctional connections in tinnitus remains unknown.

A Granger causality analysis (GCA) study is employed to identify directionality in altered effective connectivity between the whole brain and the NAc as well as the vmPFC among subjects, providing scientific evidence for in-depth research. GCA has been applied broadly to expose the causal effects among brain regions in other neurological or psychiatric disorders, such as Alzheimer's disease (Zhong et al., 2014), mild cognitive impairment (Yu et al., 2017), depression (Guo et al., 2015), and presbycusis (Chen et al., 2019). In the current study, fMRI combined with the GCA method was used to collect and process BOLD data to precisely determine the directionality of altered resting-state directional connectivity (Jiao et al., 2011; Stephan and Roebroeck, 2012). Specific seed regions are stipulated in the NAc considering the potential role of the NAc within the frontostriatal gating circuit in tinnitus. It is hypothesized that disruption of the directional connectivity in the NAc in patients with chronic tinnitus would be observed by utilizing the GCA method. Moreover, the disrupted frontostriatal connectivity would be associated with specific tinnitus characteristics, such as tinnitus distress and duration. To our knowledge, this is the first study to use fMRI in combination with the GCA method to detect the directional connectivity of the NAc in chronic tinnitus patients.

MATERIALS AND METHODS

Subjects

Fifty chronic tinnitus patients and 55 healthy subjects (all right-handed, with at least 8 years of education) were recruited through community health screening or newspaper advertisements. No subject was excluded from the fMRI analysis due to excessive head motion during scanning. The patients and controls were paired into matched groups in terms of age, sex, and education. There were 18 left-sided and 16 right-sided tinnitus patients as well as 16 tinnitus patients who experienced bilateral tinnitus or tinnitus originating within the head. The Iowa version of the Tinnitus Handicap Questionnaires (THQ) (Kuk et al., 1990) and a pure tone audiometry (PTA) examination were used to assess the tinnitus severity, tinnitus distress, and the hearing threshold. All participants had clinically normal hearing (hearing thresholds < 25 dB) at the frequencies of 0.25, 0.5, 1, 2, 4, and 8 kHz. There were no statistically significant differences in auditory thresholds between the tinnitus group and the control group (see **Figure 1** for average hearing thresholds). According to the self-rating depression scale (SDS) and the self-rating anxiety scale (SAS) (overall scores < 50, respectively), none of the participants had depression or anxiety (Zung, 1971, 1986).

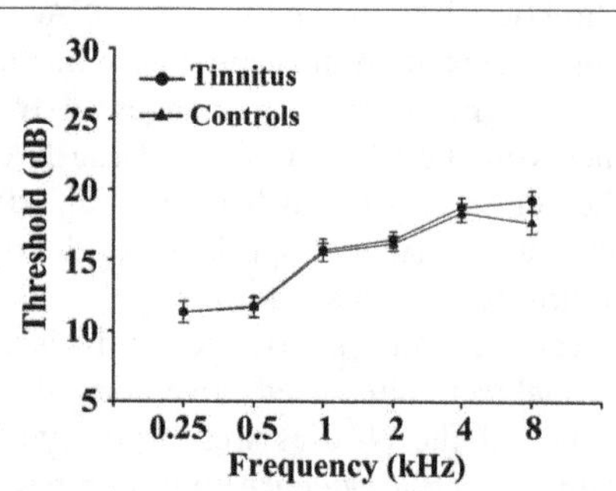

FIGURE 1 | Mean hearing thresholds of the chronic tinnitus and control groups. Data are presented as mean ± SD.

In accordance with a previous study (Khalfa et al., 2002), the Hyperacusis Questionnaire was applied to exclude participants with hyperacusis in the current study. Moreover, consistent with the previous diagnostic criteria (Lopez-Escamez et al., 2015), patients with Meniere's disease were also excluded from the study. Other exclusion criteria for the study included the following: (1) pulsatile tinnitus, hyperacusis, or Meniere's diseases; (2) a past history of severe alcoholism, smoking, or head injury; (3) stroke, Alzheimer's disease, Parkinson's disease, epilepsy, major depression, or other neurological or psychiatric illness; (4) major medical illness (e.g., cancer, anemia, and thyroid dysfunction); (5) severe visual loss; and (6) any contraindications for MRI scanning. The characteristics of the chronic tinnitus patients and healthy subjects are summarized in **Table 1**. The study was approved by the Ethics Committee of Nanjing Medical University, and informed consent was obtained from each participant.

MRI Scanning

A 3.0-T MRI scanner (Ingenia, Philips Medical Systems, Netherlands) with an eight-channel receiver array head coil was used to generate magnetic resonance images. Foam padding and earplugs were used to reduce the head motion and scanner noise. From the manufacturer's data, approximately 32 dB of scanner noise may be attenuated by the earplugs (Hearos Ultimate Softness Series, United States). All participants were instructed to remain awake, keep their eyes closed, and stay motionless without thinking of anything in particular during scanning. Structural T1-weighted images were acquired in a high-resolution three-dimensional turbo fast echo (3D-TFE) scan with the following parameters: repetition time (TR)/echo time (TE) = 8.1/3.7 ms; slices = 170; thickness = 1 mm; gap = 0 mm; flip angle (FA) = 8°; acquisition matrix = 256 × 256; and field of view (FOV) = 256 mm × 256 mm. A total of 5 min 29 s was spent in scanning the structural sequence. Functional images were collected axially using a gradient-recalled echo-planar imaging sequence as follows: TR = 2,000 ms; TE = 30 ms; slices = 36; thickness = 4 mm; gap = 0 mm; FOV = 240 mm × 240 mm;

TABLE 1 | Demographic and clinical characteristics of chronic tinnitus patients and healthy controls.

	Tinnitus patients (n = 50)	Healthy controls (n = 55)	p-value
Age (year)	50.20 ± 11.19	46.82 ± 11.99	0.139
Gender (male: female)	18:32	21:34	0.817
Education levels (years)	12.50 ± 2.93	12.674 ± 3.04	0.768
Tinnitus duration (months)	37.71 ± 34.58	–	–
THQ score	52.22 ± 15.08	–	–
Hearing thresholds (left)	16.79 ± 2.76	16.87 ± 2.55	0.890
Hearing thresholds (right)	16.60 ± 3.37	16.95 ± 2.35	0.569
Hearing thresholds (average)	16.69 ± 2.68	16.91 ± 1.62	0.642

Data are represented as mean ± SD. The PTA from both ears was averaged. PTA, pure tone audiometry; THQ, tinnitus handicap questionnaires.

acquisition matrix = 64 × 64; and FA = 90°. A total of 8 min 8 s was spent on the fMRI sequence.

Data Preprocessing

Data Processing & Analysis for Resting-State Brain Imaging (DPABI_V2.3_170105) with the following stages was applied for data analysis (Yan et al., 2016). The first 10 volumes were discarded to reduce deviation, and the remaining 230 consecutive volumes were used for data analysis. Slice timing and realignment for head motion correction were performed. Subjects were excluded if they exhibited a head motion with >2.0-mm translation or a 2.0° rotation in any direction. The Montreal Neurological Institute (MNI) template (resampling voxel size = 3 mm × 3 mm × 3 mm) and an isotropic Gaussian kernel [full width at half maximum (FWHM) = 6 mm] were employed to spatially normalize, detrend, and filter (0.01–0.08 Hz) the data.

With the WFU_PickAtlas software[1], the bilateral NAc were set as seed regions. Moreover, REST-GCA in the REST toolbox was applied to analyze the effective connectivity (Zang et al., 2012). The current study established the seed time series x by the time series of the bilateral NAc and the time series y by the time series of all voxels in the brain. The linear direct influence of x on y ($F_{x \to y}$) and of y on x ($F_{y \to x}$) was calculated on the basis of the voxel across the brain. Thus, two Granger causality maps were generated according to the influence measures for each subject. The residual-based F was normalized (F') and standardized to the Z score for each voxel ($Z_{x \to y}$ and $Z_{y \to x}$, subtracting the global mean F' values, divided by the standard deviation).

Structural Analysis

Structural images were processed using the VBM8 toolbox software in SPM8[2]. Imaging preprocessing was performed in accordance with the optimized VBM protocol previously described by Good et al. (2001) including spatial normalization, segmentation, modulation, and smoothing. In SPM8, the image is rearranged to the front and back joint axis. After rearrangement, the images were divided into GM, WM, and cerebrospinal fluid using the full-automatic algorithm in VBM8. The segmented images were used to create a custom DARTEL template, which was then normalized to the MNI space. The resulting GM and WM images were smoothed using a 10-mm FWHM Gaussian kernel. GM and WM volumes were calculated by estimating these segments. Brain parenchyma volume was calculated as the sum of GM and WM volumes. The voxel-wise GM volume was used in the following statistical analysis as covariates for GCA calculations.

Statistical Analysis

The mean values of the $Z_{x \to y}$ and $Z_{y \to x}$ maps were computed several times to analyze the effective connectivity of the bilateral NAc between groups. On the basis of the above results, four Granger causality maps, including two for each direction and two for each group (the left NAc with $Z_{x \to y}$ and $Z_{y \to x}$ and the right NAc with $Z_{x \to y}$ and $Z_{y \to x}$ for both the patients and healthy controls), were acquired. Thus, to determine the differences between tinnitus patients and healthy controls, in which the covariates were age, sex, and education, these Granger causality maps were entered into a voxel-wise two-sample t-test. To exclude potential effects of GM volume differences, the voxel-wise GM volume maps were also obtained as covariates. The voxel-wise results for group differences were corrected for multiple comparisons using 3dClustSim[3] determined by Monte Carlo simulation. A combined threshold of $p < 0.001$ and a minimum cluster size of 40 voxels were set, yielding a corrected threshold of $p < 0.01$.

Demographic data were compared by using between-group t-tests and χ^2 tests (statistical significance set at $p < 0.05$). The clusters of the significant differences in the effective connectivity of the bilateral NAc between groups were extracted to investigate the association between the clinical characteristics and the fMRI data. Partial correlations in SPSS software (version 19.0; SPSS, Chicago, IL, United States) were used to correlate the mean z values within these clusters with the characteristics of each tinnitus patient. After correction for age, sex, education, and hearing thresholds, $p < 0.05$ was considered statistically significant. Bonferroni correction for multiple comparisons was applied in the correlation analysis.

RESULTS

Structural Data

After VBM analysis, there were no significant differences in the comparisons of the whole-brain volumes (GM volume, WM volume, and brain parenchyma volume) between chronic tinnitus patients and healthy controls ($p > 0.05$). After Monte Carlo simulation correction, no suprathreshold voxel-wise difference in the GM and WM volume between the chronic tinnitus patients and healthy controls was observed.

Directional Connectivity From the NAc

In contrast to healthy controls, patients with chronic tinnitus demonstrated significantly increased directional connectivity from the left NAc to the left inferior frontal gyrus (IFG). Interestingly, decreased directional connectivity was detected in the left cuneus. In addition, significantly enhanced directional connectivity from the right NAc to the left middle frontal gyrus (MFG) and right orbitofrontal cortex (OFC) was also observed in chronic tinnitus patients. In contrast, reduced directional connectivity was observed in the right cuneus in chronic tinnitus patients (**Figures 2A,B** and **Table 2**).

Directional Connectivity to the NAc

Compared with the controls, chronic tinnitus patients showed enhanced directional connection from the left middle temporal gyrus (MTG) and right MFG to the left NAc. In addition, in patients with tinnitus, the right MTG and the right IFG showed increased directional connectivity to the right NAc

[1] http://www.ansir.wfubmc.edu
[2] http://www.fil.ion.ucl.ac.uk/spm
[3] https://afni.nimh.nih.gov/pub/dist/doc/program_help/3dClustSim.html

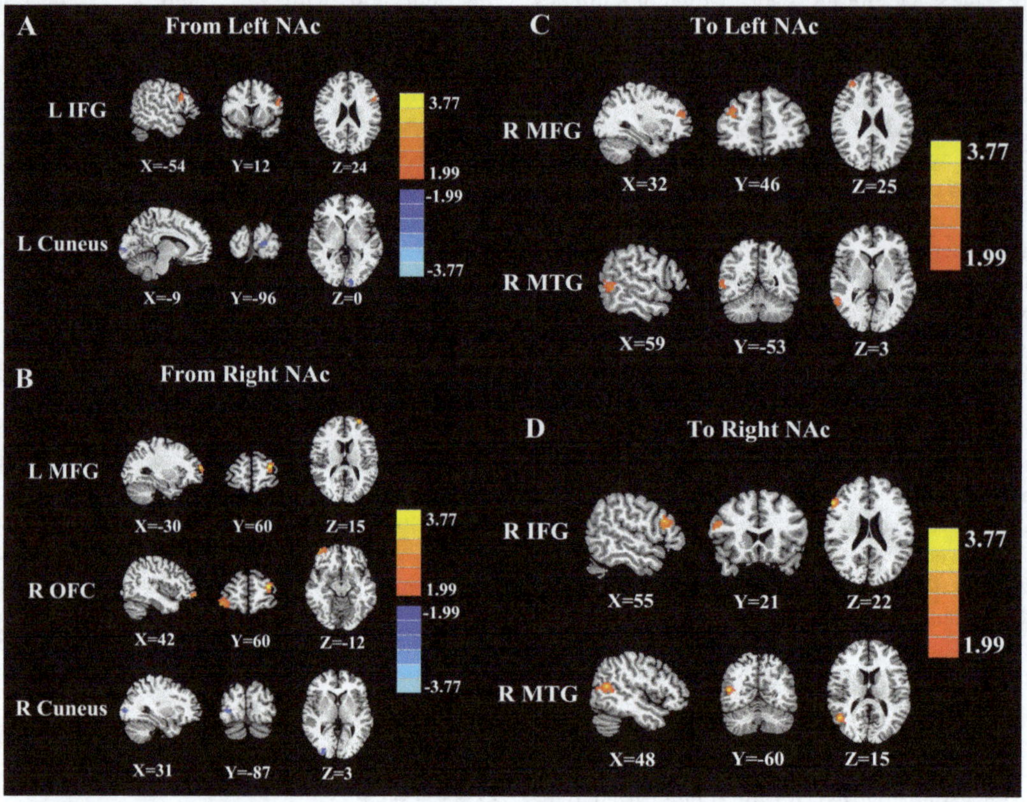

FIGURE 2 | Directional functional connectivity of the bilateral NAc in chronic tinnitus patients compared with healthy controls ($p < 0.01$ corrected by 3dClustSim). **(A)** Reduced directional connectivity from the left NAc to the left IFG and left cuneus. **(B)** Decreased directional connectivity from the right NAc to the left MFG, right OFC, and right cuneus. **(C)** Reduced directional connectivity from the right MFG and right MTG to the left NAc. **(D)** Decreased directional connectivity from the right IFG and right MTG to the right NAc.

TABLE 2 | Abnormal directional connectivity from the NAc to the other brain regions in tinnitus patients.

Brain region	BA	MNI coordinates *x, y, z* (mm)	*T* score	Cluster size
Seed: Left NAc				
L inferior frontal gyrus	45	−54, 12, 24	2.8621	44
L cuneus	17	−9, −96, 0	−2.6429	41
Seed: Right NAc				
L middle frontal gyrus	10	−30, 60, 15	4.1236	59
R orbitofrontal cortex	11	42, 60, −12	3.3899	75
R cuneus	17	31, −87, 3	−3.0587	45

Thresholds were set at a corrected p < 0.01, determined by Monte Carlo simulation. BA, Brodmann's area; MNI, Montreal neurological institute; NAc, nucleus accumbens; cluster size is in cubic millimeters.

TABLE 3 | Abnormal directional connectivity from the other brain regions to the NAc in tinnitus patients.

Brain region	BA	MNI coordinates *x, y, z* (mm)	*T* score	Cluster size
Seed: Left NAc				
R middle frontal gyrus	10	32, 46, 25	3.9302	65
R middle temporal gyrus	21	59, −53, 3	3.3662	75
Seed: Right NAc				
R inferior frontal gyrus	45	55, 21, 22	3.0863	51
R middle temporal gyrus	21	48, −60, 15	3.3322	93

Thresholds were set at a corrected p < 0.01, determined by Monte Carlo simulation. BA, Brodmann's area; MNI: Montreal neurological institute; NAc, nucleus accumbens; cluster size is in cubic millimeters.

when compared with that in healthy controls (**Figures 2C,D** and **Table 3**). No reduction in directional connectivity with the NAc was observed.

Correlation Analysis

Pearson's correlation analyses revealed that THQ scores were positively correlated with the increased directional connectivity from the right NAc to the left MFG ($r = 0.357$, $p = 0.015$) and from the right MFG to the left NAc ($r = 0.626$, $p < 0.001$). In addition, **Figure 3** shows a positive association between the enhanced directional connectivity from the right NAc to the right OFC and the tinnitus duration ($r = 0.599$, $p < 0.001$). These correlations were corrected for age, sex, education, and hearing thresholds. Other measures of increased or decreased directional connectivity were independent of tinnitus duration or

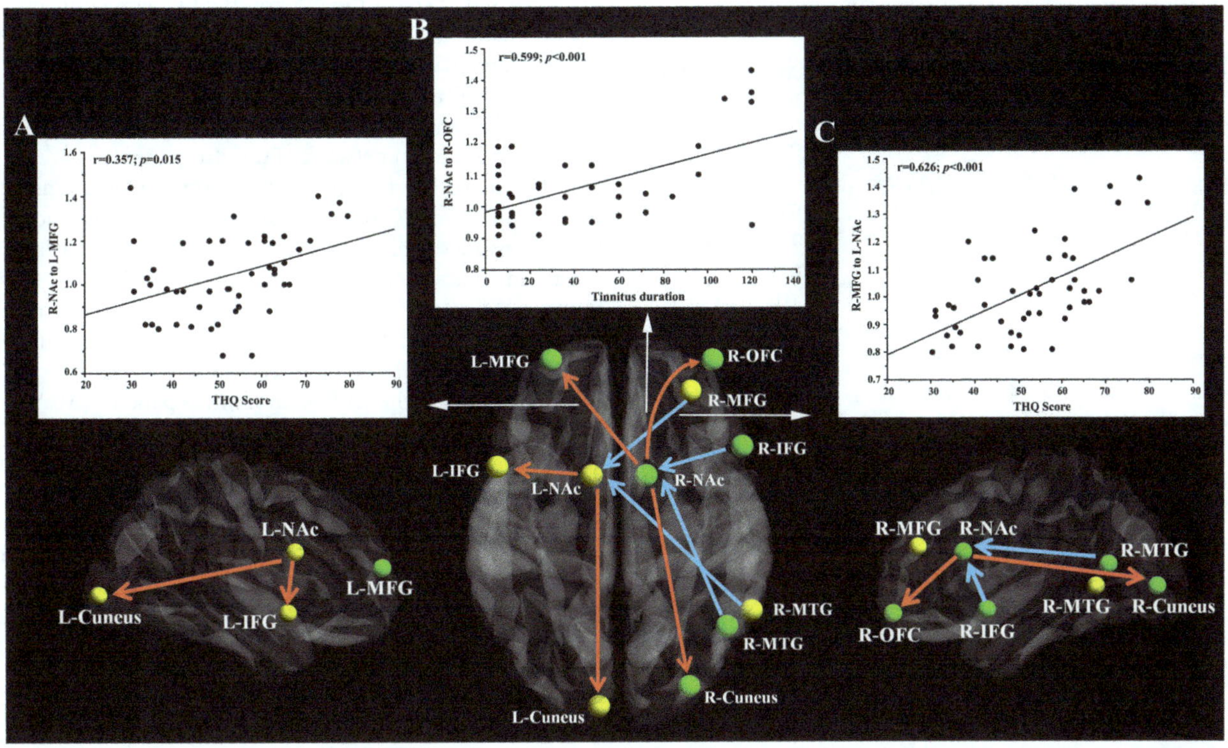

FIGURE 3 | The directional functional connectivity networks of the bilateral NAc. The red line represents the directional functional connectivity from the bilateral NAc to the other brain regions; the blue line represents the directional functional connectivity from the other brain regions to the bilateral NAc. **(A)** Positive correlation between the increased directional connectivity from the right NAc to left MFG and the THQ score ($r = 0.357$, $p = 0.015$). **(B)** Positive correlation between the increased directional connectivity from the right NAc to right OFC and the tinnitus duration ($r = 0.599$, $p < 0.001$). **(C)** Positive correlation between the enhanced directional connectivity from the right MFG to left NAc and the THQ score ($r = 0.626$, $p < 0.001$).

THQ scores. None of the disrupted directional connectivity was correlated with SAS or SDS score (**Table 4**).

DISCUSSION

In this study, resting-state fMRI combined with GCA was used to investigate the directional connectivity between the NAc and all brain regions in chronic tinnitus patients compared with healthy controls. NAc was selected as the seed region of the brain networks, as it plays an important role in establishing the significant directional connectivity patterns in the study of tinnitus. Hullfish et al. (2019) studied whether the NAc and the extended frontal striatum network participate in the pathological process of tinnitus by using resting-state fMRI. Moreover, NAc is also implicated in the pathologies of several other disorders, namely, reward deficiency syndromes, including addiction, attention deficit hyperactivity disorder, and schizophrenia (Blum et al., 2000). However, no study has observed the altered directional functional connectivity from this core region in the frontostriatal network. We note that our approach of GCA is not a conceptual innovation but is an effective solution for investigating altered directional connectivity. Our fMRI study is the first to refer to this method and settle on the NAc as the seed region of tinnitus. To provide evidence for NAc-related neural network intercorrelations and particularly emphasize the core role of the NAc and the vmPFC in tinnitus neural circuits, specifically interactions in the frontostriatal gating system, we will discuss our results combined with those of the current literature (Rauschecker et al., 2015).

Reductions in GM volumes in the NAc, vmPFC, superior frontal gyrus, superior temporal gyrus, cingulate cortex, hippocampus, and occipital lobe in tinnitus patients have been reported by previous studies (Muhlau et al., 2006; Schneider et al., 2009; Leaver et al., 2011, 2012; Boyen et al., 2013; Adjamian et al., 2014). However, we did not detect any significant differences of GM volume between our tinnitus patients and controls. It is possible that the absence of any hearing loss in our tinnitus population may be one reason for the different results. In addition, the magnetic resonance (MR) technique and analytical method should also be taken into account.

Prior studies found that the NAc receives excitatory input from the neocortex, which ends on GABAergic spiny projection neurons directly and via inhibitory interneurons (Tepper et al., 2004). Moreover, a direct GABAergic projection from the basal ganglia back to the frontal cortex can be also detected (Saunders et al., 2015). In addition, the NAc receives modulatory input from dopaminergic structures. Dopaminergic activity has been linked to valuation, motivation, and learning in the NAc (Salamone and Correa, 2012; Guitart-Masip et al., 2014). It has therefore been

TABLE 4 | Correlation coefficients and significance between the abnormal directional connectivity and tinnitus characteristics in tinnitus patients.

Brain region	Tinnitus duration	THQ	SAS	SDS
L-NAc to L-IFG	r = 0.108	r = 0.112	r = −0.149	r = 0.051
	p = 0.477	p = 0.401	p = 0.323	p = 0.736
L-NAc to L-cuneus	r = 0.180	r = 0.068	r = −0.276	r = −0.115
	p = 0.232	p = 0.652	p = 0.063	p = 0.446
R-NAc to L-MFG	r = 0.080	r = 0.357	r = 0.132	r = −0.051
	p = 0.597	p = 0.015*	p = 0.384	p = 0.712
R-NAc to R-OFC	r = 0.599	r = 0.118	r = −0.025	r = 0.007
	p < 0.001*	p = 0.435	p = 0.867	p = 0.963
R-MFG to L-NAc	r = 0.099	r = 0.626	r = −0.032	r = −0.051
	p = 0.514	p < 0.001*	p = 0.834	p = 0.735
R-MTG to L-NAc	r = 0.245	r = −0.030	r = −0.026	r = −0.184
	p = 0.119	p = 0.841	p = 0.862	p = 0.221
R-MFG to R-NAc	r = 0.225	r = −0.013	r = 0.029	r = −0.158
	p = 0.128	p = 0.932	p = 0.851	p = 0.293
R-MTG to R-NAc	r = 0.205	r = −0.138	r = 0.064	r = −0.134
	p = 0.171	p = 0.360	p = 0.672	p = 0.375

$p < 0.05$. THQ, tinnitus handicap questionnaires; SAS, self-rating anxiety scale; SDS, self-rating depression scale; NAc, nucleus accumbens; IFG, inferior frontal gyrus; MFG, middle frontal gyrus; OFC, orbitofrontal cortex; MTG, middle temporal gyrus; L, left; R, right.

claimed that dopamine and the NAc particularly relate to the valuation of tinnitus, which may influence the development of tinnitus into a chronic condition. We hypothesize that enhanced directional connectivity of NAc may increase the dopamine activity that will maintain the tinnitus perception.

Previous studies on tinnitus have provided evidence for decreased functional connectivity in the default mode network (DMN) (Husain and Schmidt, 2014; Chen et al., 2015, 2018a; Hinkley et al., 2015; Schmidt et al., 2017). In addition, in patients with chronic tinnitus, abnormal functional connectivity in limbic–auditory circuits plays a pivotal role in pathogenesis (Rauschecker et al., 2010; Leaver et al., 2011; Gunbey et al., 2017). More specifically, the subcallosal area in the limbic system is composed of the NAc and extends anteriorly toward the vmPFC (Rauschecker et al., 2010; Leaver et al., 2011; Middleton and Tzounopoulos, 2012; Adjamian et al., 2014; Carpenter-Thompson et al., 2014; De Ridder et al., 2014; Hinkley et al., 2015; Meyer et al., 2016; Hullfish et al., 2019). Therefore, Rauschecker et al. (2010) proposed a model in which the NAc and vmPFC participated in the elimination of the tinnitus signal at the level of the thalamus. Our results regarding NAc bidirectional functional connectivity were consistent with the outcomes above. The hyperactivity in the NAc and altered auditory–limbic networks may be responsible for the increased interactions between the NAc and auditory regions (Leaver et al., 2011; Adjamian et al., 2014; Rauschecker et al., 2015). Schmidt et al. (2017) found decreased DMN–precuneus connectivity and proposed correlations between interrupted connectivity and chronic tinnitus as well as tinnitus severity, which is in accordance with our result that there was decreased effective connectivity from the NAc to the bilateral cuneus. In addition, it was found that tinnitus distress was positively correlated with the increased effect of the NAc on the bilateral connection with the MFG and that the effective connection between the NAc and the OFC and MFG was enhanced. The overlapping regions of the MFG and OFC all include Brodmann's area 10, which specifically refers to the vmPFC, reflecting an interwoven relationship with the NAc in the brain network of tinnitus patients.

It is noteworthy that there were strong interactions between the NAc and vmPFC regions in tinnitus. Previous studies noted that a dysfunctional frontostriatal system can be attributed to the anomalous structure and function of the NAc and vmPFC in tinnitus patients (Rauschecker et al., 2015; Leaver et al., 2016a; Sedley et al., 2016; Hullfish et al., 2019; Tzounopoulos et al., 2019). Moreover, GM volume reduction was also detected in the subcallosal area of the vmPFC in tinnitus patients (Muhlau et al., 2006; Leaver et al., 2011; Rauschecker et al., 2015). In addition, several studies demonstrated that limbic brain regions in tinnitus are affected by functional plasticity (Lockwood et al., 1998; Mirz et al., 2000; Plewnia et al., 2007). Complementing these findings, an event-related fMRI study was the first to reveal the stimulus-evoked hyperactivity of the NAc in tinnitus patients (Leaver et al., 2011). The sgACC/vmPFC region of highly distressed tinnitus patients showed specific functional connectivity that was related to tinnitus loudness (Vanneste et al., 2014). The latest resting-state fMRI study on tinnitus utilizing NAc as a seed region revealed that NAc-related connectivity was significantly reduced, while frontostriatal connections, such as NAc–vmPFC, were most likely negatively correlated with age and mean hearing loss (Hullfish et al., 2019). Accordingly, the significantly altered effective connectivity of NAc was observed, providing effective support for the previous hypothesis of NAc–vmPFC interactions.

Beyond the discussions mentioned above, converging evidence has shown that tinnitus, as a relatively circumscribed condition, may facilitate a better understanding of the common mechanisms in limbic dysregulations of many similar disorders (Leaver et al., 2011). An analogous study was conducted, since tinnitus and chronic pain have a high degree of similarity not only in terms of sensory perception disorder and the influence of behavior but also in their pathophysiological dysfunction mechanism in the neural hierarchy (Apkarian et al., 2011; Rauschecker et al., 2015). fMRI studies on chronic pain also showed structural and functional abnormities (May, 2011; Wasan et al., 2011; Howard et al., 2012; Liu et al., 2013; Smallwood et al., 2013; Cauda et al., 2014). In addition, Rauschecker et al. (2010, 2015) concluded that chronic pain showed obvious similarity in part of the top-down modulation of sensory signals, as well as the evaluation process, and therefore proposed that the vmPFC and the NAc are crucial in the frontostriatal gating mechanism in both sensory modalities, which is consistent with our result showing bilateral altered directional connections. The intrinsic NAc–vmPFC–TRN noise cancelation system was considered the formation mechanism of tinnitus (Rauschecker et al., 2010; Sedley et al., 2016). The inhibitory signal from the NAc–vmPFC system to the TRN decreases when it becomes abnormal. Once the noise-canceling system becomes inefficient or invalid, the extra noise will stop (Rauschecker et al., 2010). Increased directional connectivity from the NAc to the IFG and MFG was observed in our study. Aberrant intrinsic connections seem to exist in frontostriatal thalamic circuits, although there is no evidence in our results indicating direct decreased connectivity to the TRN in the thalamus. Moreover, increased connectivity instead of decreased connectivity has been found in regard to the altered directional connectivity to the NAc. Based on our results and the noise-canceling mechanism, we hypothesize that with a reduced inhibitory signal, the MGN-TRN not only fails to cancel the phantom sound but also feeds back more signal to the NAc through the amygdala, which may explain the increased directional connectivity from the NAc.

Several limitations must be acknowledged in this study. First, our ability to detect the relationship between abnormal directional connectivity and tinnitus characteristics may be reduced because of our small sample size. Additional longitudinal studies involving more subjects are required in the future. Furthermore, only the NAc was selected as the seed region to investigate the directional connectivity in tinnitus. For initial consideration, this study just would like to explore more deeply about the NAc-related connectivity in tinnitus and see whether any directional NAc-related connectivity has correlation with tinnitus-related distress, based on the study of Hullfish et al. (2019). Therefore, other critical seed regions were not included in our directional connectivity analysis. We admit that the selection of the seed region is not data driven, which will result in a biased conclusion. Other data-driven methods, such as independent component analysis (ICA) and principal component analysis (PCA), will be used for generating the seed regions in our future study. The current GCA approach can be extended to other regions within the frontostriatal gating circuit, such as the sgACC. Previous structural MRI and fMRI studies have suggested the critical role of the sgACC in tinnitus patients (Rauschecker et al., 2015; Meyer et al., 2016; Hullfish et al., 2019). Disruption of the descending projection from sgACC to the TRN might prevent the suppression of irrelevant sensory signals, such as those that result in a phantom percept, which might raise the intensity of such percepts (Rauschecker et al., 2015). Our prior study has also identified the relationship between tinnitus distress and abnormal functional connectivity in the ACC, especially the dorsal and ventral ACC (Chen et al., 2018b). However, the role of sgACC has not been demonstrated in this study. In addition, the NAc–sgACC interaction involved in the frontostriatal gating circuit has not been confirmed in the study of Hullfish et al. (2019). Therefore, the exact role of the sgACC on the neuropathological mechanism underlying chronic tinnitus will require exploration in further studies. Moreover, the subjects in the current study showed no obvious hearing loss or hyperacusis, which is not representative of all tinnitus patients. Finally, the auditory pathway is likely to be activated by scanner noise, which is nearly impossible to completely eliminate even with earplugs or active noise reduction (Rondinoni et al., 2013). This uncertainty should be taken into consideration when interpreting the resting-state fMRI data in future research.

CONCLUSION

To our knowledge, this is the first fMRI study to apply the GCA method to explore the directional connectivity of the NAc in chronic tinnitus patients. The current study showed that tinnitus distress correlates with bidirectionally enhanced effective connectivity between the NAc and the prefrontal cortex. Taken together, these results help elucidate the neural basis of frontostriatal gating control of tinnitus sensation, which may play a pivotal role in the neuropathological features of tinnitus.

ETHICS STATEMENT

The studies involving human participants were reviewed and approved by the Ethics Committee of Nanjing Medical University. The patients/participants provided their written informed consent to participate in this study.

AUTHOR CONTRIBUTIONS

J-JX and JC designed the experiment, collected the data, performed the analysis, and wrote the manuscript. YF, WY, HC, and YW helped to collect the data and perform the analysis. Y-CC and XY contributed to the discussion and manuscript revision.

REFERENCES

Adjamian, P., Hall, D. A., Palmer, A. R., Allan, T. W., and Langers, D. R. (2014). Neuroanatomical abnormalities in chronic tinnitus in the human brain. *Neurosci. Biobehav. Rev.* 45, 119–133. doi: 10.1016/j.neubiorev.2014.05.013

Apkarian, A. V., Hashmi, J. A., and Baliki, M. N. (2011). Pain and the brain: specificity and plasticity of the brain in clinical chronic pain. *Pain* 152(3 Suppl.), S49–S64. doi: 10.1016/j.pain.2010.11.010

Baguley, D., McFerran, D., and Hall, D. (2013). Tinnitus. *Lancet* 382, 1600–1607. doi: 10.1016/s0140-6736(13)60142-60147

Barkhof, F., Haller, S., and Rombouts, S. A. R. B. (2014). Resting-state functional MR imaging:a new window to the brain. *Radiology* 272, 29–49. doi: 10.1148/radiol.14132388

Barry, K. M., Paolini, A. G., Robertson, D., and Mulders, W. H. (2015). Modulation of medial geniculate nucleus neuronal activity by electrical stimulation of the nucleus accumbens. *Neuroscience* 308, 1–10. doi: 10.1016/j.neuroscience.2015.09.008

Bauer, C. A. (2018). Tinnitus. *N. Engl. J. Med.* 378, 1224–1231. doi: 10.1056/NEJMcp1506631

Biswal, B., Yetkin, F. Z., Haughton, V. M., and Hyde, J. S. (1995). Functional connectivity in the motor cortex of resting human brain using Echo-PlanarMRI. *Magn. Reson. Med.* 34, 537–541. doi: 10.1002/mrm.1910340409

Blum, K., Braverman, E. R., Holder, J. M., Lubar, J. F., Monastra, V. J., Miller, D., et al. (2000). The reward deficiency syndrome: a biogenetic model for the diagnosis and treatment of impulsive, addictive and compulsive behaviors. *J. Psychol. Drugs* 32(Suppl.1), 1–112. doi: 10.1080/02791072.2000.10736099

Boyen, K., Langers, D. R., de Kleine, E., and van Dijk, P. (2013). Gray matter in the brain: differences associated with tinnitus and hearing loss. *Hear. Res.* 295, 67–78. doi: 10.1016/j.heares.2012.02.010

Carpenter-Thompson, J. R., Akrofi, K., Schmidt, S. A., Dolcos, F., and Husain, F. T. (2014). Alterations of the emotional processing system may underlie preserved rapid reaction time in tinnitus. *Brain Res.* 1567, 28–41. doi: 10.1016/j.brainres.2014.04.024

Cauda, F., Palermo, S., Costa, T., Torta, R., Duca, S., Vercelli, U., et al. (2014). Gray matter alterations in chronic pain: a network-oriented meta-analytic approach. *Neuroimage Clin.* 4, 676–686. doi: 10.1016/j.nicl.2014.04.007

Chen, G.-D., Radziwon, K. E., Kashanian, N., Manohar, S., and Salvi, R. (2014). Salicylate-induced auditory perceptual disorders and plastic changes in nonclassical auditory centers in rats. *Neural. Plast.* 2014, 1–18. doi: 10.1155/2014/658741

Chen, Y.-C., Feng, Y., Xu, J.-J., Mao, C.-N., Xia, W., Ren, J., et al. (2016). Disrupted brain functional network architecture in chronic tinnitus patients. *Front. Aging Neurosci.* 8:174. doi: 10.3389/fnagi.2016.00174

Chen, Y.-C., Liu, S., Lv, H., Bo, F., Feng, Y., Chen, H., et al. (2018b). Abnormal resting-state functional connectivity of the anterior cingulate cortex in unilateral chronic tinnitus patients. *Front. Neurosci.* 12:9. doi: 10.3389/fnins.2018.00009

Chen, Y. C., Chen, H., Bo, F., Xu, J. J., Deng, Y., Lv, H., et al. (2018a). Tinnitus distress is associated with enhanced resting-state functional connectivity within the default mode network. *Neuropsychiatr. Dis. Treat* 14, 1919–1927. doi: 10.2147/NDT.S164619

Chen, Y. C., Xia, W., Luo, B., Muthaiah, V. P., Xiong, Z., Zhang, J., et al. (2015). Frequency-specific alternations in the amplitude of low-frequency fluctuations in chronic tinnitus. *Front. Neural. Circ.* 9:67. doi: 10.3389/fncir.2015.00067

Chen, Y.-C., Yong, W., Xing, C., Feng, Y., Haidari, N. A., Xu, J.-J., et al. (2019). Directed functional connectivity of the hippocampus in patients with presbycusis. *Brain Imag. Behav.* doi: 10.1007/s11682-019-00162-z [Epub ahead of print].

Crippaa, A., Lanting, C. P., Dijk, P. V., and Roerdink, J. B. T. M. (2010). A diffusion tensor imaging study on the auditory system and tinnitus. *Open Neuroimag. J.* 4, 16–25. doi: 10.2174/1874440001004010016

De Ridder, D., Vanneste, S., Weisz, N., Londero, A., Schlee, W., Elgoyhen, A. B., et al. (2014). An integrative model of auditory phantom perception: tinnitus as a unified percept of interacting separable subnetworks. *Neurosci. Biobehav. Rev.* 44, 16–32. doi: 10.1016/j.neubiorev.2013.03.021

Eggermont, J. J. (2007). Correlated neural activity as the driving force for functional changes in auditory cortex. *Hear. Res.* 229, 69–80. doi: 10.1016/j.heares.2007.01.008

Eggermont, J. J., and Roberts, L. E. (2004). The neuroscience of tinnitus. *Trends Neurosci.* 27, 676–682. doi: 10.1016/j.tins.2004.08.010

Galazyuk, A. V., Wenstrup, J. J., and Hamid, M. A. (2012). Tinnitus and underlying brain mechanisms. *Curr. Opin. Otolaryngol. Head. Neck. Surg.* 20, 409–415. doi: 10.1097/MOO.0b013e3283577b81

Good, C. D., Johnsrude, I. S., Ashburner, J., Henson, R. N., Friston, K. J., and Frackowiak, R. S. (2001). A voxel-based morphometric study of ageing in 465 normal adult human brains. *Neuroimage* 14(1 Pt 1), 21–36. doi: 10.1006/nimg.2001.0786

Guitart-Masip, M., Duzel, E., Dolan, R., and Dayan, P. (2014). Action versus valence in decision making. *Trends Cogn. Sci.* 18, 194–202. doi: 10.1016/j.tics.2014.01.003

Gunbey, H. P., Gunbey, E., Aslan, K., Bulut, T., Unal, A., and Incesu, L. (2017). Limbic-auditory interactions of tinnitus: an evaluation using diffusion tensor imaging. *Clin. Neuroradiol.* 27, 221–230. doi: 10.1007/s00062-015-0473-470

Guo, W., Liu, F., Zhang, Z., Liu, J., Yu, M., Zhang, J., et al. (2015). Unidirectionally affected causal connectivity of cortico-limbic-cerebellar circuit by structural deficits in drug-naive major depressive disorder. *J. Affect. Disord.* 172, 410–416. doi: 10.1016/j.jad.2014.10.019

Hinkley, L. B., Mizuiri, D., Hong, O., Nagarajan, S. S., and Cheung, S. W. (2015). Increased striatal functional connectivity with auditory cortex in tinnitus. *Front. Hum. Neurosci.* 9:568. doi: 10.3389/fnhum.2015.00568

Howard, M. A., Sanders, D., Krause, K., O'Muircheartaigh, J., Fotopoulou, A., Zelaya, F., et al. (2012). Alterations in resting-state regional cerebral blood flow demonstrate ongoing pain in osteoarthritis: an arterial spin-labeled magnetic resonance imaging study. *Arth. Rheum.* 64, 3936–3946. doi: 10.1002/art.37685

Hullfish, J., Abenes, I., Yoo, H. B., De Ridder, D., and Vanneste, S. (2019). Frontostriatal network dysfunction as a domain-general mechanism underlying phantom perception. *Hum. Brain Mapp.* 40, 2241–2251. doi: 10.1002/hbm.24521

Husain, F. T., and Schmidt, S. A. (2014). Using resting state functional connectivity to unravel networks of tinnitus. *Hear. Res.* 307, 153–162. doi: 10.1016/j.heares.2013.07.010

Jiao, Q., Lu, G., Zhang, Z., Zhong, Y., Wang, Z., Guo, Y., et al. (2011). Granger causal influence predicts BOLD activity levels in the default mode network. *Hum. Brain Mapp.* 32, 154–161. doi: 10.1002/hbm.21065

Khalfa, S., Dubal, S., Veuillet, E., Perez-Diaz, F., Jouvent, R., and Collet, L. (2002). Psychometric normalization of a hyperacusis questionnaire. *ORL J. Otorhinolaryngol. Relat. Spec.* 64, 436–442. doi: 10.1159/000067570

Kim, J. Y., Kim, Y. H., Lee, S., Seo, J. H., Song, H. J., Cho, J. H., et al. (2012). Alteration of functional connectivity in tinnitus brain revealed by resting-state fMRI? A pilot study. *Int. J. Audiol.* 51, 413–417. doi: 10.3109/14992027.2011.652677

Knipper, M., Van Dijk, P., Nunes, I., Ruttiger, L., and Zimmermann, U. (2013). Advances in the neurobiology of hearing disorders: recent developments regarding the basis of tinnitus and hyperacusis. *Prog. Neurobiol.* 111, 17–33. doi: 10.1016/j.pneurobio.2013.08.002

Kreuzer, P. M., Lehner, A., Schlee, W., Vielsmeier, V., Schecklmann, M., Poeppl, T. B., et al. (2015). Combined rTMS treatment targeting the anterior cingulate and the temporal cortex for the treatment of chronic tinnitus. *Sci. Rep.* 5:18028. doi: 10.1038/srep18028

Kuk, F. K., Tyler, R. S., Russell, D., and Jordan, H. (1990). The psychometric properties of a tinnitus handicap questionnaire. *Ear Hear.* 11, 434–445. doi: 10.1097/00003446-199012000-00005

Langers, D. R., de Kleine, E., and van Dijk, P. (2012). Tinnitus does not require macroscopic tonotopic map reorganization. *Front. Syst. Neurosci.* 6:2. doi: 10.3389/fnsys.2012.00002

Leaver, A. M., Renier, L., Chevillet, M. A., Morgan, S., Kim, H. J., and Rauschecker, J. P. (2011). Dysregulation of limbic and auditory networks in tinnitus. *Neuron* 69, 33–43. doi: 10.1016/j.neuron.2010.12.002

Leaver, A. M., Seydell-Greenwald, A., and Rauschecker, J. P. (2016a). Auditory-limbic interactions in chronic tinnitus: challenges for neuroimaging research. *Hear. Res.* 334, 49–57. doi: 10.1016/j.heares.2015.08.005

Leaver, A. M., Turesky, T. K., Seydell-Greenwald, A., Morgan, S., Kim, H. J., and Rauschecker, J. P. (2016b). Intrinsic network activity in tinnitus investigated using functional MRI. *Hum. Brain Mapp.* 37, 2717–2735. doi: 10.1002/hbm.23204

Leaver, A. M., Seydell-Greenwald, A., Turesky, T. K., Morgan, S., Kim, H. J., and Rauschecker, J. P. (2012). Cortico-limbic morphology separates tinnitus from tinnitus distress. *Front. Syst. Neurosci.* 6:21. doi: 10.3389/fnsys.2012.00021

Liu, J., Hao, Y., Du, M., Wang, X., Zhang, J., Manor, B., et al. (2013). Quantitative cerebral blood flow mapping and functional connectivity of postherpetic neuralgia pain: a perfusion fMRI study. *Pain* 154, 110–118. doi: 10.1016/j.pain.2012.09.016

Lockwood, A. H., Salvi, R. J., Coad, M. L., Towsley, M. L., Wack, D. S., and Murphy, B. W. (1998). The functional neuroanatcomy of tinnitus evidence for limbic system links arid neural plasticity. *Neurology* 50, 114–120. doi: 10.1212/wnl.50.1.114

Lopez-Escamez, J. A., Carey, J., Chung, W. H., Goebel, J. A., Magnusson, M., Mandala, M., et al. (2015). Diagnostic criteria for Meniere's disease. *J. Vestib. Res.* 25, 1–7. doi: 10.3233/ves-150549

May, A. (2011). Structural brain imaging: a window into chronic pain. *Neuroscientist* 17, 209–220. doi: 10.1177/1073858410396220

Meyer, M., Neff, P., Liem, F., Kleinjung, T., Weidt, S., Langguth, B., et al. (2016). Differential tinnitus-related neuroplastic alterations of cortical thickness and surface area. *Hear. Res.* 342, 1–12. doi: 10.1016/j.heares.2016.08.016

Middleton, J. W., and Tzounopoulos, T. (2012). Imaging the neural correlates of tinnitus: a comparison between animal models and human studies. *Front. Syst. Neurosci.* 6:35. doi: 10.3389/fnsys.2012.00035

Mirz, F., Gjeddek, A., Ishizu, O., and Pedersen, C. B. (2000). Cortical networks subserving the perception of tinnitus—a PET study. *Acta Otolaryngol. Suppl.* 543, 241–243. doi: 10.1080/000164800454503

Muhlau, M., Rauschecker, J. P., Oestreicher, E., Gaser, C., Rottinger, M., Wohlschlager, A. M., et al. (2006). Structural brain changes in tinnitus. *Cereb. Cortex* 16, 1283–1288. doi: 10.1093/cercor/bhj070

Plewnia, C., Reimold, M., Najib, A., Brehm, B., Reischl, G., Plontke, S. K., et al. (2007). Dose-dependent attenuation of auditory phantom perception (tinnitus) by PET-guided repetitive transcranial magnetic stimulation. *Hum. Brain Mapp.* 28, 238–246. doi: 10.1002/hbm.20270

Raichle, M. E., MacLeod, A. M., Snyder, A. Z., Powers, W. J., Gusnard, D. A., et al. (2000). a default mode of brain function. *Proc Natl. Acad. Sci. U.S.A.* 98, 676–682.

Rauschecker, J. P., Leaver, A. M., and Mühlau, M. (2010). Tuning out the noise Limbic-auditory interactions in tinnitus. *Neuron* 66, 819–826. doi: 10.1016/j.neuron.2010.04.032

Rauschecker, J. P., May, E. S., Maudoux, A., and Ploner, M. (2015). Frontostriatal gating of tinnitus and chronic pain. *Trends Cogn. Sci.* 19, 567–578. doi: 10.1016/j.tics.2015.08.002

Rondinoni, C., Amaro, E. Jr., Cendes, F., Dos Santos, A., and Salmon, C. (2013). Effect of scanner acoustic background noise on strict resting-state fMRI. *Braz. J. Med. Biol. Res.* 46, 359–367. doi: 10.1590/1414-431x2013 2799

Salamone, J. D., and Correa, M. (2012). The mysterious motivational functions of mesolimbic dopamine. *Neuron* 76, 470–485. doi: 10.1016/j.neuron.2012.10.021

Saunders, A., Oldenburg, I. A., Berezovskii, V. K., Johnson, C. A., Kingery, N. D., Elliott, H. L., et al. (2015). A direct GABAergic output from the basal ganglia to frontal cortex. *Nature* 521:85. doi: 10.1038/nature14179

Schmidt, S. A., Carpenter-Thompson, J., and Husain, F. T. (2017). Connectivity of precuneus to the default mode and dorsal attention networks: a possible invariant marker of long-term tinnitus. *Neuroimage Clin.* 16, 196–204. doi: 10.1016/j.nicl.2017.07.015

Schneider, P., Andermann, M., Wengenroth, M., Goebel, R., Flor, H., Rupp, A., et al. (2009). Reduced volume of Heschl's gyrus in tinnitus. *Neuroimage* 45, 927–939. doi: 10.1016/j.neuroimage.2008.12.045

Sedley, W., Friston, K. J., Gander, P. E., Kumar, S., and Griffiths, T. D. (2016). An integrative tinnitus model based on sensory precision. *Trends Neurosci.* 39, 799–812. doi: 10.1016/j.tins.2016.10.004

Shargorodsky, J., Curhan, G. C., and Farwell, W. R. (2010). Prevalence and characteristics of tinnitus among US adults. *Am. J. Med.* 123, 711–718. doi: 10.1016/j.amjmed.2010.02.015

Smallwood, R. F., Laird, A. R., Ramage, A. E., Parkinson, A. L., Lewis, J., Clauw, D. J., et al. (2013). Structural brain anomalies and chronic pain: a quantitative meta-analysis of gray matter volume. *J. Pain* 14, 663–675. doi: 10.1016/j.jpain.2013.03.001

Song, J. J., De Ridder, D., Van de Heyning, P., and Vanneste, S. (2012). Mapping tinnitus-related brain activation: an activation-likelihood estimation metaanalysis of PET studies. *J. Nucl. Med.* 53, 1550–1557. doi: 10.2967/jnumed.112.102939

Song, J. J., Vanneste, S., and De Ridder, D. (2015). Dysfunctional noise cancelling of the rostral anterior cingulate cortex in tinnitus patients. *PLoS One* 10:e0123538. doi: 10.1371/journal.pone.0123538

Stephan, K. E., and Roebroeck, A. (2012). A short history of causal modeling of fMRI data. *Neuroimage* 62, 856–863. doi: 10.1016/j.neuroimage.2012.01.034

Tepper, J. M., Koós, T., and Wilson, C. J. (2004). GABAergic microcircuits in the neostriatum. *Trends Neurosci.* 27, 662–669. doi: 10.1016/j.tins.2004.08.007

Tzounopoulos, T., Balaban, C., Zitelli, L., and Palmer, C. (2019). Towards a mechanistic-driven precision medicine approach for tinnitus. *J. Assoc. Res. Otolaryngol.* 20, 115–131. doi: 10.1007/s10162-018-00709-709

Vanneste, S., Congedo, M., and De Ridder, D. (2014). Pinpointing a highly specific pathological functional connection that turns phantom sound into distress. *Cereb. Cortex* 24, 2268–2282. doi: 10.1093/cercor/bht068

Vanneste, S., and De Ridder, D. (2012). The auditory and non-auditory brain areas involved in tinnitus. an emergent property of multiple parallel overlapping subnetworks. *Front. Syst. Neurosci.* 6:31. doi: 10.3389/fnsys.2012.00031

Wasan, A. D., Loggia, M. L., Chen, L. Q., Napadow, V., Kong, J., and Gollub, R. L. (2011). Neural correlates of chronic low back pain measured by arterial spin labeling. *Anesthesiology* 115,364–374.

Yan, C.-G., Wang, X.-D., Zuo, X.-N., and Zang, Y.-F. (2016). DPABI: data processing & analysis for (resting-state) brain imaging. *Neuroinformatics* 14, 339–351. doi: 10.1007/s12021-016-9299-4

Yu, E., Liao, Z., Mao, D., Zhang, Q., Ji, G., Li, Y., et al. (2017). Directed functional connectivity of posterior cingulate cortex and whole brain in Alzheimer's disease and mild cognitive impairment. *Curr. Alzheimer Res.* 14, 628–635. doi: 10.2174/1567205013666161201201000

Zang, Z.-X., Yan, C.-G., Dong, Z.-Y., Huang, J., and Zang, Y.-F. (2012). Granger causality analysis implementation on MATLAB: a graphic user interface toolkit for fMRI data processing. *J. Neurosci. Methods* 203, 418–426. doi: 10.1016/j.jneumeth.2011.10.006

Zhong, Y., Huang, L., Cai, S., Zhang, Y., von Deneen, K. M., Ren, A., et al. (2014). Altered effective connectivity patterns of the default mode network in Alzheimer's disease: an fMRI study. *Neurosci. Lett.* 578, 171–175. doi: 10.1016/j.neulet.2014.06.043

Zung, W. (1986). "Zung self-rating depression scale and depression status inventory," in *Assessment of Depression*, eds N. Sartorius, and T. A. Ban, (Berlin: Springer), 221–231. doi: 10.1007/978-3-642-70486-4_21

Zung, W. W. (1971). A rating instrument for anxiety disorders. *Psychosomatics* 12, 371–379. doi: 10.1016/s0033-3182(71)71479-0

6

Brain Structural and Functional Reorganization in Tinnitus Patients without Hearing Loss After Sound Therapy: A Preliminary Longitudinal Study

Qian Chen[1], Han Lv[1], Zhaodi Wang[2], Xuan Wei[1], Pengfei Zhao[1], Zhenghan Yang[1], Shusheng Gong[2] and Zhenchang Wang[1*]*

[1] Department of Radiology, Beijing Friendship Hospital, Capital Medical University, Beijing, China, [2] Department of Otolaryngology Head and Neck Surgery, Beijing Friendship Hospital, Capital Medical University, Beijing, China

***Correspondence:**
Han Lv
chrislvhan@126.com
Zhenchang Wang
cjr.wzhch@vip.163.com

Sound therapy is one of the most common first-line treatments for idiopathic tinnitus. We aimed to investigate the brain structural and functional alterations between patients with idiopathic tinnitus without hearing loss (HL) and healthy controls (HCs) and between patients before and after sound therapy (narrow band noise). Structural and resting-state functional images were acquired from 13 tinnitus patients without HL and 18 HCs before and after 6 months of narrow band sound therapy (only patients received the treatment). Voxel-based morphometry (VBM) and independent component analysis (ICA) were conducted to separately investigate the brain structural and functional changes. Associations between brain changes and clinical variables were also performed. After the treatment, the % improvement of THI score was −1.30% (± 63.40%). Compared with HCs, tinnitus patients showed gray matter and white matter atrophy in the left middle temporal gyrus at baseline, and the gray matter volume was further reduced after the treatment. The patients also showed increased white matter volume in the cingulum (cingulate), right calcarine, left rolandic operculum, and left parietal and frontal lobes. Additionally, compared with HCs, tinnitus patients exhibited positive [medial visual network (mVN) and sensorimotor network (SMN), mVN and auditory network (AN)] and negative [mVN and lateral visual network (lVN)] internetwork functional connectivity (FC) at baseline and negative [left frontoparietal network (LFPN) and dorsal attention network (DAN), AN and posterior default mode network (pDMN)] internetwork FC after the narrow band sound therapy. The patients also showed negative [LFPN and right frontoparietal network (RFPN), LFPN and RFPN, anterior default mode network (aDMN) and AN, aDMN and DAN] internetwork FC after the treatment when compared with baseline. Our findings suggest that although the outcomes of idiopathic tinnitus patients without HL were not very good when the improvement of THI scores was used as an evaluation indicator, the patients experienced significant differences in auditory-related and non-auditory-related brain reorganization before and after the narrow band sound therapy, that is, sound therapy may have a significant effect on brain reorganization in patients with idiopathic tinnitus. This study may provide some new useful information for the understanding of mechanisms underlying idiopathic tinnitus.

Keywords: tinnitus without hearing loss, structural and functional reorganization, voxel-based morphometry, independent component analysis, clinical variables

INTRODUCTION

Tinnitus is a phantom sound without an external source, which affects 10–15% of the adult population, and it seriously affects the quality of patients' lives (Sereda et al., 2018). Prior studies have shown that tinnitus is caused by alterations in the brain (Eggermont and Roberts, 2004) and is associated with specific learning processes allowing increased awareness and continuous appraisal (i.e., tinnitus sensitization and centralization) (Zenner and Zalaman, 2004; Noreña and Farley, 2013). Moreover, many studies to date have shown significant brain structural and functional remodeling in tinnitus patients (Chen et al., 2015, 2020, 2021; Ryu et al., 2016; Schmidt et al., 2017). Therefore, it is very important to reverse tinnitus-related abnormal brain neural activity or reorganization.

To date, many treatment modalities have been applied to tinnitus patients, such as drug therapy, cognitive behavioral therapy (CBT), tinnitus counseling, cochlear implants (CIs), tinnitus retraining therapy, hearing aids, brain stimulation, and sound therapy (Langguth et al., 2013; Zenner et al., 2017; Sereda et al., 2018; Bae et al., 2020). There is no satisfying treatment that can benefit all patients (Langguth et al., 2013). However, of the abovementioned treatment methods, sound therapy, such as using a noise generator with an unmodulated frequency or involving the use of a recorded noise or a special noise source or mask device (Jastreboff, 1999; Oishi et al., 2013), has been widely suggested for the management of tinnitus in many studies (Jastreboff, 1999; Oishi et al., 2013; Han et al., 2019a,b; Lv et al., 2020). Meanwhile, according to meta-analytic evidence (Sereda et al., 2018), sound therapy is the first-line treatment method in UK audiology departments for tinnitus patients (together with hearing aids and information and advice) (Hobson et al., 2012; Hoare et al., 2014; Sereda et al., 2015; Tutaj et al., 2018) and was even listed as an option in the clinical guidelines (Henry et al., 2002; Tunkel et al., 2014). During this treatment, the generated sound will be set based on tinnitus features, including its pitch, loudness, and minimum masking level. This sound reduces the contrast between the tinnitus and the environment, diminishes sensitivity to tinnitus, and promotes habituation to the tinnitus sensation (Makar et al., 2017). Narrowband noise is the most commonly used and effective sound therapy method (Henry et al., 2002). However, to the best of our knowledge, few studies to date have explored the effect of sound therapy on brain remodeling in idiopathic tinnitus. Almost all studies have focused only on alterations in brain function after treatment. These studies have suggested that sound therapy achieved good outcomes when taking improvements in tinnitus handicap inventory (THI) scores as an evaluation standard (Han et al., 2019a,b; Lv et al., 2020). For example, Han et al. (2019b) and Lv et al. (2020) have indicated that sound therapy significantly changed or even had a normalizing effect on the abnormal functional connectivity (FC) in the brains of patients with idiopathic tinnitus and that the changed FC was correlated with the severity of tinnitus.

Moreover, although there are many studies on brain structural and functional changes in tinnitus patients at present (Aldhafeeri et al., 2012; Seydell-Greenwald et al., 2014; Chen et al., 2015; Ryu et al., 2016; Han et al., 2020), many of these subjects had different degrees of hearing loss (HL) (Aldhafeeri et al., 2012; Seydell-Greenwald et al., 2014; Ryu et al., 2016; Han et al., 2020). Although some researchers have noticed that HL may have an impact on the results, their studies were mainly on brain reorganization in patients without any treatment (Husain et al., 2011; Benson et al., 2014; Schmidt et al., 2017). To date, there are few studies on the changes in both brain structure and function in tinnitus patients without HL after sound therapy.

Therefore, based on the above studies, to explore the brain alterations between tinnitus patients and healthy controls (HCs) and between patients before and after sound therapy, in the present study, we combined voxel-based morphometry (VBM) and independent component analysis (ICA) in patients with tinnitus in the early stage (duration less than 48 months) without HL before and after sound therapy and further explored their relationships with clinical variables. We defined subjects with a duration of fewer than 48 months being in the early stage, which is consistent with our previous studies (Liu et al., 2018; Chen et al., 2020).

MATERIALS AND METHODS

Participants

Thirteen patients with untreated persistent idiopathic tinnitus and 18 HCs were enrolled in this study. All the patients had persistent idiopathic tinnitus, and the duration had been persistent for more than 6 months and less than 48 months, without any history of associated brain diseases confirmed by conventional magnetic resonance imaging (MRI), no preexisting mental or cognitive disorder, and no MRI contradictions. Tinnitus was present as a single high/low-pitched sound and 2

Abbreviations: HL, hearing loss; VBM, voxel-based morphometry; ICA, independent component analysis; HC, healthy control; FC, functional connectivity; CBT, cognitive behavioral therapy; CI, cochlear implant; THI, tinnitus handicap inventory; CSF, cerebrospinal fluid; GMV, gray matter volume; WMV, white matter volume; MNI, Montreal Neurological Institute; RSN, resting-state network; ROI, region of interest; MTG, middle temporal gyrus.

high/low-pitched sounds without any rhythm. All the patients were defined as tinnitus without HL based on audiogram results, which was defined as more than 25 dB HL at frequencies ranging from 250 to 8 kHz (0.250, 0.500, 1, 2, 3, 4, 6, and 8 kHz) in a pure-tone audiometry (PTA) examination. All the patients in this study were without pulsatile tinnitus, sudden deafness, Ménière's disease, hyperacusis on physical examination, otosclerosis, and other neurological diseases. We asked all the patients to complete the THI (Newman et al., 1996) and a visual analog scale (VAS) to assess the severity of disease at the time of admission. We also evaluated the severity of depression and distress of the patients at that time. Moreover, we assessed the hearing of the HCs, and all of them had normal hearing. Other exclusion criteria for the tinnitus patients were also applied with the HCs.

The study protocol was approved by the institutional review board (IRB) of Beijing Friendship Hospital, Capital Medical University, Beijing, China. All the subjects were informed of the purpose of the study and gave written consent in accordance with the Declaration of Helsinki. The registration number of the study on ClinicalTrials.gov is NCT03764826.

Sound Therapy and Clinical Evaluation

The sound therapy applied is a customized personal sound therapy based on patients' tinnitus features. We used the special tinnitus therapeutic instrument: eMasker® (Micro-DSP Technology Co., Ltd), which is a customized personal sound therapy device based on tinnitus characteristic test results. We advise patients to use it in a quiet environment to achieve the best therapeutic effect. First, to characterize the tinnitus and prepare for treatment, the audiologists in our group examined all the patients for tinnitus loudness matching, pitch matching, minimum masking level, and residual inhibition. Then, we applied narrow band noise (that was used for treatment) to treat tinnitus for 6 months, 20 min each time, three times per day. The loudness of sound we applied for each patient was set as 5 dB over the tinnitus loudness. The frequency was set as a 1 kHz narrow band while setting the tinnitus frequency as the middle point of the delivered sound (i.e., tinnitus frequency $\pm$ 0.5 kHz, for example, tinnitus frequency = 3 kHz, low sound cut = 2.5 kHz, high sound cut = 3.5 kHz). In this procedure, we used the THI scores to assess the severity of tinnitus before and after treatment. In our study, consistent with prior research, a reduction in THI scores to 16 points or a reduction of 17 points or more was considered effective treatment (Zeman et al., 2011). Therefore, we defined the primary outcome of this study as THI score changes. The HCs were not given any particular kind of sound exposure during the study. We also calculated $^{\Delta}$ THI scores and improvement in THI scores in all patients with tinnitus, which were defined as follows: $^{\Delta}$ THI score = THI on admission—THI follow-up; % improvement in THI score = (THI score at 6 months follow-up—THI score on admission) $\div$ THI score on admission $\times$ 100%.

Image Acquisition

Structural and functional imaging data of the idiopathic tinnitus patients at baseline (without any treatment) and after treatment (6 months) and from HCs were obtained using a 3.0T MRI system (Prisma, Siemens, Erlangen, Germany) with a 64-channel phase-array head coil. During the scanning process, we used tight but comfortable foam padding to minimize head motion and earplugs to reduce scanner noise. All the participants were asked to stay awake, close their eyes, breathe evenly, and try to avoid specific thoughts. We used a conventional brain axial T2 sequence before the structural and functional scans to exclude any visible brain abnormalities. Using a 3D magnetization-prepared rapid gradient-echo sequence (MP-RAGE), we obtained high-resolution three-dimensional (3D) structural T1-weighted images. The parameters were as follows: repetition time (TR) = 2,530 ms; echo time (TE) = 2.98 ms; inversion time (TI) = 1,100 ms; FA = 7°; number of slices = 192; slice thickness = 1 mm, bandwidth = 240 Hz/Px; field of view (FOV) = 256 $\times$ 256 mm^2; and matrix = 256 $\times$ 256, resulting in an isotropic voxel size of 1 $\times$ 1 $\times$ 1 mm^3. In addition, we also obtained resting-state functional images of all participants using an echo-planar imaging (EPI) sequence. The scanning parameters were as follows: 33 axial slices with a slice thickness = 3.5 mm and interslice gap = 1 mm, TR = 2,000 ms; TE = 30 ms; FA = 90°; bandwidth = 2,368 Hz/Px; FOV = 224 $\times$ 224 mm^2; and matrix = 64 $\times$ 64. The latter parameters resulted in an isotropic voxel size of 3.5 $\times$ 3.5 $\times$ 3.5 mm^3. The total number of volumes acquired was 240.

Processing of Structural Images and Voxel-Based Morphometry Analysis

We performed postprocessing of the structural data using CAT12[1] implemented in Statistical Parametric Mapping (SPM) software (version 12)[2]. SPM 12 was installed in MATLAB 2016a (Math Works, Natick, MA, United States). First, all the structural images were screened for movement artifacts. Next, the structural images were segmented into gray matter, white matter, and cerebrospinal fluid (CSF) areas using the unified standard segmentation option in SPM12. The individual gray matter and white matter components were then normalized into the standard Montreal Neurological Institute (MNI) space using the Diffeomorphic Anatomical Registration through Exponentiated Lie algebra (DARTEL) algorithm (Ashburner, 2007) after segmentation. The normalized gray matter and white matter components were modulated to generate the relative gray matter volume (GMV) and white matter volume (WMV) by multiplying by the non-linear part of the deformation field at the DARTEL step. The Gaussian kernel used to smooth the resulting GMV and WMV images was 6 mm full-width at half-maximum (FWHM).

Preprocessing of Resting-State Functional Images

We used the batch-processing tool Data Processing and Analysis for (Resting-State) Brain Imaging (DPABI)[3] (Yan et al., 2016) to preprocess the resting-state functional MRI (rs-fMRI) data,

[1] http://www.neuro.uni-jena.de
[2] https://www.fil.ion.ucl.ac.uk/spm
[3] http://www.rfmri.org/dpabi

which is based on SPM12. First, to allow for steady-state magnetization and stabilization of the subject, we removed the first 10 volumes of each functional time series of all the participants. After that, we conducted slice timing correction on the remaining 230 volumes. Head motion between volumes was evaluated and corrected using rigid body registration, and we excluded datasets with maximum translation exceeding 2.5 mm, maximum rotation exceeding 2.5° or mean framewise displacement (FD) >0.3 (Yan et al., 2013). Next, based on the standard stereotaxic coordinate system, we spatially normalized the corrected fMRI images to an MNI template brain. Then, each voxel was resampled to isotropic 3 mm × 3 mm × 3 mm. After that, to remove the possible variances from the time course of each voxel (including the WM and CSF signal and Friston-24 head motion parameters), the 26 nuisance covariates were regressed out. Finally, the Gaussian smoothing kernel for the rs-fMRI images was a 6-mm FWHM.

ICA Analysis

We performed ICA through GIG-ICA using GIFT software (version 3.0b)[4]. The main steps included data reduction, application of the ICA algorithm, and back-reconstruction for each subject. In the present study, we performed group independent component analysis (GICA) 100 times on tinnitus patients and HCs using 20 and 30 components separately. During this process, through visual inspection and previous reports (see the "Results" section for details), we identified nine components as meaningful resting-state networks (RSNs). We also obtained the individual-level components using back-reconstruction and transformed the subject-specific spatial maps to z scores.

Intranetwork Functional Connectivity Analysis

The main process was consistent with a previous study (Chen et al., 2018). To generate a sample-specific spatial map for each component, each ICA component was entered into a random-effect one-sample t-test using a family wise error (FWE) correction ($p < 0.05$) with a cluster size of >100 voxels (Song et al., 2013; Wang et al., 2014). We compared the differences in intranetwork FC between the tinnitus patients and HCs at baseline and after treatment using a two-sample t-test and applied a paired t-test to compare intranetwork FC between patients before and after treatment [false discovery rate (FDR) corrected $p < 0.05$]. Using a general linear model (GLM), we extracted and compared intranetwork FC of each region of interest (ROI) with a significant difference between groups, with age and sex serving as covariates. For the ROI-based analyses, we used Cohen's d (Parker and Hagan-Burke, 2007) to determine the effect size of each comparison.

Internetwork Functional Connectivity Analysis

During the process of the internetwork FC analysis, first, by averaging the time courses of all voxels within the sample-specific RSN mask of each subject, we calculated the mean time course of each RSN. Then, we calculated Pearson's correlation coefficients of the mean time courses between all pairs of RSNs for each subject and then converted them to z-values using Fisher's r-to-z transformation to improve normality. For each group, individual z-values were entered into a random-effect one-sample t-test to determine whether the correlation between each pair of RSNs was statistically significant ($p < 0.05$). Intergroup comparisons were carried out only if the internetwork FC of each group was statistically significant ($p < 0.05$). We performed GLM with age and sex as covariates to determine whether the pairs of internetwork FC were significantly different ($p < 0.05$) between the patients and HCs at baseline and after treatments using a two-sample t-test and between the patients before and after treatment using a paired t-test.

Statistical Analyses

During the statistical analysis process, we assessed all the data for normality using the Kolmogorov–Smirnov test. If the data were identified as not normally distributed, we applied non-parametric tests. First, we applied the voxel wise two-sample t-test and paired t-test in SPM12 to compare the whole-brain GMV and WMV differences between the tinnitus patients and HCs at baseline and after treatment and between the patients before and after narrow band sound therapy (voxel-level uncorrected $p < 0.001$, non-stationary cluster-level FWE correction with $p < 0.05$), and age and sex served as nuisance covariates. Next, the mean GMV, WMV, and FC values of each cluster that showed statistical

TABLE 1 | Demographic and clinical data of the tinnitus patients and healthy controls.

Demographic	Tinnitus (baseline, n = 13)	Tinnitus (6 months, n = 13)	Control (n = 18)	P-value
Age, years	42.23 (± 13.98)		45.33 (± 9.64)	0.470[a]
gender	6 males, 7 females		9 males, 9 females	0.561[b]
THI score	53.38 (± 28.10)	45.85 (± 25.16)	NA	0.379[c]
△ THI score	7.54 (± 29.78)		NA	NA
% improvement of THI score	−1.30% (±63.40%)		NA	
Duration, months	≥6 and ≤48		NA	NA
Type[#]	7: 2: 3: 1		NA	NA
Tinnitus pitch	250~8,000 Hz		NA	NA
Laterality	3 right, 4 left, 6 bilateral		NA	NA
Normal hearing	All		All	NA

THI, Tinnitus Handicap Inventory, △ THI score = $THI_{baseline} - THI_{treated}$, NA: not applicable.
[a]Two-sample t-tests.
[b]Chi-square test.
[c]Paired-samples t-tests.
[#]1 single high-pitched sound vs. 1 single low-pitched sound vs. 2 high pitched sounds vs. 2 low pitched sounds.

[4]http://mialab.mrn.org/software/gift/

significance were extracted for subsequent analyses. Then, we conducted a partial correlation analysis to explore any potential associations between brain alterations (intra/internetwork level) and clinical variables in tinnitus patients after removing age and sex effects (FDR $p < 0.05$). The last steps were performed using IBM SPSS Statistics version 23.0 (IBM Inc., Armonk, NY, United States).

GMV, WMV, and FC results were presented using MRIcron[5], BrainNet Viewer[6] (Xia et al., 2013) and xjView[7].

RESULTS

Demographic Data

Table 1 shows detailed demographic data of the 13 tinnitus patients with persistent idiopathic tinnitus characteristics and 18 HCs. We acquired the THI scores before and after narrow band sound therapy for all patients. In this study, the outcome of tinnitus patients was considered poor after sound therapy when taking THI score improvements as the evaluative measurement.

[5]https://www.nitrc.org/projects/mricron
[6]http://www.nitrc.org/projects/bnv/
[7]https://www.alivelearn.net/xjview/

Brain Structural Changes Between the Patients and HCs at Baseline and After Treatment and Between the Patients Before and After Treatment

Compared with the HCs, the tinnitus patients showed decreased GMV (**Figure 1** and **Table 2**) and WMV (**Figure 2** and **Table 2**) in the left middle temporal gyrus (MTG) at baseline, and the GMV was even further reduced after treatment (non-stationary cluster-level FWE correction with $p < 0.05$) (although the trend in the WMV reductions showed a decrease, the P-value was uncorrected). Additionally, the patients showed increased WMV in the cingulum (cingulate), left parietal and frontal lobes, right calcarine, and left rolandic operculum after treatment compared with the baseline (non-stationary cluster-level FWE correction with $p < 0.05$) (**Figure 3** and **Table 2**).

Resting-State Network Functional Connectivity Changes Between the Patients and HCs at Baseline and After Treatment and Between the Patients Before and After Treatment

The nine RSNs identified in our study were as follows: the auditory network (AN), the anterior (aDMN), and posterior

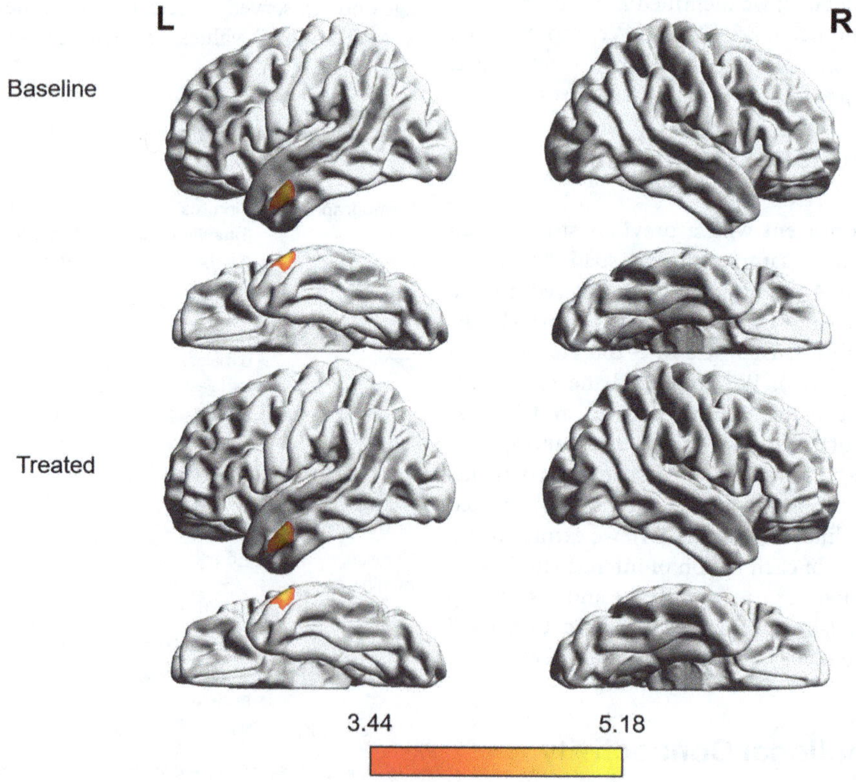

FIGURE 1 | Intergroup differences in GMV between tinnitus patients without HL and HCs before and after sound therapy. At baseline, compared with the HCs, the patients with tinnitus without HL exhibited reduced GMV in the left MTG. After sound therapy (treated), the tinnitus patients continued to show decreased GMV in the same region, and the volume of gray matter was further reduced (corrected at the non-stationary cluster level with FWE $P < 0.05$). HL, hearing loss, HC, healthy control, MTG, middle temporal gyrus, FWE, family wise error, GMV, gray matter volume. The color bar represents the extent of reduction in GMV.

TABLE 2 | Difference in gray/white matter volume between the tinnitus patients and healthy controls and between patients before and after sound therapy.

Anatomical region	MNI coordinate			Voxel size	Peak *T*-value
	x	y	z		
Gray matter (FWE cluster *p* < 0.05)					
Gray matter volume (baseline)					
Tinnitus patients < Healthy controls					
Left middle temporal gyrus	−65	−3	−24	690	5.06
Gray matter volume (after treatment)					
Tinnitus patients < Healthy controls					
Left middle temporal gyrus	−65	−3	−23	831	5.18
White matter					
White matter volume (baseline)					
Tinnitus patients < Healthy controls					
Left middle temporal gyrus (FWE cluster *p* < 0.05)	−60	2	−29	373	5.39
White matter volume (after treatment)					
Tinnitus patients < Healthy controls					
Left middle temporal gyrus (uncorrected)	−60	2	−29	362	5.49
White matter volume (FWE cluster *P* < 0.05)					
Tinnitus patients (baseline) < Tinnitus patients (after treatment)					
Cingulum_Mid_L (aal)	−8	−27	39	110	8.40
Calcarine_R (aal)	24	−51	15	65	7.98
Cingulum_Mid_R (aal)	8	−30	44	115	6.50
Rolandic_Oper_L (aal)	−45	−6	15	113	6.06
Left parietal and frontal lobe	−29	−41	44	1,345	8.04

MNI, Montreal Neurological Institute; FWE, family wise error; L, left; R, right.

(pDMN) default mode networks, the left (LFPN) and right (RFPN) frontoparietal networks, the medial (mVN) and lateral (lVN) visual networks, the sensorimotor network (SMN), and the dorsal attention network (DAN) (**Figures 4A–C**). The locations of these RSNs were in line with some prior studies (Mantini et al., 2007; Smith et al., 2009; Du et al., 2015; Ma et al., 2016).

Altered Functional Connectivity Within and Between Resting-State Networks

We found that the tinnitus patients exhibited a decreased (i.e., positive) (mVN and lVN, $p = 0.007$) or an increased (i.e., less negative) (mVN and SMN, $p = 0.018$; mVN and AN, $p = 0.035$) internetwork FC at baseline when compared with HCs (**Figure 4A** and **Table 3**). Additionally, compared with the HCs, the patients showed a decreased (i.e., positive) (AN and pDMN, $p = 0.008$; DAN and LFPN, $p = 0.005$) internetwork FC after treatment (**Figure 4B** and **Table 3**). Meanwhile, tinnitus patients also exhibited an increased (i.e., less negative) (LFPN and pDMN, $p = 0.023$; LFPN and RFPN, $p = 0.030$; aDMN and AN, $p = 0.037$; aDMN and DAN, $p = 0.008$) internetwork FC after treatment compared with baseline (**Figure 4C** and **Table 3**). However, we did not observe any intranetwork FC changes between the patients and HCs at baseline or after treatment or between the patients before and after treatment within the nine RSNs.

Correlations Between the Brain Structural and Functional Changes and Extent of THI Score Changes

We performed partial correlations between the GMV, WMV, and internetwork FC values and the THI scores, $^{\Delta}$ THI scores, % improvement in THI scores, and other clinical variables (such as duration and VAS scores) in patients with tinnitus after controlling for age and sex. We did not detect any associations among these variables ($p > 0.05$).

DISCUSSION

In the present study, all the patients had poor outcomes after the treatment when using improvements or changes in THI scores as the evaluation standard, which define a THI score reduced to 16 points or a reduction of 17 points or more as an effective treatment or good outcome (Zeman et al., 2011). Moreover, in the classic frequencies (from 250 – 8 kHz: 0.250, 0.500, 1, 2, 3, 4, 6, and 8 kHz), all the patients in this study were identified as tinnitus without HL, which is in line with one of our previous studies (Chen et al., 2020), although we cannot eliminate the possibility of hidden HL currently. Combining VBM and ICA analyses, we found significant brain gray/white matter atrophy in the auditory-related cortex at baseline, and the GMV was further reduced after sound therapy. Additionally, patients showed increased WMV in some regions that are not directly related to auditory function after treatment compared with baseline. More importantly, tinnitus patients showed significantly changes in internetwork FC in auditory-related and non-auditory-related networks at baseline or after sound therapy when compared with HCs or in the comparison of the patients before and after treatment. Therefore, although the idiopathic tinnitus patients group without HL with poor outcomes, narrow band sound therapy may have a significant effect on brain reorganization in patients with tinnitus. In this study, we chose narrow band noise as the applied sound therapy as it is a commonly used kind of sound therapy with high cost-effectiveness (Henry et al., 2002). It promotes habituation to the tinnitus sensation, diminishes the sensitivity of tinnitus, and reduces the contrast between tinnitus and the environment (Lv et al., 2020).

Auditory-Related Brain Structural and Functional Alterations Between the Patients and HCs and Between the Patients Before and After Sound Therapy

The temporal gyrus is closely related to auditory function, especially the posterior MTG, which is part of the auditory primary cortex. Studies have shown that tinnitus can cause significant cortical changes in the MTG (Boyen et al., 2013; Pereira-Jorge et al., 2018). For example, Boyen et al. (2013) found that the change in gray matter in the auditory primary cortex (including the MTG) was correlated with tinnitus rather than with HL, and they speculated that the continuous sensation of an internal sound, such as the tinnitus percept, may cause the changes in the MTG. Consistent with previous studies, our

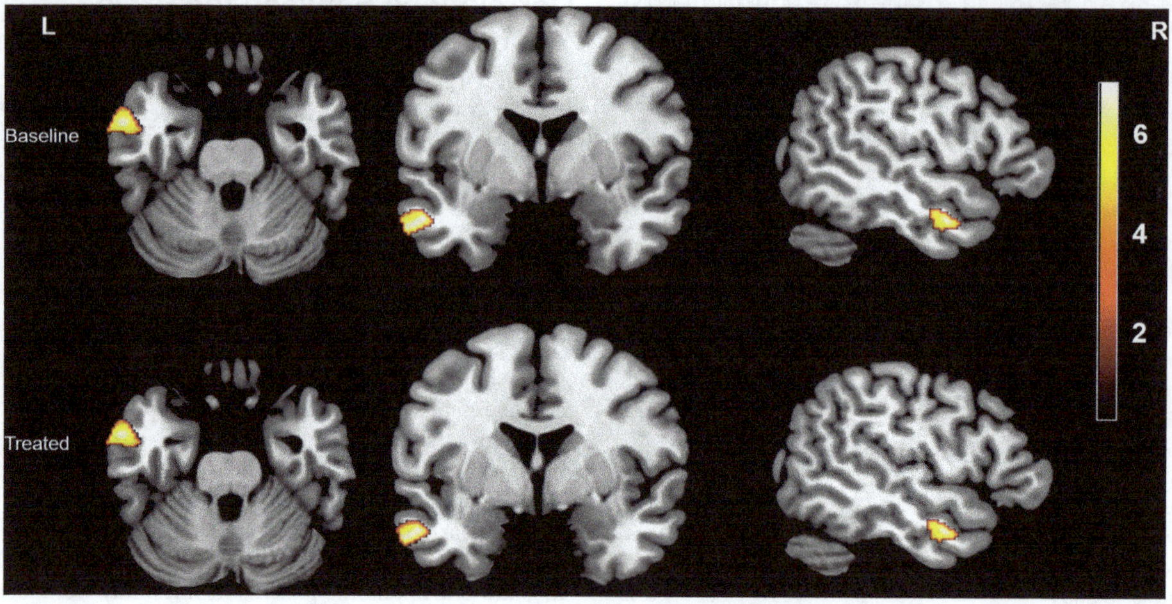

FIGURE 2 | Intergroup differences in WMV between the tinnitus patients without HL and HCs before and after sound therapy. At baseline, compared with the HCs, the patients with tinnitus without HL exhibited reduced WMV in the left MTG (corrected at non-stationary cluster level with FWE $p < 0.05$). After sound therapy (treated), the brain region with decreased WMV was still the same area, but the trend in the WMV reduction had diminished (uncorrected). HL, hearing loss, HC, healthy control, MTG, middle temporal gyrus, FWE, family wise error, WMV, white matter volume. The color bar represents the extent of reduction in WMV.

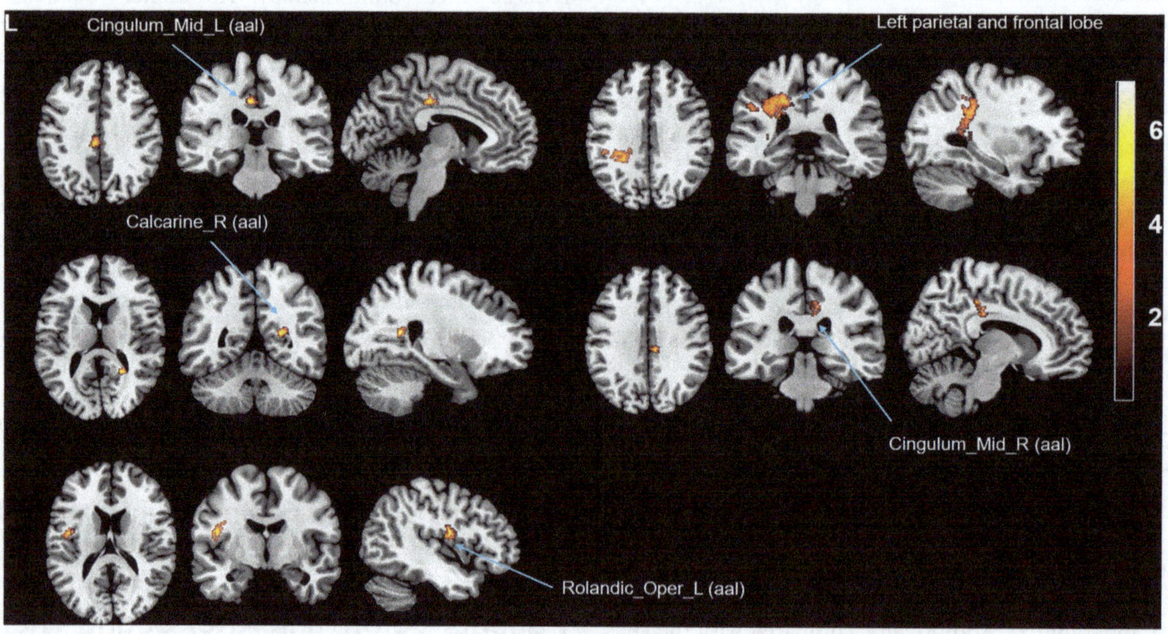

FIGURE 3 | Intergroup differences in WMV between the tinnitus patients before and after sound therapy. Compared with baseline, after sound therapy, the patients with tinnitus exhibited increased WMV in the cingulum (cingulate), right calcarine, left rolandic operculum, and left parietal and frontal lobes (corrected at the non-stationary cluster level with FWE $p < 0.05$). FWE, family wise error, WMV, white matter volume. The color bar represents the extent of reduction in WMV.

findings suggested that tinnitus without HL can cause significant brain structural changes in the auditory cortex, although we cannot eliminate the possible effect of hidden or slight HL on the brain alterations. More interestingly, after the narrow band sound therapy, we found that the GMV in the MTG was further reduced, while the trend for further decreases in WMV in the same area was diminished, but the *P*-value with the WMV was uncorrected.

In addition to the auditory-related brain structural changes, we also observed increased (i.e., negative) internetwork FC between the AN and mVN in the patients with tinnitus than

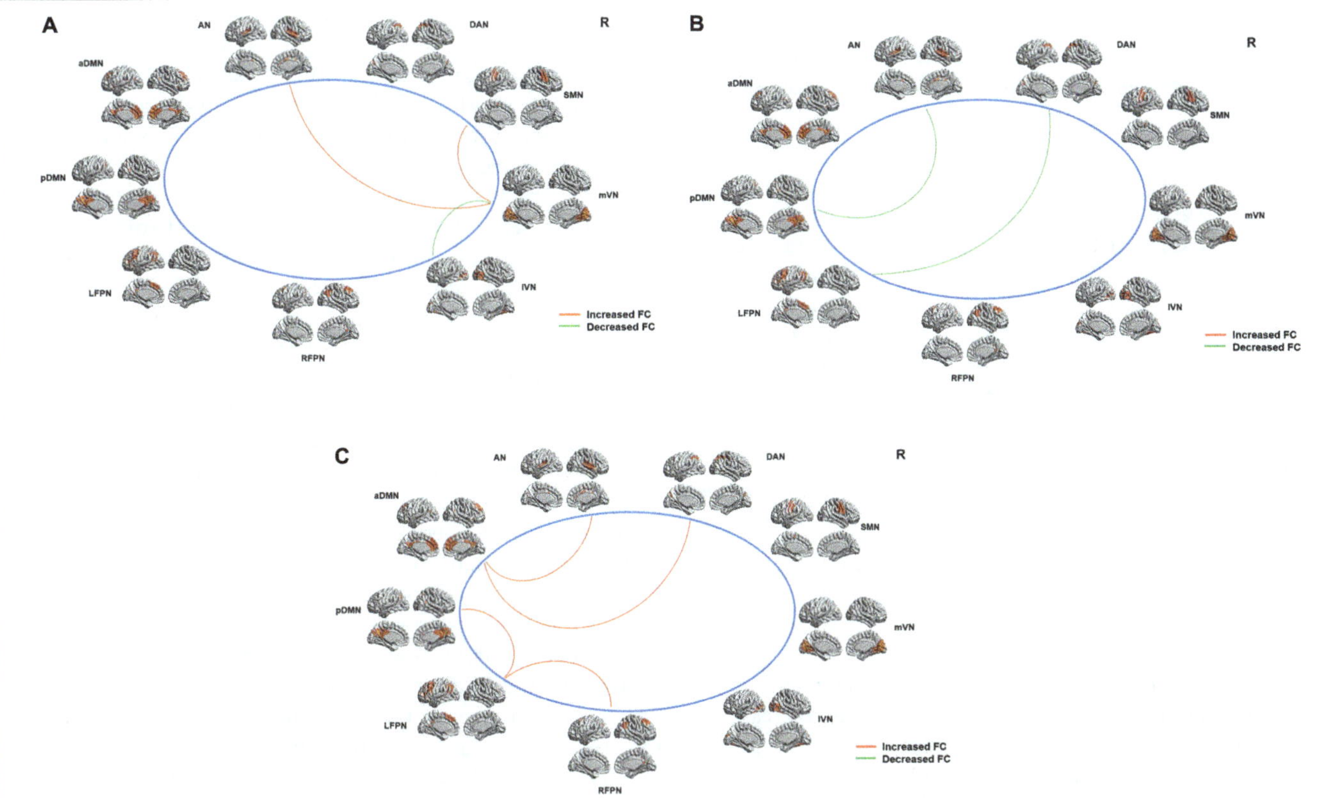

FIGURE 4 | Intergroup differences in internetwork FC between the tinnitus patients and HCs and between the patients before and after sound therapy. **(A)** Compared with the HCs, the tinnitus patients exhibited a decreased (i.e., positive) (mVN and lVN) or an increased (i.e., less negative) (mVN and SMN; mVN and AN) internetwork FC at baseline. **(B)** Compared with HCs, tinnitus patients showed a decreased (i.e., positive) (AN and pDMN; DAN and LFPN) internetwork FC after sound therapy. **(C)** Compared with the patients at baseline, the tinnitus patients exhibited increased (i.e., negative) (LFPN and pDMN; LFPN and RFPN; aDMN and AN; aDMN and DAN) internetwork FC after sound therapy. AN, auditory network; aDMN, anterior default mode network; pDMN, posterior default mode network; LFPN, left frontoparietal network; RFPN, right frontoparietal network; lVN, lateral visual network; mVN, medial visual network; SMN, sensorimotor network; DAN, dorsal attention network; FC, functional connectivity, HC, healthy control.The red line represents positive FC; the green line represents negative FC.

the HCs before treatment. The AN and VN are independent processing systems for auditory and visual functions. In tinnitus patients, the increased internetwork FC between the two processing networks may reflect abnormal large-scale functional interactions between them. The FC changes between AN and mVN at baseline may be a compensatory effect caused by tinnitus, as phantom auditory sensations also activate visual areas (Zhou et al., 2019). However, after sound therapy, we did not find any network-level FC changes between the AN and VN; meanwhile, we found decreased level (i.e., positive) and increased levels (i.e., negative) internetwork FC between the DMN and AN in patients when compared with the HCs or patients at baseline. The DMN, including the medial prefrontal cortex and anterior cingulum (cingulate) cortex as well as the posterior cingulum (cingulate) cortex and precuneus, is associated with both cognitive and emotional control (Whitfield-Gabrieli et al., 2011). Moreover, it is most active at rest and shows reduced activity when a subject enters a task-based state involving attention or goal-directed behavior (Shulman et al., 1997). The DMN connectivity changes in our study after treatment were consistent with some studies that reported DMN dysfunction (Schmidt et al., 2013; Lanting et al., 2016). Lanting et al. (2016) believed that the DMN somehow plays a role in "hearing" internally generated sound (whether it is meaningful, e.g., in schizophrenia patients, or meaningless, e.g., in tinnitus patients).

Combined with previous studies, these findings indicated that significant differences exist in the abnormal changes in auditory-related brain structure and function before and after the narrow band sound therapy (compared with HCs or patients at baseline).

Non-Auditory-Related Brain Structural and Functional Alterations Between the Patients and HCs and Between the Patients Before and After Sound Therapy

In addition to the auditory-related structural and functional changes, we also observed a significant increase in WMV in the cingulum (cingulate), right calcarine, left rolandic operculum, and the left parietal and frontal lobes in the patients after treatment compared with baseline. The Cingulum (cingulate) plays a large role in several large-scale networks in which tinnitus is involved; that is, tinnitus emerges as a function of several large-scale networks that bind together many aspects of salience, memory, perception, distress, and audition

TABLE 3 | Intergroup differences in the inter-network functional connectivity.

Functional connectivity	Baseline (HCs-Patients)		Treated (HCs-Patients)		Patients $_{pre}$ – Patients $_{pos}$	
	t	*p*	*t*	*p*	*t*	*p*
mVN-SMN	**−2.511**	**0.018**	−0.285	0.778	0.511	0.614
mVN-AN	**−2.219**	**0.035**	0.842	0.407	0.219	0.829
mVN-lVN	**2.904**	**0.007**	0.637	0.529	−0.448	0.658
LFPN-pDMN	0.162	0.873	−0.150	0.882	**−2.404**	**0.023**
LFPN-RFPN	0.999	0.326	1.504	0.143	**−2.312**	**0.030**
aDMN-AN	−0.671	0.508	0.772	0.446	**−2.216**	**0.037**
aDMN-DAN	−0.044	0.966	−0.023	0.982	**−2.904**	**0.008**
pDMN-AN	0.500	0.621	**2.836**	**0.008**	0.218	0.830
LFPN-DAN	0.500	0.623	**3.033**	**0.005**	−0.079	0.937

mVN, medial vision network; SMN, sensorimotor network; AN, auditory network; lVN, lateral network; LFPN, left frontoparietal network; RFPN, right frontoparietal network; aDMN, anterior default mode network; pDMN, posterior default mode network; DAN, dorsal attention network; HCs, healthy controls.
The bold values indicate significant differences between the tinnitus patients and HCs at baseline and after sound therapy and the differences between the tinnitus patients before and after the treatment ($p < 0.05$).

(De Ridder et al., 2011; Ridder et al., 2011; Schecklmann et al., 2012; Meyer et al., 2016). We believe that the increase in WMV in the cingulum (cingulate) indicates that tinnitus is closely related to dysfunction of the limbic system, which is in line with one of our prior studies (Chen et al., 2020). The calcarine cortex is an important part of the primary visual cortex, and it is the main relay station that transfers the signals coming from the retina. Some studies have shown that there is a close or even direct connection between the auditory and visual regions/subnetworks (Iurilli et al., 2012; Ibrahim et al., 2016). Thus, changes in the calcarine cortex may result from patients attending to phantom auditory sensations and having the visual areas contemporaneously activated (Zhou et al., 2019). Additionally, we found increased WMV in the rolandic operculum, which may correlate with tinnitus-related distress (Krick et al., 2015). Additionally, Job et al. (2012) found overactivity in the rolandic operculum; they speculated that this region was associated with middle ear proprioception, and changes in this region may suggest a hypothesis that tinnitus could arise as a proprioceptive illusion associated with widespread emotional and somatosensory dysfunction. Meanwhile, we found an increase in WMV in the left parietal and frontal lobes as the main parts of the frontoparietal network (FPN), and we believe that these areas play a large role in the process of decision-making and cognitive control (Vincent et al., 2008).

In addition to these changes in brain white matter, we also found significant differences from before to after sound therapy in the interactions among several RSNs that are not directly related to auditory function. For instance, at baseline, we found increased (i.e., less negative) and decreased (i.e., positive) internetwork FC between the mVN and the SMN and lVN, respectively. The VN and SMN are two independent systems that separately process visual and sensorimotor functions and play a role in the limbic system. A previous study on stroke suggested that the significantly changed internetwork FC between the two networks may reflect abnormal large-scale functional interactions among functional networks (Wang et al., 2014). Additionally, the vision network is divided into the mVN and lVN. The mVN includes primary visual areas, while the lVN encompasses non-primary regions of the visual cortex (Beckmann et al., 2005). We speculated that because of the increased compensatory stimulation between the auditory and visual networks caused by tinnitus, the functional interaction within the visual network is weakened. Although the exact mechanism underlying abnormal internetwork FC remains unclear, it may be the result of impairments in the thalamus, as mentioned above (Lv et al., 2020). After the treatment, we found decreased (i.e., positive) internetwork FC between the LFPN and DAN and increased (i.e., negative) internetwork FC between the LFPN and RFPN and among the LFPN, DMN, and DAN. According to a previous ICA study, the FPN is a lateralized network and has been commonly identified as an independent RSN (Smith et al., 2009). It primarily consists of two main parts: the dorsolateral prefrontal cortex and the posterior parietal cortex (several cognition/language areas), and it supports decision-making and cognitive control functions (Vincent et al., 2008). Few studies have reported tinnitus-related changes in the LFPN or RFPN (Lanting et al., 2016). Studies on stroke have proven that weakened connectivity of the FPN may represent a functional disconnection (Nomura et al., 2010) in brain regions that may underlie the cognitive impairments observed in these patients (Stebbins et al., 2008; Gottesman and Hillis, 2010). Therefore, the increased or decreased internetwork FC among the LFPN, RFPN, and DAN indicated that after tinnitus, the brain activity and functional connections in brain regions related to executive control, advanced cognition, and language are in an abnormal or dysfunctional state when compared with baseline. Meanwhile, we also observed increased internetwork FC between the DMN and DAN. The DAN is involved in visual attention (Gitelman, 2003), and the increased FC in our study was consistent with Schmidt et al. (2013), as they suggested that this increase in FC could be a compensatory attempt to handle the phantom stimulus, by delegating that process to non-attention-processing regions, such as the limbic system (Golm et al., 2013; Ooms et al., 2013).

These results suggest that in addition to auditory-related brain reorganization, there were also significant differences in the abnormal changes in non-auditory-related brain reorganization before and after sound therapy (narrow band noise). However, in the present study, we failed to find any intranetwork FC changes in tinnitus patients before and after sound therapy, which may have been due to the small sample size. Studies with a larger sample size are needed in the future. Although patients in this study with different sided tinnitus, the brain changes we found were only seen on the left side in some regions and on the right side in other areas, which is consistent with some previous studies (Husain et al., 2011; Chen et al., 2017, 2020; Liu et al., 2018; Besteher et al., 2019; Han et al., 2019a). We speculated the reason may be that many brain areas can be divided into several subregions based on their functions and the function of the right or left side of some regions in the brain is different while the exact mechanism is still not very clear.

Limitations

There are several limitations in our study. First, the sample size of our study was relatively small, and we recruited only right-handed subjects. Second, as a longitudinal study, we scanned the HCs only once. In future studies, we need to follow up with the HCs for the same period (6 months) as the patients and scan them twice (at baseline and after 6 months of follow-up). Third, in this study, we recruited only tinnitus patients without HL and HCs. We will recruit tinnitus patients with and without HL in future studies. Fourth, we didn't apply any sham therapy on patients and HCs, which we will apply to them in future studies. Fifth, the definition of tinnitus patients without HL was that there is no HL in the generally recognized frequencies (250–8 kHz: 0.250, 0.500, 1, 2, 3, 4, 6, and 8 kHz); thus, we cannot eliminate the possibility of hidden or slight HL in other frequency ranges currently.

CONCLUSION

In conclusion, we found that significant differences exist in auditory-related and non-auditory-related brain functional and structural alterations in tinnitus patients without HL before and after sound therapy (narrowband stimulation), especially changes in white matter and internetwork FC, although the outcome of all the patients may not be very good after the treatment. Therefore, we supposed that sound therapy, especially the narrow band noise, may have a significant effect on brain reorganization in patients with idiopathic tinnitus without HL. It may advance the understanding of the neural pathophysiological mechanisms of idiopathic tinnitus after sound therapy.

ETHICS STATEMENT

The studies involving human participants were reviewed and approved by the Institutional Review Board (IRB) of Beijing Friendship Hospital, Capital Medical University. The patients/participants provided their written informed consent to participate in this study. Written informed consent was obtained from the individual(s) for the publication of any potentially identifiable images or data included in this article.

AUTHOR CONTRIBUTIONS

QC was responsible for (1) study conception; (2) the acquisition, analysis, and interpretation of data; (3) drafting of the manuscript; (4) final approval of the version of the manuscript to be published; and (5) agreement to be accountable for all aspects of the work. ZDW, XW, PZ, ZY, and SG were responsible for (1) data analysis; (2) final approval of the version of the manuscript to be published; and (3) agreement to be accountable for all aspects of the work. HL was responsible for (1) revising the manuscript; (2) final approval of the version of the manuscript to be published; and (3) agreement to be accountable for all aspects of the work. ZCW was responsible for (1) study design; (2) manuscript revision; (3) final approval of the version of the manuscript to be published; and (4) agreement to be accountable for all aspects of the work. All authors contributed to the article and approved the submitted version.

ACKNOWLEDGMENTS

We thank the patients and healthy volunteers who participated in this study and gave generously of their time.

REFERENCES

Aldhafeeri, F. M., Mackenzie, I., Kay, T., Alghamdi, J., and Sluming, V. (2012). Neuroanatomical correlates of tinnitus revealed by cortical thickness analysis and diffusion tensor imaging. *Neuroradiology* 54, 883–892. doi: 10.1007/s00234-012-1044-6

Ashburner, J. (2007). A fast diffeomorphic image registration algorithm. *Neuroimage* 38, 95–113. doi: 10.1016/j.neuroimage.2007.07.007

Bae, E. B., Lee, J. H., and Song, J. (2020). Single-session of combined tDCS-TMS may increase therapeutic effects in subjects with tinnitus. *Front. Neurol.* 11:160. doi: 10.3389/fneur.2020.00160

Beckmann, C. F., DeLuca, M., Devlin, J. T., and Smith, S. M. (2005). Investigations into resting-state connectivity using independent component analysis. *Philos. Trans. R. Soc. Lond. B Biol. Sci.* 360, 1001–1013. doi: 10.1098/rstb.2005.1634

Benson, R. R., Gattu, R., and Cacace, A. T. (2014). Left hemisphere fractional anisotropy increase in noise-induced tinnitus: a diffusion tensor imaging (DTI) study of white matter tracts in the brain. *Hear. Res.* 309, 8–16. doi: 10.1016/j.heares.2013.10.005

Besteher, B., Gaser, C., Ivanšić, D., Guntinas-Lichius, O., Dobel, C., and Nenadić, I. (2019). Chronic tinnitus and the limbic system: reappraising brain structural effects of distress and affective symptoms. *NeuroImage Clin.* 24:101976. doi: 10.1016/j.nicl.2019.101976

Boyen, K., Langers, D. R. M., de Kleine, E., and van Dijk, P. (2013). Gray matter in the brain: differences associated with tinnitus and hearing loss. *Hear. Res.* 295, 67–78. doi: 10.1016/j.heares.2012.02.010

Chen, Q., Lv, H., Wang, Z., Wei, X., Zhao, P., Yang, Z., et al. (2021). Outcomes at 6 months are related to brain structural and white matter microstructural reorganization in idiopathic tinnitus patients treated with sound therapy. *Hum. Brain Mapp.* 42, 753–765. doi: 10.1002/hbm.25260

Chen, Q., Wang, Z., Lv, H., Zhao, P., Yang, Z., Gong, S., et al. (2020). Reorganization of brain white matter in persistent idiopathic tinnitus patients without hearing loss: evidence from baseline data. *Front. Neurosci.* 14:591. doi: 10.3389/fnins.2020.00591

Chen, Q., Zheng, W., Chen, X., Li, X., Wang, L., Qin, W., et al. (2018). Whether visual-related structural and functional changes occur in brain of patients with acute incomplete cervical cord injury: a multimodal based MRI study. *Neuroscience* 393, 284–294. doi: 10.1016/j.neuroscience.2018.10.014

Chen, Y., Li, X., Liu, L., Wang, J., Lu, C., Yang, M., et al. (2015). Tinnitus and hyperacusis involve hyperactivity and enhanced connectivity in auditory-limbic-arousal-cerebellar network. *eLife* 4:e06576. doi: 10.7554/eLife.06576

Chen, Y., Xia, W., Chen, H., Feng, Y., Xu, J., Gu, J., et al. (2017). Tinnitus distress is linked to enhanced resting-state functional connectivity from the limbic system to the auditory cortex. *Hum. Brain Mapp.* 38, 2384–2397. doi: 10.1002/hbm.23525

De Ridder, D., Vanneste, S., and Congedo, M. (2011). The distressed brain: a group blind source separation analysis on tinnitus. *PLoS One* 6:e24273. doi: 10.1371/journal.pone.0024273

Du, Y., Pearlson, G. D., Liu, J., Sui, J., Yu, Q., He, H., et al. (2015). A group ICA based framework for evaluating resting fMRI markers when disease categories are unclear: application to schizophrenia, bipolar, and schizoaffective disorders. *Neuroimage* 122, 272–280. doi: 10.1016/j.neuroimage.2015.07.054

Eggermont, J. J., and Roberts, L. E. (2004). The neuroscience of tinnitus. *Trends Neurosci.* 27, 676–682. doi: 10.1016/j.tins.2004.08.010

Gitelman, D. R. (2003). Attention and its disorders. *Br. Med. Bull.* 65, 21–34. doi: 10.1093/bmb/65.1.21

Golm, D., Schmidt-Samoa, C., Dechent, P., and Kröner-Herwig, B. (2013). Neural correlates of tinnitus related distress: an fMRI-study. *Hear. Res.* 295, 87–99. doi: 10.1016/j.heares.2012.03.003

Gottesman, R. F., and Hillis, A. E. (2010). Predictors and assessment of cognitive dysfunction resulting from ischaemic stroke. *Lancet Neurol.* 9, 895–905. doi: 10.1016/S1474-4422(10)70164-2

Han, J. J., Ridder, D. D., Vanneste, S., Chen, Y., Koo, J., and Song, J. (2020). Pre-treatment ongoing with hearing aids. *Front. Neurosci.* 14:410. doi: 10.3389/fnins.2020.00410

Han, L., Na, Z., Chunli, L., Yuchen, C., Pengfei, Z., Hao, W., et al. (2019a). Baseline functional connectivity features of neural network nodes can predict improvement after sound therapy through adjusted narrow band noise in tinnitus patients. *Front. Neurosci.* 13:614. doi: 10.3389/fnins.2019.00614

Han, L., Yawen, L., Hao, W., Chunli, L., Pengfei, Z., Zhengyu, Z., et al. (2019b). Effects of sound therapy on resting-state functional brain networks in patients with tinnitus: a graph-theoretical-based study. *J. Magn. Resonance Imag.* 50, 1731–1741. doi: 10.1002/jmri.26796

Henry, J. A., Schechter, M. A., Nagler, S. M., and Fausti, S. A. (2002). Comparison of tinnitus masking and tinnitus retraining therapy. *J. Am. Acad. Audiol.* 13, 559–581.

Hoare, D. J., Edmondson-Jones, M., Sereda, M., Akeroyd, M. A., and Hall, D. (2014). Amplification with hearing aids for patients with tinnitus and co-existing hearing loss. *Cochrane Database Syst. Rev.* D10151. doi: 10.1002/14651858.CD010151.pub2

Hobson, J., Chisholm, E., and El, R. A. (2012). Sound therapy (masking) in the management of tinnitus in adults. *Cochrane Database Syst. Rev.* 11:D6371. doi: 10.1002/14651858.CD006371.pub3

Husain, F. T., Medina, R. E., Davis, C. W., Szymko-Bennett, Y., Simonyan, K., Pajor, N. M., et al. (2011). Neuroanatomical changes due to hearing loss and chronic tinnitus: a combined VBM and DTI study. *Brain Res.* 1369, 74–88. doi: 10.1016/j.brainres.2010.10.095

Ibrahim, L. A., Mesik, L., Ji, X., Fang, Q., Li, H., Li, Y., et al. (2016). Cross-modality sharpening of visual cortical processing through Layer-1-Mediated inhibition and disinhibition. *Neuron* 89, 1031–1045. doi: 10.1016/j.neuron.2016.01.027

Iurilli, G., Ghezzi, D., Olcese, U., Lassi, G., Nazzaro, C., Tonini, R., et al. (2012). Sound-driven synaptic inhibition in primary visual cortex. *Neuron* 73, 814–828. doi: 10.1016/j.neuron.2011.12.026

Jastreboff, P. J. (1999). Tinnitus retraining therapy. *Br. J. Audiol.* 33, 68–70.

Job, A., Pons, Y., Lamalle, L., Jaillard, A., Buck, K., Segebarth, C., et al. (2012). Abnormal cortical sensorimotor activity during "Target" sound detection in subjects with acute acoustic trauma sequelae: an fMRI study. *Brain Behav.* 2, 187–199. doi: 10.1002/brb3.21

Krick, C. M., Grapp, M., Daneshvar-Talebi, J., Reith, W., Plinkert, P. K., and Bolay, H. V. (2015). Cortical reorganization in recent-onset tinnitus patients by the Heidelberg model of music therapy. *Front. Neurosci.* 9:49. doi: 10.3389/fnins.2015.00049

Langguth, B., Kreuzer, P. M., Kleinjung, T., and De Ridder, D. (2013). Tinnitus: causes and clinical management. *Lancet Neurol.* 12, 920–930. doi: 10.1016/S1474-4422(13)70160-1

Lanting, C., WoźAniak, A., van Dijk, P., and Langers, D. R. M. (2016). Tinnitus-and task-related differences in resting-state networks. *Adv. Exp. Med. Biol.* 894, 175–187. doi: 10.1007/978-3-319-25474-6_19

Liu, Y., Lv, H., Zhao, P., Liu, Z., Chen, W., Gong, S., et al. (2018). Neuroanatomical alterations in patients with early stage of unilateral pulsatile tinnitus: a voxel-based morphometry study. *Neural Plast.* 2018:4756471. doi: 10.1155/2018/4756471

Lv, H., Liu, C., Wang, Z., Zhao, P., Cheng, X., Yang, Z., et al. (2020). Altered functional connectivity of the thalamus in tinnitus patients is correlated with symptom alleviation after sound therapy. *Brain Imag. Behav.* 14, 2668–2678. doi: 10.1007/s11682-019-00218-0

Ma, Y., Shaik, M. A., Kozberg, M. G., Kim, S. H., Portes, J. P., Timerman, D., et al. (2016). Resting-state hemodynamics are spatiotemporally coupled to synchronized and symmetric neural activity in excitatory neurons. *Proc. Natl. Acad. Sci. U.S.A.* 113, E8463–E8471. doi: 10.1073/pnas.1525369113

Makar, S. K., Mukundan, G., and Gore, G. (2017). Treatment of tinnitus: a scoping review. *Int. Tinnitus J.* 21, 144–156. doi: 10.5935/0946-5448.20170027

Mantini, D., Perrucci, M. G., Del, G. C., Romani, G. L., and Corbetta, M. (2007). Electrophysiological signatures of resting state networks in the human brain. *Proc. Natl. Acad. Sci. U.S.A.* 104, 13170–13175. doi: 10.1073/pnas.0700668104

Meyer, M., Neff, P., Liem, F., Kleinjung, T., Weidt, S., Langguth, B., et al. (2016). Differential tinnitus-related neuroplastic alterations of cortical thickness and surface area. *Hear. Res.* 342, 1–12. doi: 10.1016/j.heares.2016.08.016

Newman, C. W., Jacobson, G. P., and Spitzer, J. B. (1996). Development of the tinnitus handicap inventory. *Arch. Otolaryngol. Head Neck Surg.* 122, 143–148.

Nomura, E. M., Gratton, C., Visser, R. M., Kayser, A., Perez, F., and D'Esposito, M. (2010). Double dissociation of two cognitive control networks in patients with focal brain lesions. *Proc. Natl. Acad. Sci. U.S.A.* 107, 12017–12022. doi: 10.1073/pnas.1002431107

Noreña, A. J., and Farley, B. J. (2013). Tinnitus-related neural activity: theories of generation, propagation, and centralization. *Hear. Res.* 295, 161–171. doi: 10.1016/j.heares.2012.09.010

Oishi, N., Oishi, N., Shinden, S., Shinden, S., Kanzaki, S., Kanzaki, S., et al. (2013). Effects of tinnitus retraining therapy involving monaural noise generators. *Eur. Arch. OtoRhinoLaryngol.* 270, 443–448. doi: 10.1007/s00405-012-1951-5

Ooms, E., Vanheule, S., Meganck, R., Vinck, B., Watelet, J., and Dhooge, I. (2013). Tinnitus, anxiety and automatic processing of affective information: an explorative study. *Eur. Arch. OtoRhinoLaryngol.* 270, 823–830. doi: 10.1007/s00405-012-2044-1

Parker, R. I., and Hagan-Burke, S. (2007). Useful effect size interpretations for single case research. *Behav. Ther.* 38, 95–105. doi: 10.1016/j.beth.2006.05.002

Pereira-Jorge, M. R., Andrade, K. C., Palhano-Fontes, F. X., Diniz, P. R. B., Sturzbecher, M., Santos, A. C., et al. (2018). Anatomical and functional MRI changes after one year of auditory rehabilitation with hearing aids. *Neural Plast.* 2018, 1–13. doi: 10.1155/2018/9303674

Ridder, D. D., Elgoyhen, A. B., Romo, R., and Langguth, B. (2011). Phantom percepts: tinnitus and pain as persisting aversive memory networks. *Proc. Natl. Acad. Sci. U.S.A.* 108, 8075–8080. doi: 10.1073/pnas.1018466108

Ryu, C., Park, M. S., Byun, J. Y., Jahng, G., and Park, S. (2016). White matter integrity associated with clinical symptoms in tinnitus patients: a tract-based spatial statistics study. *Eur. Radiol.* 26, 2223–2232. doi: 10.1007/s00330-015-4034-3

Schecklmann, M., Lehner, A., Poeppl, T. B., Kreuzer, P. M., Hajak, G., Landgrebe, M., et al. (2012). Cluster analysis for identifying sub-types of tinnitus: a positron emission tomography and voxel-based morphometry study. *Brain Res.* 1485, 3–9. doi: 10.1016/j.brainres.2012.05.013

Schmidt, S. A., Akrofi, K., Carpenter-Thompson, J. R., and Husain, F. T. (2013). Default mode, dorsal attention and auditory resting state networks exhibit differential functional connectivity in tinnitus and hearing loss. *PLoS One* 8:e76488. doi: 10.1371/journal.pone.0076488

Schmidt, S. A., Carpenter-Thompson, J., and Husain, F. T. (2017). Connectivity of precuneus to the default mode and dorsal attention networks: a possible invariant marker of long-term tinnitus. *NeuroImage Clin.* 16, 196–204. doi: 10.1016/j.nicl.2017.07.015

Sereda, M., Hoare, D. J., Nicholson, R., Smith, S., and Hall, D. A. (2015). Consensus on hearing aid candidature and fitting for mild hearing loss, with and without tinnitus: delphi review. *Ear Hear.* 36, 417–429. doi: 10.1097/AUD.0000000000000140

Sereda, M., Xia, J., El Refaie, A., Hall, D. A., and Hoare, D. J. (2018). Sound therapy (using amplification devices and/or sound generators) for tinnitus. *Cochrane Database Syst. Rev.* 12:D13094. doi: 10.1002/14651858.CD013094.pub2

Seydell-Greenwald, A., Raven, E. P., Leaver, A. M., Turesky, T. K., and Rauschecker, J. P. (2014). Diffusion imaging of auditory and auditory-limbic connectivity in tinnitus: preliminary evidence and methodological challenges. *Neural Plast.* 2014:145943. doi: 10.1155/2014/145943

Shulman, G. L., Fiez, J. A., Corbetta, M., Buckner, R. L., Miezin, F. M., Raichle, M. E., et al. (1997). Common blood flow changes across visual tasks: II. Decreases in cerebral cortex. *J. Cogn. Neurosci.* 9, 648–663. doi: 10.1162/jocn.1997.9.5.648

Smith, S. M., Fox, P. T., Miller, K. L., Glahn, D. C., Fox, P. M., Mackay, C. E., et al. (2009). Correspondence of the brain's functional architecture during activation and rest. *Proc. Natl. Acad. Sci. U.S.A.* 106, 13040–13045. doi: 10.1073/pnas.0905267106

Song, J., Qin, W., Liu, Y., Duan, Y., Liu, J., He, X., et al. (2013). Aberrant functional organization within and between resting-state networks in AD. *PLoS One* 8:e63727. doi: 10.1371/journal.pone.0063727

Stebbins, G. T., Nyenhuis, D. L., Wang, C., Cox, J. L., Freels, S., Bangen, K., et al. (2008). Gray matter atrophy in patients with ischemic stroke with cognitive impairment. *Stroke* 39, 785–793. doi: 10.1161/STROKEAHA.107.507392

Tunkel, D. E., Bauer, C. A., Sun, G. H., Rosenfeld, R. M., Chandrasekhar, S. S., Cunningham, E. R., et al. (2014). Clinical Practice Guideline. *Otolaryngol. Head Neck Surg.* 151, S1–S40. doi: 10.1177/0194599814545325

Tutaj, L., Hoare, D. J., and Sereda, M. (2018). Combined amplification and sound generation for Tinnitus. *Ear Hear.* 39, 412–422. doi: 10.1097/AUD.0000000000000516

Vincent, J. L., Kahn, I., Snyder, A. Z., Raichle, M. E., and Buckner, R. L. (2008). Evidence for a frontoparietal control system revealed by intrinsic functional connectivity. *J. Neurophysiol.* 100, 3328–3342. doi: 10.1152/jn.90355.2008

Wang, C., Qin, W., Zhang, J., Tian, T., Li, Y., Meng, L., et al. (2014). Altered functional organization within and between resting-state networks in chronic subcortical infarction. *J. Cereb. Blood Flow Metab.* 34, 597–605. doi: 10.1038/jcbfm.2013.238

Whitfield-Gabrieli, S., Moran, J. M., Nieto-Castañón, A., Triantafyllou, C., Saxe, R., and Gabrieli, J. D. E. (2011). Associations and dissociations between default and self-reference networks in the human brain. *NeuroImage* 55, 225–232. doi: 10.1016/j.neuroimage.2010.11.048

Xia, M., Wang, J., and He, Y. (2013). BrainNet Viewer: a network visualization tool for human brain connectomics. *PLoS One* 8:e68910. doi: 10.1371/journal.pone.0068910

Yan, C. G., Cheung, B., Kelly, C., Colcombe, S., Craddock, R. C., Di Martino, A., et al. (2013). A comprehensive assessment of regional variation in the impact of head micromovements on functional connectomics. *Neuroimage* 76, 183–201. doi: 10.1016/j.neuroimage.2013.03.004

Yan, C. G., Wang, X. D., Zuo, X. N., and Zang, Y. F. (2016). DPABI: data processing & analysis for (Resting-State) brain imaging. *Neuroinformatics* 14, 339–351. doi: 10.1007/s12021-016-9299-4

Zeman, F., Koller, M., Figueiredo, R., Aazevedo, A., Rates, M., Coelho, C., et al. (2011). Tinnitus handicap inventory for evaluating treatment effects: which changes are clinically relevant? *Otolaryngol. Head Neck Surg.* 145, 282–287. doi: 10.1177/0194599811403882

Zenner, H., Delb, W., Kröner-Herwig, B., Jäger, B., Peroz, I., Hesse, G., et al. (2017). A multidisciplinary systematic review of the treatment for chronic idiopathic tinnitus. *Eur. Arch. Otorhinolaryngol.* 274, 2079–2091. doi: 10.1007/s00405-016-4401-y

Zenner, H., and Zalaman, I. M. (2004). Cognitive tinnitus sensitization: behavioral and neurophysiological aspects of tinnitus centralization. *Acta Otolaryngol.* 124, 436–439. doi: 10.1080/00016480410016333

Zhou, G., Shi, X., Wei, H., Qu, L., Yu, Y., Zhou, Q., et al. (2019). Disrupted intraregional brain activity and functional connectivity in unilateral acute tinnitus patients with hearing loss. *Front. Neurosci.* 13:1010. doi: 10.3389/fnins.2019.01010

7

Reorganization of Brain White Matter in Persistent Idiopathic Tinnitus Patients without Hearing Loss: Evidence From Baseline Data

Qian Chen[1†], Zhaodi Wang[2†], Han Lv[1], Pengfei Zhao[1], Zhenghan Yang[1], Shusheng Gong[2] and Zhenchang Wang[1*]*

[1] *Department of Radiology, Beijing Friendship Hospital, Capital Medical University, Beijing, China,* [2] *Department of Otolaryngology Head and Neck Surgery, Beijing Friendship Hospital, Capital Medical University, Beijing, China*

***Correspondence:**
Shusheng Gong
gongss1962@163.com
Zhenchang Wang
cjr.wzhch@vip.163.com

† These authors have contributed equally to this work

It remains unknown whether tinnitus or tinnitus-related hearing loss (HL) could indirectly impair or reshape the white matter (WM) of the human brain. We aim to explore the possible brain WM change in tinnitus patients without HL and further to investigate their associations with clinical variables. Structural and diffusion tensor imaging (DTI) of 20 idiopathic tinnitus patients without HL and 22 healthy controls (HCs) were obtained. Voxel-based morphometry (VBM) and tract-based spatial statistics (TBSS) analysis were conducted to investigate the differences in WM volume and integrity between patients and HCs, separately. We extracted WM parameters to determine a sensitive imaging index to differentiate the idiopathic tinnitus patients from the HCs in the early stage. Correlations between the clinical variables and WM indices were also performed in patients. Compared with the controls, the tinnitus patients without HL exhibited significant decreased fractional anisotropy (FA) in the body and genu of corpus callosum (CC), left cingulum (LC) and right cingulum (RC), and right superior longitudinal fasciculus (RSLF) and increase in mean diffusivity (MD) in the body of CC in WM. Moreover, the patients also showed decreases in WM axial diffusivity (AD) in LC, left superior longitudinal fasciculus (LSLF), and right interior cerebellar peduncle (ICP) and increases in radial diffusivity (RD) in the body and genu of CC and RSLF ($p < 0.05$, voxel-level FWE corrected). Furthermore, the increased RD value of the genu of CC is closely associated with the tinnitus handicap inventory (THI) subscale scores. No WMV changes were detected in tinnitus patients. We combined the altered WM integrity index of body and genu of CC and LC and RSLF as an index to differentiate the two groups and reached a sensitivity of 100% and a specificity of 77.3%. Our findings suggest that tinnitus without HL is associated with significant alterations of WM integrity. These changes may be irrespective of the duration and other clinical performance. The combination of diffusion indices of body and genu of CC and LC and RSLF might be used as the potential useful imaging index for the diagnosis of persistent idiopathic tinnitus without HL in the early stage.

Keywords: tinnitus without hearing loss, brain white matter, reorganization, tract-based spatial statistics, clinical variables

---

Abbreviations: AD, axial diffusivity; BDI, Beck Depression Inventory; CC, corpus callosum; CSF, cerebrospinal fluid; FA, fractional anisotropy; HC, healthy control; HL, hearing loss; ICP, interior cerebellar peduncle; LC, left cingulum; MD, mean diffusivity; MNI, Montreal Neurological Institute; RC, right cingulum; RD, radial diffusivity; SLF, superior longitudinal fasciculus; THI, Tinnitus Handicap Inventory; WM, white matter; WMV, white matter volume.

INTRODUCTION

Tinnitus, as a perception of sound without an external source, is regarded as a problem of the central nervous system (CNS) (Eggermont and Roberts, 2004). Previous studies have proved that tinnitus can cause significant brain functional and structural changes, which are closely related to the patient's clinical performance (Ryu et al., 2016; Schmidt et al., 2018; Han et al., 2019). Most of this research has focused on the cortical or resting-state functional alterations (Leaver et al., 2011; Chen et al., 2015a; Liu et al., 2018; Lv et al., 2018), indicating cortical functional changes in some auditory-related areas and altered interactions between multiple auditory-related areas and limbic-related regions in tinnitus. However, studies on brain white matter (WM) changes of the tinnitus are relatively small. Considering the role of the link between the auditory cortex and the limbic system in the generation and maintenance of tinnitus, examining the WM connectivity between these systems may be very important for us to understand the pathophysiology of the disorder.

Currently, there have been a few non-invasive structural studies on brain WM change in tinnitus patients with diverse results (Crippa et al., 2010; Husain et al., 2011; Aldhafeeri et al., 2012; Benson et al., 2014; Seydell-Greenwald et al., 2014; Ryu et al., 2016; Schmidt et al., 2018). Lee et al. (2007) find significantly reduced fractional anisotropy (FA) in superior longitudinal fasciculus in tinnitus patients. Aldhafeeri et al. (2012) also report that tinnitus causes decreased FA in some brain regions or WM fiber bundles, which may be associated with patients' cognitive deficits, negative emotional suffering, or the imbalance between the two hemispheres in terms of excitation and inhibition. Using tract-based spatial statistics (TBSS) analysis, the study conducted by Seydell-Greenwald et al. (2014) indicates tinnitus-related FA and mean diffusivity (MD) changes in auditory cortical WM, which were correlated with age and hearing loss. Additionally, Ryu et al. (2016) find that the tinnitus group also has higher MD and axial diffusivity (AD) in WM under the auditory cortex and limbic system, and the changed diffusion indices are correlated with patients' depression. All the studies above prove that tinnitus can result in changes in brain WM integrity, but none of them has made it clear whether the alterations are due to tinnitus or hearing loss (HL).

To date, several studies have analyzed the effect of tinnitus-related HL. For example, Husain et al. (2011) assess WM integrity and find profound changes in the tracts near the auditory cortex in subjects with HL. More specifically, their analyses reveal reduced FA in their HL groups in some auditory or limbic system–related bundles. They speculate these changes could reflect that HL–related sensory deprivation or compensatory mechanisms cause damage to WM tracts or even an expansion of other fibers into these regions. Other research also performs a comparison between groups of subjects with and without tinnitus that are purposely matched with respect to HL (Benson et al., 2014). They also find that the FA elevated in some important hearing or limbic system related tracts and interpret this as the consequence of large-scale changes in excitatory and inhibitory neurotransmission. All of these studies only focus on FA as a measure of tract integrity although, in fact, the interpretation may be problematic due to the high likelihood of crossing fibers and partial-volume effects in the assessed voxels (Seydell-Greenwald et al., 2014).

On the contrary, some research even fails to find any WM changes in tinnitus. An early study investigates the WM connections between the auditory cortex and subcortical nuclei in tinnitus and finds stronger auditory-limbic connectivity in patients, but the employed statistical criteria of their study is lenient as no corrections for multiple comparisons are made (Crippa et al., 2010). Also, Schmidt et al. (2018) even find that there are no differences in diffusion indices in patients when compared with controls, and the severity and duration do not affect FA values as well. They speculate this may be due to the differences in imaging parameters, which do not have the sensitivity to detect the changes.

Based on the above studies, whether tinnitus can cause any change in brain WM and the possible change is due to tinnitus or tinnitus-related HL remains unclear. Therefore, in the present study, we combined used TBSS and VBM to investigate possible changes in brain WM of tinnitus patients without HL and to further explore their relationship with clinical variables. It has been proven that 3–4 years is a kind of turning point in the efficacy of treatment of tinnitus (De Ridder et al., 2007; Plewnia et al., 2007; Langguth et al., 2008). Compared with patients in the early stage of disease (less than 48 months), patients' brain structure and function with long duration is significantly changed, and this might be the reason why it is difficult for them to be successfully treated (Schlee et al., 2009; Vanneste et al., 2011a,b,c; Liu et al., 2018). Thus, we defined subjects with duration less than 48 months as in the early stage. As prior studies only chose one or two diffusion indices of DTI (Seydell-Greenwald et al., 2014; Ryu et al., 2016; Schmidt et al., 2018), in order to improve the sensitivity of diffusion tensor imaging (DTI) parameters, we apply the four diffusion indices (FA, MD, AD, and radial diffusivity: RD) of DTI to measure the WM integrity of the tinnitus patients.

MATERIALS AND METHODS

Subjects

A total of 20 patients with untreated persistent idiopathic tinnitus were enrolled in this study. (We defined the patients who were diagnosed with idiopathic tinnitus without any treatment as baseline, and after 6 months of sound therapy, as post-treatment.) Twenty-two right-handed healthy volunteers were recruited as healthy controls (HCs). All the patients met the inclusion criteria: persistent idiopathic tinnitus ($\geq$ 6 months persistently and $\leq$ 48 months) without any history of associated brain diseases confirmed by conventional MRI, no preexisting mental illness or cognitive disorder affecting the structural outcome, and no contradictions to MRI. Tinnitus was present as a single high-/low-pitched sound and two high/low pitched sounds without any rhythm. Based on audiogram results, all the subjects were without hearing loss, which was defined as more than 25 dB hearing loss at frequencies ranging from 250 to 8 kHz (0.250, 0.500, 1, 2, 3, 4, 6, and 8 kHz) in a pure tone audiometry (PTA) examination. We excluded patients with the following criteria: pulsatile tinnitus, hyperacusis on physical examination, otosclerosis, sudden deafness, Ménière's disease, and other neurological diseases. All the patients were asked to fill in the tinnitus handicap inventory (THI) (Newman et al., 1996) and visual analog scale (VAS) to assess the severity of disease at the time of MRI acquisition. A Beck depression inventory (BDI) was also administered to evaluate the depression at that time. We also evaluated the hearing condition of healthy controls by the audiologists using the questionnaire. Other exclusion criteria for HCs were the same as above.

All the participants were informed of the purpose of the study and gave written consent. The current study was approved by the institutional review board (IRB) of Beijing Friendship Hospital, Capital Medical University (Beijing, China), and was in accordance with the Declaration of Helsinki. The registration number of our study on ClinicalTrials.gov is NCT02774122.

Image Acquisition

Images were obtained using a 3.0T MRI system (Prisma, Siemens, Erlangen, Germany) with a 64-channel phase-array head coil. The conventional brain axial T2 sequence was acquired prior to the DTI scan to exclude any abnormality in the brain. The DTI experiments were performed using a single-shot, gradient-echo, echo-planar imaging sequence with the following imaging parameters: TR = 8500 ms, TE = 63 ms, matrix = 128 × 128, acquisition voxel size 2 mm × 2 mm × 2 mm, FOV = 224 mm × 224 mm, non-zero b value = 1000 s/mm^2, gradient directions = 64, slice thickness = 2 mm, and bandwidth = 2232 Hz/Px. A total of 74 contiguous slices parallel to the anterior commissure–posterior commissure line were acquired. High-resolution three-dimensional (3-D) structural T1-weighted images were acquired using a 3-D magnetization-prepared rapid gradient-echo sequence (MP-RAGE) with the following parameters: TR = 2530 ms; TE = 2.98 ms; inversion time (TI) = 1100 ms; FA = 7°; number of slices = 192; slice thickness = 1 mm, bandwidth = 240 Hz/Px; FOV = 256 mm × 256 mm; and matrix = 256 × 256; resulting in an isotropic voxel size of 1 mm × 1 mm × 1 mm.

During the scanning process, tight but comfortable foam padding minimized head motion, and earplugs reduced imaging noise. The participants were asked to close their eyes, stay awake, breathe evenly, and try to avoid specific thoughts.

Image Analysis

Data Processing and Diffusion Tensor Imaging (DTI)

Post-processing was performed using TBSS implemented with the FSL 5.0.3 software package (Centre for FMRIB, Oxford University, Oxford, United Kingdom)[1] (Smith et al., 2006). The following post-processing steps were included: All DTI images were visually checked to eliminate images with apparent artifacts caused by the following: eddy current corrections were applied, and motion artifacts were removed using affine alignment. Next, the non-brain tissues were removed using the brain extract tool (BET); this process reduces the computation times of the DTI fitting and tracking processes and improves the accuracy of the spatial registration. After that, the diffusion tensor of each voxel was fitted using a linear least squares algorithm, and the FA, MD, AD, and RD maps were calculated based on the eigenvalues of diffusion tensors (Raya et al., 2012). For the TBSS analysis, the main procedures were as follows: the entire FA data set was non-linearly coregistered to the Montreal Neurological Institute (MNI) FA template in the FSL database. Next, a mean FA skeleton from the mean FA images of all of the subjects was derived and represented the center of the WM tracts common to the group. An FA threshold of 0.2 was used to involve only the major white matter pathways while eliminating peripheral tracts that are susceptible to misregistration. Finally, each aligned FA map was then projected back onto the skeleton to generate a subject-specific FA skeleton. The processes of non-linear warping and skeleton projection of the FA maps were also applied to MD, AD, and RD maps.

Structural Data Processing and Whole Brain Voxel-Based Morphometry Analysis

We did the post-processing of structural data using SPM12. First, all the structural images were checked to make sure no apparent artifacts were caused by factors, such as head motion, susceptibility artifacts, and instrument malfunction. Then, the images were manually reoriented to place the anterior commissure at the origin and the anterior-posterior commissure in the horizontal plane. Next, the structural images were segmented into GM, WM, and cerebrospinal fluid (CSF) areas using the unified standard segmentation option in SPM12. The individual WM and GM components were then normalized into the standard MNI space using the diffeomorphic anatomical registration through exponentiated lie algebra (DARTEL) algorithm (Ashburner, 2007) after segmentation. The normalized WM component was modulated to generate the relative white matter volume (WMV) by multiplication by the non-linear part of the deformation field at the DARTEL step. The resulting WMV images were then smoothed with a 6-mm full-width at half maximum Gaussian kernel.

Statistical Analyses

For DTI data, TBSS using a non-parametric permutation test (5000 permutations) was performed to compare the DTI indices between the tinnitus patients and the HCs. The permutation test was performed with a fixed-effect general linear model (GLM) with age and gender as nuisance covariates. Statistical significance was set at $p < 0.05$ and corrected for multiple comparisons using the threshold-free cluster enhancement (TFCE) method. For T1 MP-RAGE images, using the GLM in SPM12, a voxel-wise two-sample t test was applied to compare the WMV differences in the whole brain between the tinnitus patients and the HCs (voxel-level uncorrected $P < 0.001$, non-stationary cluster-level FWE correction with $P < 0.05$), and age and gender served as nuisance covariates. Next, the regions that exhibited alterations in the DTI indices and WMV in tinnitus patients defined as the regions of interest (ROIs) and the mean values of each ROI of each

[1] https://fsl.fmrib.ox.ac.uk/fsl/fslwiki/

subject were extracted for subsequent analyses. Finally, partial correlation analysis was performed to explore any potential associations between the patients' clinical variables (such as the duration, THI scores, BDI scores, and VAS scores) and the indices after removing age and gender effects. Moreover, to test the laterality of tinnitus, we did a one-way ANOVA and *post hoc* analysis among these three different-sided tinnitus groups using the extracted mean values of each ROI that exhibited significant alterations in the DTI indices. The last steps were performed using IBM SPSS Statistics version 23.0 (IBM Inc., Armonk, NY, United States). All data in this study were assessed by Kolmogorov–Smirnov test for normality. Data identified as not normally distributed were analyzed using non-parametric tests.

RESULTS

Demographics and Clinical Characteristics

Table 1 provides detailed demographic and clinical data of 20 patients with persistent idiopathic tinnitus and 22 healthy controls. We didn't find the significant differences of gender and age between the tinnitus and HC groups (both *Ps* > 0.01).

Brain WM Changes Between the Tinnitus Patients and HCs and Among Tinnitus Subgroups

Compared with the HCs, we found that the tinnitus patients exhibited significant decreases in white matter FA in the body and genu of the corpus callosum (CC), left cingulum (LC) and right cingulum (RC), right superior longitudinal fasciculus (RSLF), and increase in MD in the body of CC. Moreover, the patients also showed decreases in WM AD in LC, left superior longitudinal fasciculus (LSLF), right interior cerebellar peduncle (ICP), and increases in RD in the body and genu of CC and RSLF (voxel-level FWE correction with $p < 0.05$) (**Figure 1** and **Table 2**). No significant differences in WMV were found between the tinnitus and HCs. We also found that there were no significant differences among the three different sided tinnitus subgroups (**Supplementary Material**). In addition, partial correlation analyses revealed that the RD value of the genu of CC was positively correlated with a subscale of the THI score

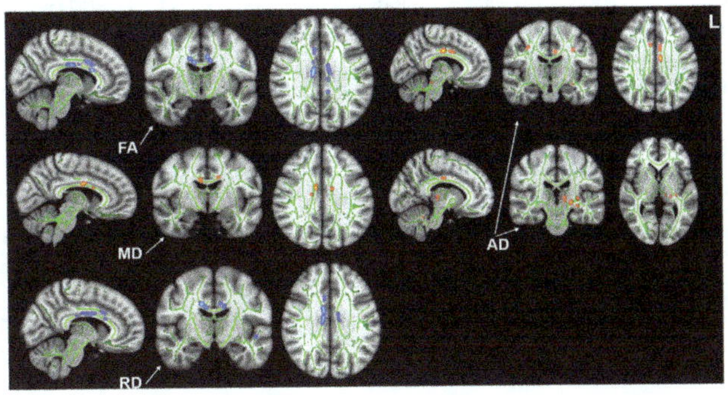

FIGURE 1 | Intergroup differences in white matter integrity between the tinnitus patients and HCs. Patients showed significant decreases of FA in the body and genu of CC, bilateral cingulum, right SLF, and increase of MD in the body of CC. Patients also showed decreases of AD in left cingulum, left SLF, right ICP, and increases of RD in the body and genu of CC and right SLF ($p < 0.05$, voxel-level FWE corrected). HC, healthy control; FA, fractional anisotropy; MD, mean diffusivity; AD, axial diffusivity; RD, radial diffusivity; CC, corpus callosum; SLF, superior longitudinal fasciculus; ICP, interior cerebellar peduncle.

($r = -0.481$, $p = 0.032$; uncorrected; **Figure 2**). No correlations were found between the brain white matter changes and tinnitus duration and other clinical variables.

The Combination of Four Diffusion Parameters of Brain WM Integrity as Diagnostic Index

Figure 3A and **Table 3** show the sensitivity and specificity of the diffusion indices of the four different white-matter tracts for the tinnitus group and controls. Using the cutoff value of 0.864, 0.818, 0.627, and 0.768, we differentiated the two groups with a sensitivity of 100% and specificity of 86.4% using the body of CC and with a sensitivity of 100% and specificity of 81.8% using the genu of CC and with a sensitivity of 90% and specificity of 72.7% using the LC and with a sensitivity of 95% and specificity of 81.8% using the RSLF separately. The area under the curve (AUC) for the ROC were 0.927 (95% confidence intervals from 0.832 to 1) and 0.943 (95% confidence intervals from 0.871 to 1) and 0.920 (95% confidence intervals from 0.841 to 1) and 0.945 (95% confidence intervals from 0.884 to 1) separately.

TABLE 1 | Demographic and Clinical Data of 20 Patients with persistent Idiopathic Tinnitus and 22 Healthy Controls.

Demographic	Tinnitus (n = 20)	Control (n = 22)	*P*-value
Age, years	39.7 (±12.53)	43.7 (±10.47)	0.437
gender	8 males	10 males	0.509
Tinnitus Handicap Inventory	50.5 (±24.34)	NA	NA
Duration, months	≥6 months & ≤48 months	NA	NA
Type[#]	13: 3: 3: 1	NA	NA
Tinnitus pitch	250 ~ 8,000 Hz	NA	NA
Laterality	5 right, 6 left, 9 bilateral	NA	NA
Normal hearing	All	All	NA

NA, not applicable. [#]*1 single high-pitched sound vs. 1 single low-pitched sound vs. 2 high pitched sounds vs. 2 low pitched sounds.*

TABLE 2 | Regions of significant clusters with changed FA, MD, AD, and RD values in the tinnitus patients compared with the HCs according to the TBSS voxel-based analysis (FWE voxel $p < 0.05$).

Cluster Index	Location of clusters	Volume (mm^3)	Mean DTI value		*p* value
			Tinnitus	Control	
FA					
1	Body of CC	141	4.2906	3.3838	0.002
2	Genu of CC	36	1.4034	1.2008	0.011
3	LC	24	0.6656	0.5560	0.003
4	RC	20	0.4924	0.3463	0.002
5	RSLF	11	0.5047	0.4761	0.01
MD					
1	Body of CC	10	0.0024	0.0026	0.022
AD					
1	LC	23	0.0028	0.0026	0.026
2	LSLF	8	0.0012	0.0011	0.005
3	RICP	6	0.0012	0.0011	0.004
RD					
1	Body of CC	60	0.0016	0.0024	0.019
2	Genu of CC	19	0.00069	0.00089	0.014
3	RSLF	10	0.00050	0.00054	0.001

FA, fractional anisotropy; MD, mean diffusivity; AD, axial diffusivity; RD, radial diffusivity; CC, corpus callosum; LC, left cingulum; RC, right cingulum; RSLF, right superior longitudinal fasciculus; LSLF, left superior longitudinal fasciculus; RICP, right interior cerebellar peduncle; FWE, family wise error; TBSS = tract-based spatial statistics.

Figure 3B and **Table 3** show the sensitivity and specificity of the combination of four diffusion indices of these white matter tracts for the tinnitus group and controls. Using this cutoff value, 0.773, we differentiated the two groups by a sensitivity of 100% and a specificity of 77.3%. The AUC for the ROC was 0.973 (95% confidence intervals from 0.934 to 1).

DISCUSSION

By performing TBSS analysis, the present study shows significant increased FA and AD and decreased MD and RD in the distributed WM of the tinnitus patients' brain; all of these WM tracts are closely related to the information transmission between brain regions or even between hemispheres direct or indirect, especially the auditory information. Moreover, we find that the combination of diffusion indices of several main white-matter tracts could be used to differentiate the persistent tinnitus from controls in the early stage. For the patients, all of them were tested as tinnitus without HL in the classical frequencies in this study. To date, several studies have analyzed HL-related brain reorganization but with inconsistent findings (Crippa et al., 2010; Husain et al., 2011, 2015; Seydell-Greenwald et al., 2014; Schmidt et al., 2018). For example, Husain et al. (2011) assessed the WM integrity and found profound changes in the tracts near the auditory cortex in subjects with HL. More specifically, their analyses revealed reduced FA in their HL groups in some auditory or limbic system–related bundles, which may reflect that HL-related sensory deprivation or compensatory mechanisms caused damage to WM tracts or even an expansion of other fibers into these regions. Other research on tinnitus and tinnitus-related HL found that the FA elevated in some important hearing or limbic system–related tracts and interpreted this as the consequence of large-scale changes in excitatory and inhibitory neurotransmission (Benson et al., 2014). Also, Seydell-Greenwald et al. (2014) found that tinnitus is associated with changes that might reflect increases in auditory and auditory-limbic connectivity while hearing loss is associated with changes in diffusion measures that may reflect decreases in anatomical connectivity of central auditory pathways. Moreover, Schmidt et al. (2018) found no changes in brain white matter between subgroups or compared with HCs. Thus, to investigate the possible tinnitus-caused brain white matter changes and eliminate the effect of hearing loss on the results, all the patients were tinnitus without HL, we believe that the changes in brain white matter integrity may be caused by tinnitus (although we can't eliminate possible hidden or slight hearing loss in other frequency ranges). Combined with the previous studies, our findings may advance the understanding of the neural pathophysiological mechanisms of tinnitus from the perspective of WM microstructure.

Brain WM Microstructural Abnormality in Tinnitus Patients

To our knowledge, there are only a few studies that have investigated the brain WM changes in tinnitus so far (Lee et al., 2007; Crippa et al., 2010; Husain et al., 2011; Aldhafeeri et al., 2012; Benson et al., 2014; Seydell-Greenwald et al., 2014; Ryu et al., 2016; Schmidt et al., 2018). Our present study demonstrates a significantly decreased FA and increased RD in the main part (body and genu) of CC WM. For the DTI indices, FA is considered to be the largest in regions in which strongly myelinated fiber tracts run in parallel, permitting free

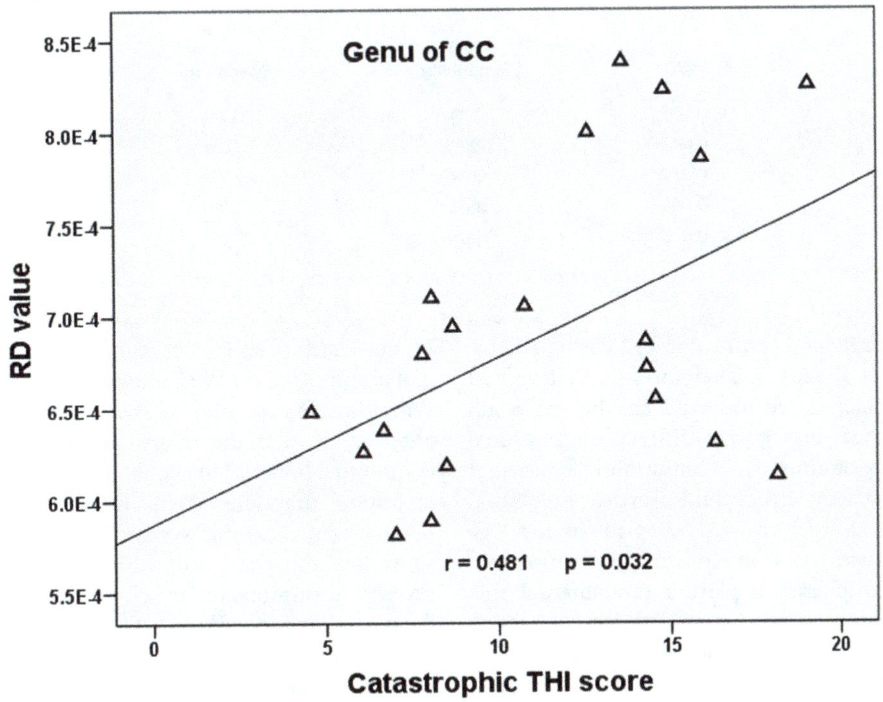

FIGURE 2 | Correlation between diffusion metrics and clinical scale scores in tinnitus patients. Pearson correlation showed positive association between the RD of the genu of CC and the catastrophic THI score ($r = -0.481$, $p = 0.032$; uncorrected). RD, radial diffusivity; CC, corpus callosum; THI, Tinnitus Handicap Inventory.

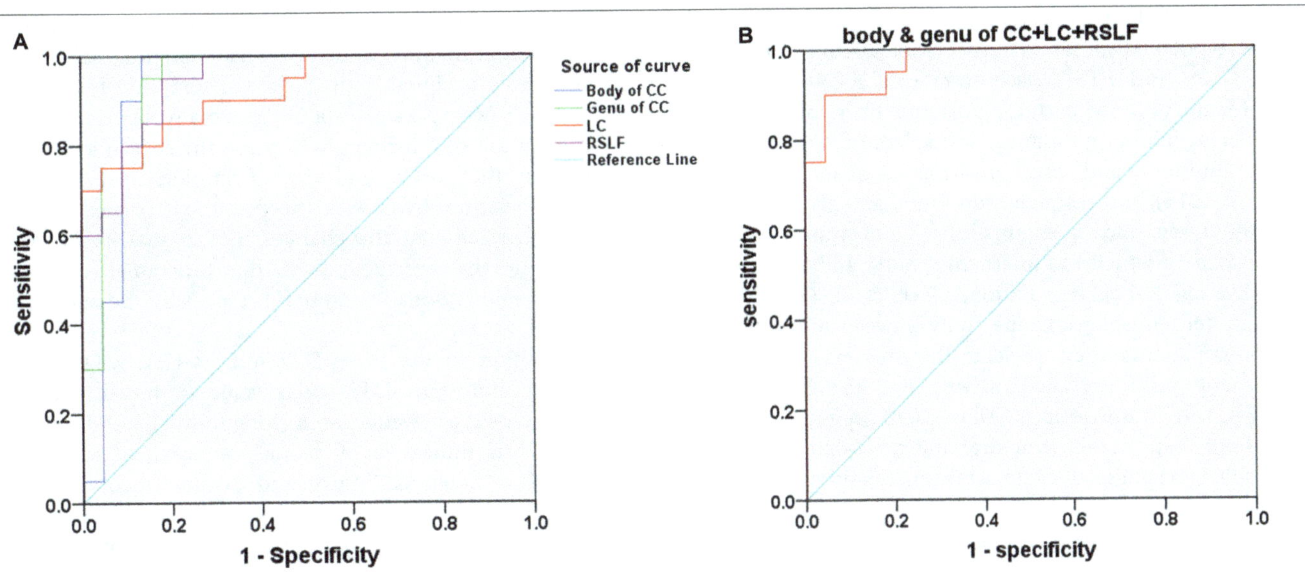

FIGURE 3 | (A) Receiver operating characteristic (ROC) curve for uncorrected diffusion metrics in different WM bundles of patients with tinnitus and HCs. An optimal diffusion metric cutoff value of these four bundles was determined at a sensitivity of 100, 100, 90, and 95% and specificity of 86.4, 81.8, 72.7, and 81.8% separately. The area under the curve (AUC) for the ROC were 0.927, 0.943, 0.920, and 0.945 separately (95% confidence intervals from 0.832 to 1, 0.871 to 1, 0.841 to 1, and 0.884 to 1 separately). **(B)** ROC curve for the combination of four diffusion indices in these different WM tracts of patients with tinnitus and HCs. An optimal diffusion metric cutoff value was determined at a sensitivity of 100% and specificity of 77.3%. The AUC for the ROC was 0.973 (95% confidence intervals from 0.934 to 1).

diffusion along but preventing diffusion perpendicular to the fibers. Thus, reductions in myelination or in the number of parallel fibers result in lower FA (Seydell-Greenwald et al., 2014). In addition, RD and MD may also mainly reflect abnormalities in myelination (Bledsoe et al., 2018) although RD may also be affected by axonal loss (Jones et al., 2013) or differences in axonal packing density or diameter (Alexander et al., 2007) although MD to some extent is considered to be inversely

TABLE 3 | Results of receiver operator characteristic (ROC) curve analysis of the combination of four diffusion parameters of brain white matter integrity as a possible diagnostic index.

Brain white matter integrity	AUC	Sensitivity	Specificity	*P* value	Cutoff
Body of CC	0.927	100%	86.4%	0.000	0.864
Genu of CC	0.943	100%	81.8%	0.000	0.818
LC	0.920	90%	72.7%	0.000	0.627
RSLF	0.945	95%	81.8%	0.000	0.768
Body & genu of CC + LC + RSLF	0.973	100%	77.3%	0.000	0.773

ROC, receiver operator characteristic; CC, corpus callosum; LC, left cingulum; RSLF, right superior longitudinal fasciculus; AUC, area under curve.

related to membrane density and sensitive to cellularity, edema, or necrosis (Alexander et al., 2011). Therefore, we believe that the FA, MD, and RD changes we observed can be the result of demyelination or axonal loss or the differences in axonal packing density caused by tinnitus. More importantly, consistent with prior studies (Aldhafeeri et al., 2012; Seydell-Greenwald et al., 2014), we found changes in WM integrity in the CC. As the largest white matter tract and the major commissure connecting the two hemispheres, it plays a fundamental role in integrating information and mediating complex behaviors (Quigley et al., 2003; van der Knaap and van der Ham, 2011; Hinkley et al., 2012; Roland et al., 2017). The importance of it (especially the anterior part of the CC, such as the genu of it) is embodied in interhemispheric and intrahemispheric communication and the consequent integration of cognitive, emotional, and motor functions. Reduced WM integrity of the CC was reported in some emotional and cognitive disorders such as bipolar disorder (Wang et al., 2008), ADHD (Cao et al., 2010), and PTSD (Jackowski et al., 2008). Moreover, except for the anterior part, the posterior fibers of CC crossing the posterior midbody, isthmus, and splenium transfer somatic sensory, auditory, and visual information (Fabri et al., 2014; Xue et al., 2018), and research even found an enlarged posterior part (the body and splenium) of CC in tinnitus patients, the CC area in which the interhemispheric auditory pathways cross (Diesch, 2012). In addition, Chen et al. (2015b) found stronger interhemispheric connectivity between auditory cortices in tinnitus patients; they speculate that this may be caused by tinnitus and tinnitus-related distress, and the CC played an important role in this process. All of these suggest that tinnitus can not only cause brain structural and functional changes, but also result in changes of brain white matter integrity, and the changed FA and RD of WM in the CC might be caused by the demyelination or axonal loss of persistent tinnitus; then it causes an imbalance between the two hemispheres in terms of simultaneous excitation and inhibition (Aldhafeeri et al., 2012). Also, we found the RD value of the genu of CC positively correlated with the subscale of THI score (catastrophic). A few studies have explored the correlations between WM changes and clinical variables but with controversial results. Several studies found no significant correlations between WM changes and age and clinical performances in tinnitus patients (Lee et al., 2007; Aldhafeeri et al., 2012). However, Ryu et al. (2016) reported that WM integrity in tinnitus patients was associated with depression symptoms, and this finding indicates the WM change in the auditory-limbic circuit attributable to tinnitus and the global influence on WM integrity by tinnitus-related emotional symptoms. As mentioned above, genu is the main part of the anterior CC and the role of it embodied in interhemispheric communication and the consequent integration of cognitive and emotional functions. Thus, this association may indicate the involvement of limbic system dysfunction in tinnitus and also show that the change of white matter may be related to the severity of tinnitus, for which we need to expand the sample in the future for further research on this.

Additionally, a significant decrease in FA and increase in RD was observed in the right superior longitudinal fasciculus (SLF) and an only decreased AD was observed in the left SLF. The SLF is considered to be the major association fiber tract that connects the auditory and frontal cortices, which is consist with three components (I, II, and III) and projects from the frontotemporal and frontoparietal regions in a bidirectional manner, and the inferior longitudinal fasciculus interconnects occipital with ipsilateral temporal lobes (Catani et al., 2002; Makris et al., 2005). The main function of SLF is the integration of information between the speech and auditory regions in the cortex and the integration of auditory and visual association areas with the prefrontal cortex. Therefore, we hypothesized that the changes in SLF may result at least partially in the destruction of the functional connections between some regions in the brain, especially the auditory and prefrontal cortex.

In addition to the three DTI indices (FA, MD, and RD), AD is an important DTI scalar value to measure the WM microstructure as well. As a longitudinal diffusion along axons, AD is indicative of axonal damage and is negatively correlated with axonal injury and positively correlated with axonal repair. Also, studies have proved that AD is usually associated with WM axonal injury in animal models (Song et al., 2003; Alexander et al., 2011) and humans (Smith et al., 2006). In the present study, we found decreased FA and AD in LC and only decreased FA in RC. The cingulum bundle is a prominent WM tract that interconnects frontal, parietal, and medial temporal sites while also linking subcortical nuclei to the cingulate gyrus, which is a major structure in the limbic system and involved in various cognitive functions, including memory, attention, learning, motivation, emotion, and pain perception (Bubb et al., 2018; Jang and Seo, 2018). In addition, DTI reconstructions often suggest a corresponding increase in parietal-temporal connections within the human parahippocampal cingulum bundle (Bubb et al., 2018). Moreover, some structural and functional studies also showed that, as an important aspect of the limbic system, the cingulum (also known as cingulate, including the anterior cingulate and posterior cingulate) plays a key role in several large-scale networks that tinnitus involved in, that is tinnitus emerges as a function of several large-scale networks that bind together various aspects of perception, salience, memory, distress, and audition (De Ridder et al., 2011; Ridder et al., 2011; Schecklmann et al., 2012; Meyer et al., 2016). Therefore, the WM integrity changes in the cingulum suggest that tinnitus is closely related to the limbic system dysfunction.

Together with some previous research (Schlee et al., 2008; Landgrebe et al., 2009; Husain et al., 2011; Leaver et al., 2011; Maudoux et al., 2012; Chen et al., 2015a), all of these findings support the hypotheses that the limbic system plays an important role in the generation of tinnitus, and tinnitus can stress and change neuronal activity and plasticity in the limbic system, which neesd to be further studied in the future. However, no WMV changes found in tinnitus patients, we speculated the reason may be that tinnitus in the early stage may only cause changes in WM integrity, but not have resulted in changes in WMV; further research on this is needed in the future.

The Combination of Four Diffusion Parameters of Brain WM Integrity as a Diagnostic Index

To date, the pathological changes of WM integrity in the body and genu of CC, the LC, and the SLF have been consistently reported in previous studies but in a separate way (Lee et al., 2007; Aldhafeeri et al., 2012; Benson et al., 2014; Seydell-Greenwald et al., 2014; Ryu et al., 2016). As mentioned above, all these fiber bundles are part of or closely related to the limbic system, and more importantly, they play a role in the onset and development of tinnitus, such as transmitting information between the prefrontal cortices and auditory cortices. Therefore, in the current study, by using the combination of the altered white matter integrity index of body and genu of CC and LC and RSLF as a possible diagnostic index, we could differentiate the two groups at the cutoff value of 0.773 yielding a sensitivity of 100%, specificity of 77.3%, and the AUC value of 0.973. It was an interesting result that could be used as valuable imaging indices for the early diagnosis of persistent idiopathic tinnitus.

Limitations

Several issues should be noticed in the future. First, the sample size was relatively small, and only right-handed subjects were recruited. Second, as a cross-sectional study, we did not conduct this work as a longitudinal study. Future long-term follow-up studies are necessary to document the full-time course of WM microstructure reorganization in tinnitus. Third, as a pilot study, only tinnitus patients without HL and HCs were recruited in our study. In the future, we will try to design more strict experiments, including tinnitus patients with HL, and that's exactly what we're doing recently. Fourth, the definition of tinnitus patients without hearing loss is that there is no hearing loss in the generally recognized frequencies from 250 to 8 kHz; further studies are needed in the future with more accurate instruments to eliminate some possible hidden or slight hearing loss in other frequency ranges.

CONCLUSION

In conclusion, we identified that tinnitus without HL can result in significant alterations in brain white matter microstructure, and some of the changes were related to the tinnitus severity. The changes in patients' WM integrity suggested that there is a close relationship between tinnitus and the limbic system. Moreover, the combination of diffusion parameters of body and genu of CC and LC and RSLF could be used as a valuable imaging index for the diagnosis of early persistent idiopathic tinnitus without HL. These findings added new evidence for the understanding of pathophysiological mechanism of tinnitus.

ETHICS STATEMENT

The studies involving human participants were reviewed and approved by the Institutional Review Board (IRB) of Beijing Friendship Hospital, Capital Medical University. The patients/participants provided their written informed consent to participate in this study.

AUTHOR CONTRIBUTIONS

QC and ZW were responsible for study conception, acquisition, analysis and interpretation of data, drafting of the manuscript, final approval of the version of the manuscript to be publish, and agreement to be accountable for all aspects of the work. HL, PZ, and ZY were responsible for data analysis, final approval of the version of the manuscript to be publish, and agreement to be accountable for all aspects of the work. SG was responsible for revising the manuscript, final approval of the version of the manuscript to be publish, and agreement to be accountable for all aspects of the work. ZW was responsible for study design, manuscript revision, final approval of the version of the manuscript to be publish, and agreement to be accountable for all aspects of the work. All authors contributed to the article and approved the submitted version.

ACKNOWLEDGMENTS

The authors thank the patients and healthy volunteers who participated in this study and gave generously of their time.

REFERENCES

Aldhafeeri, F. M., Mackenzie, I., Kay, T., Alghamdi, J., and Sluming, V. (2012). Neuroanatomical correlates of tinnitus revealed by cortical thickness analysis and diffusion tensor imaging. *Neuroradiology* 54, 883–892. doi: 10.1007/s00234-012-1044-6

Alexander, A. L., Hurley, S. A., Samsonov, A. A., Adluru, N., Hosseinbor, A. P., Mossahebi, P., et al. (2011). Characterization of cerebral white matter properties using quantitative magnetic resonance imaging stains. *Brain Connect.* 1, 423–446. doi: 10.1089/brain.2011.0071

Alexander, A. L., Lee, J. E., Lazar, M., and Field, A. S. (2007). Diffusion tensor imaging of the brain. *Neurotherapeutics* 4, 316–329. doi: 10.1016/j.nurt.2007.05.011

Ashburner, J. (2007). A fast diffeomorphic image registration algorithm. *Neuroimage* 38, 95–113. doi: 10.1016/j.neuroimage.2007.07.007

Benson, R. R., Gattu, R., and Cacace, A. T. (2014). Left hemisphere fractional anisotropy increase in noise-induced tinnitus: a diffusion tensor imaging (DTI) study of white matter tracts in the brain. *Hear. Res.* 309, 8–16. doi: 10.1016/j.heares.2013.10.005

Bledsoe, I. O., Stebbins, G. T., Merkitch, D., and Goldman, J. G. (2018). White matter abnormalities in the corpus callosum with cognitive impairment in Parkinson disease. *Neurology* 91, e2244–e2255. doi: 10.1212/WNL.0000000000006646

Bubb, E. J., Metzler-Baddeley, C., and Aggleton, J. P. (2018). The cingulum bundle: anatomy, function, and dysfunction. *Neurosci. Biobehav. Rev.* 92, 104–127. doi: 10.1016/j.neubiorev.2018.05.008

Cao, Q., Sun, L., Gong, G., Lv, Y., Cao, X., Shuai, L., et al. (2010). The macrostructural and microstructural abnormalities of corpus callosum in children with attention deficit/hyperactivity disorder: a combined morphometric and diffusion tensor MRI study. *Brain Res.* 1310, 172–180. doi: 10.1016/j.brainres.2009.10.031

Catani, M., Howard, R. J., Pajevic, S., and Jones, D. K. (2002). Virtual in vivo interactive dissection of white matter fasciculi in the human brain. *Neuroimage* 17, 77–94. doi: 10.1006/nimg.2002.1136

Chen, Y., Li, X., Liu, L., Wang, J., Lu, C., Yang, M., et al. (2015a). Tinnitus and hyperacusis involve hyperactivity and enhanced connectivity in auditory-limbic-arousal-cerebellar network. *eLife* 4:e06576. doi: 10.7554/eLife.06576

Chen, Y., Xia, W., Feng, Y., Li, X., and Zhang, J. (2015b). Altered interhemispheric functional coordination in chronic tinnitus patients. *Biomed. Res. Intern.* 2015, 1–8. doi: 10.1155/2015/345647

Crippa, A., Lanting, C., Dijk, P. V., and Roerdink, J. B. T. M. (2010). A diffusion tensor imaging study on the auditory system and tinnitus. *Open Neuroimaging J.* 4, 16–25. doi: 10.2174/1874440001004010016

De Ridder, D., De Mulder, G., Menovsky, T., Sunaert, S., and Kovacs, S. (2007). Electrical stimulation of auditory and somatosensory cortices for treatment of tinnitus and pain. *Prog. Brain Res.* 166, 377–388. doi: 10.1016/S0079-6123(07)66036-1

De Ridder, D., Vanneste, S., and Congedo, M. (2011). The distressed brain: a group blind source separation analysis on tinnitus. *PLoS One* 6:e24273. doi: 10.1371/journal.pone.0024273

Diesch, E. (2012). Structural changes of the corpus callosum in tinnitus. *Front. Syst. Neurosci.* 6:17. doi: 10.3389/fnsys.2012.00017

Eggermont, J. J., and Roberts, L. E. (2004). The neuroscience of tinnitus. *Trends Neurosci.* 27, 676–682. doi: 10.1016/j.tins.2004.08.010

Fabri, M., Pierpaoli, C., Barbaresi, P., and Polonara, G. (2014). Functional topography of the corpus callosum investigated by DTI and fMRI. *World J. Radiol.* 6, 895–906. doi: 10.4329/wjr.v6.i12.895

Han, L., Na, Z., Chunli, L., Yuchen, C., Pengfei, Z., Hao, W., et al. (2019). Baseline functional connectivity features of neural network nodes can predict improvement after sound therapy through adjusted narrow band noise in tinnitus patients. *Front. Neurosci.* 13:614. doi: 10.3389/fnins.2019.00614

Hinkley, L. B., Marco, E. J., Findlay, A. M., Honma, S., Jeremy, R. J., Strominger, Z., et al. (2012). The role of corpus callosum development in functional connectivity and cognitive processing. *PLoS One* 7:e39804. doi: 10.1371/journal.pone.0039804

Husain, F. T., Akrofi, K., Carpenter-Thompson, J. R., and Schmidt, S. A. (2015). Alterations to the attention system in adults with tinnitus are modality specific. *Brain Res.* 1620, 81–97. doi: 10.1016/j.brainres.2015.05.010

Husain, F. T., Medina, R. E., Davis, C. W., Szymko-Bennett, Y., Simonyan, K., Pajor, N. M., et al. (2011). Neuroanatomical changes due to hearing loss and chronic tinnitus: a combined VBM and DTI study. *Brain Res.* 1369, 74–88. doi: 10.1016/j.brainres.2010.10.095

Jackowski, A. P., Douglas-Palumberi, H., Jackowski, M., Win, L., Schultz, R. T., Staib, L. W., et al. (2008). Corpus callosum in maltreated children with posttraumatic stress disorder: a diffusion tensor imaging study. *Psychiatry Res* 162, 256–261. doi: 10.1016/j.pscychresns.2007.08.006

Jang, S. H., and Seo, J. P. (2018). Diffusion tensor tractography studies on injured anterior cingulum recovery mechanisms: a mini-review. *Front. Neurol.* 9:1073. doi: 10.3389/fneur.2018.01073

Jones, D. K., Knösche, T. R., and Turner, R. (2013). White matter integrity, fiber count, and other fallacies: the do's and don'ts of diffusion MRI. *Neuroimage* 73, 239–254. doi: 10.1016/j.neuroimage.2012.06.081

Landgrebe, M., Langguth, B., Rosengarth, K., Braun, S., Koch, A., Kleinjung, T., et al. (2009). Structural brain changes in tinnitus: grey matter decrease in auditory and non-auditory brain areas. *Neuroimage* 46, 213–218. doi: 10.1016/j.neuroimage.2009.01.069

Langguth, B., Kleinjung, T., Frank, E., Landgrebe, M., Sand, P., Dvorakova, J., et al. (2008). High-frequency priming stimulation does not enhance the effect of low-frequency rTMS in the treatment of tinnitus. *Exp. Brain Res.* 184, 587–591. doi: 10.1007/s00221-007-1228-1

Leaver, A. M., Renier, L., Chevillet, M. A., Morgan, S., Kim, H. J., and Rauschecker, J. P. (2011). Dysregulation of limbic and auditory networks in tinnitus. *Neuron* 69, 33–43. doi: 10.1016/j.neuron.2010.12.002

Lee, Y., Bae, S., Lee, S., Lee, J., Lee, K., Kim, M., et al. (2007). Evaluation of white matter structures in patients with tinnitus using diffusion tensor imaging. *J. Clin. Neurosci.* 14, 515–519. doi: 10.1016/j.jocn.2006.10.002

Liu, Y., Lv, H., Zhao, P., Liu, Z., Chen, W., Gong, S., et al. (2018). Neuroanatomical alterations in patients with early stage of unilateral pulsatile tinnitus: a voxel-based morphometry study. *Neural Plast.* 2018, 1–7. doi: 10.1155/2018/4756471

Lv, H., Zhao, P., Liu, Z., Liu, X., Ding, H., Liu, L., et al. (2018). Lateralization effects on functional connectivity of the auditory network in patients with unilateral pulsatile tinnitus as detected by functional MRI. *Prog. Neuro Psychopharmacol. Biol. Psychiatry* 81, 228–235. doi: 10.1016/j.pnpbp.2017.09.020

Makris, N., Kennedy, D. N., McInerney, S., Sorensen, A. G., Wang, R., Caviness, V. S., et al. (2005). Segmentation of subcomponents within the superior longitudinal fascicle in humans: a quantitative, in vivo, DT-MRI study. *Cereb. Cortex* 15, 854–869. doi: 10.1093/cercor/bhh186

Maudoux, A., Lefebvre, P., Cabay, J. E., Demertzi, A., Vanhaudenhuyse, A., Laureys, S., et al. (2012). Connectivity graph analysis of the auditory resting state network in tinnitus. *Brain Res.* 1485, 10–21. doi: 10.1016/j.brainres.2012.05.006

Meyer, M., Neff, P., Liem, F., Kleinjung, T., Weidt, S., Langguth, B., et al. (2016). Differential tinnitus-related neuroplastic alterations of cortical thickness and surface area. *Hear. Res.* 342, 1–12. doi: 10.1016/j.heares.2016.08.016

Newman, C. W., Jacobson, G. P., and Spitzer, J. B. (1996). Development of the tinnitus handicap inventory. *Archiv. Otolaryngol. Head Neck Surg.* 122:143.

Plewnia, C., Reimold, M., Najib, A., Reischl, G., Plontke, S. K., and Gerloff, C. (2007). Moderate therapeutic efficacy of positron emission tomography-navigated repetitive transcranial magnetic stimulation for chronic tinnitus: a randomised, controlled pilot study. *J. Neurol. Neurosurg. Psychiatry* 78, 152–156. doi: 10.1136/jnnp.2006.095612

Quigley, M., Cordes, D., Turski, P., Moritz, C., Haughton, V., Seth, R., et al. (2003). Role of the corpus callosum in functional connectivity. *Am. J. Neuroradiol.* 24:208.

Raya, J. G., Horng, A., Dietrich, O., Krasnokutsky, S., Beltran, L. S., Storey, P., et al. (2012). Articular cartilage: in vivo diffusion-tensor imaging. *Radiology* 262, 550–559. doi: 10.1148/radiol.11110821

Ridder, D. D., Elgoyhen, A. B., Romo, R., and Langguth, B. (2011). Phantom percepts: tinnitus and pain as persisting aversive memory networks. *Proc. Natl. Acad. Sci. U.S.A.* 108, 8075–8080. doi: 10.1073/pnas.1018466108

Roland, J. L., Snyder, A. Z., Hacker, C. D., Mitra, A., Shimony, J. S., Limbrick, D. D., et al. (2017). On the role of the corpus callosum in interhemispheric functional connectivity in humans. *Proc. Natl. Acad. Sci. U.S.A.* 114, 13278–13283. doi: 10.1073/pnas.1707050114

Ryu, C., Park, M. S., Byun, J. Y., Jahng, G., and Park, S. (2016). White matter integrity associated with clinical symptoms in tinnitus patients: a tract-based spatial statistics study. *Eur. Radiol.* 26, 2223–2232. doi: 10.1007/s00330-015-4034-3

Schecklmann, M., Lehner, A., Poeppl, T. B., Kreuzer, P. M., Hajak, G., Landgrebe, M., et al. (2012). Cluster analysis for identifying sub-types of tinnitus: a positron emission tomography and voxel-based morphometry study. *Brain Res.* 1485, 3–9. doi: 10.1016/j.brainres.2012.05.013

Schlee, W., Hartmann, T., Langguth, B., and Weisz, N. (2009). Abnormal resting-state cortical coupling in chronic tinnitus. *BMC Neurosci.* 10:11. doi: 10.1186/1471-2202-10-11

Schlee, W., Weisz, N., Bertrand, O., Hartmann, T., and Elbert, T. (2008). Using auditory steady state responses to outline the functional connectivity in the tinnitus brain. *PLoS One* 3:e3720. doi: 10.1371/journal.pone.0003720

Schmidt, S. A., Zimmerman, B., Bido Medina, R. O., Carpenter-Thompson, J. R., and Husain, F. T. (2018). Changes in gray and white matter in subgroups within the tinnitus population. *Brain Res.* 1679, 64–74. doi: 10.1016/j.brainres.2017.11.012

Seydell-Greenwald, A., Raven, E. P., Leaver, A. M., Turesky, T. K., and Rauschecker, J. P. (2014). Diffusion imaging of auditory and auditory-limbic connectivity in tinnitus: preliminary evidence and methodological challenges. *Neural Plast.* 2014, 1-16. doi: 10.1155/2014/145943

Smith, S. M., Jenkinson, M., Johansen-Berg, H., Rueckert, D., Nichols, T. E., Mackay, C. E., et al. (2006). Tract-based spatial statistics: voxelwise analysis of multi-subject diffusion data. *Neuroimage* 31, 1487–1505. doi: 10.1016/j.neuroimage.2006.02.024

Song, S. K., Sun, S. W., Ju, W. K., Lin, S. J., Cross, A. H., and Neufeld, A. H. (2003). Diffusion tensor imaging detects and differentiates axon and myelin degeneration in mouse optic nerve after retinal ischemia. *Neuroimage* 20, 1714–1722. doi: 10.1016/j.neuroimage.2003.07.005

van der Knaap, L. J., and van der Ham, I. J. M. (2011). How does the corpus callosum mediate interhemispheric transfer? a review. *Behav. Brain Res.* 223, 211–221. doi: 10.1016/j.bbr.2011.04.018

Vanneste, S., Heyning, P. V., and Ridder, D. D. (2011a). Contralateral parahippocampal gamma-band activity determines noise-like tinnitus laterality: a region of interest analysis. *Neuroscience* 199, 481–490. doi: 10.1016/j.neuroscience.2011.07.067

Vanneste, S., Plazier, M., van der Loo, E., Van de Heyning, P., and De Ridder, D. (2011b). The difference between uni- and bilateral auditory phantom percept. *Clin. Neurophysiol.* 122, 578–587. doi: 10.1016/j.clinph.2010.07.022

Vanneste, S., van de Heyning, P., and De Ridder, D. (2011c). The neural network of phantom sound changes over time: a comparison between recent-onset and chronic tinnitus patients. *Eur. J. Neurosci.* 34, 718–731. doi: 10.1111/j.1460-9568.2011.07793.x

Wang, F., Kalmar, J. H., Edmiston, E., Chepenik, L. G., Bhagwagar, Z., Spencer, L., et al. (2008). Abnormal corpus callosum integrity in bipolar disorder: a diffusion tensor imaging study. *Biol. Psychiatry* 64, 730–733. doi: 10.1016/j.biopsych.2008.06.001

Xue, C., Shi, L., Hui, S. C. N., Wang, D., Lam, T. P., Ip, C. B., et al. (2018). Altered white matter microstructure in the corpus callosum and its cerebral interhemispheric tracts in adolescent idiopathic scoliosis: diffusion tensor imaging analysis. *Am. J. Neuroradiol.* 39, 1177–1184. doi: 10.3174/ajnr.A5634

8

Prefrontal-Temporal Pathway Mediates the Cross-Modal and Cognitive Reorganization in Sensorineural Hearing Loss with or without Tinnitus: A Multimodal MRI Study

*Ying Luan, Congxiao Wang, Yun Jiao, Tianyu Tang, Jian Zhang and Gao-Jun Teng**

Jiangsu Key Laboratory of Molecular and Functional Imaging, Department of Radiology, Zhongda Hospital, Medical School of Southeast University, Nanjing, China

Correspondence:
Gao-Jun Teng
gjteng@vip.sina.com

Objective: Hearing loss, one main risk factor of tinnitus and hyperacusis, is believed to involve significant central functional abnormalities. The recruitment of the auditory cortex in non-auditory sensory and higher-order cognitive processing has been demonstrated in the hearing-deprived brain. The dorsolateral prefrontal cortex (dlPFC), which has dense anatomical connections with the auditory pathway, is known to play a crucial role in multi-sensory integration, auditory regulation, and cognitive processing. This study aimed to verify the role of the dlPFC in the cross-modal reorganization and cognitive participation of the auditory cortex in long-term sensorineural hearing loss (SNHL) by combining functional and structural measurements.

Methods: Thirty five patients with long-term bilateral SNHL and 35 matched healthy controls underwent structural imaging, resting-state functional magnetic resonance imaging (rs-fMRI), diffusion tensor imaging (DTI), and neuropsychological assessments. Ten SNHL patients were with subjective tinnitus.

Results: No differences in gray matter volume, spontaneous neural activity, or diffusion characteristics in the dlPFC were found between the SNHL and control groups. The functional connectivity (FC) between the dlPFC and the auditory cortex and visual areas, such as the cuneus, fusiform, lingual cortex, and calcarine sulcus was increased in patients with SNHL. ANOVA and *post hoc* tests revealed similar FC alterations in the SNHL patients with and without tinnitus when compared with the normal hearing controls, and SNHL patients with and without tinnitus showed no difference in the dlPFC FC. The FC in the auditory cortex was associated with the symbol digit modality test (SDMT) scores in the SNHL patients, which reflect attentional function, processing speed, and visual working memory. Hearing-related FC with the dlPFC was found in the lingual cortex. A tract-based spatial statistics (TBSS) analysis revealed decreased fractional anisotropy (FA) values, mainly in the temporal inferior fronto-occipital fasciculus (IFOF), which showed remarkable negative correlations with the mean hearing thresholds in SNHL.

Conclusion: Higher functional coupling between the dlPFC and auditory and visual areas, accompanied by decreased FA along the IFOF connecting the frontal cortex and the occipito-temporal area, might mediate cross-modal plasticity via top-down regulation and facilitate the involvement of the auditory cortex in higher-order cognitive processing following long-term SNHL.

Keywords: sensorineural hearing loss, dorsolateral prefrontal cortex, multimodal MRI, resting-state functional connectivity, tract-based spatial statistics, cross-modal reorganization, cognition, tinnitus

INTRODUCTION

Approximately half a billion people are suffering from disabling hearing deprivation, accounting for 6–8% of the global population (Wilson et al., 2017). Hearing loss is associated with several common hearing disorders, such as tinnitus and hyperacusis (Eggermont and Roberts, 2004; Knipper et al., 2013). Since the most discussed pathology of tinnitus and hyperacusis is the elevated central auditory gain as a response to the loss of peripheral auditory input, hearing loss is one of the main risk factors to develop these hearing impairments (Knipper et al., 2013). The exploration of the neural abnormalities of hearing loss might be essential to develop a better understanding of the neural mechanisms underlying tinnitus, hyperacusis or other hearing disorders. Previous research indicates that widespread functional reorganization, within both the central auditory system and the non-auditory brain, is involved in hearing loss. The association between hearing loss and the raised risk of cognitive and emotional impairments has been widely accepted (Smith and Pichora-Fuller, 2015; Rutherford et al., 2018). No specific treatment has been proven effective for hearing loss. Hearing aids and cochlear implants are two major ways to partially restore the perception of environmental sounds and speech, but they are of limited value, particularly with regard to the cognitive decline, affective disorders, and social isolation that occur in cases of severe or profound hearing loss (Dawes et al., 2015; Rutherford et al., 2018).

Cross-modal plasticity is an intrinsic ability of the central multi-sensory brain, and refers to the recruitment of resources from the deprived modality into the intact sensory processing; it is known as a compensatory adaption of wide-ranging brain circuits (Glick and Sharma, 2017). Cross-modal reorganization has been well-documented in hearing loss. A functional near-infrared spectroscopy study revealed a stronger response in the auditory cortex elicited by visual motion stimulation in deaf patients compared to normal-hearing controls (Dewey and Hartley, 2015). The N1 visual evoked potential was reported in the temporal lobe in patients with hearing loss, although they had received cochlear implants (Buckley and Tobey, 2011). The auditory cortex in patients with early moderate hearing loss also shows robust activation to somatosensory stimuli (Cardon and Sharma, 2018). However, the exact principles of where and how the cross-modal organization happens following hearing loss remain poorly understood. Although it has been proposed that this reorganization might result from changes in local connectivity, supported by altered sensory maps, recent opinions emphasize the promising role of long-ranging connections in cross-modal reorganization. Besides, those studies on cross-modal activation overlooked the spontaneous functional architecture associated with hearing deprivation, as revealed by a recent study that showed cross-modal functional coupling patterns were different between resting state and sensory stimuli (Pelland et al., 2017).

Apart from low-level sensory processing, accumulating evidence has indicated that the deprived auditory cortex is also recruited for higher-order cognitive functions. Language stimuli-evoked activation in the superior temporal gyrus (STG) of deaf patients shows enhanced functional coupling with frontal areas, which correlates with the language learning function (Que et al., 2018). Activation in the auditory cortex was also elicited during the visual working memory task in patients with early hearing loss, suggesting that the functional modification related to hearing loss might not be explained by a bottom-up mechanism only (Ding et al., 2015). These results indicate that cross-modal reorganization might also rely on interactions with the fronto-parietal areas, which are thought to process higher-order cognitive functions.

The dorsolateral PFC (dlPFC) plays a crucial role in top-down regulation (O'Reilly, 2010), multi-sensory integration (Fuster et al., 2000), and cognitive function, including working memory (Wang et al., 2015), decision making (Philiastides et al., 2011), and response inhibition (Gläscher et al., 2012). Anatomically, the dlPFC receives multiple sensory afferents from the sensory cortices (Jones and Powell, 1970; Romanski et al., 1999), which support its multi-sensory integration, notably for sight and sound. The dlPFC also directly projects axons to the thalamic reticular nucleus (TRN), including the auditory portion, which is involved in negative regulation of auditory thalamo-cortical communication (Zikopoulos and Barbas, 2006). The dense connections between the dlPFC and the sensory areas provide a convenient circuit for cross-modal plasticity and top-down regulation (Morrone, 2010). Hence, we hypothesize that the dlPFC might mediate the recruitment of the auditory cortex in cross-modal plasticity and higher-order cognitive functions in hearing loss.

To verify our hypotheses, we evaluated the structural and functional properties of the dlPFC by combining multimodal magnetic resonance imaging (MRI) techniques. We aimed to determine whether the functional coupling pattern of the dlPFC changes following long-term sensorineural hearing loss (SNHL) with and without accompanying tinnitus, with a particular focus on the multiple sensory areas, and its relevance to hearing perception and higher-order cognitive performance. We further evaluated the properties of the white matter microstructure of the prefrontal-temporal pathway using a tract-based spatial statistics (TBSS) approach. We aimed to identify the dlPFC as a potential biomarker underlying the cross-modal reorganization and cognitive participation of the auditory cortex related to SNHL.

MATERIALS AND METHODS

Participants

Thirty-five patients with long-term bilateral SNHL were recruited for this study (all right-handed, 21 men and 14 women, 31–69 years old). All of these SNHL patients reported consistent hearing loss over the duration from the onset age of 3–42 years. Hearing loss was caused due to a clinical history of ototoxic drug application in one case of the SNHL subjects, others had no clear etiology. Ten of these SNHL patients were accompanied by mild subjective tinnitus. Thirty-five age-, sex-, and education-matched normal-hearing controls were also included in this study (all right-handed, 17 men and 18 women, age range: 32–69 years). All participants were Chinese Han. The criteria for the inclusion of the patients with long-term bilateral SNHL were as follows: (1) age range: 20–70 years; (2) clinically diagnosed SNHL with a disease duration above 3 years; (3) post-lingual hearing loss; (4) bilateral hearing loss with mean hearing thresholds above 25 dB HL for both ears. The criteria of exclusion for both the SNHL and control groups were as follows: clinically diagnosed Meniere's disease and acoustic neuroma, a clinical history of head injury, cancer, stroke or otologic surgery, poorly controlled diabetes or hypertension, seizures, Multiple Sclerosis, Parkinson's disease, Alzheimer's disease, depression, schizophrenia, and other neuropsychiatric diseases. This research was approved by the Ethics Committee of Affiliated Zhongda Hospital of Southeast University. A written informed consent was obtained from each of the participants before the experiment. All procedures were performed in accordance with the Declaration of Helsinki.

Audiological Assessment

The hearing thresholds were measured at the frequency of 250, 500, 1000, 2000, 4000, and 8000 Hz via pure tone audiometry using a GSI-61 audiometer. The monaural mean hearing threshold was computed as the averaged value of the air conduction thresholds at 500, 1000, 2000, and 4000 Hz. The binaural mean hearing threshold was calculated by averaging the monaural mean hearing thresholds. Acoustic immittance was performed to exclude hearing loss due to conductive deafness. All subjects in the control group had mean thresholds <25 dB HL for both ears. All subjects in the SNHL group had mean thresholds >25 dB for both ears.

Neuropsychological Assessment

A series of neuropsychological assessments that covered the relevant cognitive or emotional domains were conducted with all participants. The tests for each participant took approximately 1 h to complete and were administered by the same researcher in the same order. For cognitive assessment, the general cognitive state was evaluated by the Mini Mental State Examination (MMSE) (Galea and Woodward, 2005). The functions involving attention, visual scanning, and working memory, and the processing seed were assessed by the Symbol Digit Modalities Test (SDMT) (Smith, 1982). The episodic memory of verbal information was assessed by the Auditory Verbal Learning Test (AVLT) (Schmidt, 1996), comprising an immediate recall, a 5-min delayed recall, and a 20-min delayed recall test. For emotional assessment, possible depression, and anxiety states were determined via the Hamilton Depression Rating Scale (HAM-D) (Hamilton, 1960) and the Self-Rating Anxiety Scale (SAS) (Zung, 1971), respectively.

MRI Data Acquisition

All participants underwent brain structural, resting state fMRI (rs-fMRI), and diffusion tensor imaging (DTI) scanning in a Siemens 3.0 T MRI scanner (Siemens, Erlangen, Germany) with a 12-channel head coil at the Department of Radiology, Affiliated Zhongda Hospital of Southeast University. Soft foam padding was used to alleviate head motion; earplugs and a headphone were used to alleviate the noise during scanning. The participants were instructed to keep their head still, eyes closed, and avoid thinking about anything in particular during the MRI scanning. Structural images were acquired using a high-resolution three-dimensional magnetization-prepared rapid gradient-echo (3D MPRAGE) T1-weighted sequence. The sequence parameters were as follows: repetition time: 1900 ms, echo time: 2.48 ms, flip angle: 9.0°, inversion time: 900 ms, slice number: 176, slice thickness: 1.0 mm, field of view: 250 mm × 250 mm, matrix: 256 × 256. Functional raw data were obtained using a gradient-recalled echo-planar imaging (GRE-EPI) sequence in an interleaved order. The sequence parameters were as follows: repetition time: 1900 ms, echo time: 2.48 ms, flip angle: 90.0°, slice number: 32, slice thickness: 4.0 mm, the field of view: 240 mm × 240 mm, matrix: 64 × 64, volumes number: 240. The DTI raw data were acquired using a single-shot echo planar imaging sequence (EPI) with the following parameters: repetition time: 5800 ms, echo time: 82 ms, flip angle: 90°, slice number: 31, slice thickness: 4.0 mm, *b*-values: 0 and 1000 s/mm^2, acquired resolution: 2 mm × 2 mm × 2 mm, direction: 30, matrix: 128 × 128.

Structural Data Analyses

To avoid the impact of structural damage on the functional measurements, we computed the volume of gray matter (GM) and white matter (WM) for each participant using the voxel-based morphometry (VBM) method via the SPM8 toolbox. The T1-weighted images of each subject were segmented into the GM, WM, and cerebro-spinal fluid and then non-linearly normalized to the standard Montreal Neurological Institute (MNI) space. The images after normalization were smoothed with an 8-mm full-width at half-maximum (FWHM) Gaussian kernel. The whole-brain GM and WM volumes were calculated by estimating the segments. The voxel-based between-group difference in GM and WM was determined via analysis of variance (ANOVA) using a general linear model (GLM) with age, sex, and education included as nuisance covariates of no interest. Significant differences were determined to have a

p-value threshold <0.05 corrected by the false discovery rate (FDR) method for multiple comparison correction. The region of interest (ROI)-based VBM analysis was used to compare the regional GM volume between two groups. The ROIs were defined from the Brodmann template as the bilateral dlPFC. The subject-specific GM data within the ROI were exacted from the normalized and smoothed GM images.

Functional Data Preprocessing and Analyses

The Statistical Parametric Mapping software (SPM8[1]) and the Data Processing and Analysis for Brain Imaging V2.3 (DPABI[2]) toolbox were used to preprocess the fMRI data including the following steps: exclusion of the first 10 volumes; slice-timing for correcting the differences in acquisition time between slices; realignment for head motion correction; spatial normalization to a standard template in the MNI space using a DARTAL approach followed by reslicing into 3 mm × 3 mm × 3 mm voxel size; spatial smoothing with a Gaussian kernel size of 6 mm × 6 mm × 6 mm FWHM; linear detrending; nuisance covariate regression for the white matter and cerebrospinal fluid signal and the head motion parameters; bandpass filter with the frequency window from 0.01 to 0.1 Hz. Subjects were excluded if their head motion exceeded 2.0 mm in the x, y, z plane, or 2.0° of axial rotation. No participant was excluded in the current study due to head motion.

Functional Connectivity and Hearing-Related Functional Connectivity Analyses

The seed-based functional connectivity (FC) analysis was implemented using the Resting-state fMRI Data Analysis Toolkit (REST[3]). The region of interest (ROI) in the left and right dlPFC was defined using the Wake Forest University (WFU) PickAtlas software[4] (Macaluso and Driver, 2001) from the Brodmann template. The mean time series for each ROI were extracted and the Pearson's correlation coefficients were calculated between the mean time series of the ROIs and each voxel across the brain. Fisher's r-to-z transformation was implemented for each voxel to improve normality. The FC z-score map was generated for each participant. The between-group differences between the SNHL and control groups were determined by the ANOVA analysis using a GLM with age, sex, and education as the nuisance covariates of no interest. Differences with a $p < 0.05$ were deemed statistically significant, using an FDR method for multiple comparison correction. A one-way ANOVA was performed to determine the main effect of group on dlPFC FC among SNHL without tinnitus, SNHL with tinnitus and control groups, with age, sex, and education as the nuisance covariates of no interest. Then the two-sample t-tests masked by the ANOVA main effect results were used to identify (1) SNHL patients without tinnitus vs. controls, (2) SNHL patients with tinnitus vs. healthy controls, and (3) SNHL patients without tinnitus vs. SNHL patients with tinnitus. Differences with a $p < 0.05/3$ were deemed statistically significant for *post hoc* two-sample t-tests, using an FDR method for multiple comparison correction. A hearing-related FC map was calculated by correlating the binaural mean hearing thresholds with the FC z-scores of each voxel, with the ROI set at the left and right dlPFC, respectively, in all SNHL patients, with age, sex, and education as the covariates. Significant differences were considered with a cluster threshold of $p < 0.05$ using the Gaussian Random Field method at a voxel height of $p < 0.001$.

Amplitude of Low-Frequency Fluctuation Calculation

The whole brain amplitude of low-frequency fluctuation (ALFF) was calculated for each participant using the REST software. The preprocessed time series of each voxel was transformed to a power spectrum via a fast-Fourier transform. The square root of the power spectrum was calculated at each frequency and averaged across a low-frequency (0.01–0.1 Hz) domain to acquire the amplitude (Zou et al., 2015). Then the individual ALFF map was transferred into a z-score map by subtracting the averaged ALFF value. The mean ALFF z-scores were extracted from the bilateral dlPFC for each participant.

Diffusion Imaging Preprocessing and Analyses

The DTI data processing was performed using the FMRIB Software Library (FSL[5]). The skulls were removed using the brain extraction tool of FSL. FMRIB's Diffusion Toolbox was used to correct head motion and the distortions resulting from the eddy currents, estimate the diffusion tensor, and generate the fractional anisotropy (FA) map and mean diffusion (MD) maps for each participant. Finally, the individual FA and MD maps were directly registered to the high-resolution FMRIB58 template in a 1 mm × 1 mm × 1 mm standard MNI152 space using a non-linear algorithm.

Diffusion Measurements of the dlPFC

The normalized FA and MD maps were spatially smoothed with a Gaussian kernel size of 6 mm × 6 mm × 6 mm FWHM. Again, the averaged FA and MD values of the bilateral dlPFC were obtained from each of the participants referring to the Brodmann template.

Tract-Based Spatial Statistics

The TBSS analysis was employed following the pipeline of FSL. Briefly, the mean WM tract skeleton was generated in the normalized space with the threshold of FA >0.2, representing the central fiber bundles across all participants. Then all FA maps were projected to the mean FA skeleton. The voxelwise FA values in the WM skeleton were compared between the SNHL group and the control group using a randomization test with 5000 permutations in FSL, with age, sex, and education included as covariates. The statistical significance was set at $p < 0.05$ and we corrected for multiple comparisons using the threshold-free cluster enhancement method (TFCE).

[1] http://www.fil.ion.ucl.ac.uk/spm/

[2] http://rfmri.org/dpabi/

[3] http://www.restfmri.net/forum/

[4] http://www.ansir.wfubmc.edu

[5] http://www.fmrib.ox.ac.uk/fsl

Statistical Analyses

Group differences in age, education, mean hearing thresholds, results of neuropsychological tests, GM volume, ALFF, FA values and MD values in ROIs between SNHL patients and healthy controls were determined with a Student's *t*-test. Group differences in age, education, and mean hearing thresholds among the SNHL with tinnitus, SNHL without tinnitus and healthy control group were determined with one-way ANOVA. Group difference in sex was determined by the chi-square test (SPSS, 19 software, Chicago, IL, United States). Differences with $p < 0.05$ were considered to be statistically significant. The correlations between the functional or structural parameters and clinical variants in the SNHL group were assessed using a partial correlation analysis, controlling for age, sex, and education. Differences with $p < 0.05$ were considered to be statistically significant. To determine the power of the differences observed from the seed-based FC analysis, we used the receiver operating characteristic (ROC) curve analysis and calculated the area under the curve. All data are presented as the mean ± standard deviation (SD).

RESULTS

Demographic, Hearing, and Neuropsychological Characteristics

Thirty five patients with SNHL and 35 healthy controls were included. All of the SNHL subjects had a history of long-term consistent hearing loss when this study was conducted. The mean duration of auditory deprivation in the SNHL subjects was 9.29 ± 8.95 years. Most of them acquired the hearing loss with no clear cause. There was no difference in age, sex, education, handedness, or ethnicity between the SNHL group and control group. The mean hearing thresholds of the left and right side were above 40 dB HL in the SNHL group (**Figure 1**). There was no significant difference between the two sides ($p = 0.109$). The mean hearing thresholds of both sides in the control group were significantly lower than in the SNHL group and were within the normal range (<20 dB HL). There was no significant difference between the two sides ($p = 0.622$). Relative to healthy controls, patients with SNHL presented significantly increased SAS and HAM-D scores, and significantly decreased AVLT-5 scores. No other between-group difference was found with regard to the MMSE, AVLT, AVLT-20, or SDMT tests. The detailed demographic, hearing, and neuropsychological results are shown in **Table 1**.

Among the 35 long-term SNHL patients, 10 subjects were accompanied by subjective tinnitus. As illustrated in **Table 2**, there was no significant difference among the SNHL patients with tinnitus, SNHL patients without tinnitus, and healthy controls in age ($F = 0.835$, $p = 0.438$), gender ($\chi^2 = 1.485$, $p = 0.476$) or education ($F = 0.775$, $p = 0.465$). *Post hoc* Least-Significance Difference (LSD) tests revealed no significant difference in the left mean hearing threshold ($p = 0.263$), right mean hearing threshold ($p = 0.901$), or bilateral mean hearing threshold ($p = 0.440$) between the SNHL patients with tinnitus and SNHL patients without tinnitus.

Structural Results

No significant difference in the GM or WM volumes of the whole brain was observed between the SNHL and control groups at a threshold of $p < 0.05$ corrected by FDR.

Regional Multimodal Measurements of the dlPFC

As illustrated by **Table 3**, no significant difference in the ALFF, GM volume, FA, or MD value was detected in the SNHL group when compared to the control group for both the left and right dlPFC.

Seed-Based FC With Bilateral dlPFC

The FC patterns of the left and right dlPFC were significantly different between the SNHL and control groups, as presented in **Figure 2A** and **Table 4**. When the ROI was set to the left dlPFC, the right superior temporal gyrus (STG), supplementary motor area (SMA), and several visual areas, including the right cuneus, calcarine sulcus, and left fusiform gyrus, showed significantly enhanced FC in the SNHL group. When the ROI was set to the right dlPFC, the right STG and left lingual gyrus showed significantly enhanced FC in the SNHL group. In the SNHL group, the SDMT scores were positively correlated

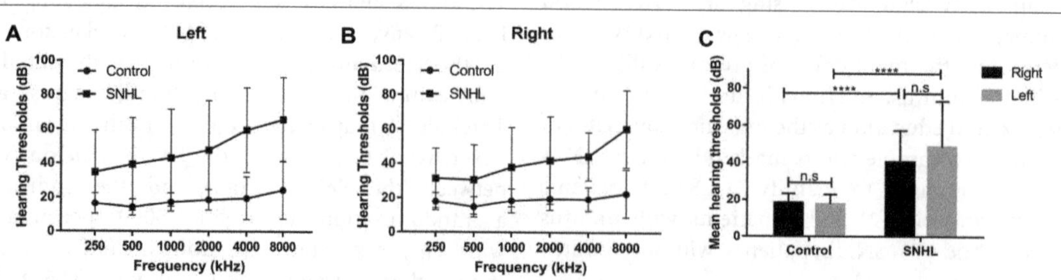

FIGURE 1 | The hearing thresholds of **(A)** right side and **(B)** left side at 250, 500, 1000, 2000, 4000, and 8000 Hz in the control and SNHL groups. **(C)** No side differences in mean hearing thresholds are shown for either group. The mean hearing thresholds for each side in patients with SNHL are significantly higher than in healthy controls. The data are shown as mean ± standard deviation. ****$p < 0.0001$.

TABLE 1 | Demographic, clinical, and neuropsychological characteristics of the patients with SNHL and healthy controls.

	SNHL patients (n = 35)	Healthy controls (n = 35)	t/χ^2	P-value
Age (years)	54.49 ± 9.45	55.97 ± 7.80	−0.717	0.476
Gender (M/F)	21/14	17/18	0.921	0.337
Education (years)	11.09 ± 3.28	11.51 ± 3.46	−0.531	0.597
Handedness (R/L)	35/0	35/0		
Mean PTA of right ear (dB HL)	40.28 ± 16.98	18.12 ± 5.20	7.319	<0.0001****
Mean PTA of left ear (dB HL)	48.48 ± 24.59	17.46 ± 5.44	7.253	<0.0001****
Averaged PTA of both ears (dB HL)	44.38 ± 19.03	17.78 ± 4.89	7.954	<0.0001****
Duration of hearing loss (years)	9.29 ± 8.95	–	–	–
Neuropsychological tests				
MMSE	29.49 ± 0.83	29.83 ± 0.47	−1.929	0.058
AVLT	17.09 ± 3.53	17.28 ± 5.43	−0.162	0.872
AVLT-5	6.11 ± 2.10	7.17 ± 1.54	−2.259	0.027*
AVLT-20	6.06 ± 2.27	6.50 ± 2.05	−0.812	0.420
SDMT	37.66 ± 12.13	40.86 ± 8.24	−1.209	0.231
HAM-D	6.20 ± 3.90	4.21 ± 2.47	2.481	0.016*
SAS	31.14 ± 7.98	27.41 ± 4.02	2.418	0.019*

*All data are presented as mean ± standard deviation. *p < 0.05, ****p < 0.0001. M/F, male/female; R/L, right/left; PTA, pure tone audiometry from 0.5 to 4 kHz; MMSE, Mini Mental State Examination; AVLT, Auditory Verbal Learning Test; AVLT-5, Auditory Verbal Learning Test 5-min recall; AVLT-20, Auditory Verbal Learning Test 20-min recall; SDMT, Symbol Digit Modalities Test; HAM-D, Hamilton Depression Rating Scale; SAS, Self-Rating Anxiety Scale.*

TABLE 2 | Demographical and clinical comparisons of the SNHL subgroups and control group.

	SNHL patients without tinnitus (n = 25)	SNHL patients with tinnitus (n = 10)	Healthy controls (n = 35)	Significance, p-value
Age (years)	55.48 ± 9.79	52.00 ± 8.50	55.97 ± 7.80	$F = 0.835, p = 0.438^a$
Gender (M/F)	16/9	5/5	17/18	$\chi^2 = 1.485, p = 0.476$
Education (years)	10.68 ± 3.19	12.10 ± 3.48	11.51 ± 3.46	$F = 0.775, p = 0.465^a$
Handedness (R/L)	25/0	10/0	35/0	–
Mean PTA of right ear (dB HL)	40.46 ± 17.65	39.84 ± 16.05	18.12 ± 5.20	$p = 0.901^b$
Mean PTA of left ear (dB HL)	50.72 ± 24.19	42.89 ± 25.99	17.46 ± 5.44	$p = 0.263^b$
Averaged PTA of both ears (dB HL)	45.59 ± 18.62	41.37 ± 20.74	17.78 ± 4.89	$p = 0.440^b$

[a]ANOVA: SNHL without tinnitus, SNHL with tinnitus and healthy controls. χ^2 test: SNHL without tinnitus, SNHL with tinnitus and healthy controls. [b]Post hoc Least-Significance Difference (LSD) test: SNHL without tinnitus and SNHL with tinnitus.

with left dlPFC-seeded FC in the right cuneus and STG, and with right dlPFC-seeded FC in the right STG (**Figures 2B–D**), after controlling for the effects of age, sex, and education. The area under the receiver operating characteristic curve (AUC) of the temporal and occipital clusters with significant between-group differences in the FC with the left (**Figure 3A**) and right (**Figure 3B**) dlPFC were all above 0.75.

To further determine the effect of tinnitus associated with hearing loss on the dlPFC FC changes, we divided the SNHL patients into two subgroups and compared the dlPFC among the SNHL patients without tinnitus, SNHL patients with tinnitus and healthy controls (**Figure 4**). When the ROI was set to the left dlPFC, right STG, SMA, and several visual areas, including right fusiform, calcarine, and cuneus, and left lingual gyrus, fusiform gyrus, and calcarine sulcus, showed significantly enhanced FC when comparing the SNHL patients without tinnitus with healthy controls. Left lingual gyrus and fusiform gyrus showed significantly enhanced FC when comparing the SNHL patients with tinnitus with healthy controls. No significant difference was observed when comparing the SNHL patients without tinnitus with SNHL patients with tinnitus. When the ROI was set to the right dlPFC, the right STG and left lingual gyrus showed significantly increased FC when comparing the SNHL patients without tinnitus with healthy controls. Left lingual gyrus showed significantly increased FC when comparing the SNHL patients with tinnitus with healthy controls. No significant difference was observed when comparing the SNHL patients without tinnitus with SNHL patients with tinnitus.

Hearing-Related dlPFC-Seeded FC

In patients with long-term SNHL, several brain regions showed hearing-related FC with the dlPFC. **Table 5** presents the cluster size, cluster coordinates, and statistics. **Figure 5A** shows the anatomical locations of the significant clusters. FC in the left lingual gyrus and right anterior prefrontal cortex (aPFC) with the left dlPFC exhibited significant positive correlations with the binaural mean hearing thresholds with age, sex, and education considered as nuisance covariates. The mean FC z-scores in the left lingual gyrus were extracted and were found to be positively associated with the binaural mean hearing thresholds ($p < 0.0001$, **Figure 5B**), controlling for the effects of age, sex, and education.

TABLE 3 | Multimodal measurements of the bilateral dlPFC.

Metrics	SNHL patients	Healthy controls	*t*	*P*-value
Left dlPFC				
ALFF *z*-score	−0.0178 ± 0.1323	0.0300 ± 0.2434	−1.023	0.310
GM volume	0.2978 ± 0.0363	0.2959 ± 0.0388	0.224	0.824
FA value	0.0699 ± 0.0028	0.0702 ± 0.0039	−0.412	0.682
MD value	0.0007 ± 0.0001	0.0007 ± 0.0001	1.709	0.092
Right dlPFC				
ALFF *z*-score	−0.0905 ± 0.1466	−0.0622 ± 0.2103	−0.653	0.516
GM volume	0.3225 ± 0.0425	0.3249 ± 0.0368	−0.243	0.809
FA value	0.0862 ± 0.0034	0.0875 ± 0.0046	−1.297	0.200
MD value	0.0007 ± 0.0001	0.0007 ± 0.0001	0.863	0.391

Data are shown as mean ± standard deviation. dlPFC, dorsolateral prefrontal cortex; ALFF, amplitude of low-frequency fluctuation; GM, gray matter; FA, fractional anisotropy; MD, mean diffusion.

Similarly, the FC in the right lingual gyrus and right aPFC with the right dlPFC exhibited significant positive correlations with the binaural mean hearing thresholds, with age, sex, and education considered as nuisance covariates in patients with SNHL. The mean FC *z*-scores in the right lingual gyrus were extracted and positively associated with the binaural mean hearing thresholds ($p < 0.0001$, **Figure 5C**), controlling for the effects of age, sex, and education.

Comparison of FA Values Between Patients With SNHL and Controls Using TBSS

Several clusters with altered FA values were found in patients with SNHL compared with healthy controls (**Figure 6A**). The patients with SNHL showed reduced FA values within the WM skeleton in the bilateral inferior fronto-occipital fasciculus (IFOF), inferior longitudinal fasciculus (ILF), and superior longitudinal fasciculus (SLF), particularly in the temporal part near the auditory cortex. The mean FA value extracted from the significant cluster in the right temporal lobe exhibited a negative correlation with binaural mean hearing thresholds in

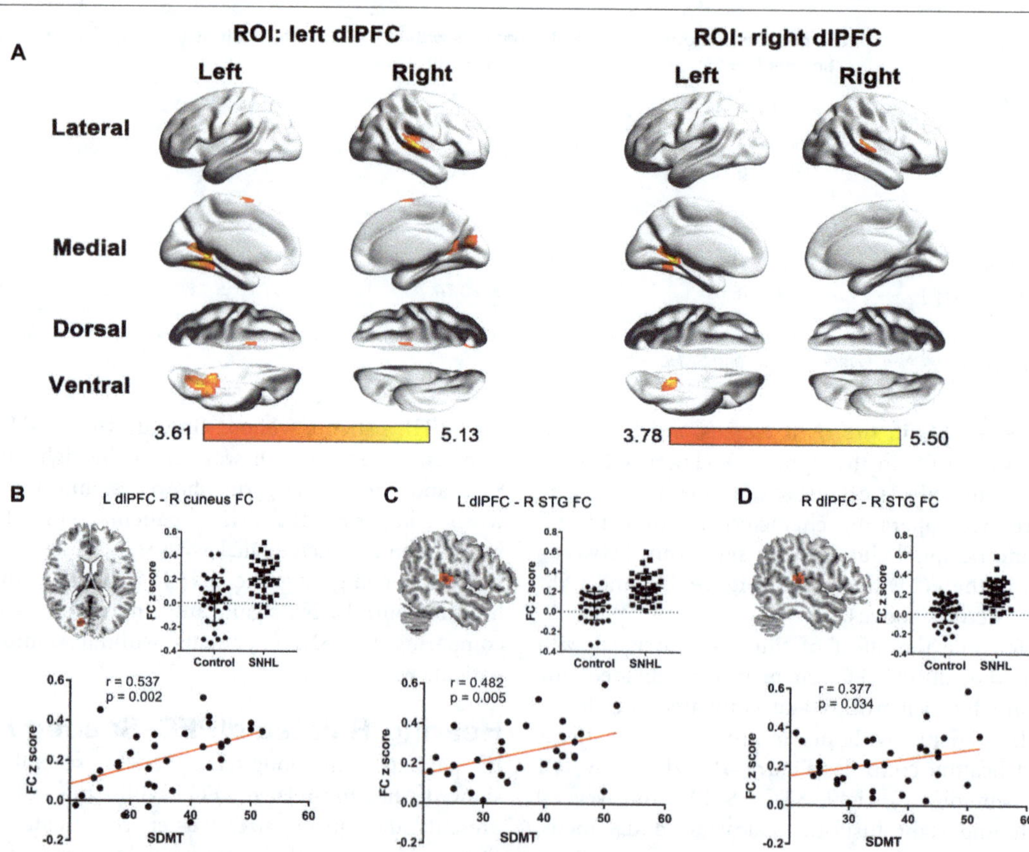

FIGURE 2 | **(A)** The between-group difference distribution map of FC with the seed set to the left and right dlPFC independent of age, sex, or education ($p < 0.05$, corrected by FDR). Significantly increased FC is present in the red-yellow heat scales. The color bar below shows the *t*-scores obtained from the between-group comparisons. The SDMT scores are positively correlated with the left dlPFC-seeded FC in the right cuneus **(B)**, left dlPFC-seeded FC in the right STG **(C)**, and the right dlPFC-seeded FC in the right STG **(D)** in patients with SNHL, after controlling for age, sex, and education. FC, functional connectivity; dlPFC, dorsolateral prefrontal cortex; FDR, false discovery rate; SDMT, Symbol Digit Modalities Test; STG, superior temporal gyrus; ROI, region of interest; L, left; R, right.

TABLE 4 | Differences in FC in patients with SNHL compared with healthy controls when the ROI was set at the left and right dlPFC.

Brain region	BA	Voxel size	Peak MNI coordinates (mm)			Peak *t*-values
			X	*Y*	*Z*	
Left dlPFC						
SNHL patients > healthy controls						
Right cuneus	18	28	15	−81	18	4.3364
Right calcarine sulcus	17	25	27	−51	6	4.4442
Right superior temporal gyrus	22/41/42	87	51	−30	6	5.0824
Supplementary motor area	6	42	6	0	75	4.4006
Left fusiform gyrus	37	118	−21	−45	−3	5.1345
Right dlPFC						
SNHL patients > Healthy controls						
Right superior temporal gyrus	41/42	40	51	−27	6	5.3037
Left lingual gyrus	18	36	−21	−45	−3	5.5005

FC, functional connectivity; ROI, region of interest; BA, Brodmann's area; MNI, Montreal Neurological Institute.

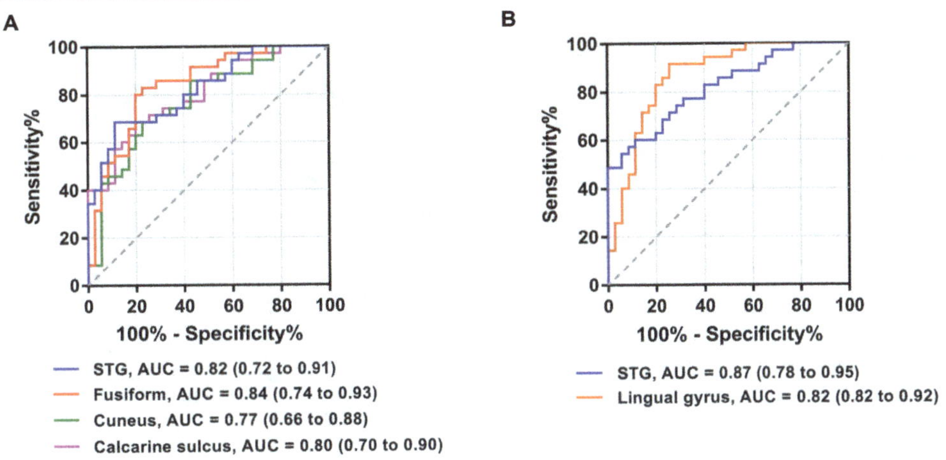

FIGURE 3 | Receiver operating characteristic curves for differentiating patients with SNHL and healthy controls based on the significant FC with the left dlPFC **(A)** and right dlPFC **(B)**. AUC, area under the receiver operating characteristic curve.

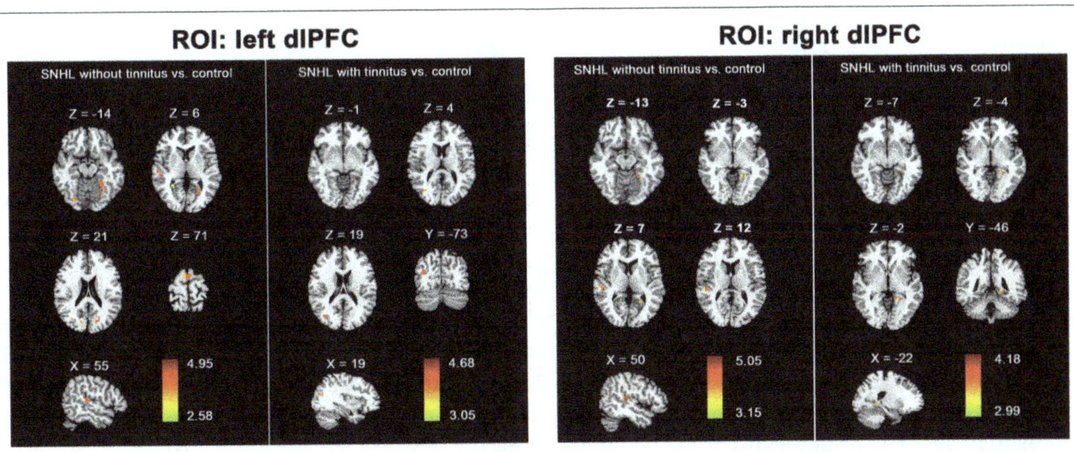

FIGURE 4 | The between-group difference distribution map of FC with the seed set to the left and right dlPFC among the SNHL without tinnitus, SNHL with tinnitus, and healthy controls, independent of age, sex, or education ($p < 0.05/3$, corrected by FDR). Significantly increased FC is present in the red-yellow heat scales. The color bars show the t scores obtained from the between-group comparisons.

TABLE 5 | Hearing-related FC with the dlPFC in patients with SNHL.

Brain region	BA	Voxel size	Peak MNI coordinates (mm)			Peak *z*-values
			X	*Y*	*Z*	
Left dlPFC						
Left lingual gyrus	18	109	−18	−96	−3	4.1467
Right anterior prefrontal cortex	10	33	24	63	9	3.7206
Right dlPFC						
Right lingual gyrus	18	44	21	−81	−12	5.2721
Right anterior prefrontal cortex	10	74	27	57	24	3.9782

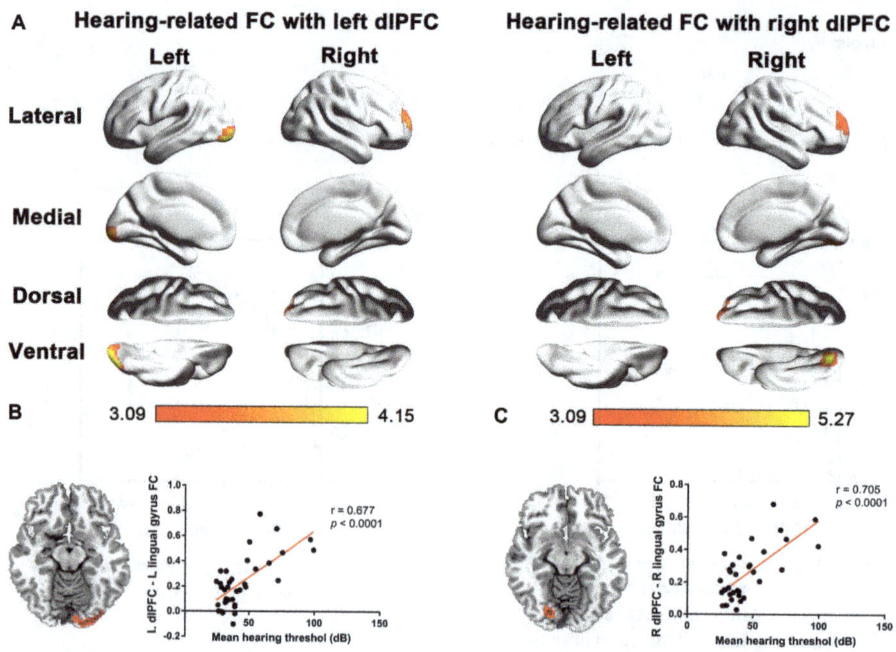

FIGURE 5 | (A) Voxel-wise hearing-related FC patterns with the left and right dlPFC in patients with SNHL, independent of age, sex, and education. Significant positive correlations are presented in the red-yellow heat scales. The color bar below shows the *z*-scores. The scatterplots show the correlations in the patients with SNHL between the binaural mean hearing thresholds with the mean left dlPFC-seeded FC in the left lingual gyrus **(B)** and the mean right dlPFC-seeded FC in the right lingual gyrus **(C)**, which were shown to be significant by the voxel-wise correlation analysis, after controlling for the effects of age, sex, and education.

patients with SNHL (**Figure 6B**), controlling the effects of age, sex, and education.

DISCUSSION

Recruitment of the auditory cortex into cross-modal and higher-order cognitive processing has been reported following hearing deprivation. We hypothesized that the connectivity between the dlPFC and auditory cortex or other brain areas might play a role in this. We assessed both local properties and long-ranging connectivity properties of the dlPFC by combining functional and structural measurements. The results showed that no ALFF, GM volume, FA, or MD changes occurred in the dlPFC. However, the distant functional coupling between the dlPFC and auditory cortex and multiple visual areas were remarkably increased in patients with SNHL independent of tinnitus. The long-ranging FC between the dlPFC and auditory cortex is associated with cognitive performance linking attentional function, information processing speed, and visual working memory in the subjects with SNHL. Higher levels of hearing loss contribute to stronger dlPFC-visual cortex coupling. Decreased FA values within the mean WM skeleton were observed in several central fiber bundles in SNHL, particularly in the temporal lobe near auditory cortex, which is associated with the degree of hearing loss.

In line with our local measurement results, most previous functional and structural imaging studies did not report significant regional changes of spontaneous neural activity, GM volume, or WM microstructure properties in the dlPFC in hearing loss (Li et al., 2012; Hribar et al., 2014; Lin et al., 2014; Rachakonda et al., 2014; Yang et al., 2014; Wang et al., 2016). Therefore, we speculate that the way by which the dlPFC regulates functional reorganization following SNHL is more likely via long-ranging connectivity rather than local functional

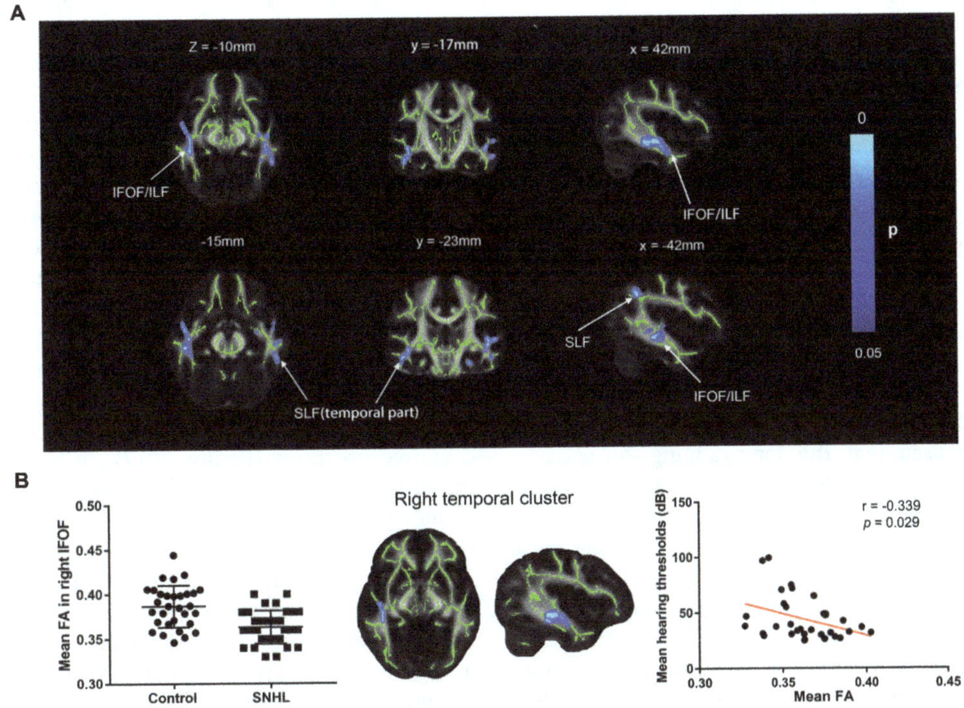

FIGURE 6 | (A) Distribution map of the FA value that was significantly lower in the SNHL group compared with the control group based on the TBSS analysis. The mean FA skeleton (green) is overlaid with the blue clusters denoting significantly decreased FA values in patients with SNHL. The color bar on the left presents the *p*-value. The mean FA values in the significant cluster of the right temporal lobe are positively correlated with the binaural mean hearing thresholds in patients with SNHL, after controlling for the effects of the age, sex, and education **(B)**. FA, fractional anisotropy; IFOF, inferior fronto-occipital fasciculus; ILF, inferior longitudinal fasciculus; SLF, superior longitudinal fasciculus.

or structural alterations. However, one recent rs-fMRI study reported increased ALFF in the dlPFC in patients with severe congenital hearing loss (Xia et al., 2017). This discrepancy could be related to the differences in the patients that were focused on, since in the current study, we recruited patients who acquired SNHL late and with a relatively wide range of hearing loss.

Prior behavioral, neuroimaging, and electrophysiological studies have provided convincing evidence of cross-modal plasticity following sensory modality deprivation, such as hearing loss and blindness; however, there is still much debate about where and how this kind of functional reorganization happens (Xia et al., 2017). Cross-modal plasticity and multisensory integration are influenced by bottom-up cochlear hearing loss (Sharma, 2014, 2017) and top-down regulation from cortical areas (Levin et al., 2007). One of the most robust candidates is the prefrontal top-down attentional control. The human brain has a limited capacity for information processing and can make a selection from the considerable inputs from the multiple sensory environments for dominant sensory stimuli. The competition among these sensory signals relies upon a bottom-up processing by which the salience stimuli evokes a robust cortical response, and a top-down regulation by which neural activity is biased toward a specific pattern relevant to the current behavioral intention (Kastner et al., 1998; Moore and Zirnsak, 2017). Selective attention regulates normal sensory processing. In cases of sensory deprivation, cross-modal reorganization is also mediated by the attentional transition from the deprived modality to the retained modalities via top-down modulation from the prefrontal cortex (PFC) (Morrone, 2010). Hearing loss can contribute to auditory attention deficits (Nagarkar and Panda, 2007; Park et al., 2016). A previous study revealed a cascade-of-control model during attention-demanding tasks, in which the dlPFC performs the top-down attentional control prior to the attentional selection modulated by the dorsal anterior cingulate cortex (dACC) (Silton et al., 2010). The dlPFC is one of the most described top-down control PFC regions in earlier studies (MacDonald et al., 2000; Dosenbach et al., 2006, 2008). Besides, cross-modal plasticity is assumed to rely on both multimodal brain structure and the unimodal brain areas. For example, visuo-tactile stimuli could elicit activation in the visual cortex when the tactile stimuli was on the same side as the visual target. The visual cortex also exhibited higher effective connectivity from the multimodal inferior parietal area and somatosensory cortex in the spatially congruent bimodal tasks. These findings indicate that the inferior parietal area, which is involved in the spatial and attentional processing, integrates the bimodal information and mediates the recruitment of the visual cortex to the sensory stimuli in cross-modal plasticity of spatial attention (Macaluso et al., 2000). Similar to the inferior parietal region, the dlPFC is also a multimodal brain area. In particular, the dlPFC is rich in audio-visual associative cells, supporting the involvement of the dlPFC in audio-visual association and integration (Fuster et al., 2000). The lesion of the dlPFC leads to deficiencies in discriminating auditory and visual stimuli (Petrides, 1986). Based on this notion, we proposed that the hypersynchrony of the dlPFC with both the auditory and visual cortices might reflect the adaptive reorganization of the audio-visual integration under circumstances of hearing loss, which facilitates the participation of the auditory cortex in visual processing. Besides, our voxelwise correlation analyses revealed that the hearing-related dlPFC FC was also located in the visual cortex, indicating that the reinforced functional integration between the dlPFC and the visual cortex was owing to the loss of peripheral hearing. Taken together, these findings suggest that hearing loss leads to cross-modal reorganization between the auditory and visual modalities, which is probably mediated by the dlPFC.

It has been proposed that the long-ranging connectivity between the PFC and the multiple sensory areas might mediate the recruitment of the deprived sensory cortices into high-order cognitive functions. The dlPFC has dense anatomical connections with the auditory cortex. In normal hearing subjects, these kinds of connections regulate auditory processing through attention control (Knight et al., 1995). The dlPFC lesions contribute to reduced attention effects during an auditory selective attention task (Knight et al., 1981). However, when SNHL is present, the innervation from the high-order cognitive circuit, such as the prefrontal areas, might lead the auditory cortex to participate more in higher-order cognitive functions. Moreover, the connections between the auditory cortex and the prefrontal multimodal areas are greater than other sensory cortices, such as the visual cortex (Beer et al., 2011; Yeterian et al., 2012). The takeover by prefrontal high-order cognitive areas in the auditory cortex might thus be a major pattern of functional reorganization in SNHL (Bedny, 2017). Findings from several recent studies on hearing loss have supported this hypothesis. The STG exhibited robust activation during a visual working memory task in deaf individuals, and this predicted the speed and accuracy of their working memory performances. Moreover, deaf individuals had stronger effective connectivity from the prefrontal eye field to the STG, implying the effects of the PFC on the participation of the auditory cortex in working memory processing (Ding et al., 2015). Resting-state FC between the STG and dorsal anterior cingulate cortex also predicted spatial working memory performances in patients with hearing loss (Ding et al., 2016). Apart from working memory, the auditory cortex is also implicated in language processing in hearing loss. A word recognition task led to enhanced activity in the auditory cortex, dlPFC, and inferior frontal cortex in older adults with hearing loss (Kuchinsky et al., 2016). Greater activation was also observed in the auditory cortex which depended on the degree of hearing loss during a sign language task (Lambertz et al., 2005). Larger and stronger response in auditory cortex to both natural speech and unintelligible speech understanding tasks was correlated with their speech understanding performances in the hearing loss patients, even though they already had the cochlear implants which partially restored their hearing (Olds et al., 2016). A recently proposed theory of cognitive pluripotency in the sensory cortices might account for these findings. During development, the auditory cortex is pluripotent, with the capability of performing a variety of low-level auditory and high-level cognitive functions based on its intrinsic physiology, including the local and long-ranging connectivity among the auditory pathway, other sensory cortices, and prefrontal high-order cognitive areas. The functional specialization depends on the input during development, confined by experience and connectivity (Gao and Suga, 2000). Under normal conditions, the dominant function of auditory cortex is processing the information in the acoustic signal, which is transmitted along the hierarchical bottom-up auditory processing system (Irvine, 2007). Altered information transmission causes cortical specialization. The loss of auditory input leads the intrinsic long-ranging connectivity from the prefrontal areas to recruit the auditory cortex into a series of cognitive processes (Bedny, 2017). In order to assess whether the dlPFC is involved in high-order cognitive takeover in the auditory cortex in SNHL, we correlated the elevated dlPFC FC in the STG with the SDMT performances in patients with SNHL. The finding of their association was in line with the previous theory that the long-ranging connectivity linking the prefrontal areas and auditory cortex contributes to functional modification in the auditory deprived brain. Previous event-related fMRI studies revealed activation in the fronto-parietal network and visual areas during SDMT tests, including the dlPFC, cuneus, and lingual gyrus (Forn et al., 2009, 2013; Akbar et al., 2016; Dobryakova et al., 2016). The SDMT requires the visual tracking, scanning, and attention regulated by the visual areas, as well as the attentional control, memory coding, working memory, and inferential reasoning involving the dlPFC (Silva et al., 2018). In the current study, the enhanced FC between the dlPFC and cuneus was also associated with the SDMT performances in the patients with SNHL, suggesting that the stronger functional integration between the dlPFC and visual cortex also contributed to faster information processing speed in SNHL. We propose that this result might be due to the hearing loss caused by the reinforced attention shift from the auditory modality to the visual modality, which was implicated in SDMT processing.

Regarding the seed-based FC results, remarkably enhanced dlPFC FC was mainly located in the STG and the visual cortex, including the cuneus, lingual gyrus, calcarine sulcus, and the fusiform gyrus. All of these abnormalities of dlPFC FC presented fair to excellent distinguishing power ($0.7 < AUC < 1$) when differentiating patients with SNHL from healthy controls, indicating that the dlPFC might be a potential imaging marker to identify patients with SNHL with cross-modal and higher-order cognitive reorganization in the auditory cortex. In addition, after we divided the SNHL patients into two subgroups according to whether they were accompanied by tinnitus, these two subgroups showed similar FC changes (i.e., increased dlPFC FC in the auditory and visual areas) when compared with the healthy controls, and no between-group difference. These findings indicate that the accompanying tinnitus makes negligible impacts on the hearing loss-related functional reorganization between the dlPFC with auditory, and visual areas. Tinnitus is generally accepted to be associated with the maladaptive plasticity of the auditory deafferentation caused by auditory deprivation (De Ridder et al., 2014). Previous functional imaging studies revealed the hyperactivity in the auditory area and the coactivation of some other brain areas, such as dlPFC (Vanneste et al., 2010). Electrophysiologic study has indicated that the tinnitus might be associated with the dysfunction in the dlPFC-dependent top-down inhibitory auditry modulation (Norena et al., 1999). However, we did not find additional impacts made by the tinnitus on the dlPFC FC beyond the SNHL. One of the possible explanations might be that the effects of the relatively mild tinnitus did not overweigh the profound effects of long-term bilateral hearing loss on the dlPFC FC pattern. Another interpretation might be the very limited sample size of the SNHL patients accompanied by the tinnitus and the heterogeneity of the tinnitus characteristics.

It is also important to understand the neural mechanisms underlying such reorganization in the auditory cortex in SNHL and distinguish the structural aspects from the functional aspects. Although the pathological substrates of DTI damage are still not clear, developing quantitative evaluations of the DTI metrics will provide a powerful tool to understand the microstructural features of the WM in the central brain. FA, a DTI measurement of the directional diffusion of water within the WM tracts, depends on the anatomical characteristics of the axonal microstructure (Scholz et al., 2009). A reduced FA value was observed in the bilateral IFOF, ILF, and SLF, particularly within the temporal lobe near the STG, in the SNHL group. These results were consistent with prior DTI studies conducted on deaf individuals (Kim et al., 2009; Husain et al., 2011; Stevens et al., 2017). The IFOF connects the lateral frontal cortex with the occipital and temporal lobes, the ILF links the ipsilateral occipital and temporal lobes, and the SLF connects the fronto-parietal and fronto-temporal areas (Catani et al., 2002). The temporal cortex facilitates these main WM tracts to communicate with the fronto-parietal and occipital regions. The reduced FA value in the temporal WM near the auditory cortex is speculated to be associated with the disuse in the auditory cortex due to the loss of the peripheral auditory input; lower FA with greater magnitudes of hearing loss found in the current study might support this assumption. Since the FA value is known to reflect the fiber density, fiber amount, and the degree of myelination (Schmithorst et al., 2005), one interpretation for the neural basis of such plasticity might be that the loss of peripheral auditory input resulted in the disuse-driven WM microstructural alterations in the temporal lobe near auditory cortex, such as axonal loss and demyelination (Song et al., 2002; Kim et al., 2009). In addition to the WM integrity damages of the fiber tracts, the FA value could also be affected by the distribution patterns of the WM fibers. Hence, another possible explanation might be the compensatory mechanism, which means other fibers expanding into this region result in more disordered WM tracts (Husain et al., 2011). Such compensation might provide the neuroanatomical substrate for cross-modal reorganization and the cognitive recruitment of the auditory cortex (Shiell and Zatorre, 2016; Karns et al., 2017). Although the exact underlying mechanism of both resting-state FC and the FA changes is difficult to understand, one possible interpretation might be that the functional connectivity is largely constrained by the structural connectivity (Sporns et al., 2009; Supekar et al., 2009). A previous study has indicated the association between neural activity and myelination by addressing the cellular substrates (Demerens et al., 1996). Hence, the intrinsic WM connectivity between the frontal and temporal areas, as an infrastructure, might mediate the functional coupling changes.

Surprisingly, we found that the functional abnormality of the STG was particularly located in the right side, even though the patients recruited in the current study all had bilateral SNHL. This might be due to the tendency of their higher hearing loss to be on the left side. Another possible explanation might be related to the specification of hemisphere dominance. Phonetic and language processing is left hemisphere dominant in the primary auditory cortex, and pitch processing is right hemisphere dominant in the primary auditory cortex (Zatorre et al., 1992). Prior studies indicate the important role of the left STG in sign language in individuals with hearing loss (MacSweeney et al., 2002; Sakai et al., 2005). Our patients with SNHL mostly had mild to moderate hearing loss, and none of these patients use sign language. We suggested that the right STG would be the predominately influenced area in the functional reorganization related to the loss of auditory input. Consistent with our finding, a previous study also found regional homogeneity in the right STG, but not the left STG, was altered in individuals with acquired bilateral hearing loss (Li et al., 2013).

Several limitations of this study must be acknowledged. First, because of the cross-sectional nature of this study, we were unable to track the dynamic progression of the SNHL. Further longitudinal studies will address this question. Second, although the total pool of subjects in the SNHL and the control groups was more than 30, the sample size was not large enough to divide the patients into different subgroups according to different cognitive or emotional states or by the severity or frequency of characteristics of hearing loss. We were able to partially overcome this problem by performing correlation analyses. Third, the blood-oxygen-level dependent (BOLD) signal is a reflection of local cerebral blood changes and is not a direct measure of neural activity. Combining rs-MRI with other non-invasive techniques, such as electroencephalography or magnetoencephalography, might be helpful to better understand the brain-wise neurophysiological mechanisms underlying SNHL and the cognitive associated with SNHL. Finally, the neuropsychological tests applied in the current study were relatively rudimentary. Future research will address the neural mechanisms underlying the more specific higher-order functions related to SNHL.

In summary, the current study substantiated the role of the prefrontal area, particularly the dlPFC, in the recruitment of the auditory area into cross-sensory and higher-order processing through a top-down control in conditions of long-term bilateral SNHL, by providing combined functional and structural neuroimaging evidence. Our findings enhance the understanding of cortical pluripotency and the underlying mechanisms of cross-modal reorganization and cognitive participation in the deprived auditory cortex.

AUTHOR CONTRIBUTIONS

YL conducted the experiments, recruited the participants, analyzed the data, and wrote the manuscript. CW helped with the integration of the data. YJ and TT helped with the analyses of the data. JZ helped the data collection. G-JT directed this study, designed the research, and gave key advice.

REFERENCES

Akbar, N., Banwell, B., Sled, J. G., Binns, M. A., Doesburg, S. M., Rypma, B., et al. (2016). Brain activation patterns and cognitive processing speed in patients with pediatric-onset multiple sclerosis. *J. Clin. Exp. Neuropsychol.* 38, 393–403. doi: 10.1080/13803395.2015.1119255

Bedny, M. (2017). Evidence from blindness for a cognitively pluripotent cortex. *Trends Cogn. Sci.* 21, 637–648. doi: 10.1016/j.tics.2017.06.003

Beer, A. L., Plank, T., and Greenlee, M. W. (2011). Diffusion tensor imaging shows white matter tracts between human auditory and visual cortex. *Exp. Brain Res.* 213, 299–308. doi: 10.1007/s00221-011-2715-y

Buckley, K., and Tobey, E. (2011). Cross-modal plasticity and speech perception in pre- and postlingually deaf cochlear implant users. *Ear Hear.* 32, 2–15. doi: 10.1097/AUD.0b013e3181e8534c

Cardon, G., and Sharma, A. (2018). Somatosensory cross-modal reorganization in adults with age-related, early-stage hearing loss. *Front. Hum. Neurosci.* 12:172. doi: 10.3389/fnhum.2018.00172

Catani, M., Howard, R. J., Pajevic, S., and Jones, D. K. (2002). Virtual in vivo interactive dissection of white matter fasciculi in the human brain. *Neuroimage* 17, 77–94. doi: 10.1006/nimg.2002.1136

Dawes, P., Emsley, R., Cruickshanks, K., Moore, D., Fortnum, H., Edmondson-Jones, M., et al. (2015). Hearing loss and cognition: the role of hearing AIDS, social isolation and depression. *PLoS One* 10:e0119616. doi: 10.1371/journal.pone.0119616

De Ridder, D., Vanneste, S., and Freeman, W. (2014). The Bayesian brain: phantom percepts resolve sensory uncertainty. *Neurosci. Biobehav. Rev.* 44, 4–15. doi: 10.1016/j.neubiorev.2012.04.001

Demerens, C., Stankoff, B., Logak, M., Anglade, P., Allinquant, B., Couraud, F., et al. (1996). Induction of myelination in the central nervous system by electrical activity. *Proc. Natl. Acad. Sci. U.S.A.* 93, 9887–9892. doi: 10.1073/pnas.93.18.9887

Dewey, R., and Hartley, D. (2015). Cortical cross-modal plasticity following deafness measured using functional near-infrared spectroscopy. *Hear. Res.* 325, 55–63. doi: 10.1016/j.heares.2015.03.007

Ding, H., Ming, D., Wan, B., Li, Q., Qin, W., and Yu, C. (2016). Enhanced spontaneous functional connectivity of the superior temporal gyrus in early deafness. *Sci. Rep.* 6:23239. doi: 10.1038/srep23239

Ding, H., Qin, W., Liang, M., Ming, D., Wan, B., Li, Q., et al. (2015). Cross-modal activation of auditory regions during visuo-spatial working memory in early deafness. *Brain* 138(Pt 9), 2750–2765. doi: 10.1093/brain/awv165

Dobryakova, E., Costa, S. L., Wylie, G. R., DeLuca, J., and Genova, H. M. (2016). Altered effective connectivity during a processing speed task in individuals with multiple sclerosis. *J. Int. Neuropsychol. Soc.* 22, 216–224. doi: 10.1017/s1355617715001034

Dosenbach, N., Visscher, K., Palmer, E., Miezin, F., Wenger, K., Kang, H., et al. (2006). A core system for the implementation of task sets. *Neuron* 50, 799–812. doi: 10.1016/j.neuron.2006.04.031

Dosenbach, N. U., Fair, D. A., Cohen, A. L., Schlaggar, B. L., and Petersen, S. E. (2008). A dual-networks architecture of top-down control. *Trends Cogn. Sci.* 12, 99–105. doi: 10.1016/j.tics.2008.01.001

Eggermont, J. J., and Roberts, L. E. (2004). The neuroscience of tinnitus. *Trends Neurosci.* 27, 676–682. doi: 10.1016/j.tins.2004.08.010

Forn, C., Belloch, V., Bustamante, J., Garbin, G., Parcet-Ibars, M., Sanjuan, A., et al. (2009). A symbol digit modalities test version suitable for functional MRI studies. *Neurosci. Lett.* 456, 11–14. doi: 10.1016/j.neulet.2009.03.081

Forn, C., Ripolles, P., Cruz-Gomez, A. J., Belenguer, A., Gonzalez-Torre, J. A., and Avila, C. (2013). Task-load manipulation in the Symbol Digit Modalities Test: an alternative measure of information processing speed. *Brain Cogn.* 82, 152–160. doi: 10.1016/j.bandc.2013.04.003

Fuster, J., Bodner, M., and Kroger, J. (2000). Cross-modal and cross-temporal association in neurons of frontal cortex. *Nature* 405, 347–351. doi: 10.1038/35012613

Galea, M., and Woodward, M. (2005). Mini-mental state examination (MMSE). *Aust. J. Physiother.* 51:198. doi: 10.1016/S0004-9514(05)70034-9

Gao, E., and Suga, N. (2000). Experience-dependent plasticity in the auditory cortex and the inferior colliculus of bats: role of the corticofugal system. *Proc. Natl. Acad. Sci. U.S.A.* 97, 8081–8086. doi: 10.1073/pnas.97.14.8081

Gläscher, J., Adolphs, R., Damasio, H., Bechara, A., Rudrauf, D., Calamia, M., et al. (2012). Lesion mapping of cognitive control and value-based decision making in the prefrontal cortex. *Proc. Natl. Acad. Sci. U.S.A.* 109, 14681–14686. doi: 10.1073/pnas.1206608109

Glick, H., and Sharma, A. (2017). Cross-modal plasticity in developmental and age-related hearing loss: clinical implications. *Hear. Res.* 343, 191–201. doi: 10.1016/j.heares.2016.08.012

Hamilton, M. (1960). A rating scale for depression. *J. Neurol. Neurosurg. Psychiatry* 23, 56–62. doi: 10.1136/jnnp.23.1.56

Hribar, M., Suput, D., Carvalho, A. A., Battelino, S., and Vovk, A. (2014). Structural alterations of brain grey and white matter in early deaf adults. *Hea. Res.* 318, 1–10. doi: 10.1016/j.heares.2014.09.008

Husain, F. T., Medina, R. E., Davis, C. W., Szymko-Bennett, Y., Simonyan, K., Pajor, N. M., et al. (2011). Neuroanatomical changes due to hearing loss and chronic tinnitus: a combined VBM and DTI study. *Brain Res.* 1369, 74–88. doi: 10.1016/j.brainres.2010.10.095

Irvine, D. R. (2007). Auditory cortical plasticity: Does it provide evidence for cognitive processing in the auditory cortex? *Hear. Res.* 229, 158–170. doi: 10.1016/j.heares.2007.01.006

Jones, E., and Powell, T. (1970). An anatomical study of converging sensory pathways within the cerebral cortex of the monkey. *Brain* 93, 793–820. doi: 10.1093/brain/93.4.793

Karns, C. M., Stevens, C., Dow, M. W., Schorr, E. M., and Neville, H. J. (2017). Atypical white-matter microstructure in congenitally deaf adults: a region of interest and tractography study using diffusion-tensor imaging. *Hear. Res.* 343, 72–82. doi: 10.1016/j.heares.2016.07.008

Kastner, S., De Weerd, P., Desimone, R., and Ungerleider, L. (1998). Mechanisms of directed attention in the human extrastriate cortex as revealed by functional MRI. *Science* 282, 108–111. doi: 10.1126/science.282.5386.108

Kim, D. J., Park, S. Y., Kim, J., Lee, D. H., and Park, H. J. (2009). Alterations of white matter diffusion anisotropy in early deafness. *Neuroreport* 20, 1032–1036. doi: 10.1097/WNR.0b013e32832e0cdd

Knight, R. T., Grabowecky, M. F., and Scabini, D. (1995). Role of human prefrontal cortex in attention control. *Adv. Neurol.* 66, 21–36.

Knight, R. T., Hillyard, S. A., Woods, D. L., and Neville, H. J. (1981). The effects of frontal cortex lesions on event-related potentials during auditory selective attention. *Electroencephalogr. Clin. Neurophysiol.* 52, 571–582. doi: 10.1016/0013-4694(81)91431-0

Knipper, M., Van Dijk, P., Nunes, I., Ruttiger, L., and Zimmermann, U. (2013). Advances in the neurobiology of hearing disorders: recent developments regarding the basis of tinnitus and hyperacusis. *Prog. Neurobiol.* 111, 17–33. doi: 10.1016/j.pneurobio.2013.08.002

Kuchinsky, S. E., Vaden, K. I. Jr., Ahlstrom, J. B., Cute, S. L., Humes, L. E., Dubno, J. R., et al. (2016). Task-related vigilance during word recognition in noise for older adults with hearing loss. *Exp. Aging Res.* 42, 50–66. doi: 10.1080/0361073X.2016.1108712

Lambertz, N., Gizewski, E. R., de Greiff, A., and Forsting, M. (2005). Cross-modal plasticity in deaf subjects dependent on the extent of hearing loss. *Brain Res. Cogn. Brain Res.* 25, 884–890. doi: 10.1016/j.cogbrainres.2005.09.010

Levin, H., Koval, M., and Everling, S. (2007). Top-down control-signal dynamics in anterior cingulate and prefrontal cortex neurons following task switching. *Neuron* 53, 453–462. doi: 10.1016/j.neuron.2006.12.023

Li, J., Li, W., Xian, J., Li, Y., Liu, Z., Liu, S., et al. (2012). Cortical thickness analysis and optimized voxel-based morphometry in children and adolescents with prelingually profound sensorineural hearing loss. *Brain Res.* 1430, 35–42. doi: 10.1016/j.brainres.2011.09.057

Li, Y., Booth, J. R., Peng, D., Zang, Y., Li, J., Yan, C., et al. (2013). Altered intra- and inter-regional synchronization of superior temporal cortex in deaf people. *Cereb. Cortex* 23, 1988–1996. doi: 10.1093/cercor/bhs185

Lin, F. R., Ferrucci, L., An, Y., Goh, J. O., Doshi, J., Metter, E. J., et al. (2014). Association of hearing impairment with brain volume changes in older adults. *Neuroimage* 90, 84–92. doi: 10.1016/j.neuroimage.2013.12.059

Macaluso, E., and Driver, J. (2001). Spatial attention and crossmodal interactions between vision and touch. *Neuropsychologia* 39, 1304–1316. doi: 10.1016/S0028-3932(01)00119-1

Macaluso, E., Frith, C., and Driver, J. (2000). Modulation of human visual cortex by crossmodal spatial attention. *Science* 289, 1206–1208. doi: 10.1126/science.289.5482.1206

MacDonald, A., Cohen, J., Stenger, V., and Carter, C. (2000). Dissociating the role of the dorsolateral prefrontal and anterior cingulate cortex in cognitive control. *Science* 288, 1835–1838. doi: 10.1126/science.288.5472.1835

MacSweeney, M., Woll, B., Campbell, R., McGuire, P. K., David, A. S., Williams, S. C., et al. (2002). Neural systems underlying British Sign Language and audio-visual English processing in native users. *Brain* 125, 1583–1593. doi: 10.1093/brain/awf153

Moore, T., and Zirnsak, M. (2017). Neural mechanisms of selective visual attention. *Annu. Rev. Psychol.* 68, 47–72. doi: 10.1146/annurev-psych-122414-033400

Morrone, M. C. (2010). Brain development: critical periods for cross-sensory plasticity. *Curr. Biol.* 20, R934–R936. doi: 10.1016/j.cub.2010.09.052

Nagarkar, A., and Panda, N. (2007). Intervention strategies in children with cochlear implants having attention deficit hyperactivity disorder. *Int. J. Pediatr. Otorhinolaryngol.* 71, 985–988. doi: 10.1016/j.ijporl.2007.02.020

Norena, A., Cransac, H., and Chery-Croze, S. (1999). Towards an objectification by classification of tinnitus. *Clin. Neurophysiol.* 110, 666–675. doi: 10.1016/S1388-2457(98)00034-0

Olds, C., Pollonini, L., Abaya, H., Larky, J., Loy, M., Bortfeld, H., et al. (2016). Cortical activation patterns correlate with speech understanding after cochlear implantation. *Ear Hear.* 37:e160. doi: 10.1097/AUD.0000000000000258

O'Reilly, R. C. (2010). The What and How of prefrontal cortical organization. *Trends Neurosci.* 33, 355–361. doi: 10.1016/j.tins.2010.05.002

Park, S., Ahn, M., and Min, B. (2016). Top-down and bottom-up neurodynamic evidence in patients with tinnitus. *Hear. Res.* 342, 86–100. doi: 10.1016/j.heares.2016.10.002

Pelland, M., Orban, P., Dansereau, C., Lepore, F., Bellec, P., and Collignon, O. (2017). State-dependent modulation of functional connectivity in early blind individuals. *Neuroimage* 147, 532–541. doi: 10.1016/j.neuroimage.2016.12.053

Petrides, M. (1986). The effect of periarcuate lesions in the monkey on the performance of symmetrically and asymmetrically reinforced visual and auditory go, no-go tasks. *J. Neurosci.* 6, 2054–2063. doi: 10.1523/JNEUROSCI.06-07-02054.1986

Philiastides, M., Auksztulewicz, R., Heekeren, H., and Blankenburg, F. (2011). Causal role of dorsolateral prefrontal cortex in human perceptual decision making. *Curr. Biol.* 21, 980–983. doi: 10.1016/j.cub.2011.04.034

Que, M., Jiang, X., Yi, C., Gui, P., Jiang, Y., Zhou, Y., et al. (2018). Language and sensory neural plasticity in the superior temporal cortex of the deaf. *Neural Plast.* 2018:9456891. doi: 10.1155/2018/9456891

Rachakonda, T., Shimony, J. S., Coalson, R. S., and Lieu, J. E. (2014). Diffusion tensor imaging in children with unilateral hearing loss: a pilot study. *Front. Syst. Neurosci.* 8:87. doi: 10.3389/fnsys.2014.00087

Romanski, L. M., Tian, B., Fritz, J., Mishkin, M., Goldman-Rakic, P. S., and Rauschecker, J. P. (1999). Dual streams of auditory afferents target multiple domains in the primate prefrontal cortex. *Nat. Neurosci.* 2, 1131–1136. doi: 10.1038/16056

Rutherford, B. R., Brewster, K., Golub, J. S., Kim, A. H., and Roose, S. P. (2018). Sensation and psychiatry: linking age-related hearing loss to late-life depression and cognitive decline. *Am. J. Psychiatry* 175, 215–224. doi: 10.1176/appi.ajp.2017.17040423

Sakai, K. L., Tatsuno, Y., Suzuki, K., Kimura, H., and Ichida, Y. (2005). Sign and speech: amodal commonality in left hemisphere dominance for comprehension of sentences. *Brain* 128, 1407–1417. doi: 10.1093/brain/awh465

Schmidt, M. (1996). *Rey Auditory Verbal Learning Test: A Handbook.* Los Angeles, CA: Western Psychological Services.

Schmithorst, V. J., Wilke, M., Dardzinski, B. J., and Holland, S. K. (2005). Cognitive functions correlate with white matter architecture in a normal pediatric population: a diffusion tensor MRI study. *Hum. Brain Mapp.* 26, 139–147. doi: 10.1002/hbm.20149

Scholz, J., Klein, M. C., Behrens, T. E., and Johansen-Berg, H. (2009). Training induces changes in white-matter architecture. *Nat. Neurosci.* 12, 1370–1371. doi: 10.1038/nn.2412

Sharma, A. (2014). Cross-modal re-organization in adults with early stage hearing loss. *PLoS One* 9:e90594. doi: 10.1371/journal.pone.0090594

Sharma, A. (2017). Cross-modal plasticity in developmental and age-related hearing loss: clinical implications. *Hear. Res.* 343, 191–201. doi: 10.1016/j.heares.2016.08.012

Shiell, M. M., and Zatorre, R. J. (2016). White matter structure in the right planum temporale region correlates with visual motion detection thresholds in deaf people. *Hear. Res.* 343, 64–71. doi: 10.1016/j.heares.2016.06.011

Silton, R. L., Heller, W., Towers, D. N., Engels, A. S., Spielberg, J. M., Edgar, J. C., et al. (2010). The time course of activity in dorsolateral prefrontal cortex and anterior cingulate cortex during top-down attentional control. *Neuroimage* 50, 1292–1302. doi: 10.1016/j.neuroimage.2009.12.061

Silva, P. H. R., Spedo, C. T., Barreira, A. A., and Leoni, R. F. (2018). Symbol digit modalities test adaptation for magnetic resonance imaging environment: a systematic review and meta-analysis. *Mult. Scler. Relat. Disord.* 20, 136–143. doi: 10.1016/j.msard.2018.01.014

Smith, A. (1982). *Symbol Digit Modalities Test (SDMT): Manual.* Los Angeles, CA: Western Psychological Services.

Smith, S., and Pichora-Fuller, M. (2015). Associations between speech understanding and auditory and visual tests of verbal working memory: effects of linguistic complexity, task, age, and hearing loss. *Front. Psychol.* 6:1394. doi: 10.3389/fpsyg.2015.01394

Song, S.-K., Sun, S.-W., Ramsbottom, M. J., Chang, C., Russell, J., and Cross, A. H. (2002). Dysmyelination revealed through MRI as increased radial (but unchanged axial) diffusion of water. *Neuroimage* 17, 1429–1436. doi: 10.1006/nimg.2002.1267

Sporns, O., Cammoun, L., Gigandet, X., Thiran, J., Meuli, R., and Hagmann, P. (2009). Predicting human resting-state functional connectivity from structural connectivity. *Proc. Natl. Acad. Sci. U.S.A.* 106, 2035–2040. doi: 10.1073/pnas.0811168106

Stevens, C., Dow, M., Schorr, E., and Neville, H. (2017). Atypical white-matter microstructure in congenitally deaf adults: a region of interest and tractography study using diffusion-tensor imaging. *Hear. Res.* 343, 72–82. doi: 10.1016/j.heares.2016.07.008

Supekar, K., Menon, V., and Dougherty, R. (2009). Resting-state functional connectivity reflects structural connectivity in the default mode network. *Cereb. Cortex* 19, 72–78. doi: 10.1093/cercor/bhn059

Vanneste, S., Plazier, M., der Loo, E., de Heyning, P. V., Congedo, M., and De Ridder, D. (2010). The neural correlates of tinnitus-related distress. *Neuroimage* 52, 470–480. doi: 10.1016/j.neuroimage.2010.04.029

Wang, L., Li, X., Hsiao, S., Lenz, F., Bodner, M., Zhou, Y., et al. (2015). Differential roles of delay-period neural activity in the monkey dorsolateral prefrontal cortex in visual-haptic crossmodal working memory. *Proc. Natl. Acad. Sci. U.S.A.* 112, E214–E219. doi: 10.1073/pnas.1410130112

Wang, X., Xu, P., Li, P., Wang, Z., Zhao, F., Gao, Z., et al. (2016). Alterations in gray matter volume due to unilateral hearing loss. *Sci. Rep.* 6:25811. doi: 10.1038/srep25811

Wilson, B. S., Tucci, D. L., Merson, M. H., and O'Donoghue, G. M. (2017). Global hearing health care: new findings and perspectives. *Lancet* 390, 2503–2515. doi: 10.1016/S0140-6736(17)31073-5

Xia, S., Song, T., Che, J., Li, Q., Chai, C., Zheng, M., et al. (2017). Altered brain functional activity in infants with congenital bilateral severe sensorineural hearing loss: a resting-state functional MRI study under sedation. *Neural Plast.* 2017:8986362. doi: 10.1155/2017/8986362

Yang, M., Chen, H. J., Liu, B., Huang, Z. C., Feng, Y., Li, J., et al. (2014). Brain structural and functional alterations in patients with unilateral hearing loss. *Hear. Res.* 316, 37–43. doi: 10.1016/j.heares.2014.07.006

Yeterian, E. H., Pandya, D. N., Tomaiuolo, F., and Petrides, M. (2012). The cortical connectivity of the prefrontal cortex in the monkey brain. *Cortex* 48, 58–81. doi: 10.1016/j.cortex.2011.03.004

Zatorre, R. J., Evans, A. C., Meyer, E., and Gjedde, A. (1992). Lateralization of phonetic and pitch discrimination in speech processing. *Science* 256, 846–849. doi: 10.1126/science.1589767

Zikopoulos, B., and Barbas, H. (2006). Prefrontal projections to the thalamic reticular nucleus form a unique circuit for attentional mechanisms. *J. Neurosci.* 26, 7348–7361. doi: 10.1523/JNEUROSCI.5511-05.2006

Zou, Q., Miao, X., Liu, D., Wang, D., Zhuo, Y., and Gao, J. (2015). Reliability comparison of spontaneous brain activities between BOLD and CBF contrasts in eyes-open and eyes-closed resting states. *Neuroimage* 121, 91–105. doi: 10.1016/j.neuroimage.2015.07.044

Zung, W. W. (1971). A rating instrument for anxiety disorders. *Psychosomatics* 12, 371–379. doi: 10.1016/S0033-3182(71)71479-0

9

Altered Topological Patterns of Gray Matter Networks in Tinnitus: A Graph-Theoretical-Based Study

Xiaofeng Lin[1,2†], Yueyao Chen[3†], Mingxia Wang[4], Chao Song[5], Bingling Lin[6], Xiaoping Yuan[5], Qingyu Liu[5], Haidi Yang[7] and Ningyi Jiang[1,2*]*

[1] *Department of Nuclear Medicine, Sun Yat-sen Memorial Hospital, Sun Yat-sen University, Guangzhou, China,* [2] *Department of Nuclear Medicine, The Seventh Affiliated Hospital, Sun Yat-sen University, Shenzhen, China,* [3] *Department of Radiology, Shenzhen Traditional Chinese Medicine Hospital, Shenzhen, China,* [4] *Department of Hearing and Speech Sciences, Xinhua College of Sun Yat-sen University, Guangzhou, China,* [5] *Department of Radiology, Sun Yat-sen Memorial Hospital, Sun Yat-sen University, Guangzhou, China,* [6] *Department of Radiology, Peking University Shen Zhen Hospital, Shenzhen, China,* [7] *Department of Otolaryngology, Sun Yat-sen Memorial Hospital, Sun Yat-sen University, Guangzhou, China*

***Correspondence:**
Ningyi Jiang
ningyij@163.net
Haidi Yang
yanghd@mail.sysu.edu.cn

† These authors have contributed equally to this work and share first authorship

Objective: Tinnitus is a prevalent hearing disorder, which could have a devastating impact on a patient's life. Functional studies have revealed connectivity pattern changes in the tinnitus brains that suggested a change of network dynamics as well as topological organization. However, no studies have yet provided evidence for the topological network changes in the gray matter. In this research, we aim to use the graph-theoretical approach to investigate the changes of topology in the tinnitus brain using structural MRI data, which could provide insights into the underlying anatomical basis for the neural mechanism in generating phantom sounds.

Methods: We collected 3D MRI images on 46 bilateral tinnitus patients and 46 age and gender-matched healthy controls. Brain networks were constructed with correlation matrices of the cortical thickness and subcortical volumes of 80 cortical/subcortical regions of interests. Global network properties were analyzed using local and global efficiency, clustering coefficient, and small-world coefficient, and regional network properties were evaluated using the betweenness coefficient for hub connectivity, and interregional correlations for edge properties. Between-group differences in cortical thickness and subcortical volumes were assessed using independent sample *t*-tests, and local efficiency, global efficiency, clustering coefficient, sigma, and interregional correlation were compared using non-parametric permutation tests.

Results: Tinnitus was found to have increased global efficiency, local efficiency, and cluster coefficient, indicating generally heightened connectivity of the network. The small-world coefficient remained normal for tinnitus, indicating intact small-worldness. Betweenness centrality analysis showed that hubs in the amygdala and parahippocampus were only found for tinnitus but not controls. In contrast, hubs in the auditory cortex, insula, and thalamus were only found for controls but not tinnitus. Interregional correlation analysis further found in tinnitus enhanced connectivity between the auditory cortex and prefrontal lobe, and decreased connectivity of the insula with anterior cingulate gyrus and parahippocampus.

Conclusion: These findings provided the first morphological evidence of altered topological organization of the brain networks in tinnitus. These alterations suggest that heightened efficiency of the brain network and altered auditory-limbic connection for tinnitus, which could be developed in compensation for the auditory deafferentation, leading to overcompensation and, ultimately, an emotional and cognitive burden.

Keywords: tinnitus, structural analysis, graph theory, centrality, hub, edge

INTRODUCTION

Subjective tinnitus (henceforth referred to as tinnitus), also known as "ringing in the ears," refers to the perception of sound in the absence of corresponding external source. It is a prevalent condition that affects approximately 10–15% of the adult population (Jastreboff, 1990; Heller, 2003; Shargorodsky et al., 2010), among whom an estimated 5–15% of the condition can become chronic and have a substantial negative impact on the quality of the patients' lives (Dobie, 2003; Heller, 2003).

Current theories concerning the etiology of tinnitus mainly include a bottom-up deafferentation process following a hearing loss from cochlear damage, and a top–down maladaptive compensational mechanism (Rauschecker et al., 2010), resulting in hyperactivity in the auditory pathway (Eggermont and Roberts, 2004; Soleymani et al., 2011). A proposed model further suggested that the tinnitus sensation might be perceived only when aberrant neuronal activity in the primary auditory cortex is transmitted to a global workplace involving frontal, parietal, and limbic regions (De Ridder et al., 2011). The limbic system, with the thalamus, in particular, was proposed to play an inhibitory role in eliminating the noise signal transmitted to the global workplace (De Ridder et al., 2011). When the limbic regions become dysfunctional, noise-cancelation breaks down and the tinnitus signal pervades to the conscious perception (Rauschecker et al., 2010; Leaver et al., 2011). This model has been supported by empirical evidence from functional and structural imaging studies. For instance, using tract-based spatial statistics in diffusion tensor imaging data, one study found that the mean diffusion was significantly higher in the left superior, middle and inferior temporal white matter for tinnitus than control, which suggested enhanced connectivity between Heschl's gyrus and limbic regions (Ryu et al., 2016). Furthermore, the compromised auditory representation could also be compensated with enhanced auditory memory retrieval through parahippocampal regions, thus sustaining the memory of the phantom sounds (Yoo et al., 2016b). These regions could constitute a complex network in maintaining and enhancing the symptoms, which is involved in not only auditory representation but also attention, memory, and emotion (Weisz et al., 2007; Leaver et al., 2011; Auerbach et al., 2014).

In recent years, connectome analysis of the brain has gained increasing popularity, given its ability in unraveling the complex network organization, and various network-based approaches such as graph-theoretical methods have been developed accordingly (Bullmore and Sporns, 2009; Lv et al., 2018). They have also been applied in tinnitus, which indeed helps find topological changes in their neural network properties (Mohan et al., 2016; Kandeepan et al., 2019). For instance, one study used a graph-theoretical approach to investigate the lagged phase functional connectivity in tinnitus using resting-state EEG and found that the topology of the patients' network had increased regularity in low-frequency carrier oscillations, whereas decreased regularity in the high-frequency oscillations, which suggested maladaptive top-down modulation in compensation for the auditory deafferentation (Mohan et al., 2016). Another study using a graph-theoretical approach to investigate the relation between tinnitus distress and functional network activities found that tinnitus distress was strongly correlated within and between the right executive control network and the other four resting-state networks (Kandeepan et al., 2019). However, current topologic analyses on tinnitus neural networks have all been based on functional data. As far as we know, no studies have yet used topologic analysis approaches on structural data of tinnitus. Given that neural adaptation and age could lead to morphometric changes of the brain (Yoo et al., 2016b), it is likely that the topological changes seen in the functional neural networks of tinnitus could be accompanied with structural changes. Indeed, there has been structural evidence supporting changes in multiple brain regions in tinnitus (Mühlau et al., 2006; Simonetti and Oiticica, 2015), such as the Heschl's gyrus (Schneider et al., 2009), and limbic regions such as thalamus (Mühlau et al., 2006) and parahippocampal cortex (Besteher et al., 2019).

In this study, we set out to explore network topology in tinnitus using structural MRI data with graph-theoretical techniques. We hypothesize that topologic characteristics could be seen in the structural networks of tinnitus, which is likely to involve both global and regional network changes, mainly auditory and limbic areas. Hence, we used several graph-theoretical based methods to assess the network properties of the brain, including global properties such as global efficiency (Eglob), local efficiency (Eloc), clustering coefficient (CC) and small-world coefficient (sigma), as well as regional properties including betweenness-centrality (BC) and interregional connectivity.

In graph theory, a network is defined as a set of nodes and the edges connecting them (Rubinov and Sporns, 2010; Bassett and Bullmore, 2017). Graph-theoretical studies have assessed structurally defined networks based on features such as gray matter volume, cortical thickness, surface area, and white matter connections between gray matter regions (Chen et al., 2008; Bassett and Bullmore, 2017). In the current study, a seed-based approach is adopted, where the nodes of a network correspond to anatomically segmented brain structures [regions of interest (ROI)], and the edges are defined by the strength of correlation between regional volume cortical thickness (Bassett and Bullmore, 2009; Rubinov and Sporns, 2010). Using these measurements, we assessed the topology of the brain networks by many properties, such as its functional segregation (CC and Eloc), functional integration (Eglob), small-worldness (sigma), centrality (BC) and edge (interregional connectivity analysis) (Rubinov and Sporns, 2010; Mijalkov et al., 2017). A more detailed introduction to these metrics can be found in Chap. 2.4.

MATERIALS AND METHODS

Subjects

Tinnitus patients were recruited from Sun Yat-sen Memorial Hospital of Sun Yat-sen University in Guangzhou. In this study, we only recruited bilateral tinnitus patients, to avoid the possible confounding effect brought upon by laterality of the tinnitus. Inclusion criteria for the tinnitus group were as follows: (i) age between 18 and 60 years; (ii) all patients described their tinnitus as bilateral or originated within the head; (iii) tinnitus duration of more than 6 months; (iv) normal hearing level or mild hearing loss. To avoid confounding effects of severe hearing loss to the brain, hearing thresholds were controlled below 40 dB HL.

Exclusion criteria included objective tinnitus, Ménière's disease, otosclerosis, chronic headache, severe alcoholism, smoking, head injury, stroke, Alzheimer's disease, Parkinson's disease, epilepsy, major depression or other neurological, psychiatric illness or major physical illnesses (e.g., cancer, anemia, and thyroid dysfunction). Moreover, we used the Hyperacusis Questionnaire to exclude participants with hyperacusis in the current study (Khalfa et al., 2002).

A total of forty-six patients with bilateral subjective tinnitus were eventually recruited for this study (all right-handed, 31 men and 15 women). Forty-six healthy subjects (all right-handed, 26 men and 20 women) with normal hearing were also recruited through a routine community physical examination and newspaper advertisements. All the subjects provided written informed consent before they participated in the study protocol, and the research was approved by The Research Ethics Committee of the Sun Yat-sen memorial hospital, Sun Yat-sen University.

Audiological and Behavioral Assessments

All participants were screened for the extent of hearing loss using pure tone audiometry by the British Society of Audiology procedures at frequencies of 0.25, 0.5, 1, 2, 4, and 8 kHz (British Society of Audiology, 2012). Hearing thresholds were measured separately for the two ears. The hearing level for each ear was calculated as the numerical average of hearing thresholds of all the frequencies. Also, according to the self-rating depression scale (SDS) and the self-rating anxiety scale (SAS) (overall scores < 60, respectively), none of the participants had major depression or anxiety (Zung, 1971).

All tinnitus patients were interviewed to determine their tinnitus laterality and duration and for qualities of their tinnitus tone (pure tone-like tinnitus or noise-like tinnitus). Frequency and loudness of their perceived tinnitus tones were tested using audiometric tinnitus matching analysis. Depending on whether a patient perceives a pure tone or narrow-band noise, a pure tone or a narrow band noise at or around 1 kHz (1/3 of an octave above and below the center frequency) was presented contralateral to the (worse) tinnitus ear at 10 dB above their hearing threshold. The matching analysis was performed on the (better) tinnitus ear following the procedures recommended by the American Academy of Audiology (Henry and Meikle, 2000). The severity of tinnitus and related distress was assessed by the tinnitus handicap inventory (THI) (Newman et al., 1996) and visual analog scale (VAS) (Dawes and Haslock, 1982) (see **Supplementary Table 1** for a sample).

Image Acquisition and Preprocessing

We acquired structural T1 weighted MR images of all participants with a Philips 3-Tesla MR scanner (Achieva, Philips Medical Systems, Netherlands) with an 8-channel receiver array head coil. Structural images were acquired with a three-dimensional turbo fast echo (3D-TFE) T1WI sequence with high resolution (repetition time (TR) = 8.1 ms, echo time (TE) = 3.7 ms, slices = 170 (sagittal plane), thickness = 1 mm; gap = 0 mm; flip angle (FA) = 8°; acquisition matrix = 256 × 256; field of view (FOV) = 256 mm × 256 mm; and 1- mm isotropic resolution).

Image preprocessing was performed using the FreeSurfer software (version 5.3.0[1]) developed at the Martinos Center for Biomedical Imaging (Massachusetts General Hospital, Harvard Medical School) on a 64-bit Linux ubuntu 14.0. Preprocessing steps included removal of non-brain tissue using a watershed/surface deformation procedure (Ségonne et al., 2004), automated transformation to Tailarach space, intensity normalization (Sled et al., 1998), segmentation of subcortical gray/white matter tissue, tessellation of the gray matter – white matter boundary, automated correction of topology (Ségonne et al., 2007) and surface deformation (Fischl and Dale, 2000).

In the current study, we chose two measurements to construct the neural network: cortical thickness (CT) and subcortical volume. CT was chosen because it reflects the size, density, and arrangement of cells (neurons, neuroglia, and nerve fibers), which was found to show correlation with functional changes in development and disease (Narr et al., 2005; Chen et al., 2008; Bethlehem et al., 2017). This technique is known to be more robust than the widely used volumetry, as it is less sensitive to position errors and spatial variances (MacDonald et al., 2000) while also providing more precise measurements (Fischl and Dale, 2000; Pereira et al., 2012). Furthermore, subcortical areas could also contain important nodes that contribute to the generation of tinnitus (Rauschecker et al., 2010; Leaver et al., 2011), which cannot be captured by CT. Therefore, we used a combination of subcortical volumes with CT to construct a complete brain network. This method has been used by previous studies (Yun et al., 2020; Li et al., 2017). CT is defined as the Euclidean distance between the vertices of the gray-white surfaces (Singh et al., 2008), followed by parcelation of the cerebral cortex into 68 cortical areas (34 for each hemisphere)

[1]http://surfer.nmr.mgh.harvard.edu

(Desikan et al., 2006). Subcortical volumetric analyses were performed using an automated procedure that estimates the probability of structure-classification based on prior templates in which those structures were manually identified (Fischl et al., 2002). We obtained 12 subcortical areas, including the thalamus, hippocampus, amygdala, caudate, putamen, and pallidum for each hemisphere. The anatomical labeling of the selected regions can be found in **Supplementary Table 2.**

Network Construction and Assessment

Structural networks were constructed using GAT (Graph Analysis Toolbox) (Hosseini et al., 2012). The 68 cortical ROIs and 12 subcortical ROIs obtained in the last step were regarded as nodes in the current study. Regional cortical thickness and subcortical volume from these 80 ROIs were extracted and calculated for their correlation coefficients between subjects. After controlling for confounding effects of age and gender using linear regression, the residuals were used in the graph analysis. Possible edges were defined as the correlation of the cortical thickness and subcortical volumes between every pair of these nodes. The final structural brain network for each group contained a total of 80 nodes and 3,160 (80 × 79/2) possible edges. The definition of a valid edge was calculated with an above-threshold (absolute) correlation value that was set to 1, with an invalid edge with subthreshold values (including negative correlations) set to 0 (Gong and Xu, 2012), and this constituted an undirected (i.e., symmetric) and unweighted (binary) matrix.

Given that there could be discrepancies in the low-level correlation threshold between controls and patients' brain networks (Yasuda et al., 2015), it is necessary to control the edge density (percentile of detected connections over the number of all possible connections). As there has been no established standard for a valid density, a range of different densities were used in this study. Specifically, edge density of the brain network was defined as the ratio of valid edges over total possible edges, i.e., 3160 edges, and in this study the density was controlled at a fixed range between 10 and 46%, to exclude disconnected networks and random network topology (Yasuda et al., 2015).

In this study, we used several methods to assess various global network properties of the brain, including global efficiency (Eglob), local efficiency (Eloc), clustering coefficient (CC), and small-world coefficient (sigma). Eglob and Eloc have been proposed to be able to reveal the network's capability of integrating information effectively (Bullmore and Sporns, 2012). Eglob was used to assess the ability of a network to rapidly incorporate information from distinct anatomical regions based on the length of paths. A shorter length of paths indicated stronger functional integration, which was defined as the average of the inverse of the shortest path length between pairs of nodes (the smallest number of edges of which the path passes through any two nodes) in the entire network (Latora and Marchiori, 2001). Eloc, on the other hand, characterized the resistance of a network to failure on a small scale, by quantifying how well-information is exchanged by its neighbors when a node is removed. It was calculated from the average of the inverse characteristic path length among the neighboring nodes of the node (Bullmore and Sporns, 2012). CC was used to assess the presence of clustering within a network that indicates potential functional segregation, by computing the fractions of the nodes' neighbors that were also neighbors to each other (Watts and Strogatz, 1998; Rubinov and Sporns, 2010). Finally, the small-worldness of a network, i.e., the ability of the network to reconcile the opposing demands of functional segregation and integration, was assessed with the small-world coefficient, i.e., sigma value, which was determined by the ratio of the clustering and the characteristic path length. Specifically, networks were considered to have small-world architecture if they had much higher clustering coefficients but an approximately equal characteristic path length when compared to a population of random networks with equal edge strength (Humphries and Gurney, 2008).

Regional network properties were assessed using normalized betweenness centrality (BC) and interregional correlations. The BC characterized the importance of a specific node, in which a node with high BC would indicate that it was part of "highly traveled paths." In BC, the number of shortest paths that passed through a specific node was divided by the total number of short paths in the entire network (Brandes, 2001). In the current study, we considered a node to be a hub if its BC was at least 1.5 standard deviation higher than the mean network BC (Zhang et al., 2015). Interregional correlations were used to analyze edge properties between each pair of nodes. Previous studies have found that strong functional connections commonly exist between regions with no direct structural connection, and could be reflected a certain extent by the large-scale anatomical structure of the human cerebral cortex (Honey et al., 2009). Interregional structural correlations could capture these indirect structural correlations between two regions facilitated by a third party, from which diverse factors such as pathologic changes to the connectivity patterns could be detected (Evans, 2013). In this study, interregional correlations analysis was performed by directly comparing all the edge values (correlation coefficients) between the two groups.

Statistical Analyses

Demographic and clinical data were analyzed using SPSS. 21 (IBM, Corp., Armonk, NY, United States). Demographic data were compared between the tinnitus and healthy control groups using independent-sample t-tests for continuous variables and non-parametric tests for categorical variables. Clinical data of the tinnitus group were summarized using descriptive analysis. Correlation between the cortical thickness/subcortical volume of the tinnitus patients and their clinical characteristics, such as average hearing threshold, SDS, SAS, the duration of tinnitus, THI, and VAS, was calculated using Pearson's bivariate correlation and hierarchical regression analysis.

For the analyses of structural brain images, we used the GAT software. We first performed whole-brain comparisons of cortical thickness and subcortical volumes between the tinnitus and control groups. Before the comparison, cortical thickness data were first smoothed in surface-space using a 10 mm^2 FWHM Gaussian kernel. Between-group comparisons (i.e., controls > patients) were then conducted vertex-wise across the entire cortex using independent sample t-tests, and results were thresholded at original $p < 0.001$, FDR corrected at $p < 0.05$.

For group-level network analyses, the four network property metrics (CC, Eglob, Eloc, and sigma) and interregional correlations were compared between the two groups. Specifically, metric values were subtracted for tinnitus > control and obtained a difference score for each metric. Non-parametric permutation testing was used to calculate the statistical significance of these difference scores. In each permutation, subject labels were randomly reassigned to 1 of 2 groups of the same size as the original groups, and the test statistics were calculated for each pair of randomized groups and subtracted in the same way as in the "real" data. The permutation was iterated 1000 times to form the distribution of difference scores from random data. Final results were thresholded at $p < 0.001$, FDR corrected at $p < 0.05$.

RESULTS

Demographic and Clinical Data

Between the two groups, no difference was found in either the demographic (age, gender, and education years) or clinical status (hearing thresholds, SDS and SAS scores) (see **Table 1** for more details).

Whole-Brain Structural Difference Between the Two Groups

No significant difference was found for either CT or subcortical volumes between the two groups after FDR correction. No significant correlation was found between clinical data and CT/subcortical volumes.

Global Network Properties

Figure 1 shows the analysis results of the global network measures in the two groups. CC, Eloc, and Eglob increased for both groups with increasing edge density values. At the same time, Sigma showed a generally similar pattern of small-worldness between the two groups, with fluctuations in tinnitus at density values of 0.1 and 0.13 (**Figure 1**). Group comparisons showed that tinnitus patients had significantly higher CC at network densities from 0.22 to 0.31, as well as increased Eloc and Eglob across most densities (from 0.16 to 0.37). Also, we found trends toward elevated small-world coefficients at a few network densities for the tinnitus group (**Figure 1D**). While the results of the small-world measures were rather unstable across densities, overall sigma values of the two groups were larger than 1, which indicated that the tinnitus brain maintained normal small-world characteristics with generally balanced global and local efficiency.

TABLE 1 | Demographic and clinical characteristics of study participants.

	Tinnitus	Control	t/χ^2	p-Value
Age (year)	40.9 ± 12.5	42.3 ± 14.2	0.503	0.608[a]
Gender (M/F)	31/15	26/20	1.153	0.283[b]
Education (year)	13.6 ± 3.9	14.0 ± 4.3	0.361	0.703[a]
SDS score	35.9 ± 11.3	31.9 ± 8.9	1.875	0.064[a]
SAS score	33.6 ± 13.4	29.6 ± 9.3	1.645	0.104[a]
Hearing threshold (dB HL)	20.02 ± 4.7	18.5 ± 3.0	1.866	0.065[a]
Tinnitus duration (month)	24.46 ± 12.31	NA		NA
THI score	54.59 ± 17.31	NA		NA
VAS score	2.97 ± 1.73	NA		NA

SDS, self-rating depression scale; SAS, self-rating anxiety scale; THI, Tinnitus Handicap Inventory; VAS, visual analog scale; NA, not applicable. [a]*Two-sample t-tests.* [b]*Chi-square test.*

Regional Network Analysis

The hub connectivity of the anatomic network was examined with BC separately for each group at an edge density of 22%. Eight hub regions were identified with high BC in the control group and seven in the tinnitus group (**Table 2** and **Figure 2**). Three hubs with high BC in the superior temporal gyrus (STG), bilateral insula, and thalamus were only found for the control group. In contrast, three hubs in the amygdala and parahippocampus were only found for the tinnitus group.

Interregional correlation analysis results were shown in **Table 3** and **Figure 3**. Compared with controls, the tinnitus group showed generally higher connectivity between nodes, especially the right transverse temporal gyrus (the auditory cortex) to the prefrontal lobe (caudal middle frontal, right pars orbitalis, and left frontal pole) and the sensorimotor area (right paracentral). Meanwhile, the connectivity between the orbitofrontal cortex (OFC, including the right pars orbitalis, bilateral medial orbitofrontal gyrus) and the somatosensory area (bilateral post-central gyrus and superior parietal gyrus) increased. However, decreased connections were found between the right rostral- and caudal-anterior cingulate gyrus (ACG) with the left insula, pars opercularis, lateral orbitofrontal (OFC) and posterior cingulate gyrus (PCG), as well as between the left parahippocampus and right insula.

DISCUSSION

In this study, we investigated the network topology changes in the gray matter of tinnitus patients. Multiple interesting results were found. First, the network topology of tinnitus exhibited increased CC, Eloc and Eglob, but maintained roughly similar small-worldness. Second, a different hub connection pattern was found for tinnitus that supports the existing theories on an auditory-limbic interaction. Specifically, compared with healthy controls, tinnitus patients were found with lower hub connectivity in the auditory cortex, insula and thalamus, and higher connectivity in the amygdala and parahippocampus. Finally, significantly altered interregional connections were found for tinnitus, including increased connectivity between the auditory cortex and PFC/sensorimotor region, and decreased connectivity between ACG and insula/OFC/PCG, as well as between insula and parahippocampus. To the best of our knowledge, this study is the first to investigate the topologic changes of structural network properties in the gray matter of tinnitus, and the results supported our hypothesis that altered topological morphological changes were present for tinnitus, which could underlie a maladaptive auditory-limbic interaction in the generation of their symptoms.

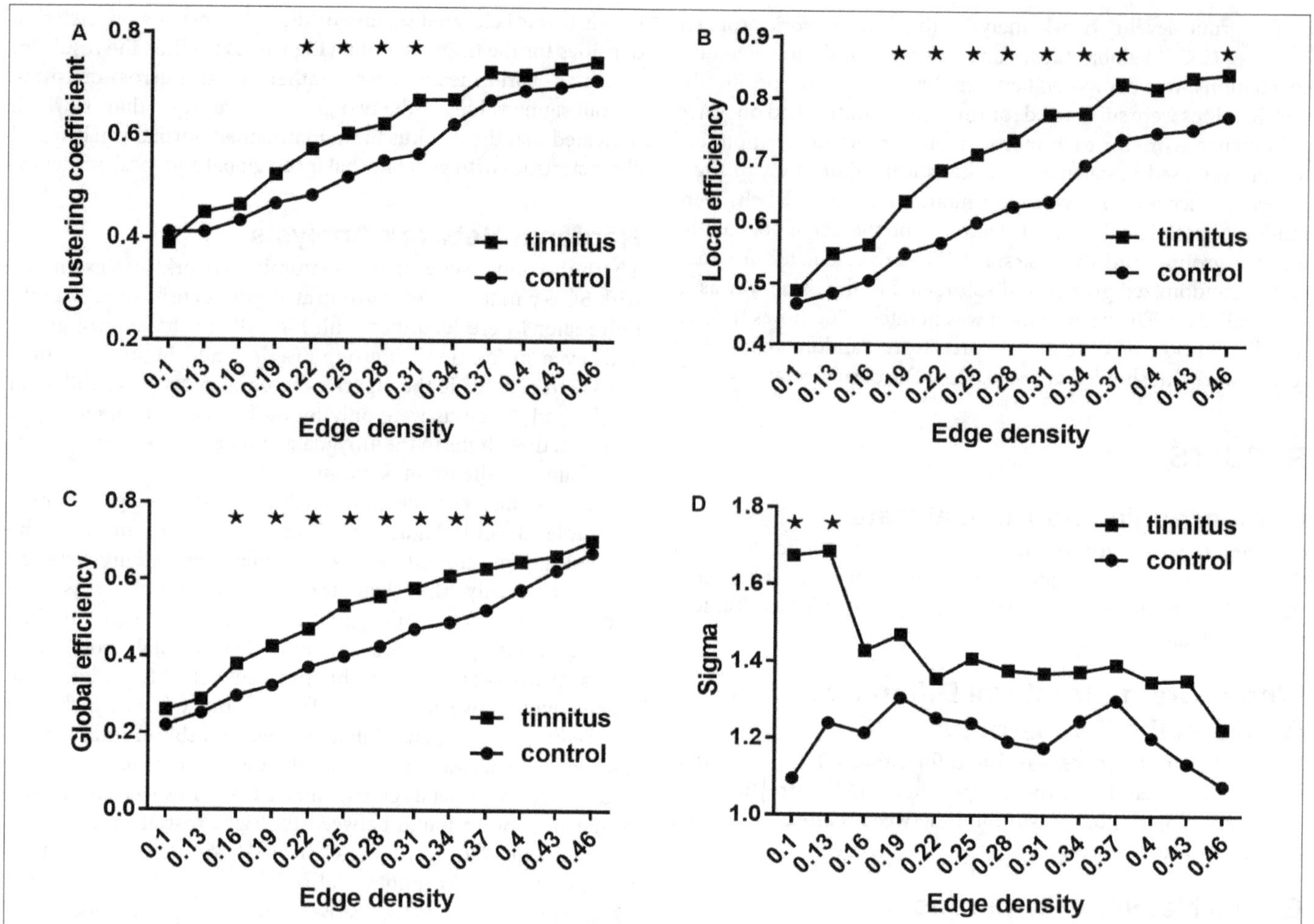

FIGURE 1 | Between-group comparisons of global network measures. **(A)** Clustering coefficient, **(B)** local efficiency, **(C)** global efficiency, and **(D)** small-world property (sigma). **(A–C)** Increased as the network density increases, and **(D)** decreases as the network density increases. ★ Represents significant values. Results shown were thresholded at $p < 0.001$, corrected for multiple comparisons using the FDR procedure.

TABLE 2 | Betweenness centrality analysis for tinnitus and control.

Group	Region	Normalized BC
Control	Right-bankssts	5.940
	Left-cuneus	4.505
	Left-temporal pole	4.501
	Right-superior temporal	3.984
	Right-posterior cingulate	3.943
	Left-insula	3.905
	Right-thalamus	2.994
	Right-insula	2.926
Tinnitus	Left-caudal anterior cingulate	7.086
	Left-posterior cingulate	5.091
	Left-rostral anterior cingulate	3.336
	Left-amygdala	3.264
	Right-parahippocampal	3.263
	Right-precuneus	3.210
	Right-frontal pole	2.596

Results shown were corrected at $p < 0.05$, FDR corrected. bankssts, banks of the superior temporal sulcus.

Abnormal Global Network Properties in Tinnitus

The increased Eglob, Eloc, and CC found for tinnitus patients in our study suggest that the neural network of tinnitus has an abnormally higher network efficiency, with faster information flow across the brain (reflected by Eglob) and a higher level of local connectedness (reflected by the CC and Eloc). This could be a reflection of a compensational mechanism for the hearing loss (Langguth et al., 2013; Noreña and Farley, 2013). Specifically, the increased Eglob indicated a more compact global network, which could involve intensified information exchange from distributed regions. This could explain the common findings of increased connectivity between auditory and distress-related regions such as the amygdala (Rauschecker et al., 2010). On the other hand, an increased Eloc and CC could indicate an enhanced neuro-synchronization in localized regions, which has indeed been found for tinnitus in regions like the auditory cortex (Eggermont, 2006), and other regions, in particular limbic regions such as bilateral anterior insula, shown by a resting-state fMRI study using the regional homogeneity (ReHo) index

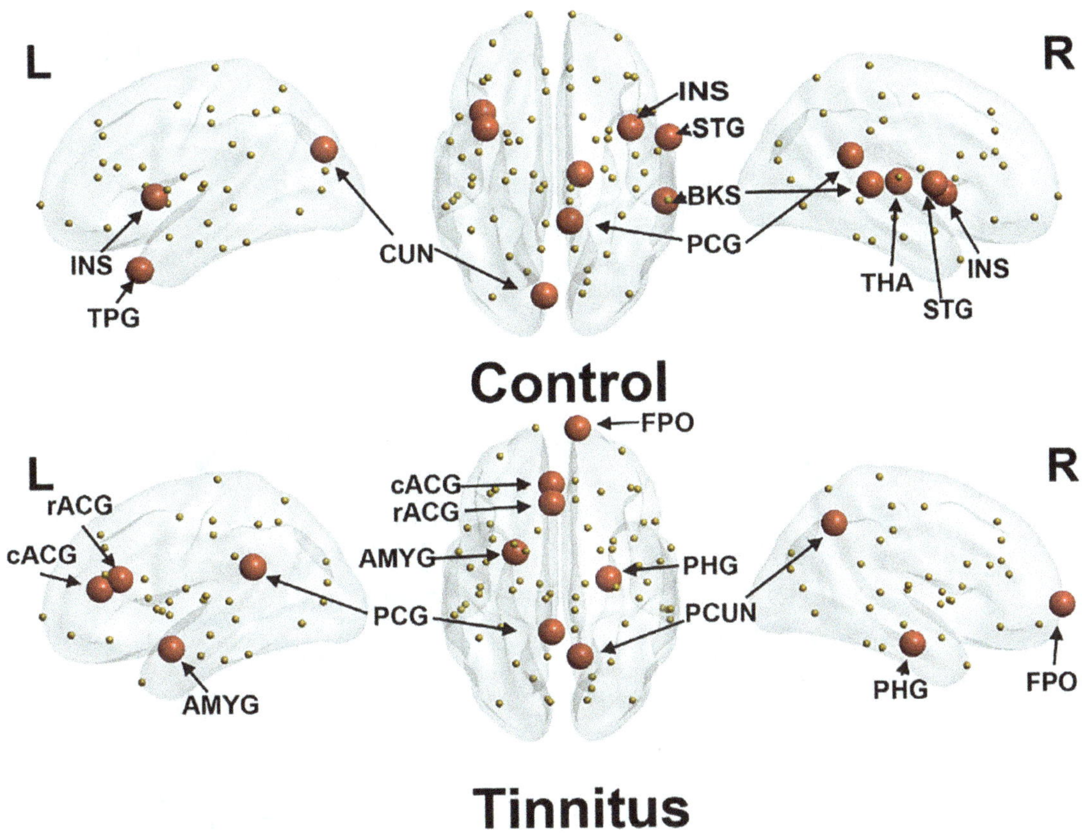

FIGURE 2 | Distribution of hub regions of control (upper panel) and tinnitus (lower panel) based on regional betweenness centrality (mean + 1.5 SD). Large red spheres represent brain hubs and small yellow spheres represent non-hub brain regions. INS, insula; TPG, temporal pole; CUN, cuneus; STG, superior temporal gyrus; PCG, posterior cingulate gyrus; BKS, bankssts; THA, thalamus; rACG, rostral anterior cingulate gyrus; cACG, caudal anterior cingulate gyrus; AMYG, amygdala; PHG, parahippocampus; PCUN, precuneus; FPO, frontal pole; L, left hemisphere; R, right hemisphere.

TABLE 3 | Interregional correlation difference of tinnitus > control.

Num	Interregional correlations		r(NC)	r(tinnitus)	z-Score
1	**Right transverse temporal –**	Left caudal middle frontal	0	0.697	4.972[a]
2	**Right transverse temporal –**	Right paracentral	0	0.414	2.975
3	**Right transverse temporal –**	Right pars orbitalis	0	0.396	2.823
4	**Right transverse temporal –**	Left frontal pole	0	0.326	2.310
5	**Right pars orbitalis –**	Right post-central	0	0.399	2.828
6	**Right pars orbitalis –**	Right superior parietal	0	0.341	2.387
7	**Right pars orbitalis –**	Left superior parietal	0	0.504	3.585
8	**Right pars orbitalis –**	Left post-central	0	0.887	6.228
9	**Right medial orbitofrontal –**	Right paracentral	0.046	0.771	5.204
10	**Right superior parietal –**	Right insula	0	0.544	3.908
11	**Left medial orbitofrontal –**	Right superior parietal	0	0.42	3.300
12	**Left medial orbitofrontal –**	Right paracentral	0	0.489	3.506
13	**Left medial orbitofrontal –**	Left post-central	0	0.343	2.429
14	**Right rostral anterior cingulate –**	Left insula	0.308	0	−2.197[b]
15	**Right rostral anterior cingulate –**	Left lateral orbitofrontal	0.664	0	−4.784
16	**Right rostral anterior cingulate –**	Left posterior cingulate	0.932	0	−6.643
17	**Right rostral anterior cingulate –**	Left pars opercularis	0.977	0.006	−6.880
18	**Right caudal anterior cingulate –**	Left insula	0.424	0	−2.998
19	**Right caudal anterior cingulate –**	Right precentral	0.985	0.014	−6.797
20	**Left transverse temporal –**	Right middle temporal	0.971	0	−6.907
21	**Left parahippocampal –**	Right insula	0.997	0.013	−6.909

NC, normal controls; r, Pearson correlation coefficient. [a]Positive values indicate stronger connections for tinnitus than control. [b]Negative values indicate weaker connections for tinnitus than control.

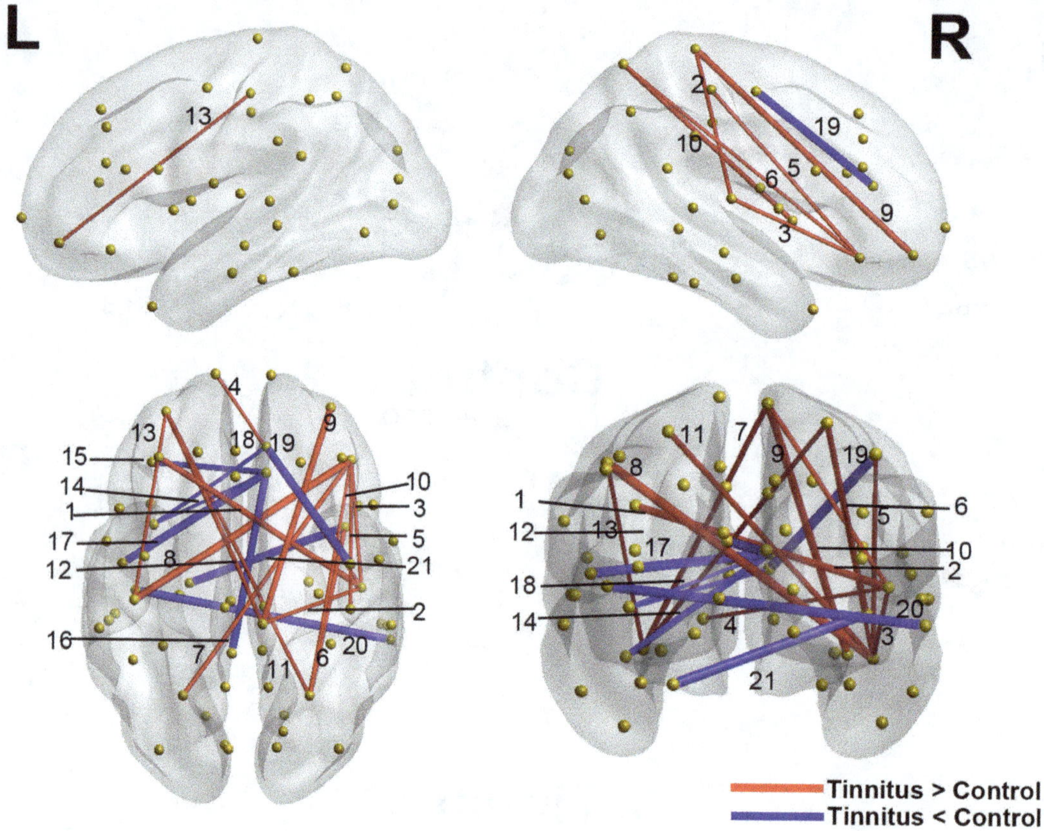

FIGURE 3 | Significant differences of interregional correlations in the tinnitus vs. control comparison. Red lines indicate increased connection (tinnitus > control), and blue lines indicate the decreased connection (tinnitus < control). Yellow spheres represent non-hub brain regions, and the width of the lines correlate with the absolute values of the Z scores for the difference between two groups. L: left hemisphere; R: right hemisphere. Results shown were corrected at $p < 0.001$, corrected for multiple comparisons using the FDR procedure. The numbering of the lines corresponds to the connections listed in **Table 3**.

(Chen et al., 2015b). Taken together, these findings indicated overcompensation in the structural networks of tinnitus, which could contribute to the development of distress, possibly through heightened local synchrony in auditory and limbic regions. On the other hand, no noticeable difference was found in the small-world property analysis between the two groups except for the two lowest densities. Both the neural networks in tinnitus and healthy controls in this study showed a small-world property (Mohan et al., 2016). This indicated a generally balanced modulation between integration and segregation was intact for the whole brain.

Pathologic Changes in Hub Node Distribution of Tinnitus Patients

Highly interesting differences were found in hub connectivity measured by BC for tinnitus and the healthy controls, respectively. First of all, as compared to healthy controls, no hub was found in the primary auditory cortex in tinnitus patients. This anomaly is interesting because it has been proposed that hyperactivity in the auditory cortex could be a compensatory mechanism in tinnitus for the deafferented areas (Chen et al., 2015a). However, increased activity does not equate to increased integrity. Given that in BC, hubs are defined as nodes with high topological values, which are critical for efficient interactions, they are consequently associated with both integrative information processing and adaptive behaviors (Crossley et al., 2014). It could be that the hyperactivity within the auditory cortex prohibits this area from communicating with other regions of the brain, thus reducing the number of its edges and thus lowered BC, i.e., compromised network integrity.

Another finding is the absence of hubs in the thalamus for tinnitus. As reflected in the BC analysis for healthy controls, the thalamus serves as an important hub in the healthy population, exchanging information with multi-sensory pathways. It has been found to play an important role in sensory gating, i.e., selectively block certain unwanted sensory signals such as noise (Rauschecker et al., 2010). Based on our results, this hub characteristic of the thalamus is lost in tinnitus patients. This finding is strongly supported by several previous models indicating a dysfunctional auditory-thalamic interaction leading to a failed noise-canceling system (Rauschecker et al., 2010; Leaver et al., 2011).

Furthermore, high BCs were found in the insula for both sides of the brain in healthy controls while not in the tinnitus patients. The insula is proposed to be responsible for converging and integrating multi-modality sensory signals and assigning subjectivity into these signals, to form feelings and emotions (Craig, 2009; Menon and Uddin, 2010). In tinnitus patients, the lack of insula as a hub could be a result of the hyperactivity in the auditory cortex driving imbalanced attentional resources in various sensory pathways, i.e., excessive attention to the unwanted auditory signals, which could disrupt the regulatory ability of the insula and eventually lead to distress (Kandeepan et al., 2019).

Finally, the amygdala and parahippocampus were found with heightened BC in tinnitus, but not in healthy controls. The amygdala was found to be associated with especially negative emotions (Derntl et al., 2009; Feinstein et al., 2011), while the parahippocampal gyrus was found to be highly involved in memory (van Strien et al., 2009). The abnormally heightened connectivity of these two areas indicated a significant association for a negative emotion-memory system in these patients. In this system, the tinnitus perception could be associated with distress by primarily the amygdala and reinforced as a persistent awareness by the memory system through the parahippocampus.

Changes in Interregional Connections in Tinnitus

Although we didn't find hubs in the auditory cortex in tinnitus patients with the BC analysis, in the interregional connectivity analysis, we found enhanced connectivity of the right transverse temporal gyrus (Heschl's gyrus) with especially bilateral frontal lobes. These frontal areas were primarily located at the lateral part of the cortex, adjacent to the dorsolateral prefrontal cortex (DLPFC). DLPFC is a crucial region in the executive control network that is proposed to be highly involved in cognitive control (Pessoa, 2014; Lehr et al., 2019), and has been used as an important target for stimulation in transcranial magnetic stimulation (TMS) and transcranial direct current stimulation (tDCS) treatment for tinnitus (Vanneste et al., 2011; De Ridder et al., 2012). Specifically, an EEG study showed that the responders to bihemispheric DLPFC tDCS differed from non-responders according to their resting brain activity in the right auditory cortex and parahippocampal area and the functional connectivity between DLPFC and the subgenual anterior cingulate cortex in particular (Vanneste et al., 2011). Combining our results and these previous findings, it is possible that there could be abnormal connections between the DLPFC and other areas of the brain, that could contribute to the distress of tinnitus, indicating a possible readaptation for the auditory loss/distress through cognitive modulation by strengthening connections with the frontal lobe.

Another interesting finding is the enhanced connectivity between the auditory cortex and the paracentral lobule in tinnitus. The paracentral lobule is adjacent to the somatosensory area (SMA), which was proposed to be involved in sensorimotor integration (Edwards et al., 2019; Umeda et al., 2019). Previous studies have found that some patients could modulate their tinnitus intensity by jaw protrusion (Lanting et al., 2010), suggesting enhanced auditory-somatosensory integration. Our finding provided structural evidence that the tinnitus brain may have an abnormally heightened exchange of auditory and somatosensory information. However, this assumption needs further testing with functional data.

Moreover, we found a decreased connectivity between the left parahippocampus and right insula. In the previous BC analysis, tinnitus was found with a lack of insula hubs and an additional hub in the parahippocampus. Combining the BC results with the current result, it shows a possible dissociation between these regions. Specifically, there could be generally compromised connectivity in the insula, resulting in the compromised modulating ability of multimodal sensory signals (Heydrich and Blanke, 2013). This change could result in a compensatory enhancement of the parahippocampal connectivity for the patients to retrieve auditory information from memory, which eventually leads to the sustaining of (phantom) auditory signals.

Finally, decreased connectivity between the ACG and left insula was also seen for the tinnitus patients. These are the two crucial nodes within the salience network (Menon and Uddin, 2010), which was proposed to assign saliency to various stimuli, and modulate dynamic interactions between various large-scale functional networks, such as the default mode network and executive control network (Uddin et al., 2017). This result is in slight disagreement with previous findings. In several previous studies, tinnitus has been proposed to have enhanced attention to especially tinnitus-related stimuli (Kandeepan et al., 2019) and was found to have more powerful activations in the salience network (Golm et al., 2013). One explanation for this discrepancy is that the enhanced functional activities found in the salience network might be a result of overcompensation from a diminished structural connection within the salience network. However, more research should be performed for this assumption.

The above findings are not only highly consistent with previous functional study findings, but they also provided empirical support for the anatomical basis for current theories of tinnitus. Current theories concerning the etiology of tinnitus mainly include a bottom–up deafferentation process following a hearing loss from cochlear damage, and a top–down maladaptive compensational mechanism (Rauschecker et al., 2010), resulting in hyperactivity in the auditory pathway (Eggermont and Roberts, 2004; Soleymani et al., 2011). A proposed model suggests that the tinnitus sensation might be perceived only when aberrant neuronal activity in the primary auditory cortex is transmitted to a global workplace involving frontal, parietal, and limbic regions (De Ridder et al., 2011), while the limbic system, in which the thalamus, in particular, plays an inhibitory role in eliminating the noise signal transmitted to global workplace. When the limbic regions become dysfunctional, noise-cancelation breaks down and the tinnitus signal pervades to the conscious perception (Rauschecker et al., 2010; Leaver et al., 2011).

Limitation

Several limitations of this study should be addressed. Firstly, the structural brain networks were constructed based on inter-regional cortical thickness/subcortical volume correlations across subjects in groups of bilateral tinnitus patients and healthy controls. Each group could only form one structural matrix, and the individual matrix cannot be obtained. Therefore, only group-level analyses could be performed and could not provide individual correlations between brain structures and clinical data. This limited the power of the interpretations. It is desirable to obtain individual-level measurements of network properties using methods such as resting-state functional MRI and diffusion-weighted imaging data. Secondly, the chain of events and the causal interactions between brain networks cannot be inferred directly from structural data. Moreover, although anatomical covariance holds great promises in revealing the structural foundation for brain disorders, its exact relation with the various factors generating the diseases is still unclear (Evans' 2013). Finally, the small sample size is another limitation of this study. Future studies should be performed on patients with more diverse symptoms and larger sample sizes. For instance, in the current analyses, no correlation was found between any clinical characteristics (such as THI scores or SDS scores) of tinnitus and their structural parameters. However, previous studies have shown different results. For instance, it has been found that the cortical thickness changes related to hearing loss overlap with those related to normal aging, and tinnitus-related distress level and subjective loudness were found negatively correlated to the thalamic volume (Yoo et al., 2016a). Since tinnitus is also considered highly correlated with hearing loss, it could be that age and tinnitus severity are also correlated, which should both show a correlation with cortical thickness. Combining the above, results in this study should be interpreted with caution, and future studies investigating causal relations in the network dynamics are strongly suggested. For instance, resting-state fMRI could be combined with structural MRI to investigate the possible topographical changes in the functional network (Salvador et al., 2005; Achard et al., 2006), building a weighted network with multi-modality approaches such as fMRI and DTI (Jiao et al., 2020), or using combined volume-based and tract-based approaches (Husain et al., 2011) along with graph-theoretical analyses to investigate the causal relationship between duration/severity and brain network topology.

CONCLUSION

In summary, by the construction of a brain network using cortical thickness and subcortical volume data, we have found alterations in the topology of structural brain networks of tinnitus. The heightened CC, Eloc and Eglob, indicated a generally more intensified information flow within both global and local properties of the tinnitus neural network, possibly as a compensatory mechanism for the deafferented signals. Subsequent regional analyses showed that hubs with high BC in the auditory cortex, insula, and thalamus were only present in the control group, but not in tinnitus. In contrast, hubs in the amygdala and parahippocampus were found for tinnitus but not in the control group. Interregional connectivity analysis showed enhanced connectivity between primarily the auditory cortex and prefrontal cortex/somatosensory areas, as well as reduced connectivity between primarily the insula and ACG/parahippocampus. Our findings provided the first anatomical evidence of gray matter network topological changes, supporting previous models of a dysfunctional auditory-limbic interaction that could be the underlying mechanism generating auditory phantom perceptions.

ETHICS STATEMENT

The studies involving human participants were reviewed and approved by The Research Ethics Committee of the Sun Yat-sen Memorial Hospital, Sun Yat-sen University. The patients/participants provided their written informed consent to participate in this study.

AUTHOR CONTRIBUTIONS

XL and YC participated in experiment design, data collection and analysis, and writing of the manuscript. CS, BL, and XY participated in data collection and analysis. MW and QL participated in the discussion and revision of the manuscript. HY and NJ are the corresponding authors of this manuscript, who have full access to all the data in the study and take responsibility for the integrity of the data and the accuracy of the data analysis.

REFERENCES

Achard, S., Salvador, R., Whitcher, B., Suckling, J., and Bullmore, E. (2006). A resilient, low-frequency, small-world human brain functional network with highly connected association cortical hubs. *J. Neurosci.* 26, 63–72. doi: 10.1523/JNEUROSCI.3874-05.2006

Auerbach, B. D., Rodrigues, P. V., and Salvi, R. J. (2014). Central gain control in tinnitus and hyperacusis. *Front. Neurol.* 5:206. doi: 10.3389/fneur.2014.00206

Bassett, D. S., and Bullmore, E. T. (2009). Human brain networks in health and disease. *Curr. Opin. Neurol.* 22, 340–347. doi: 10.1097/WCO.0b013e32832d93dd

Bassett, D. S., and Bullmore, E. T. (2017). Small-world brain networks revisited. *Neuroscientist* 23, 499–516. doi: 10.1177/1073858416667720

Besteher, B., Christian, G., Daniela, I., Orlando, G. L., Christian, D., and Igor, N. (2019). Chronic tinnitus and the limbic system: reappraising brain structural effects of distress and affective symptoms. *NeuroImage* 24, 101976. doi: 10.1016/j.nicl.2019.101976

Bethlehem, R. A. I., Romero-Garcia, R., Mak, E., Bullmore, E. T., and Baron-Cohen, S. (2017). Structural covariance networks in children with autism or ADHD. *Cereb. Cortex* 27, 4267–4276. doi: 10.1093/cercor/bhx135

Brandes, U. (2001). A faster algorithm for betweenness centrality. *J. Math. Soc.* 25, 163–177. doi: 10.1080/0022250X.2001.9990249

British Society of Audiology (2012). *Recommended Procedure Bone-Conduction Threshold Audiometry with and without Masking*. Bathgate: British Society of Audiology.

Bullmore, E., and Sporns, O. (2009). Complex brain networks: graph theoretical analysis of structural and functional systems. *Nat. Rev. Neurosci.* 10, 186–198. doi: 10.1038/nrn2575

Bullmore, E., and Sporns, O. (2012). The economy of brain network organization. *Nat. Rev. Neurosci.* 13, 336–349. doi: 10.1038/nrn3214

Chen, Y. C., Li, X., Liu, L., Wang, J., Lu, C. Q., Yang, M., et al. (2015a). Tinnitus and hyperacusis involve hyperactivity and enhanced connectivity in auditory-limbic-arousal-cerebellar network. *ELife* 4:e06576. doi: 10.7554/eLife.06576

Chen, Y. C., Zhang, J., Li, X. W., Xia, W., Feng, X., Qian, C., et al. (2015b). Altered intra- and interregional synchronization in resting-state cerebral networks associated with chronic tinnitus. *Neural Plast.* 2015, 1–11. doi: 10.1155/2015/475382

Chen, Z. J., He, Y., Rosa-Neto, P., Germann, J., and Evans, A. C. (2008). Revealing modular architecture of human brain structural networks by using cortical thickness from MRI. *Cereb. Cortex* 18, 2374–2381. doi: 10.1093/cercor/bhn003

Craig, A. D. (2009). How do you feel – now? The anterior insula and human awareness. *Nat. Rev. Neurosci.* 10, 59–70. doi: 10.1038/nrn2555

Crossley, N. A., Mechelli, A., Scott, J., Carletti, F., Fox, P. T., McGuire, P., et al. (2014). The hubs of the human connectome are generally implicated in the anatomy of brain disorders. *Brain* 137(Pt 8), 2382–2395. doi: 10.1093/brain/awu132

Dawes, P., and Haslock, I. (1982). Visual analogue scales. *Ann. Rheum. Dis.* 41, 434–435. doi: 10.1136/ard.41.4.434

De Ridder, D., Vanneste, S., and Congedo, M. (2011). The distressed brain: a group blind source separation analysis on tinnitus. *PLoS One* 6:e24273. doi: 10.1371/journal.pone.0024273

De Ridder, D., Vanneste, S., Plazier, M., Menovsky, T., van de Heyning, P., Kovacs, S., et al. (2012). Dorsolateral prefrontal cortex transcranial magnetic stimulation and electrode implant for intractable tinnitus. *World Neurosurg.* 77, 778–784. doi: 10.1016/j.wneu.2011.09.009

Derntl, B., Windischberger, C., Robinson, S., Kryspin-Exner, I., Gur, R. C., Moser, E., et al. (2009). Amygdala activity to fear and anger in healthy young males is associated with testosterone. *Psychoneuroendocrinology* 34, 687–693. doi: 10.1016/j.psyneuen.2008.11.007

Desikan, R. S., Ségonne, F., Fischl, B., Quinn, B. T., Dickerson, B. C., Blacker, D., et al. (2006). An automated labeling system for subdividing the human cerebral cortex on MRI scans into gyral based regions of interest. *NeuroImage* 31, 968–980. doi: 10.1016/j.neuroimage.2006.01.021

Dobie, R. A. (2003). Depression and tinnitus. *Otolaryngol. Clin. North Am.* 36, 383–388. doi: 10.1016/S0030-6665(02)00168-8

Edwards, L. L., King, E. M., Buetefisch, C. M., and Borich, M. R. (2019). Putting the 'Sensory' into sensorimotor control: the role of sensorimotor integration in goal-directed hand movements after stroke. *Front. Integr. Neurosci.* 13:16. doi: 10.3389/fnint.2019.00016

Eggermont, J. J. (2006). Cortical tonotopic map reorganization and its implications for treatment of tinnitus. *Acta Otolaryngol. Suppl.* 126, 9–12. doi: 10.1080/03655230600895259

Eggermont, J. J., and Roberts, L. E. (2004). The neuroscience of tinnitus. *Trends Neurosci.* 27, 676–682. doi: 10.1016/j.tins.2004.08.010

Evans, A. C. (2013). Networks of anatomical covariance. *NeuroImage* 80, 489–504. doi: 10.1016/j.neuroimage.2013.05.054

Feinstein, J. S., Ralph, A., Antonio, D., and Daniel, T. (2011). The human amygdala and the induction and experience of fear. *Curr. Biol.* 21, 34–38. doi: 10.1016/j.cub.2010.11.042

Fischl, B., and Dale, A. M. (2000). Measuring the thickness of the human cerebral cortex from magnetic resonance images. *Proc. Natl. Acad. Sci. U.S.A.* 97, 11050–11055. doi: 10.1073/pnas.200033797

Fischl, B., Salat, D. H., Busa, E., Albert, M., Dieterich, M., Haselgrove, C., et al. (2002). Whole brain segmentation: automated labeling of neuroanatomical structures in the human brain. *Neuron* 33, 341–355.

Golm, D., Schmidt-Samoa, C., Dechent, P., and Kröner-Herwig, B. (2013). Neural correlates of tinnitus related distress: an FMRI-study. *Hear. Res.* 295, 87–99. doi: 10.1016/j.heares.2012.03.003

Gong, S. C., and Xu, G. H. (2012). On the nullity of a graph with cut-points. *Linear Algebra Appl.* 436, 135–142. doi: 10.1016/j.laa.2011.06.039

Heller, A. J. (2003). Classification and epidemiology of tinnitus. *Otolaryngol. Clin. North Am.* 36, 239–248. doi: 10.1016/S0030-6665(02)00160-3

Henry, J. A., and Meikle, M. B. (2000). Psychoacoustic measures of tinnitus. *J. Am. Acad. Audiol.* 11, 138–155.

Heydrich, L., and Blanke, O. (2013). Distinct illusory own-body perceptions caused by damage to posterior insula and extrastriate cortex. *Brain* 136, 790–803. doi: 10.1093/brain/aws364

Honey, C. J., Sporns, O., Cammoun, L., Gigandet, X., Thiran, J. P., Meuli, R., et al. (2009). Predicting human resting-state functional connectivity from structural connectivity. *Proc. Natl. Acad. Sci. U.S.A.* 106, 2035–2040. doi: 10.1073/pnas.0811168106

Hosseini, S. M., Hoeft, F., and Kesler, S. R. (2012). GAT: a graph-theoretical analysis toolbox for analyzing between-group differences in large-scale structural and functional brain Networks. *PLoS One* 7:e40709. doi: 10.1371/journal.pone.0040709

Humphries, M. D., and Gurney, K. (2008). Network 'Small-World-Ness': a quantitative method for determining canonical network equivalence. *PLoS One* 3:e0002051. doi: 10.1371/journal.pone.0002051

Husain, F. T., Medina, R. E., Davis, C. W., Szymko-Bennett, Y., Simonyan, K., Pajor, N. M., et al. (2011). Neuroanatomical changes due to hearing loss and chronic tinnitus: a combined VBM and DTI study. *Brain Res.* 1369, 74–88. doi: 10.1016/j.brainres.2010.10.095

Jastreboff, P. J. (1990). Phantom auditory perception (Tinnitus): mechanisms of generation and perception. *Neurosci. Res.* 8, 221–254. doi: 10.1016/0168-0102(90)90031-9

Jiao, Y., Lin F., Wu J., Li, H., Fu, W., Huo, R., et al. (2020). Plasticity in language cortex and white matter tracts after resection of dominant inferior parietal lobule arteriovenous malformations: a combined fmri and dti study. *J. Neurosurg.* 20, 1–8. doi: 10.3171/2019.12.JNS191987

Kandeepan, S., Maudoux, A., Ribeiro de Paula, D., Zheng, J. Y., Cabay, J. E., Gómez, F., et al. (2019). Tinnitus distress: a paradoxical attention to the sound? *J. Neurol.* 266, 2197–2207. doi: 10.1007/s00415-019-09390-1

Khalfa, S., Dubal, S., Veuillet, E., Perez-Diaz, F., Jouvent, R., and Collet, L. (2002). Psychometric normalization of a hyperacusis questionnaire. *Orl* 64, 436–442. doi: 10.1159/000067570

Langguth, B., Kreuzer, P. M., Kleinjung, T., and De Ridder, D. (2013). Tinnitus: causes and clinical management. *Lancet Neurol.* 12, 920–930. doi: 10.1016/S1474-4422(13)70160-1

Lanting, C. P., de Kleine, E., Eppinga, R. N., and van Dijk, P. (2010). Neural correlates of human somatosensory integration in tinnitus. *Hear. Res.* 267, 78–88. doi: 10.1016/j.heares.2010.04.006

Latora, V., and Marchiori, M. (2001). Efficient behavior of small-world networks. *Phys. Rev. Lett.* 87:198701. doi: 10.1103/PhysRevLett.87.198701

Leaver, A. M., Renier, L., Chevillet, M. A., Morgan, S., Kim, H. J., and Rauschecker, J. P. (2011). Dysregulation of limbic and auditory networks in Tinnitus. *Neuron* 69, 33–43. doi: 10.1016/j.neuron.2010.12.002

Lehr, A., Niklas, H., Tarana, N., Walter, P., and Andrea, A. (2019). Modulation of conflict processing by theta-range TACS over the dorsolateral prefrontal cortex. *Neural Plast.* 2019:6747049. doi: 10.1155/2019/6747049

Li, W., Yang, C., Shi, F., Wu, S., Wang, Q., Nie, Y., et al. (2017). Construction of individual morphological brain networks with multiple morphometric features. *Front. Neuroanat.* 11:34. doi: 10.3389/fnana.2017.00034

Lv, H., Wang, Z., Tong, E., Williams, L. M., Zaharchuk, G., Zeineh, M., et al. (2018). Resting-state functional MRI: everything that Nonexperts have always wanted to know. *Am. J. Neuroradiol.* 39, 1390–1399. doi: 10.3174/ajnr.A5527

MacDonald, D., Kabani, N., Avis, D., and Evans, A. C. (2000). Automated 3-D extraction of inner and outer surfaces of cerebral cortex from MRI. *NeuroImage* 12, 340–356. doi: 10.1006/nimg.1999.0534

Menon, V., and Uddin, L. Q. (2010). Saliency, switching, attention and control: a network model of insula function. *Brain Struct. Funct.* 214, 655–667. doi: 10.1007/s00429-010-0262-0

Mijalkov, M., Kakaei, E., Pereira, J. B., Westman, E., Volpe, G., and Alzheimers Disease Neuroimaging Initiative (2017). BRAPH: a graph theory software for the analysis of brain connectivity. *PLoS One* 12:e0178798. doi: 10.1371/journal.pone.0178798

Mohan, A., De Ridder, D., and Vanneste, S. (2016). Graph theoretical analysis of brain connectivity in phantom sound perception. *Sci. Rep.* 6:19683. doi: 10.1038/srep19683

Mühlau, M., Rauschecker, J. P., Oestreicher, E., Gaser, C., Röttinger, M., Wohlschläger, A. M., et al. (2006). Structural brain changes in Tinnitus. *Cereb. Cortex* 16, 1283–1288. doi: 10.1093/cercor/bhj070

Narr, K. L., Toga, A. W., Szeszko, P., Thompson, P. M., Woods, R. P., Robinson, D., et al. (2005). Cortical thinning in cingulate and occipital cortices in first episode schizophrenia. *Biol. Psychiatry* 58, 32–40. doi: 10.1016/j.biopsych.2005.03.043

Newman, C. W., Jacobson, G. P., and Spitzer, J. B. (1996). Development of the Tinnitus handicap inventory. *Arch. Otolaryngol. Head Neck Surg.* 122, 143–148. doi: 10.1001/archotol.1996.01890140029007

Noreña, A. J., and Farley, B. J. (2013). Tinnitus-related neural activity: theories of generation, propagation, and centralization. *Hear. Res.* 295, 161–171. doi: 10.1016/j.heares.2012.09.010

Pereira, J. B., Ibarretxe-Bilbao, N., Marti, M. J., Compta, Y., Junqué, C., Bargallo, N., et al. (2012). Assessment of cortical degeneration in patients with parkinson's disease by voxel-based morphometry, cortical folding, and cortical thickness. *Hum. Brain Map.* 33, 2521–2534. doi: 10.1002/hbm.21378

Pessoa, L. (2014). Précis of the cognitive-emotional brain. *Behav. Brain Sci.* 43:e71. doi: 10.1017/S0140525X14000120

Rauschecker, J. P., Leaver, A. M., and Mühlau, M. (2010). Tuning out the noise: limbic-auditory interactions in Tinnitus. *Neuron* 66, 819–826. doi: 10.1016/j.neuron.2010.04.032

Rubinov, M., and Sporns, O. (2010). Complex network measures of brain connectivity: uses and interpretations. *NeuroImage* 52, 1059–1069. doi: 10.1016/j.neuroimage.2009.10.003

Ryu, C. W., Park, M. S., Byun, J. Y., Jahng, G. H., and Park, S. (2016). White matter integrity associated with clinical symptoms in tinnitus patients: a tract-based spatial statistics study. *Eur. Radiol.* 26, 2223–2232. doi: 10.1007/s00330-015-4034-3

Salvador, R., Suckling, J., Coleman, M. R., Pickard, J. D., Menon, D., and Bullmore, E. (2005). Neurophysiological architecture of functional magnetic resonance images of human brain. *Cereb. Cortex* 15, 1332–1342. doi: 10.1093/cercor/bhi016

Schneider, P., Andermann, M., Wengenroth, M., Goebel, R., Flor, H., Rupp, A., et al. (2009). Reduced volume of Heschl's gyrus in Tinnitus. *NeuroImage* 45, 927–939. doi: 10.1016/j.neuroimage.2008.12.045

Ségonne, F., Dale, A. M., Busa, E., Glessner, M., Salat, D., Hahn, H. K., et al. (2004). A hybrid approach to the skull stripping problem in MRI. *NeuroImage* 22, 1060–1075. doi: 10.1016/j.neuroimage.2004.03.032

Ségonne, F., Pacheco, J., and Fischl, B. (2007). Geometrically accurate topology-correction of cortical surfaces using nonseparating loops. *IEEE Trans. Med. Imaging* 26, 518–529. doi: 10.1109/TMI.2006.887364

Shargorodsky, J., Curhan, G. C., and Farwell, W. R. (2010). Prevalence and characteristics of Tinnitus among US adults. *Am. J. Med.* 123, 711–718. doi: 10.1016/j.amjmed.2010.02.015

Simonetti, P., and Oiticica, J. (2015). Tinnitus neural mechanisms and structural changes in the brain: the contribution of neuroimaging research. *Int. Arch. Otorhinolaryngol.* 19, 259–265. doi: 10.1055/s-0035-154 8671

Singh, V., Mukherjee, L., and Chung, M. K. (2008). Cortical surface thickness as a classifier: boosting for autism classification. *Med. Image Comput. Comput. Assist. Interv.* 11(Pt 1), 999–1007. doi: 10.1007/978-3-540-85988-8_119

Sled, J. G., Zijdenbos, A. P., and Evans, A. C. (1998). A nonparametric method for automatic correction of intensity nonuniformity in Mri data. *IEEE Trans. Med. Imaging* 17, 87–97. doi: 10.1109/42.668698

Soleymani, T., Pieton, D., Pezeshkian, P., Miller, P., Gorgulho, A. A., Pouratian, N., et al. (2011). Surgical approaches to tinnitus treatment: a review and novel approaches. *Surg. Neurol. Int.* 2:154. doi: 10.4103/2152-7806.86834

Uddin, L. Q., Nomi, J. S., Hébert-Seropian, B., Ghaziri, J., and Boucher, O. (2017). Structure and function of the human insula. *J. Clin. Neurophysiol.* 34, 300–306. doi: 10.1097/WNP.0000000000000377

Umeda, T., Isa, T., and Nishimura, Y. (2019). The somatosensory cortex receives information about motor output. *Sci. Adv.* 5:eaaw5388. doi: 10.1126/sciadv.aaw5388

van Strien, N. M., Cappaert, N. L. M., and Witter, M. P. (2009). The anatomy of memory: an interactive overview of the parahippocampal-hippocampal network. *Nat. Rev. Neurosci.* 10, 272–282. doi: 10.1038/nrn2614

Vanneste, S., Focquaert, F., Van de Heyning, P., and De Ridder, D. (2011). Different resting state brain activity and functional connectivity in patients who respond and not respond to bifrontal TDCS for Tinnitus suppression. *Exp. Brain Res.* 210, 217–227. doi: 10.1007/s00221-011-2617-z

Watts, D. J., and Strogatz, S. H. (1998). Collective dynamics of 'small-World' networks. *Nature* 393, 440–442. doi: 10.1038/30918

Weisz, N., Muller, S., Schlee, W., Dohrmann, K., Hartmann, T., and Elbert, T. (2007). The neural code of auditory phantom perception. *J. Neurosci.* 27, 1479–1484. doi: 10.1523/jneurosci.3711-06.2007

Yasuda, C. L., Chen, Z., Beltramini, G. C., Coan, A. C., Morita, M. E., Kubota, B., et al. (2015). Aberrant topological patterns of brain structural network in temporal lobe epilepsy. *Epilepsia* 56, 1992–2002. doi: 10.1111/epi.13225

Yoo, H. B., De Ridder, D., and Vanneste, S. (2016a). The importance of aging in gray matter changes within tinnitus patients shown in cortical thickness, surface area and volume. *Brain Topogr.* 29, 885–896. doi: 10.1007/s10548-016-0511-5

Yoo, H. B., De Ridder, D., and Vanneste, S. (2016b). White matter changes in tinnitus: is it all age and hearing loss? *Brain Connect.* 6, 84–93. doi: 10.1089/brain.2015.0380

Yun, J. Y., Boedhoe, P. S. W., Vriend, C., Jahanshad, N., Abe, Y., Ameis, S. H., et al. (2020). Brain structural covariance networks in obsessive-compulsive disorder: a graph analysis from the ENIGMA consortium. *Brain* 143, 684–700. doi: 10.1093/brain/awaa001

Zhang, W., Li, H., and Pan, X. (2015). Positive and negative affective processing exhibit dissociable functional hubs during the viewing of affective pictures. *Hum. Brain Map.* 36, 415–426. doi: 10.1002/hbm.22636

Zung, W. W. (1971). A rating instrument for anxiety disorders. *Psychosomatics* 12, 371–379. doi: 10.1016/S0033-3182(71)71479-0

10

Glucose Control has an Impact on Cerebral Blood Flow Alterations in Chronic Tinnitus Patients

Wenqing Xia[1†], Jinluan Cui[2†], Yong Luo[1], Jin-Jing Xu[3], Huiyou Chen[2], Xindao Yin[2], Jianhua Ma[1*] and Yuanqing Wu[3*]

[1] Department of Endocrinology, Nanjing First Hospital, Nanjing Medical University, Nanjing, China, [2] Department of Radiology, Nanjing First Hospital, Nanjing Medical University, Nanjing, China, [3] Department of Otolaryngology, Nanjing First Hospital, Nanjing Medical University, Nanjing, China

***Correspondence:**
Jianhua Ma
majianhua@china.com
Yuanqing Wu
cnnxdd@163.com

† These authors have contributed equally to this work

Purpose: Both tinnitus and type 2 diabetes mellitus (T2DM) are linked with cognitive decline and brain dysfunction. This study used arterial spin labeling (ASL) perfusion functional magnetic resonance imaging (fMRI) to examine the abnormal cerebral blood flow (CBF) patterns existed in tinnitus patients and potential relationships between the abnormal CBF and cognitive performance. The impact of T2DM on CBF alterations in tinnitus patients was further explored.

Methods: Sixty tinnitus patients and 40 non-tinnitus subjects were recruited. CBF images were collected and analyzed using ASL perfusion fMRI. Brain regions with CBF alterations between tinnitus patients and non-tinnitus controls were identified by one-way analysis of variance. Interaction effects between tinnitus and T2DM for CBF changes were also selected. Then, correlation analyses were calculated to specify the link between CBF changes and cognitive performance and between CBF changes and diabetic characteristics.

Results: Tinnitus patients showed decreased CBF, primarily in the auditory area and default mode network (DMN), compared with non-tinnitus controls. Decreased CBF in these regions was correlated with executive function and attention. The interaction effect between tinnitus and T2DM was significant in the right medial prefrontal gyrus. Additionally, CBF in the right medial prefrontal gyrus was correlated with tinnitus distress and cognitive performance. In tinnitus patients, Hemoglobin A_{1c} was associated with CBF in the right medial prefrontal gyrus.

Conclusion: Tinnitus affects brain perfusion in the auditory area and DMN. T2DM and uncontrolled glucose levels may aggravate a CBF decrease in tinnitus patients. These new findings implied that tinnitus patients may benefit from blood glucose control in terms of their cognitive function and tinnitus distress.

Keywords: tinnitus, type 2 diabetes mellitus, cognitive impairment, cerebral blood flow, magnetic resonance imaging

INTRODUCTION

Tinnitus is a common audiological disorder that affects approximately 10–15% of adult populations (Langguth et al., 2013; Nemholt et al., 2015). Metabolic disorders, such as hyperinsulinemia and diabetes, are considered as risk factors of tinnitus symptoms or comorbidities and have significant relationships with the tinnitus distress, with or without hearing loss (Taneja, 2017). Tinnitus as a symptom is mostly observed in disorders involving metabolic disturbances and diabetes mellitus (DM) (Nemati et al., 2018). Conversely, higher blood glucose level will increase the burden of tinnitus distress.

Numerous studies have demonstrated poorer cognitive performance, especially on control of attention, executive, and memory in tinnitus patients compared to individuals without tinnitus (Das et al., 2012; Pierce et al., 2012; Heeren et al., 2014); however, there are still a few investigations that reported no influence of tinnitus in the cognitive function (Husain et al., 2015). Interestingly, both clinical and animal studies suggest that type 2 DM (T2DM) is a modifiable and independent causal risk factor for the development and progression of cognitive impairment (Zuloaga et al., 2016; Pal et al., 2018). Therefore, T2DM is a potential risk factor for the cognitive decline observed in tinnitus patients. The precise correlation between hyperglycemic state and brain functioning has not been illustrated in tinnitus patients.

Cognitive deterioration may be affected by a declined CBF as a result of brain ischemia and energy depletion (Ogoh, 2017). Cerebral blood flow (CBF) can be evaluated using single-photon emission computed tomography (SPECT). Current researches using SPECT shows that tinnitus patients exhibit decreased CBF in certain brain areas (Farhadi et al., 2010; Laureano et al., 2014). Arterial spin labeling (ASL) is a non-invasive functional magnetic resonance imaging (fMRI) technique for measuring regional CBF that uses magnetically labeled blood water as an endogenous tracer (Detre et al., 1992). With higher resolution and accurate localization, ASL perfusion fMRI has been applied to detect early stages of dementia patients (Binnewijzend et al., 2013; Dolui et al., 2020), but has never been used to evaluate CBF in tinnitus patients. Regarding T2DM, our previous study shows that T2DM patients exhibited reduced CBF in widespread brain regions, primarily in the visual area and the default mode network (DMN) (Xia et al., 2015), which is later confirmed by further studies (Bangen et al., 2018; Hu et al., 2019). Further research is needed to investigate whether brain areas show CBF alterations in the tinnitus patients and to determine whether T2DM is involved in the CBF fluctuation in these regions.

Hence, hypothesis was raised that patients with tinnitus would exhibit abnormal CBF and cognitive decline compared with non-tinnitus subjects and that the comorbidity of T2DM would aggravate the abnormal brain perfusion. We also intended to explore whether diabetic characteristics would be correlated with higher CBF values in tinnitus patients.

MATERIALS AND METHODS

Participants

Study protocol was approved by the Research Ethics Committee of the Nanjing Medical University prior to study initiation. All the subjects provided written informed consent before any study procedures.

Through community health screening and newspaper advertisements, 60 patients with tinnitus and 40 non-tinnitus controls, who were all right-handed and completed at least 6 years of education, were recruited (matched for age, sex, and education) from March 2016 to November 2019. All tinnitus patients reported their tinnitus as bilateral or originating within the head. According to the World Health Organization 1999 criteria for T2DM diagnosis, 25 tinnitus patients were diagnosed with T2DM. Participants who had hearing loss (defined as thresholds ≥25 dB HL) at the frequencies of 0.25, 0.5, 1, 2, 4, and 8 kHz were excluded. Participants with hyperacusis were excluded according to Hyperacusis Questionnaire (Khalfa et al., 2002). In addition, according to previous diagnostic criteria (Lopez-Escamez et al., 2015), patients with Ménière diseases were excluded. Subjects were also excluded if they

TABLE 1 | Demographics and cognitive characteristics of tinnitus patients and non-tinnitus controls.

	Tinnitus patients (n = 58)	Non-tinnitus controls (n = 39)	p value
Age, years	49.81 ± 10.57	47.46 ± 11.69	0.307
Gender, male:female	21:37	16:23	0.632
Education levels, years	12.47 ± 3.09	13.03 ± 3.04	0.381
Tinnitus duration, months	37.07 ± 34.40	–	–
THQ score	52.50 ± 13.76	–	–
Hearing thresholds (left)	16.03 ± 3.02	16.99 ± 2.48	0.105
Hearing thresholds (right)	16.62 ± 3.16	16.67 ± 2.39	0.942
Hearing thresholds (mean)	16.10 ± 2.64	16.83 ± 1.51	0.123
Diabetes characteristics			
HbA_{1C}, % (mmol/mol)	6.53 ± 1.68	6.15 ± 1.24	0.228
Fasting glucose, mmol/L	6.48 ± 2.29	5.79 ± 1.56	0.103
Triglyceride, mmol/L	1.48 ± 0.71	1.54 ± 0.57	0.648
Total cholesterol, mmol/L	5.64 ± 1.05	5.29 ± 0.90	0.092
LDL-C, mmol/L	3.44 ± 0.70	3.24 ± 0.74	0.201
HDL-C, mmol/L	1.40 ± 0.32	1.44 ± 0.34	0.511
Cognitive performance			
MMSE	29.07 ± 1.00	28.77 ± 1.20	0.187
AVLT	34.02 ± 7.26	34.10 ± 6.72	0.954
CFT	34.22 ± 1.82	34.64 ± 1.67	0.255
CFT-delayed recall	17.38 ± 2.49	16.54 ± 2.98	0.136
TMT-A	64.72 ± 20.49	47.72 ± 12.84	<0.001*
TMT-B	155.02 ± 65.60	103.72 ± 36.09	<0.001*
CDT	3.50 ± 0.54	3.38 ± 0.59	0.322

*Data are presented as mean ± standard deviation. *p < 0.001. THQ, Tinnitus Handicap Questionnaire; LDL-C, low-density lipoprotein cholesterol; HDL-C, high-density lipoprotein cholesterol; MMSE, Mini Mental State Examination; AVLT, Auditory Verbal Learning Test; CFT, Complex Figure Test; TMT-A, Trail Making Test–Part A; TMT-B, Trail Making Test–Part B; CDT, Clock Drawing Test.*

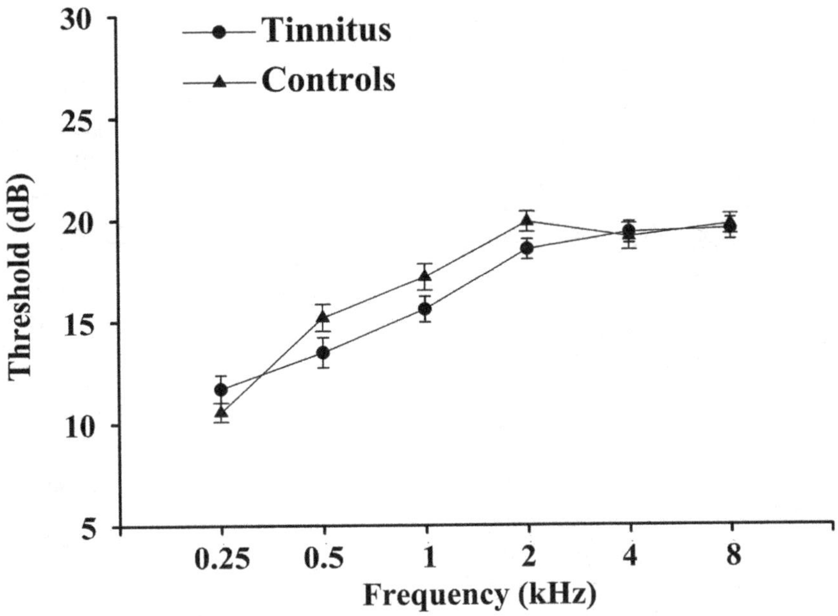

FIGURE 1 | Average hearing thresholds of chronic tinnitus patients and non-tinnitus controls. Data are presented as mean ± SEM.

had objective tinnitus, severe visual loss, a history of stroke, major medical illness, neurological or psychiatric illness such as Alzheimer disease, head injury, anemia, Parkinson disease, epilepsy, and major depression, magnetic resonance imaging (MRI) contraindications, severe heart diseases, and damaged liver/kidney function.

Clinical Data

Demographic information was collected prior to the MRI scan. Hearing thresholds were assessed by pure tone audiometry by an experienced otolaryngologist. The tinnitus distress was assessed by the Iowa version of the Tinnitus Handicap Questionnaire (THQ) (Kuk et al., 1990). After an overnight fast, venous blood samples were collected. Fasting blood glucose, hemoglobin A_{1c} (HbA_{1c}), and blood lipid levels were assessed. Cognitive performance was evaluated by the cognitive tests in a fixed order, including the Mini Mental State Examination (MMSE), Rey–Osterrieth Complex Figure Test (CFT), Auditory Verbal Learning Test, Clock Drawing Test, and Trail Making Test (TMT) Parts A and B.

Magnetic Resonance Imaging Data Acquisition

All participants were scanned using a 3.0-T MRI scanner (Ingenia, Philips Medical Systems, Netherlands). The participants were instructed to rest quietly with eyes closed and avoiding either falling asleep or making a sudden head motion and to not think of anything in particular. Three-dimensional T1-weighted images were acquired using the parameters as follows: repetition time (TR) = 8.1 ms, echo time (TE) = 3.7 ms, thickness = 1 mm, slices = 170, gap = 0 mm, flip angle (FA) = 8°, field of view (FOV) = 256 mm × 256 mm, and acquisition matrix = 256 × 256. ASL images were obtained with a pseudocontinuous ASL sequence with a two-dimensional fast spin-echo acquisition and background suppression using the parameters as follows: TR = 4,000 ms, TE = 11 ms, slice thickness = 4 mm, label duration = 1,650 ms; postlabel delay = 2,000 ms, FA = 90°, FOV = 220 mm × 220 mm, slices thickness = 4 mm, gap = 0.4 mm, and matrix = 64 × 64.

TABLE 2 | Comparisons of the brain volumes between tinnitus patients and non-tinnitus controls.

	Tinnitus patients (n = 58)	Non-tinnitus controls (n = 39)	p value
Gray matter volume (% of TIV)	31.8 ± 2.0	32.6 ± 2.0	0.071
White matter volume (% of TIV)	29.4 ± 1.5	29.7 ± 1.7	0.448
Brain parenchyma volume (% of TIV)	61.2 ± 2.9	62.2 ± 3.2	0.109

Data are expressed as mean ± SD. TIV, total intracranial volume.

TABLE 3 | Brain regions with significant differences in CBF between tinnitus patients and non-tinnitus controls.

Brain regions	BA	Peak MNI coordinates x, y, z (mm)	Peak T value	Cluster size (voxels)
R superior temporal gyrus	22	58, 6, 6	−4.2384	189
L posterior cingulate cortex	23	−5, −44, 17	−4.7829	135
R medial prefrontal gyrus	24	3, 44, −8	−4.1908	140

Thresholds were set at a corrected p < 0.01 corrected by FWE criterion. L, left; R, right.

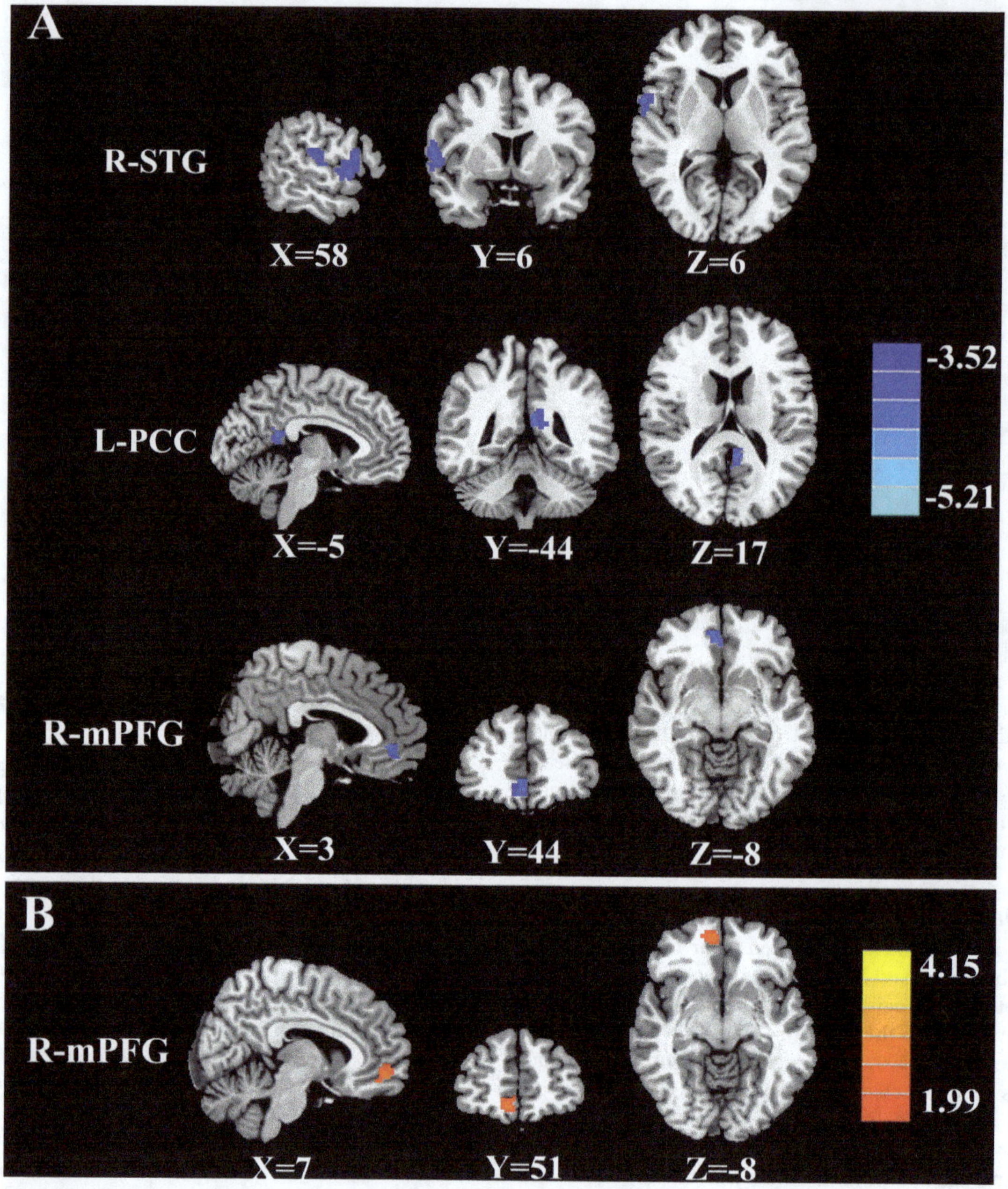

FIGURE 2 | The CBF differences between tinnitus patients and non-tinnitus controls. **(A)** The tinnitus patients exhibited decreased CBF in the right superior temporal gyrus (STG), left posterior cingulate cortex (PCC), and right medial prefrontal gyrus (mPFG) ($p < 0.01$, FWE corrected). **(B)** The interaction effect of diabetes and tinnitus in the right mPFG ($p < 0.01$, FWE corrected).

Imaging Data Processing

To estimate the whole-brain volumes, a voxel-based morphometry (VBM) approach was performed using the VBM8 toolbox[1]. We used DARTEL to improve intersubject registration of the structural images. Briefly, cerebral tissues were segmented into gray matter (GM), white matter (WM), and cerebrospinal fluid by a unified segmentation algorithm (Ashburner and Friston, 2005). Resulting GM and WM images were then normalized to the Montreal Neurological Institute (MNI) template. Smoothing was followed by using a 6-mm full width at half maximum (FWHM) Gaussian kernel. The final voxel-wise GM volume maps were later entered as covariates in the ASL analysis.

Using the ASL Perfusion MRI Signal Processing Toolbox (ASLtbx), which is based on SPM12[2] (Wang, 2012), the ASL

[1] http://dbm.neuro.uni-jena.de/vbm

[2] http://www.fil.ion.ucl.ac.uk/spm/

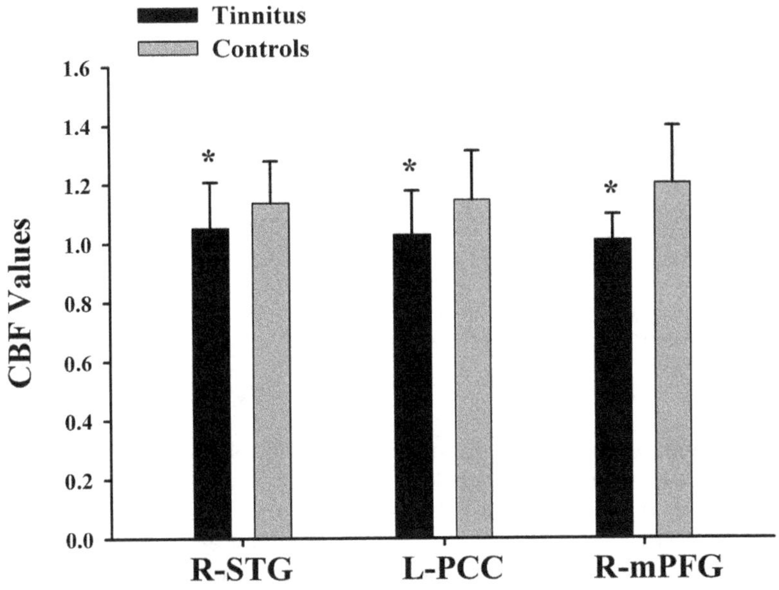

FIGURE 3 | The CBF values of chronic tinnitus patients and non-tinnitus controls in the right STG, left PCC, and right mPFG ($p < 0.01$). *Means significant difference between two groups.

data were preprocessed to generate CBF maps. Images were first rearranged and adjusted to correct head movement. Then, a non-linear transformation was performed on the CBF images of non-tinnitus subjects, which were co-registered with the positron emission tomography (PET) perfusion template in MNI space. The MNI-standard CBF template was defined as the average co-registered CBF images of the control group. Next, the CBF images of all subjects were co-registered to the MNI-standard CBF template. Every co-registered CBF was removed from the non-brain tissue, followed by a spatial smoothing using a 6-mm FWHM isotropic Gaussian. Normalization was finally performed. The CBF was divided per voxel by the average CBF (Aslan and Lu, 2010). Two tinnitus patients and one non-tinnitus control were excluded from the study because of head movement exceeding 2.0 mm of maximum translation in any of the *x*, *y*, and *z* directions or 2.0° of the maximum rotation around the three axes.

Statistical Analysis

Clinical measures were analyzed using Statistical Package for the Social Sciences (SPSS) statistics software package version 20.0. Differences between the patients with tinnitus and non-tinnitus subjects were calculated. For normally distributed variable, a Student *t* test was used. For asymmetrically distributed variable, a non-parametric Mann–Whitney *U* test was used. For categorical variable, a χ^2 test was used. The statistical significance level was set at $p < 0.05$, two-tailed.

A one-way analysis of variance (ANOVA) was then performed to determine between-group differences in brain volumes, with age, gender, and education level as the nuisance covariates. Between-group differences in CBF were also calculated via one-way ANOVA in SPM12, with age, gender, and education level as the nuisance covariates. Significant thresholds were corrected using false discovery rate criterion and set at $p < 0.01$. A full-factorial model was utilized to detect potential interaction effects between tinnitus and diabetes on CBF differences. Significant thresholds were corrected using cluster-level family-wise error (FWE), and the threshold was set at $p < 0.01$.

The relationships between abnormal CBF in certain brain areas and THQ scores, cognitive performance, and glucose levels were further calculated. First, the brain regions that showed significant differences between the two groups were extracted, and the mean *z* values of abnormal CBF region mask were calculated within each subject. Then, Pearson correlation analysis between the mean *z* values and THQ scores, cognitive performance, and glucose characteristic was performed using SPSS software. Partial correlations were calculated after correction for age, gender, and education. $P < 0.05$ was considered statistically significant.

RESULTS

A set of Chinese Han population was tested in the current study. The average age for tinnitus was 49.81 ± 10.57 years, and duration of tinnitus was 37.07 ± 34.40 months. There are

TABLE 4 | Regions showing interaction effects of tinnitus and diabetes on CBF.

Brain regions	BA	Peak MNI coordinates x, y, z (mm)	Peak *T* value	Cluster size (voxels)
R medial prefrontal gyrus	24	7, 51, −8	3.9320	95

Thresholds were set at a corrected p < 0.01 corrected by FWE criterion. R, right.

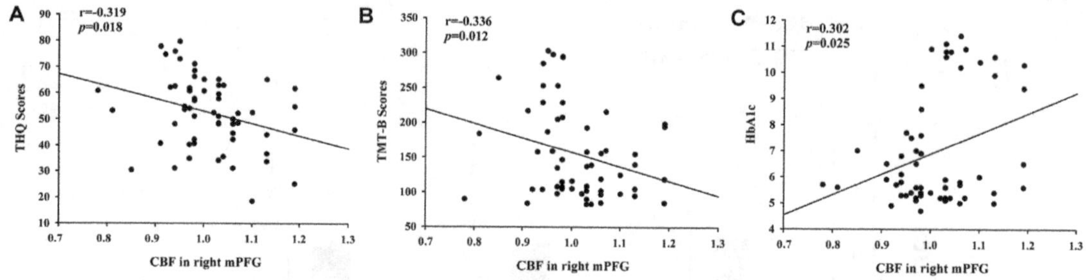

FIGURE 4 | The significant correlations between the CBF changes and the clinical data in tinnitus patients. **(A)** CBF in the right mPFG was negatively associated with THQ scores ($r = -0.319$, $p = 0.018$). **(B)** CBF in the right mPFG was negatively associated with TMT-B scores ($r = -0.336$, $p = 0.012$). **(C)** CBF in the right mPFG was positively correlated with the HbA_{1c} values ($r = 0.302$, $p = 0.025$).

no significant differences between tinnitus patients and controls in terms of age, gender, and education level. Key diabetes characteristics (i.e., HbA_{1c}, fasting glucose, and lipid levels) also did not differ meaningfully between the two groups. All subjects exhibited normal performance according to MMSE score. We detected a trend for a difference in TMT-A and TMT-B scores ($p < 0.001$) between groups (**Table 1**). There were no significant differences of auditory thresholds between tinnitus patients and non-tinnitus controls (**Figure 1**).

In the current study, none of structural changes in specific brain regions were observed between patients with chronic tinnitus and non-tinnitus controls ($p > 0.05$). Besides, the GM, WM, and BP volumes of each group were not significantly different (**Table 2**). We also did not observe any differences of the brain volumes between tinnitus patients with and without diabetes ($p > 0.05$).

The tinnitus patients displayed disrupted CBF, primarily in the auditory area and DMN, including the decreased CBF regions, namely, right superior temporal gyrus (STG), left posterior cingulate cortex (PCC), and right medial prefrontal gyrus (mPFG) ($p < 0.01$, corrected; **Table 3** and **Figure 2A**). The CBF values in each brain region for different groups are shown in **Figure 3**. The interaction effect between tinnitus and diabetes was significant in the right mPFG ($p < 0.01$, corrected; **Table 4** and **Figure 2B**). We did not observe other abnormal DMN regions in tinnitus patients with or without diabetes.

By calculating correlations between CBF in certain areas and THQ scores as well as cognitive scores (**Figure 4**), we observed that the relative CBF in the right mPFG was correlated THQ scores ($r = -0.319$, $p = 0.018$) and TMT-B scores ($r = -0.336$, $p = 0.012$). Moreover, HbA_{1c} was associated with CBF in the right mPFG in tinnitus patients ($r = 0.302$, $p = 0.025$).

DISCUSSION

The current study quantified CBF in tinnitus patients and investigated the influence of diabetes on the brain of tinnitus patients. Compared to non-tinnitus controls, tinnitus patients exhibit reduced CBF, which was directly associated with the severity of tinnitus. Interestingly, we also revealed that diabetes exacerbated CBF reduction in tinnitus patients, and poorly controlled glucose level was associated with decreased brain perfusion.

Structural alterations could contribute to aberrant brain perfusion; however, we did not detect structural alterations between tinnitus patients and non-tinnitus subjects in this study. It could be explained by the relatively younger ages and shorter duration of the tinnitus population. Considering the lack of structural change, our results indicated that CBF changes related to tinnitus can occur prior to structural abnormalities.

In our study, main effects of tinnitus were primarily in auditory and DMN regions. Self-directed attention and poor performance on memory tasks could be regarded as symptomatic of a hyperactive autobiographical memory network, known as the DMN in its "resting-state" form, which is responsible for rumination and introspection. The DMN, consisting of nodes in the PCC/anterior cingulate cortex, medial prefrontal cortex, middle temporal cortex, precuneus, and IPL, is active at rest and suspended when entering a task-based state involving attention or goal-directed behavior. Chen et al. investigate the disrupted intrinsic functional connectivity within the DMN regions in tinnitus patients (Chen et al., 2018a), which was correlated with cognitive performance (Chen et al., 2018b). Previous research also implicated a negative influence of tinnitus on verbal fluency, which could be related to a deficit in executive cognitive control (Cardon et al., 2019). Similarly, a previous systematic review indicates the presence of tinnitus negatively impacts the cognitive functioning, particularly attentional functioning (Trevis et al., 2018). Consistent with these, TMT-B test, as a reflection of execution and attention, also showed significant differences between tinnitus patients and controls and is correlated with the diminished CBF in mPFG in the current study. TMT-B score is a neurocognitive test that reflects the function of the prefrontal cortex, and it has been commonly used to define cognitive impairments, especially the executive dysfunction (Ardila et al., 2000). Medial prefrontal cortex takes charge of the ongoing supervision of information and coordinates the activities of multiple cortical regions (Krueger et al., 2007). It is also involved in auditory attention and exerts early inhibitory modulation of input to auditory cortex (Knight et al., 1989). Task MRI study has postulated that the impairment of executive function caused by prefrontal cortex changes could be an important factor in the generation and persistence of tinnitus (Araneda et al., 2017).

Previous studies have also suggested the mPFG as an important role in chronic tinnitus (Rauschecker et al., 2015; Araneda et al., 2017; Chen et al., 2018a,b). The relationships between CBF and THQ as well as CBF and TMT-B scores probably support the hypothesis that an abnormal perfusion pattern within DMN and auditory region may play a vital role in tinnitus-related cognitive impairment.

Furthermore, the mPFG works as a vital hub of the DMN and is also considered as a region vulnerable to T2DM. A neuroimaging study focusing on the brain glucose metabolic changes assessed by ^{18}F–fluorodeoxyglucose PET reported that the terrible executive function and memory impairment in T2DM correlated with reduced glucose metabolism in the medial prefrontal cortex regions (García-Casares et al., 2014). In another fMRI study exploring the diabetic DMN regions, T2DM patients showed increased connectivity in the medial prefrontal cortex (Cui et al., 2015). In addition, animal experiment also suggested that axon initial segments were significantly shortened in medial prefrontal cortex of db/db mice, a diabetic animal model, compared with controls (Yermakov et al., 2019). In the current study, higher blood glucose levels were correlated with lower CBF values in tinnitus patients, indicating that hyperglycemic state has a negative impact on the brain perfusion in tinnitus patients, and tinnitus patients may benefit from controlled glucose levels to maintain better cognitive functions.

Several limitations of this study should be summarized. First, while we presented some preliminary evidences supporting a possible relationship between the brain perfusion and the cognitive performance, as well as tinnitus distress, it is still inconclusive at this point, and more longitudinal study with bigger sample size of the relationships is required. Second, because of the limited sample size, we did not conduct subgroup analysis. However, the comparison between the left-sided, right-sided, and bilateral tinnitus could be meaningful for the mechanism of the lateralization in tinnitus. Finally, we cannot completely prevent subjects from hearing some sound during the MRI scan, although this study has attempted to minimize the amount of scanner noise with earplugs. It should still be taken into account while attempting to draw conclusions in studies involving auditory stimulation in general.

In conclusion, the current study reveals that patients with tinnitus exhibit disrupted CBF in DMN and auditory regions and that reduced CBF in tinnitus patients associated with the tinnitus distress and cognitive behavior. T2DM exacerbates CBF decline in tinnitus patients, and the better controlled glucose was positively associated with CBF values in tinnitus patients. Thus, tinnitus patients would likely benefit from glucose control in order to maintain brain perfusion and prevent the progression of tinnitus.

ETHICS STATEMENT

The studies involving human participants were reviewed and approved by the Research Ethics Committee of the Nanjing Medical University. The patients/participants provided their written informed consent to participate in this study. Written informed consent was obtained from the individual(s) for the publication of any potentially identifiable images or data included in this article.

AUTHOR CONTRIBUTIONS

WX and JC designed the study and supervised the conduct of the study. YL and J-JX contributed to the data collection. HC and XY provided methodological advice, performed the data analysis, and results interpretation. WX, JM, and YW drafted the manuscript, which all authors reviewed and approved for publication.

REFERENCES

Araneda, R., Renier, L., Dricot, L., Decat, M., Ebner-Karestinos, D., Deggouj, N., et al. (2017). A key role of the prefrontal cortex in the maintenance of chronic tinnitus: an fMRI study using a Stroop task. *Neuroimage Clin.* 17, 325–334. doi: 10.1016/j.nicl.2017.10.029

Ardila, A., Pineda, D., and Rosselli, M. (2000). Correlation between intelligence test scores and executive function measures. *Arch. Clin. Neuropsychol.* 15, 31–36. doi: 10.1016/s0887-6177(98)00159-0

Ashburner, J., and Friston, K. J. (2005). Unified segmentation. *NeuroImage* 26, 839–851. doi: 10.1016/j.neuroimage.2005.02.018

Aslan, S., and Lu, H. (2010). On the sensitivity of ASL MRI in detecting regional differences in cerebral blood flow. *Magn. Resonan. Imag.* 28, 928–935. doi: 10.1016/j.mri.2010.03.037

Bangen, K. J., Werhane, M. L., Weigand, A. J., Edmonds, E. C., Delano-Wood, L., Thomas, K. R., et al. (2018). Reduced regional cerebral blood flow relates to poorer cognition in older adults with type 2 diabetes. *Front. Aging Neurosci.* 10:270. doi: 10.3389/fnagi.2018.00270

Binnewijzend, M. A., Kuijer, J. P., Benedictus, M. R., Van Der Flier, W. M., Wink, A. M., Wattjes, M. P., et al. (2013). Cerebral blood flow measured with 3D pseudocontinuous arterial spin-labeling MR imaging in Alzheimer disease and mild cognitive impairment: a marker for disease severity. *Radiology* 267, 221–230. doi: 10.1148/radiol.12120928

Cardon, E., Jacquemin, L., Mertens, G., Van De Heyning, P., Vanderveken, O. M., Topsakal, V., et al. (2019). Cognitive performance in chronic tinnitus patients: a cross-sectional study using the RBANS-H. *Otol. Neurotol.* 40, e876–e882.

Chen, Y. C., Chen, H., Bo, F., Xu, J. J., Deng, Y., Lv, H., et al. (2018a). Tinnitus distress is associated with enhanced resting-state functional connectivity within the default mode network. *Neuropsychiatr. Dis. Treat.* 14, 1919–1927. doi: 10.2147/ndt.s164619

Chen, Y. C., Zhang, H., Kong, Y., Lv, H., Cai, Y., Chen, H., et al. (2018b). Alterations of the default mode network and cognitive impairment in patients with unilateral chronic tinnitus. *Quant. Imag. Med. Surg.* 8, 1020–1029. doi: 10.21037/qims.2018.11.04

Cui, Y., Jiao, Y., Chen, H. J., Ding, J., Luo, B., Peng, C. Y., et al. (2015). Aberrant functional connectivity of default-mode network in type 2 diabetes patients. *Eur. Radiol.* 25, 3238–3246. doi: 10.1007/s00330-015-3746-8

Das, S. K., Wineland, A., Kallogjeri, D., and Piccirillo, J. F. (2012). Cognitive speed as an objective measure of tinnitus. *Laryngoscope* 122, 2533–2538. doi: 10.1002/lary.23555

Detre, J. A., Leigh, J. S., Williams, D. S., and Koretsky, A. P. (1992). Perfusion imaging. *Magn. Resonan. Med.* 23, 37–45.

Dolui, S., Li, Z., Nasrallah, I. M., Detre, J. A., and Wolk, D. A. (2020). Arterial spin labeling versus 18F-FDG-PET to identify mild cognitive impairment. *NeuroImage Clin.* 25, 102146. doi: 10.1016/j.nicl.2019.102146

Farhadi, M., Mahmoudian, S., Saddadi, F., Karimian, A. R., Mirzaee, M., Ahmadizadeh, M., et al. (2010). Functional brain abnormalities localized in 55 chronic tinnitus patients: fusion of SPECT coincidence imaging and MRI. *J. Cereb. Blood Flow Metab.* 30, 864–870. doi: 10.1038/jcbfm.2009.254

García-Casares, N., Jorge, R. E., García-Arnés, J. A., Acion, L., Berthier, M. L., Gonzalez-Alegre, P., et al. (2014). Cognitive dysfunctions in middle-aged type 2 diabetic patients and neuroimaging correlations: a cross-sectional study. *J. Alzheimers Dis.* 42, 1337–1346. doi: 10.3233/jad-140702

Heeren, A., Maurage, P., Perrot, H., De Volder, A., Renier, L., Araneda, R., et al. (2014). Tinnitus specifically alters the top-down executive control sub-component of attention: evidence from the attention network task. *Behav. Brain Res.* 269, 147–154. doi: 10.1016/j.bbr.2014.04.043

Hu, B., Yan, L.-F., Sun, Q., Yu, Y., Zhang, J., Dai, Y.-J., et al. (2019). Disturbed neurovascular coupling in type 2 diabetes mellitus patients: evidence from a comprehensive fMRI analysis. *NeuroImage Clin.* 22:101802. doi: 10.1016/j.nicl.2019.101802

Husain, F. T., Akrofi, K., Carpenter-Thompson, J. R., and Schmidt, S. A. (2015). Alterations to the attention system in adults with tinnitus are modality specific. *Brain Res.* 1620, 81–97. doi: 10.1016/j.brainres.2015.05.010

Khalfa, S., Dubal, S., Veuillet, E., Perez-Diaz, F., Jouvent, R., and Collet, L. (2002). Psychometric normalization of a hyperacusis questionnaire. *Orl* 64, 436–442. doi: 10.1159/000067570

Knight, R. T., Scabini, D., and Woods, D. L. (1989). Prefrontal cortex gating of auditory transmission in humans. *Brain Res.* 504, 338–342. doi: 10.1016/0006-8993(89)91381-4

Krueger, F., Moll, J., Zahn, R., Heinecke, A., and Grafman, J. (2007). Event frequency modulates the processing of daily life activities in human medial prefrontal cortex. *Cereb. Cortex* 17, 2346–2353. doi: 10.1093/cercor/bhl143

Kuk, F. K., Tyler, R. S., Russell, D., and Jordan, H. (1990). The psychometric properties of a tinnitus handicap questionnaire. *Ear Hear.* 11, 434–445. doi: 10.1097/00003446-199012000-00005

Langguth, B., Kreuzer, P. M., Kleinjung, T., and De Ridder, D. (2013). Tinnitus: causes and clinical management. *Lancet Neurol.* 12, 920–930. doi: 10.1016/s1474-4422(13)70160-1

Laureano, M. R., Onishi, E. T., Bressan, R. A., Castiglioni, M. L. V., Batista, I. R., Reis, M. A., et al. (2014). Memory networks in tinnitus: a functional brain image study. *PLoS One* 9:e87839. doi: 10.1371/journal.pone.0087839

Lopez-Escamez, J. A., Carey, J., Chung, W.-H., Goebel, J. A., Magnusson, M., Mandalà, M., et al. (2015). Diagnostic criteria for Menière's disease. *J. Vestib. Res.* 25, 1–7.

Nemati, S., Hassanzadeh, R., Mehrdad, M., and Sajedi Kia, S. (2018). Hearing status in patients with Type 2 diabetes mellitus according to blood-sugar control: a comparative study. *Iran J. Otorhinolaryngol.* 30, 209–218.

Nemholt, S. S., Schmidt, J. H., Wedderkopp, N., and Baguley, D. M. (2015). Prevalence of tinnitus and/or hyperacusis in children and adolescents: study protocol for a systematic review. *BMJ Open* 5:e006649. doi: 10.1136/bmjopen-2014-006649

Ogoh, S. (2017). Relationship between cognitive function and regulation of cerebral blood flow. *J. Physiol. Sci.* 67, 345–351. doi: 10.1007/s12576-017-0525-0

Pal, K., Mukadam, N., Petersen, I., and Cooper, C. (2018). Mild cognitive impairment and progression to dementia in people with diabetes, prediabetes and metabolic syndrome: a systematic review and meta-analysis. *Soc. Psychiatry Psychiatr. Epidemiol.* 53, 1149–1160. doi: 10.1007/s00127-018-1581-3

Pierce, K. J., Kallogjeri, D., Piccirillo, J. F., Garcia, K. S., Nicklaus, J. E., and Burton, H. (2012). Effects of severe bothersome tinnitus on cognitive function measured with standardized tests. *J. Clin. Exp. Neuropsychol.* 34, 126–134. doi: 10.1080/13803395.2011.623120

Rauschecker, J. P., May, E. S., Maudoux, A., and Ploner, M. (2015). Frontostriatal gating of tinnitus and chronic pain. *Trends Cogn. Sci.* 19, 567–578. doi: 10.1016/j.tics.2015.08.002

Taneja, N. (2017). Tinnitus, hearing impair-ment and diabetes: a mini-review. *Otolaryngol. Open J.* SE, S6–S9.

Trevis, K. J., Mclachlan, N. M., and Wilson, S. J. (2018). A systematic review and meta-analysis of psychological functioning in chronic tinnitus. *Clin. Psychol. Rev.* 60, 62–86. doi: 10.1016/j.cpr.2017.12.006

Wang, Z. (2012). Improving cerebral blood flow quantification for arterial spin labeled perfusion MRI by removing residual motion artifacts and global signal fluctuations. *Magn. Resonan. Imag.* 30, 1409–1415. doi: 10.1016/j.mri.2012.05.004

Xia, W., Rao, H., Spaeth, A. M., Huang, R., Tian, S., Cai, R., et al. (2015). Blood pressure is associated with cerebral blood flow alterations in patients with T2DM as revealed by perfusion functional MRI. *Medicine* 94:e2231. doi: 10.1097/md.0000000000002231

Yermakov, L. M., Griggs, R. B., Drouet, D. E., Sugimoto, C., Williams, M. T., Vorhees, C. V., et al. (2019). Impairment of cognitive flexibility in type 2 diabetic db/db mice. *Behav. Brain Res.* 371:26.

Zuloaga, K. L., Johnson, L. A., Roese, N. E., Marzulla, T., Zhang, W., Nie, X., et al. (2016). High fat diet-induced diabetes in mice exacerbates cognitive deficit due to chronic hypoperfusion. *J. Cereb. Blood Flow Metab.* 36, 1257–1270. doi: 10.1177/0271678x15616400

11

Inhibition of Brain Area and Functional Connectivity in Idiopathic Sudden Sensorineural Hearing Loss with Tinnitus, Based on Resting-State EEG

Yuexin Cai[1,2†], Jiahong Li[1,2†], Yanhong Chen[1,2], Wan Chen[3], Caiping Dang[4,5], Fei Zhao[6,7], Wenrui Li[1,2], Guisheng Chen[1,2], Suijun Chen[1,2], Maojin Liang[1,2] and Yiqing Zheng[1,2]*

[1] Department of Otolaryngology, Sun Yat-sen Memorial Hospital, Sun Yat-sen University, Guangzhou, China, [2] Institute of Hearing and Speech-Language Science, Sun Yat-sen University, Guangzhou, China, [3] State Key Laboratory of Ophthalmology, Zhongshan Ophthalmic Center, Sun Yat-sen University, Guangzhou, China, [4] Affiliated Brain Hospital of Guangzhou Medical University, Guangzhou, China, [5] Department of Psychology, Guangzhou Medical University, Guangzhou, China, [6] Department of Speech Language Therapy and Hearing Science, Cardiff Metropolitan University, Cardiff, United Kingdom, [7] Department of Hearing and Speech Science, Xinhua College, Sun Yat-sen University, Guangzhou, China

***Correspondence:**
Yiqing Zheng
zhengyiq@mail.sysu.edu.cn;
yiqingzheng@hotmail.com

†These authors have contributed equally to this work

This study aimed to identify the mechanism behind idiopathic sudden sensorineural hearing loss (ISSNHL) in patients with tinnitus by investigating aberrant activity in areas of the brain and functional connectivity. High-density electroencephalography (EEG) was used to investigate central nervous changes in 25 ISSNHL subjects and 27 healthy controls. ISSNHL subjects had significantly reduced activity in the left frontal lobe at the alpha 2 frequency band compared with controls. Linear lagged connectivity and lagged coherence analysis showed significantly reduced functional connectivity between the temporal gyrus and supramarginal gyrus at the gamma 2 frequency band in the ISSNHL group. Additionally, a significantly reduced functional connectivity was found between the central cingulate gyrus and frontal lobe under lagged phase synchronization analysis. These results strongly indicate inhibition of brain area activity and change in functional connectivity in ISSNHL with tinnitus patients.

Keywords: tinnitus, ISSNHL, EEG, source localization, functional connectivity

INTRODUCTION

Sudden sensorineural hearing loss (SSNHL) defines rapid onset hearing loss with reduction in hearing of no less than 30 dB in at least three consecutive audiometric frequencies within 3 days (Stachler et al., 2012). SSNHL is typically accompanied by sudden onset of tinnitus, vertigo and ear fullness (Koç and Sanisoğlu, 2003). The incidence of SSNHL ranges from 3.9 to 27.5 people per 100,000/year (Nosrati-Zarenoe et al., 2010). The etiology of more than two thirds of SSNHL is unclear and considered idiopathic (Chau et al., 2010). Clinicians employ multiple treatment options to cure idiopathic SSNHL (ISSNHL), including oral and transtympanic steroid therapy (Kuhn et al., 2011). However, the therapeutic effectiveness between ISSNHL patients is highly variable. Unfortunately, some ISSNHL subjects do not improve even with high quality treatment, and indeed there may be some adverse effects (Kuhn et al., 2011). The therapeutic effectiveness of ISSNHL treatments may be improved were a better understanding of the mechanism behind ISSNHL available.

Tinnitus, a common and troublesome symptom of ISSNHL, is the perception of sound that lacks any external or internal sound source (Kang et al., 2017). The incidence of tinnitus in ISSNHL patients is between 80 and 95% (Rah et al., 2015; Nogueira-Neto et al., 2016). Tinnitus brings a series of adverse effects to ISSNHL patients, including insomnia and depression (Chen et al., 2013). Additionally, tinnitus symptoms often continue in ISSNHL patients with tinnitus even after treatment, indicating that these patients may have aberrant changes in the brain. Therefore, it is advisable that clinicians pay more attention to the treatment of tinnitus when acting to cure ISSNHL patients.

To treat ISSNHL and tinnitus subjects effectively requires an in-depth investigation into the underlying mechanism of ISSNHL. Current research shows abnormal brain area activity and network connectivity in ISSNHL patients. For example, Micarelli et al. (2017) showed that ISSNHL subjects had hypermetabolism in the right superior and medial frontal gyrus, and a relative reduction in fluorodeoxyglucose uptake in the right middle temporal, precentral and postcentral gyrus, left posterior cingulate cortex, left lingual, superior, middle temporal and middle frontal gyrus and left insula. A study by Xu et al. (2016) showed that SSNHL subjects had some increased activities between auditory and non-auditory networks, including the default mode network (DMN) and limbic system. Other studies have explored the intrinsic mechanism of chronic tinnitus with hearing impairment. It is generally believed that the generation and development of tinnitus is not only related to peripheral hearing impairment, but also correlated with abnormal neural activity (Chen et al., 2014, 2015a, 2016, 2017). A functional imaging study by Lanting et al. (2009) suggested that tinnitus patients had hyperactivity in the auditory system. Tinnitus subjects also show some aberrant neural activity in non-auditory regions, including the frontal gyrus, limbic system, cerebellum and insula (Chen et al., 2017). A number of studies have identified abnormal brain networks in tinnitus including the auditory network (Leaver et al., 2016), DMN (Leaver et al., 2016), dorsal attention network (Schmidt et al., 2013), ventral attention network (Burton et al., 2012) and visual system (Chen et al., 2015b). However, there are few studies exploring the difference of brain area and network connectivity between ISSNHL patients and healthy subjects. Therefore, our research aimed to investigate the underlying mechanism of ISSNHL and tinnitus based on resting-state electroencephalography (EEG).

Approximately 85% of tinnitus patients have an uninterrupted perception of tinnitus sound (Schecklmann et al., 2014). Resting state brain function measurement is therefore suitable for exploring the neural mechanism of tinnitus and ISSNHL. EEG investigates instantaneous electric activity of the brain by recording electrical potentials with electrodes placed on the scalp. It is a technique that is non-invasive and has high temporal resolution (Ingber and Nunez, 2011). At present, a number of methods can be used to extract useful information from multichannel EEG signals, including spectrum analysis, source localization and neural network function analysis. These analytical methods are useful to explore topological property alterations of the brain.

It is still unknown as to whether neural activity changes occur in ISSNHL patients with tinnitus. Thus, our study aim was to gain brain region activity and functional connectivity of central networks in ISSNHL and tinnitus patients based on resting-state EEG. Moreover, we explored the change in balance between excitation and inhibition of the whole brain in these patients.

MATERIALS AND METHODS

Participants

ISSNHL patients with tinnitus were recruited from the Ear, Nose and Throat clinic, Sun Yat-sen Memorial hospital, Guangzhou, China. Selection criteria for ISSNHL subjects with tinnitus were as follows:

(a) Patients had no less than 30 dB sensorineural hearing impairment associated with tinnitus in more than three consecutive audiometric frequencies that had onset within 3 days.
(b) Patients had sought clinical help due to hearing impairment and tinnitus.
(c) Subjects with middle ear surgery, pulsatile tinnitus, Ménière's disease, autoimmune hearing loss, acoustic neurinoma, central nervous system disorders, head trauma, depression or insomnia were excluded.

Data was collected before patients received any therapeutic intervention within 30 days. In this study, 25 ISSNHL subjects with tinnitus (9 males and 16 females; age mean = 46.16 years, *SD* = 13.15 years) and 27 healthy subjects (10 males and 17 females; age mean = 41.48 years, *SD* = 13.53 years) were included. All participants were told about the background and purpose of the study. A written consent form was signed by all subjects. This research was approved by the Institution Review Board of the Sun Yat-sen Memorial Hospital at Sun Yat-sen University of China.

Audiological Examinations

All participants underwent otoscopy and pure tone audiometry. Subjects were asked to sit in an acoustically shielded room for the pure tone audiometry test. Hearing thresholds of the subjects were then measured. Air conduction thresholds at 0.125, 0.25, 0.5, 1, 2, 4, and 8 kHz were measured on both ears. Bone conduction thresholds at 0.25, 0.5, 1, 2, and 4 kHz were also determined. Mean hearing threshold was calculated from hearing thresholds at 0.5, 1, 2, and 4 kHz (British Society of Audiology Recommendation, 1988; Dispenza et al., 2011; Bing et al., 2018).

Tinnitus Specific Assessments

Information about the duration and laterality of tinnitus was collected. A tinnitus pitch matching test was then performed (Teismann et al., 2011). An approximate pitch match was determined using the frequencies 0.125, 0.25, 0.5, 1, 2, 3, 4, 6, and 8 kHz. Patients were asked to compare the matching pitch and perceived tinnitus pitch; the matching pitch was adjusted based on the feedback from the subject. A more accurate matching pitch was obtained by adjusting the frequency in half-octave steps. Narrow band noise was used if a matching pure tone could not be found. After finding the best matching pitch, the initial level was set to 5 dB above the audiometric threshold to find an approximation of the tinnitus loudness. Loudness was adjusted in 1 dB steps until the patient expressed a loudness match. Tinnitus loudness was computed by subtracting the presented sound intensity level with the auditory threshold at that frequency. Finally, tinnitus severity was evaluated using a Tinnitus Handicap Inventory (THI). The THI used an increasing handicap scale from 0 to 100 to assess the level of handicap (Newman et al., 1996). Patients were asked to fill in the THI before the experiment commenced.

Data Collection

Electroencephalography signals were gained using a standard procedure. EEG signals were recorded using an EGI 128 channel system. Before the experiment, participants were informed of the aim of this study to ensure they were in a relaxed state. Participants sat in an acoustic and electrically shielded room. Their eyes were open and they were asked to view a computer screen, to blink as little as possible, not to move their head and to keep awake. A mesh electrode cap was positioned with a careful positioning of the center electrode Vref. Impedances of all electrodes were kept at no more than 50 kΩ. The recording system synchronized the EEG data, and the recording lasted for 7 min.

Preprocessing of EEG Data

Recordings were analyzed in MATLAB for R2013a using EEGLAB for v13.0.0. The whole process was a seven-step instruction as follows. (1) The sampling rate was reduced to 500 Hz. (2) ERPLAB filter was used for sag filtering to remove 50 Hz power frequency interference and the data was band-pass filtered (0.01 Hz high-pass and 100 Hz low-pass). (3) The average reference of all electrodes was used. (4) EEG data was removed with a wide range of drift periods. If the electrode signal was unstable, linear interpolation was performed on the electrode. (5) Independent component analysis algorithm (ICA) was applied to remove independent components related to artifacts. (6) The EEG data was segmented (divided into 2 s). If the amplitude of a segment at any one electrode exceeded 75 μV, then the segment would be removed. (7) Average Fourier cross-spectral matrices were computed for frequency bands, including delta (0.5–3.5 Hz), theta (4–7.5 Hz), alpha 1 (8–10 Hz), alpha 2 (10–12 Hz), beta 1 (13–18 Hz), beta 2 (18.5–21 Hz), beta 3 (21.5–30 Hz), gamma 1 (30.5–44 Hz), and gamma 2 (55–100 Hz).

Data Analysis

Source Localization

Standardized low-resolution brain electromagnetic tomography (sLORETA) was applied to analyze the activation of brain regions in each group and understand the activation distribution of central brain regions in ISSNHL patients with tinnitus in the nine frequency bands mentioned above. After performing a common mean reference transformation (Pascual-Marqui, 2002), the sLORETA algorithm was applied. Electrical neuronal activity was calculated by sLORETA as current density ($A.m^{-2}$). The LORETA-Key software was used to analyze the solution space applied in the research and correlated lead field matrix. The software revisited realistic electrode coordinates (Jurcak et al., 2007) and the lead field (Fuchs et al., 2002) applying the boundary element on the MMI-152 (Montreal Neurological Institute, Canada). According to probabilities returned by the Demon Atlas, the neocortical MNI-152 volume in 6239 voxels was divided and labeled by the sLORETA-Key anatomical template (Lancaster et al., 2000). The co-registration used the correct translation from the MNI-152 space into the Talairach and Tournoux space.

Functional Connectivity Analysis

Cross-talking between areas contributing to the source activity can be used to interpret the lagged phase coherence between two brain areas (Congedo et al., 2010). When two brain areas oscillate coherently with a phase lag, cross-talk can be interpreted as information sharing by axonal transmission. Precisely, the data were decomposed in a limited number of cosine and sine waves at the Fourier frequencies by using the discrete Fourier transform. The work of Pascual-Marqui (2007a,b) showed the significant threshold for a given lagged phase coherence value based on asymptotic results. We used sLORETA to extract current density for regions of interest with time series. Power in all 6,239 voxels was normalized to a power of 1 and log transformed at each time point. Therefore, region of interest values reflect the log transformed fraction of total power across all voxels for specific frequencies. As shown in **Table 1**, regions of interest were determined according to previous studies and the result of source localization (Raichle, 2011).

TABLE 1 | The regions of interest.

Brain region	X	Y	Z
Posterior cingulate	0	−52	27
Medial prefrontal	−1	54	27
Left lateral parietal	−46	−66	30
Right lateral parietal	49	−63	33
Left inferior temporal	−61	−24	−9
Right inferior temporal	0	−12	9
Medial dorsal thalamus	−25	−81	−33
Right posterior cerebellum	25	−81	−33
Left frontal eye field	−29	−9	54
Right frontal eye field	29	−9	54
Left posterior intraparietal sulcus	−26	−66	48
Right posterior intraparietal sulcus	26	−66	48
Left anterior intraparietal sulcus	−44	−39	45
Right anterior intraparietal sulcus	41	−39	45
Left middle temporal	−50	−66	−6
Right middle temporal	53	−63	−6
Left Visual system	−7	83	2
Right Visual system	7	83	2
Left Auditory system	−62	−30	12
Right Auditory system	59	−27	15

Statistical Analysis

To identify potential differences in resting-state ongoing cortical oscillatory activity between ISSNHL subjects and normal controls, non-parametric statistical analysis of LORETA-KEY images (statistical non-parametric mapping; SnPM) were applied to every contrast using LORETA-KEY's built-in voxel-wise randomization tests (5000 permutations). We employed at statistic for independent groups with a threshold of $P < 0.01$ (corrected for multiple comparison). A relatively strict threshold for statistical significance was applied as the number of subjects was relatively small. A correction for multiple comparisons in SnPM using 5000 random permutations has been shown to yield similar results with those acquired from a statistical parametric mapping approach using a general linear model with multiple comparisons corrections.

We compared lagged connectivity differences between two groups and used the t-statistics for independent groups with a threshold of $P < 0.05$. Additionally, LORETA-KEY's built-in voxel-wise randomization tests were used to correct for multiple comparisons for all the voxels included in the region of interest for connectivity analysis (5000 permutations).

RESULTS

Source Localization

As shown in **Figure 1**, compared with healthy controls, ISSNHL subjects demonstrated significantly reduced electric activity in the left frontal lobe (BA6; $P < 0.05$) alpha 2 frequency band. In other frequency bands, no significant difference was found between the two groups. Moreover, there was no significant difference in other brain areas.

Functional Connectivity

Functional connectivity analysis suggested significant differences between ISSNHL subjects and controls in the gamma 2 frequency

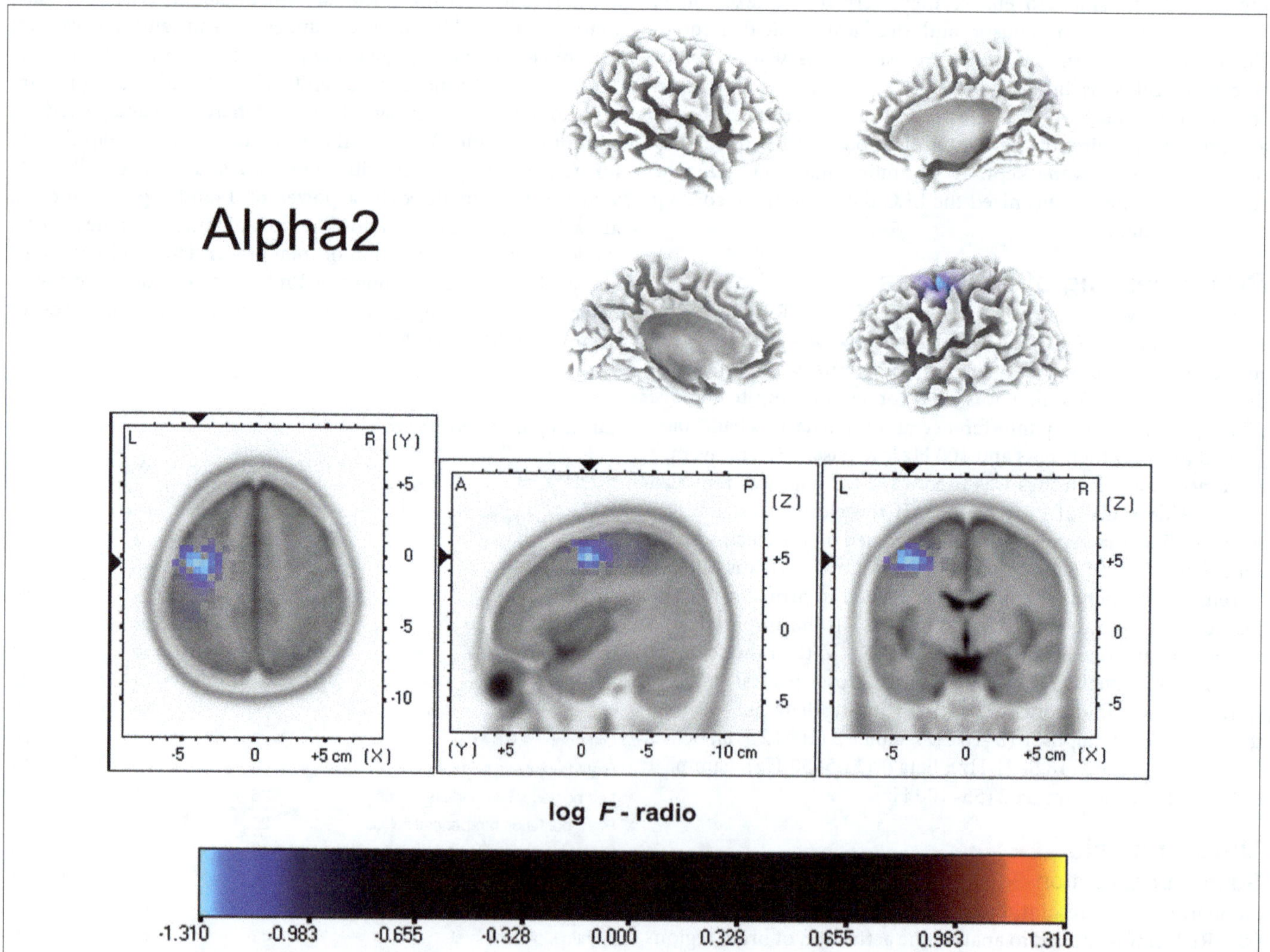

FIGURE 1 | Standardized low-resolution brain electromagnetic tomography. Compared with the healthy group, the ISSNHL group had significantly decreased activity in the left frontal lobe for the alpha 2 frequency band. Labels L, R, A and P represent left, right, anterior and posterior, respectively. Labels S and I represent superior and inferior.

band. There was significantly decreased functional connectivity between the temporal gyrus (BA20) and supramarginal gyrus (BA40) in the gamma 2 frequency band in the linear lagged connectivity and lagged coherence analysis (**Figure 2**). Additionally, there was a significantly reduced functional connectivity between the central cingulate gyrus (BA23) and right frontal lobe (BA10) for the gamma 2 frequency band under lagged phase analysis (**Figure 3**). With other frequency bands there was no significant difference between the two groups.

DISCUSSION

This study explored changes in central nervous activities in ISSNHL with tinnitus patients when compared with healthy subjects. Overall, in the alpha 2 frequency band, the neural activity of ISSNHL patients with tinnitus was abnormally decreased in the left frontal lobe (BA6). Connections between the temporal gyrus (BA20) and supramarginal gyrus (BA40) as well as between central cingulate gyrus (BA23) and right frontal

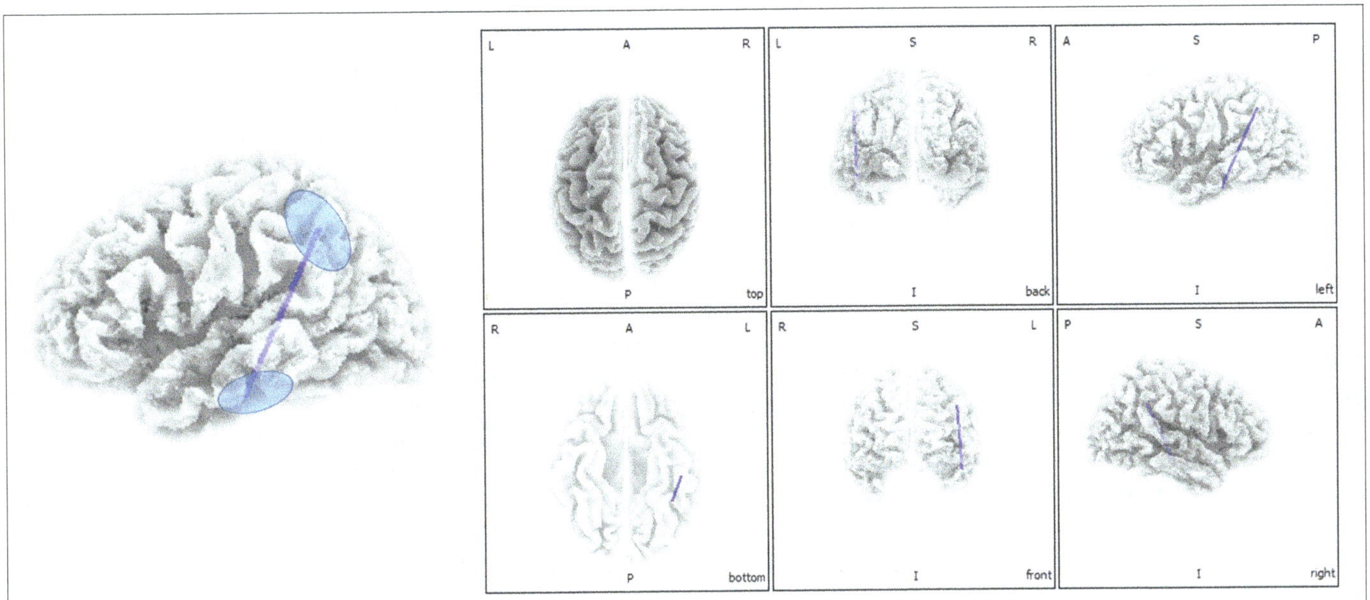

FIGURE 2 | Decreased functional connectivity between temporal gyrus and supramarginal gyrus for the gamma 2 frequency band in the linear lagged connectivity and lagged coherence analysis for ISSNHL patients with tinnitus. Labels L, R, A and P represent the left, right, anterior and posterior, respectively.

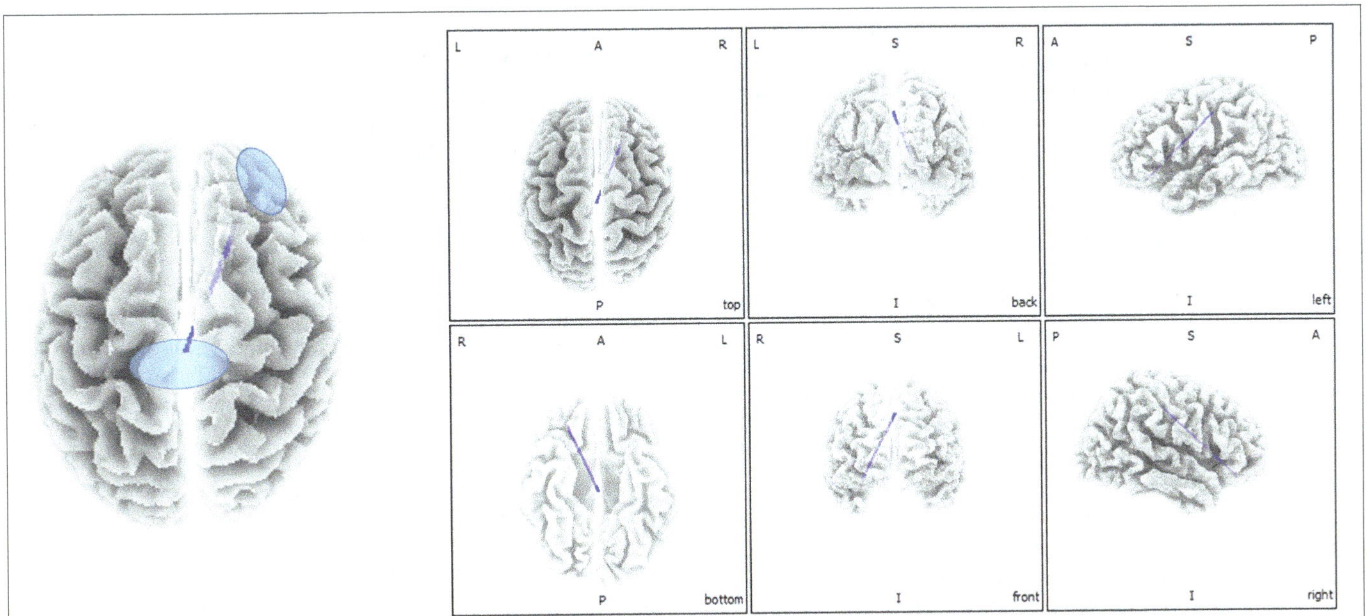

FIGURE 3 | Decreased functional connectivity between central cingulate gyrus and right frontal lobe for gamma 2 frequency band in the lagged phase analysis for ISSNHL patients with tinnitus. Labels L, R, A and P represent the left, right, anterior and posterior, respectively.

lobe (BA10) were weakened in the gamma 2 frequency band. This suggests that ISSNHL patients with tinnitus had aberrant brain area activity and functional connectivity.

Source localization analysis found that ISSNHL patients had decreased activity in the left frontal lobe (BA6) in the alpha 2 frequency band, showing similarity to the study by Micarelli et al. (2017), where ISSNHL subjects had a significant decrease of glucose metabolism in the middle frontal gyrus. It is known that the frontal lobe is one of the key areas of the DMN. Under normal circumstances, the regions of the DMN have a raised level of neuronal activity at rest (van den Heuvel and Hulshoff Pol, 2010). Activity and connectivity of the DMN are associated with the core processes of cognition, such as the integration of cognition and processing of emotion (Greicius et al., 2003), monitoring the environment (Gusnard et al., 2001) and mind-wandering (Mason et al., 2007). A study by Zhang et al. (2016) showed that long-term unilateral ISSNHL contributed to alterations of DMN, and that these alterations might influence cognitive abilities in these subjects. In addition, tinnitus as a symptom involving a perceived phantom sound, might lead to dysfunction of DMN (Chen et al., 2017). Our finding of decreased activation of the left frontal lobe might suppose that the DMN was suppressed in resting state, which consequently may activate other brain networks. It might be the reason for patients with attention and emotion issues.

Linear lagged connectivity and lagged coherence showed a weakened connection between the temporal gyrus (BA20) and supramarginal gyrus (BA40) in the gamma 2 frequency band. Previous studies by Fan et al. (2015) showed that unilateral ISSNHL patients had a significant decrease in contralateral auditory gyrus gray matter. A study by Micarelli et al. (2017) suggested a hypometabolism in the contralateral auditory gyrus in ISSNHL patients. The damage to the hair cells in ISSNHL patients causes a lack of auditory signal in the auditory network (van der Loo et al., 2009). These current results are consistent with our previous EEG microstate study (Cai et al., 2019) where there was a reduction of transition from microstate D to A in ISSNHL subjects with tinnitus that correlated with tinnitus scores. Microstate A is related to activation in the bilateral superior and middle temporal gyrus regions that are correlated with phonological processing. The supramarginal gyrus is a part of a dorsal attention network which relates to microstate D. These results indicated that generation of tinnitus in ISSNHL patients may be due to disruption of auditory and non-auditory networks.

Lagged phase synchronization showed that the connection between the central cingulate gyrus (BA23) and right frontal lobe (BA10) was decreased. Both areas are part of the DMN. The DMN is suggested to be particularly active at rest, when no tasks are performed (Mantini et al., 2007). The posterior cingulate node seems to be particularly vital, because it appears to be directly correlated with other nodes of the network and putatively acting as a mediator of intrinsic connectivity across these areas (Rosazza and Minati, 2011). This is likely because it is one of the most intensively interconnected areas in the whole brain (Cavanna and Trimble, 2006). In a task-based scenario, the network deactivated (Raichle and Snyder, 2007). Conversely, a significant increase in fluorodeoxyglucose uptake was seen in the right superior and medial frontal gyrus in ISSNHL patients (Micarelli et al., 2017). This might be a result of heterogeneity between studies. Therefore, more research is needed to understand this difference. In addition, some functional magnetic resonance imaging (fMRI) studies on tinnitus patients found aberrant functional connectivity within the DMN (Burton et al., 2012; Schmidt et al., 2013). The suppression of tinnitus would lead to a differential response pattern among the network nodes. This might result in the inhibiting effect of DMN.

In summary, the findings of our study identify specific inhibition of brain areas and functional connectivity in ISSNHL with tinnitus subjects. The inhibition of the DMN implies that ISSNHL patients have suppressed activity at resting state and are more active in involving attention or emotional behavior when compared with healthy controls. The reduced connection between the auditory system and dorsal attention network suggests decreased attention to auditory information. The brain activity is in a state of inhibition for ISSNHL patients with tinnitus.

Some limitations in this study need to be realized. ISSNHL is a heterogeneous disease. ISSNHL subjects had differences in hearing loss, laterality or accompanying symptoms (van der Loo et al., 2009). So, it was difficult to eliminate the heterogeneous factors completely even using strict inclusion and exclusion criteria. Without specific subgroups of ISSNHL with tinnitus patients, the results of our study need to be read with caution. In addition, the small sample size in the present study is unable to rule out heterogeneous factors. Therefore, we need to explain the results carefully. A further study with larger sample sizes and more subgroup comparisons is needed to investigate the underlying mechanisms in ISSNHL with tinnitus.

CONCLUSION

In this study, it was found that the central system of ISSNHL with tinnitus patients had been changed when compared with healthy controls. By using resting-state EEG and analyzing source localization and functional connectivity, we found that ISSNHL and tinnitus patients were abnormally weakened in the left frontal lobe (BA6) in the alpha 2 frequency band. The connection between the temporal gyrus (BA20) and supramarginal gyrus (BA40) is weakened in the Gamma 2 frequency band as well as the connection between the central cingulate gyrus (BA 23) and right frontal lobe (BA 10). These findings could help to make sense of the central pathogenesis in ISSNHL patients.

ETHICS STATEMENT

The studies involving human participants were reviewed and approved by Institutional Review Board of the Sun Yat-sen Memorial Hospital at Sun Yat-sen University of China. The patients/participants provided their written informed consent to participate in this study.

AUTHOR CONTRIBUTIONS

The concept and design of this research come from YxC and JL. The experiments were performed by YhC, WC, and WL. CD, GC, SC, and ML analyzed the data. FZ and YZ drafted this manuscript. All authors participated in preparing this manuscript.

ACKNOWLEDGMENTS

We thank Dr. Christopher Wigham for his contribution to proofreading.

REFERENCES

Bing, D., Ying, J., Miao, J., Lan, L., Wang, D., Zhao, L., et al. (2018). Predicting the hearing outcome in sudden sensorineural hearing loss via machine learning models. *Clin. Otolaryngol.* 43, 868–874. doi: 10.1111/coa.13068

British Society of Audiology Recommendation (1988). Descriptors for pure-tone audiograms. *Br. J. Audiol.* 22:123. doi: 10.3109/03005368809077807

Burton, H., Wineland, A., Bhattacharya, M., Nicklaus, J., Garcia, K. S., and Piccirillo, J. F. (2012). Altered networks in bothersome tinnitus: a functional connectivity study. *BMC Neurosci.* 13:3. doi: 10.1186/1471-2202-13-3

Cai, Y., Chen, S., Chen, Y., Li, J., Wang, C., Zhao, F., et al. (2019). Altered resting-state eeg microstate in idiopathic sudden sensorineural hearing loss patients with tinnitus. *Front. Neurosci.* 13:443. doi: 10.3389/fnins.2019.00443

Cavanna, A. E., and Trimble, M. R. (2006). The precuneus: a review of its functional anatomy and behavioural correlates. *Brain* 129, 564–583. doi: 10.1093/brain/awl004

Chau, J. K., Lin, J. R. J., Atashband, S., Irvine, R. A., and Westerberg, B. D. (2010). Systematic review of the evidence for the etiology of adult sudden sensorineural hearing loss. *Laryngoscope* 120:1011. doi: 10.1002/lary.20873

Chen, J., Liang, J., Ou, J., and Cai, W. (2013). Mental health in adults with sudden sensorineural hearing loss: an assessment of depressive symptoms and its correlates. *J. Psychosom. Res.* 75, 72–74. doi: 10.1016/j.jpsychores.2013.03.006

Chen, Y. C., Feng, Y., Xu, J. J., Mao, C. N., Xia, W., Ren, J., et al. (2016). Disrupted brain functional network architecture in chronic tinnitus patients. *Front. Aging Neurosci.* 8:174. doi: 10.3389/fnagi.2016.00174

Chen, Y. C., Li, X., Liu, L., Wang, J., Lu, C. Q., Yang, M., et al. (2015a). Tinnitus and hyperacusis involve hyperactivity and enhanced connectivity in auditory-limbic-arousal-cerebellar network. *Elife* 4:e06576. doi: 10.7554/eLife.06576

Chen, Y. C., Zhang, J., Li, X. W., Xia, W., Feng, X., Qian, C., et al. (2015b). Altered intra-and interregional synchronization in resting-state cerebral networks associated with chronic tinnitus. *Neural. Plast.* 2015:475382. doi: 10.1155/2015/475382

Chen, Y. C., Wang, F., Wang, J., Bo, F., Xia, W., Gu, J. P., et al. (2017). Resting-state brain abnormalities in chronic subjective tinnitus: a meta-analysis. *Front. Hum. Neurosci.* 11:22. doi: 10.3389/fnhum.2017.00022

Chen, Y. C., Zhang, J., Li, X. W., Xia, W., Feng, X., Gao, B., et al. (2014). Aberrant spontaneous brain activity in chronic tinnitus patients revealed by resting-state functional MRI. *Neuroimage Clin.* 6, 222–228. doi: 10.1016/j.nicl.2014.09.011

Congedo, M., John, R. E., De Ridder, D., Prichep, L., and Isenhart, R. (2010). On the "dependence" of "independent" group EEG sources; an EEG study on two large databases. *Brain Topogr.* 23:134. doi: 10.1007/s10548-009-0113-6

Dispenza, F., Amodio, E., De Stefano, A., Gallina, S., Marchese, D., Mathur, N., et al. (2011). Treatment of sudden sensorineural hearing loss with transtympanic injection of steroids as single therapy: a randomized clinical study. *Eur. Arch. Otorhinol.* 268, 1273–1278. doi: 10.1007/s00405-011-1523-0

Fan, W., Zhang, W., Li, J., Zhao, X., Mella, G., Lei, P., et al. (2015). Altered Contralateral auditory cortical morphology in unilateral sudden sensorineural hearing loss. *Otol. Neurotol.* 36, 1622–1627. doi: 10.1097/MAO.0000000000000892

Fuchs, M., Kastner, J., Wagner, M., Hawes, S., and Ebersole, J. S. (2002). A standardized boundary element method volume conductor model. *Clin. Neurophysiol.* 113, 702–712. doi: 10.1016/s1388-2457(02)00030-5

Greicius, M. D., Krasnow, B., Reiss, A. L., and Menon, V. (2003). Functional connectivity in the resting brain: a network analysis of the default mode hypothesis. *Proc. Natl. Acad. Sci. U. S. A.* 100, 253–258. doi: 10.1073/pnas.0135058100

Gusnard, D. A., Akbudak, E., Shulman, G. L., and Raichle, M. E. (2001). Medial prefrontal cortex and self-referential mental activity: relation to a default mode of brain function. *Proc. Natl. Acad. Sci. U. S. A.* 98, 4259–4264. doi: 10.1073/pnas.071043098

Ingber, L., and Nunez, P. L. (2011). Neocortical dynamics at multiple scales: EEG standing waves, statistical mechanics, and physical analogs. *Math. Biosci.* 229, 160–173. doi: 10.1016/j.mbs.2010.12.003

Jurcak, V., Tsuzuki, D., and Dan, I. (2007). 2007. 10/20, 10/10 and 10/5 systems revisited: their validity as relative head-surface-based positioning systems. *NeuroImage* 34, 1600–1611. doi: 10.1016/j.neuroimage.2006.09.024

Kang, W. S., Yang, C. J., Shim, M., Song, C. I., Kim, T. S., Lim, H. W., et al. (2017). Prognostic factors for recovery from sudden sensorineural hearing loss: a retrospective study. *J. Audiol. Otol.* 21, 9–15. doi: 10.7874/jao.2017.21.1.9

Koç, A., and Saniso ̆glu, O. (2003). Sudden sensorineural hearing loss: literature survey on recent studies. *J. Otolaryngol.* 32:308. doi: 10.2310/7070.2003.11288

Kuhn, M., Heman-Ackah, S. E., Shaikh, J. A., and Roehm, P. C. (2011). Sudden sensorineural hearing loss: a review of diagnosis. Treatment, and Prognosis. *Trends Amplif.* 15, 91–105. doi: 10.1177/1084713811408349

Lancaster, J. L., Woldorff, M. G., Parsons, L. M., Liotti, M., Freitas, C. S., Rainey, L., et al. (2000). Automated talairach atlas labels for functional brain mapping. *Hum. Brain Mapp.* 10, 120–131. doi: 10.1002/1097-0193(200007)10:3<120::aid-hbm30>3.0.co;2-8

Lanting, C. P., de Kleine, E., and van Dijk, P. (2009). Neural activity underlying tinnitus generation: results from PET and fMRI. *Hear. Res.* 255, 1–13. doi: 10.1016/j.heares.2009.06.009

Leaver, A. M., Turesky, T. K., Seydell-Greenwald, A., Morgan, S., Kim, H. J., and Rauschecker, J. P. (2016). Intrinsic network activity in tinnitus investigated using functional MRI. *Hum. Brain Mapp.* 37, 2717–2735. doi: 10.1002/hbm.23204

Mantini, D., Perrucci, M. G., Gratta, C. D., Romani, G. L., and Corbetta, M. (2007). Electrophysiological signatures of resting state networks in the human brain. *Proc. Natl. Acad. Sci. U. S. A.* 104, 13170–13175. doi: 10.1073/pnas.0700668104

Mason, M. F., Norton, M. I., John, D. V. H., Wegner, D. M., Grafton, S. T., and Macrae, C. N. (2007). Wandering minds: the default network and stimulus-independent thought. *Science* 315, 393–395. doi: 10.1126/science.1131295

Micarelli, A., Chiaravalloti, A., Viziano, A., Danieli, R., Schillaci, O., and Alessandrini, M. (2017). Early cortical metabolic rearrangement related to clinical data in idiopathic sudden sensorineural hearing loss. *Hear. Res.* 350, 91–99. doi: 10.1016/j.heares.2017.04.011

Newman, C. W., Jacobson, G. P., and Spitzer, J. B. (1996). Development of the tinnitus handicap inventory. *Arch. Otolaryngol Head Neck Surg.* 122:143.

Nogueira-Neto, F. B., Gallardo, F. P., Suzuki, F. A., and Penido Nde, O. (2016). Prognostic and evolutive factors of tinnitus triggered by sudden sensorineural hearing loss. *Otol. Neurotol.* 37, 627–633. doi: 10.1097/MAO.0000000000001049

Nosrati-Zarenoe, R., Hansson, M., and Hultcrantz, E. (2010). Assessment of diagnostic approaches to idiopathic sudden sensorineural hearing loss and their influence on treatment and outcome. *Acta Otolaryngol.* 130, 384–391. doi: 10.3109/00016480903161541

Pascual-Marqui, R. D. (2002). Standardized low-resolution brain electromagnetic tomography (sLORETA): technical details. *Methods Find. Exp. Clin. Pharmacol.* 24(Suppl. D), 5–12.

Pascual-Marqui, R. D. (2007a). Discrete, 3D distributed, linear imaging methods of electric neuronal activity. Part 1: exact, zero error localization. *arXiv*

Pascual-Marqui, R. D. (2007b). Instantaneous and lagged measurements of linear and nonlinear dependence between groups of multivariate time series: frequency decomposition. *arXiv*

Rah, Y. C., Park, K. T., Yi, Y. J., Seok, J., Kang, S. I., and Kim, Y. H. (2015). Successful treatment of sudden sensorineural hearing loss assures improvement of accompanying tinnitus. *Laryngoscope* 125, 1433–1437. doi: 10.1002/lary.25074

Raichle, M. E. (2011). The restless brain. *Brain Connect.* 1, 3–12. doi: 10.1089/brain.2011.0019

Raichle, M. E., and Snyder, A. Z. (2007). A default mode of brain function: a brief history of an evolving idea. *Neuroimage* 37, 1083–1090. doi: 10.1016/j.neuroimage.2007.02.041

Rosazza, C., and Minati, L. (2011). Resting-state brain networks: literature review and clinical applications. *Neurol. Sci.* 32, 773–785. doi: 10.1007/s10072-011-0636-y

Schecklmann, M., Landgrebe, M., Langguth, B., and Tri Database Study Group (2014). Phenotypic characteristics of hyperacusis in tinnitus. *PLoS One* 9:e86944. doi: 10.1371/journal.pone.0086944

Schmidt, S. A., Akrofi, K., Carpenter-Thompson, J. R., and Husain, F. T. (2013). Default mode, dorsal attention and auditory resting state networks exhibit differential functional connectivity in tinnitus and hearing loss. *PLoS One* 8:e76488. doi: 10.1371/journal.pone.0076488

Stachler, R. J., Chandrasekhar, S. S., Archer, S. M., Rosenfeld, R. M., Schwartz, S. R., Barrs, D. M., et al. (2012). Clinical practice guideline: sudden hearing loss. *Otolaryngol. Head Neck Surg.* 146, S1–S35. doi: 10.1177/0194599812436449

Teismann, H., Okamoto, H., and Pantev, C. (2011). Short and intense tailor-made notched music training against tinnitus: the tinnitus frequency matters. *PLoS One* 6:e24685. doi: 10.1371/journal.pone.002468

van den Heuvel, M. P., and Hulshoff Pol, H. E. (2010). Exploring the brain network: a review on resting-state fMRI functional connectivity. *Eur. Neuropsychopharm.* 20, 519–534. doi: 10.1016/j.euroneuro.2010.03.008

van der Loo, E., Gais, S., Congedo, M., Vanneste, S., Plazier, M., Menovsky, T., et al. (2009). Tinnitus intensity dependent gamma oscillations of the contralateral auditory cortex. *Plos One* 4:e7396. doi: 10.1371/journal.pone.0007396

Xu, H., Fan, W., Zhao, X., Li, J., Zhang, W., Lei, P., et al. (2016). Disrupted functional brain connectome in unilateral sudden sensorineural hearing loss. *Hear. Res.* 335, 138–148. doi: 10.1016/j.heares.2016.02.016

Zhang, G. Y., Yang, M., Liu, B., Huang, Z. C., Li, J., Chen, J. Y., et al. (2016). Changes of the directional brain networks related with brain plasticity in patients with long-term unilateral sensorineural hearing loss. *Neuroscience* 313, 149–161. doi: 10.1016/j.neuroscience.2015.11.042

12

Differences in Intrinsic Brain Abnormalities Between Patients with Left- and Right-Sided Long-Term Hearing Impairment

Xiaoxiao Xie[1†], Yongbo Liu[2†], Xiaowei Han[3,4†], Pei Liu[5], Hui Qiu[6], Junfeng Li[4*] and Huachen Yu[7*]

[1] Department of Radiology, The Second Affiliated Hospital and Yuying Children's Hospital of Wenzhou Medical University, Wenzhou, China, [2] Department of Radiology, Shanxi Lu'an General Hospital, Changzhi, China, [3] Graduate School, Chinese Academy of Medical Sciences, Peking Union Medical College, Beijing, China, [4] Department of Radiology, Heping Hospital of Changzhi Medical College, Changzhi, China, [5] Graduate School, Beijing University of Chinese Medicine, Beijing, China, [6] Graduate School, Changzhi Medical College, Changzhi, China, [7] Department of Orthopedics, The Second Affiliated Hospital and Yuying Children's Hospital of Wenzhou Medical University, Wenzhou, China

***Correspondence:**
Junfeng Li
lijunfengcz@163.com
Huachen Yu
huachenyu@126.com

†These authors have contributed equally to this work

Unilateral hearing impairment is characterized by asymmetric hearing input, which causes bilateral unbalanced auditory afferents and tinnitus of varying degrees. Long-term hearing imbalance can cause functional reorganization in the brain. However, differences between intrinsic functional changes in the brains of patients with left- and those with right-sided long-term hearing impairments are incompletely understood. This study included 67 patients with unilateral hearing impairments (left-sided, 33 patients; right-sided, 34 patients) and 32 healthy controls. All study participants underwent blood oxygenation level dependent resting-state functional magnetic resonance imaging and T1-weighted imaging with three-dimensional fast spoiled gradient-echo sequences. After data preprocessing, fractional amplitude of low frequency (fALFF) and functional connectivity (FC) analyses were used to evaluate differences between patients and healthy controls. When compared with the right-sided hearing impairment group, the left-sided hearing impairment group showed significantly higher fALFF values in the left superior parietal gyrus, right inferior parietal lobule, and right superior frontal gyrus, whereas it showed significantly lower fALFF values in the left Heschl's gyrus, right supramarginal gyrus, and left superior frontal gyrus. In the left-sided hearing impairment group, paired brain regions with enhanced FC were the left Heschl's gyrus and right supramarginal gyrus, left Heschl's gyrus and left superior parietal gyrus, left superior parietal gyrus and right inferior parietal lobule, right inferior parietal lobule and right superior frontal gyrus, and left and right superior frontal gyri. In the left-sided hearing impairment group, the FC of the paired brain regions correlated negatively with the duration and pure tone audiometry were in the left Heschl's gyrus and right supramarginal gyrus. In the right-sided hearing impairment group, the FC of the paired brain regions correlated negatively with the duration was in the left Heschl's gyrus and superior parietal gyrus, and with pure tone audiometry was right inferior parietal lobule and superior frontal gyrus. The intrinsic reintegration mechanisms of the brain appeared to differ between patients with left-sided hearing impairment and those with right-sided hearing impairment, and the severity of hearing impairment was associated with differences in functional integration in certain brain regions.

Keywords: unilateral hearing impairment, functional magnetic resonance imaging, fractional amplitude of low frequency fluctuation, functional connectivity, brain network

INTRODUCTION

Hearing is an important advanced function of the human brain. The mechanisms underlying hearing and hearing disorders are very complicated (Paul et al., 2017; Ungar et al., 2018). Hearing impairments can cause debilitating problems, such as poor voice location and difficulties with orientation and listening (Chen and Young, 2016; Shah et al., 2018). Unilateral hearing impairments are characterized by asymmetric auditory transmissions accompanied by tinnitus of varying degrees. This causes bilateral imbalance in auditory afferents, importantly, long-term hearing imbalance can trigger cortical reorganization of the brain (Kim et al., 2018).

The incidence of unilateral hearing impairment increases with age. Long-term unilateral hearing impairment can lead to hearing problems, as well as behavioral and psychological deficits (e.g., dysphoria and restlessness) (Paul et al., 2017). Moreover, long-term unilateral hearing impairment can lead to abnormal changes in brain function, which can cause a variety of abnormalities in brain networks involving sensory, conductive, and cognitive functions (Shah et al., 2018). Understanding these abnormal changes in brain function and related functional integration in patients with long-term unilateral hearing impairment could help to elucidate the neurological mechanisms by which impairment of brain functions may occur.

Awareness has increased over the past decade regarding how the brain remodels itself in response to hearing impairment and the mechanisms underlying the processing and integration of auditory information; this increasing awareness is due to the development and advancement of neuroimaging technologies in auditory research, such as magnetoencephalography and functional magnetic resonance imaging (fMRI) (Burton et al., 2012; Hughes et al., 2018). The complex processes of auditory information recognition and functional coding undergo restructuring in response to hearing impairment (Andoh et al., 2015). One study has suggested the presence of a frequency-sensitive coding structure in the auditory cortex of the human brain (Chang et al., 2016). The dominance of the contralateral hemisphere disappears when a unilateral auditory stimulus is presented (Andoh and Zatorre, 2011). Previous studies have shown that the pattern of auditory conduction on the side of hearing impairment can significantly affect the lateralization pattern of the auditory cortex (Chen and Young, 2016). In unilateral hearing impairment, uniaural sound conduction is present, which produces asymmetric activation patterns of unilateral neurons in the auditory network of the brain, thereby leading to dominant contralateral functional activity of the auditory projection. In addition, in long-term unilateral hearing impairment, activation of the auditory cortex tends to shift to a more symmetrical and synchronous mode of auditory conduction. Thus far, some studies in neuroimaging have confirmed that a subset of functional networks of the brain associated with integration of auditory networks may change in patients with unilateral hearing impairment. The function and structure of the auditory systems are reorganized in patients with unilateral hearing impairment (Bertolero et al., 2015). Recent studies have shown that the remodeling of hearing function occurs in patients with unilateral hearing impairment (Zhang et al., 2017a); moreover, this correlates with the patients' mental states (Kompus et al., 2012; Firszt et al., 2017). However, changes in functional activity in different regions of the brain, as well as abnormal functional connectivity (FC) patterns that could develop due to unilateral hearing impairment, remain unexplored.

In resting-state fMRI (R-fMRI), the amplitude of low frequency fluctuation (ALFF) and fractional amplitude of low frequency fluctuation (fALFF) reflect spontaneous activity in the brain (Jing et al., 2013). At low frequencies, fALFF is more sensitive and specific than ALFF, and can more accurately reflect the strength of functional activity in the brain (Zou et al., 2008). FC, defined as the correlation between a temporal series and the corresponding functionally activated events, is another method of quantification (van de Ven et al., 2004). Both fALFF and FC have been used as reliable and sensitive indicators in healthy subjects and in patients with various neurological and psychiatric diseases, such as Alzheimer's disease and depression. Additionally, some neuroimaging studies have used these methods and have reported that patients with hearing impairment exhibit abnormal intrinsic functional activities in the brain, which are involved in the auditory network (Leaver and Rauschecker, 2016). However, these quantitative methods have not been used in patients with unilateral hearing impairment, and the relationship between quantified spontaneous neurological activity, as determined by these two methods, and clinical measurements of unilateral hearing impairment has not been studied. Furthermore, regions of functional activity in patients with unilateral hearing impairment, as well as subsequent changes in functional networks that are caused by unilateral hearing impairment, remain unclear. Finally, the correlation between these changes and the degree of hearing impairment is unknown.

The purpose of our study was to explore differences in the intrinsic functional changes in the brain between patients with left- and right-sided hearing impairment using fALFF and FC. In this study, we hypothesized that patients with long-term unilateral hearing impairment would exhibit abnormal intrinsic functional activity in relevant areas of the brain and reconstruction of related functional networks. We also hypothesized that this would partially explain differences between patients and healthy controls. We tested this hypothesis using R-fMRI with fALFF and FC analysis. Furthermore, we analyzed the correlation between altered FC and the duration of illness and pure tone audiometry (PTA) scores in patients with left- and right-sided hearing impairments.

MATERIALS AND METHODS

Participants

This study included 67 patients with unilateral hearing impairments caused by idiopathic hearing loss. All patients were right-handed and aged between 28 and 54 years. Left-sided hearing impairment was present in 33 patients (19 men; 14 women), and right-sided hearing impairment was present in 34 patients (19 men; 15 women). Thirty-two healthy, right-handed controls, aged between 24 and 56 years, were also recruited (18 men; 14 women). Patients were excluded for the following reasons: (1) congenital brain dysplasia or accidental brain trauma with structural deformation of the brain or loss of consciousness; (2) addiction or dependence on special substances (history of drug use, analgesic drug intake or alcohol abuse); (3) other neurological or psychiatric diseases, or somatic diseases that may lead to central nervous system dysfunction; (4) active breast-feeding or pregnancy; and (5) refusal to undergo magnetic resonance scanning. A previous study showed that cortical remodeling occurs in patients who have had unilateral hearing impairment for more than 2 years (Schmithorst et al., 2014). Hence, all patients included in this study had been diagnosed with unilateral long-term hearing loss for at least 2.5 years by two senior otologists. The degree of hearing was evaluated using mean PTA thresholds, which were measured and calculated using the same audiometer at thresholds of 500, 1000, 2000, and 4000 Hz to reflect the listening levels of the participants. The affected ears of the patients had moderate to severe hearing impairments (PTA score > 55 dB). The unaffected ears of the patients and the healthy controls had normal hearing (PTA score ≤ 25 dB). The study was approved by the local ethics committee of our hospital, and written informed consent was obtained from each participant.

Data Acquisition

The participants underwent MRI using a 3.0T MR scanner (General Electric, Discovery MR750, Milwaukee, WI, United States) with a matched eight-channel phased array head coil, and parallel imaging of the brain was employed. The scan protocol included the following: (1) scout images; (2) T2-weighted images; (3) resting-state blood oxygenation level dependent fMRI with single-shot gradient recalled echo-planar echo imaging sequences (GRE-EPI); and (4) three-dimensional T1-weighted images with three-dimensional fast spoiled gradient-echo sequences (3D FSPGR). The parameters of the GRE-EPI included slice thickness of 3.5 mm, slice spacing of 0.7 mm, repetition time of 2000 ms, echo time of 30 ms, flip angle of 90°, matrix size of 64×64, field of view of 240×240 mm^2, and number of excitations of 1, 34 slices, and 240 time points. The parameters of the 3D FSPGR included slice thickness of 1.0 mm, repetition time of 6.7 ms, echo time of Min Full, acquisition matrix of 256×256, field of view of 256×256 mm^2, and number of excitations of 1. Participants were instructed to rest in the supine position with their eyes closed and to breathe calmly. Their heads were fixed to minimize movement, and they were provided with soft earplugs, and electrostatic headphones for both ears. They were also instructed to remain awake and not to think of anything specific.

Data Processing and Analysis

Data Pre-processing

SPM12[1] was used for data processing and analysis (Eickhoff et al., 2005). The preprocessing procedure included the following steps: (1) The data format was converted from DICOM to NIFTI, and the first five time points were removed. (2) The slice-timing was corrected. (3) The head motion was corrected in all subjects (the standard was less than 2.5 mm or 2.5°), and three translation and three rotation parameters were obtained using the head motion. (4) Spatial normalization was performed. Functional images were co-registered with corresponding T1 structural images that were segmented and warped into the anatomical Montreal Neurological Institute template; they were then transformed at a resolution of 3-mm isotropic resolution into the standard Montreal Neurological Institute space. (5) Smoothing was performed with a full width at half maximum of 4. (6) The linear drift was removed. (7) Covariate regression was performed, and six head-motion parameters, white matter, cerebrospinal fluid, and global signals were removed by applying linear regression. (8) Band-pass filtering was performed (frequencies were set at 0.01 to 0.08 Hz) to remove the effects of low-frequency drifts and high-frequency noise after fALFF calculation.

fALFF and FC Analysis

Fractional amplitude of low frequency fluctuation values from each voxel were obtained from preprocessed data. Differences between the left- and right-sided hearing impairment groups and the healthy controls were analyzed and compared to identify regions between the groups. These coordinates were used as the centers of 4-mm-sized spherical seed brain regions of interest (ROIs) that were created using the wfu_pickatlas tool in SPM12. First, FC analysis was performed by calculating the time serial correlation coefficients between each ROI and all the other non-ROI voxels (voxel-wise) in each

[1] https://www.fil.ion.ucl.ac.uk/spm/software/spm12/

participant. The z-values were obtained for further statistical analysis from these correlation coefficients using Fisher's z translation. Intergroup mean comparisons of overall FC of each brain region were conducted between left- and right-sided hearing impairment groups. In addition, the FC between two ROIs (paired ROIs) was calculated, and intergroup multiple comparisons were analyzed.

Statistical Analysis

One-way analysis of variance was used to compare age and level of education among the three groups. Two-sample t-tests were used to compare the duration of illness and PTA scores between the left- and right-sided hearing impairment groups. The chi-square test was applied to compare sex distributions. Demographic and clinical data were analyzed using SPSS (version 23.0, SPSS, Inc., Chicago, IL, United States).

One-way analysis of covariance was performed to examine group differences in fALFF values. Age, sex, and level of education were incorporated as covariates. *Post hoc* tests were conducted to identify variations between each pair of groups. Intergroup comparisons of the overall FC of each brain region were conducted by independent two-sample t-tests. Multiple comparisons of FC between each pair of ROIs were performed, and false discovery rate correction was used for multiple comparison correction in the resulting data with a threshold of 0.05 (Song et al., 2017). The z-values of abnormal FC were extracted and used for Pearson correlation analysis with duration of illness and PTA scores of the patients. The differences were considered statistically significant if the value of P was less than 0.05.

RESULTS

Clinical Data

There were no significant differences in sex, age, or level of education between patients with hearing impairment and healthy controls ($P > 0.05$). The duration of illness was comparable ($P > 0.05$) between patients with left-sided hearing impairment (mean ± standard deviation: 38.50 ± 12.57 months) and those with right-sided hearing impairment (mean ± standard deviation: 37.50 ± 11.72 months). There were no significant differences in the PTA of the affected ear between the left-sided hearing impairment group (mean ± standard deviation: 76.20 ± 24.28 dB) and right-sided hearing impairment group (mean ± standard deviation: 75.60 ± 23.11 dB) ($P > 0.05$; **Table 1**).

TABLE 1 | Demographic and clinical data of unilateral hearing impairment and healthy control patients.

Protocols	Patients		HCs (32)	*P*-value
	Left (33)	Right (34)		
Gender (M/F)	19/14	19/15	18/14	0.694[a]
Age (years)	46.15 ± 11.32	45.48 ± 10.67	44.45 ± 10.39	0.125[b]
Education (years)	10.5 ± 1.36	11.20 ± 3.27	11.05 ± 1.77	0.351[b]
Duration (months)	38.50 ± 12.57	37.50 ± 11.72	/	0.362[c]
PTA of affected ear (dB HL)	76.2 ± 24.28	75.6 ± 23.11	/	0.434[c]

HCs, healthy control patients; PTA, pure tone audiometry; [a]P-value was obtained using a Pearson Chi-square test (two-tailed) among three groups; [b]P-value was obtained using one-way ANOVA (two-tailed) among three groups; [c]P-value was obtained using the independent two sample t-test (two-tailed).

Difference in fALFF Between Left- and Right-Sided Hearing Impairment Groups

The fALFF values in the left triangular portion of the inferior frontal gyrus, left middle temporal gyrus, left calcarine, left and right thalami, right middle occipital gyrus, and right superior frontal gyrus were significantly higher in the left-sided hearing impairment group than in the healthy control group (**Table 2**).

The fALFF values in the right inferior temporal gyrus, right parahippocampal gyrus, left and right thalami, left triangular portion of the inferior frontal gyrus, left caudate, and left inferior parietal lobule were significantly higher in the right-sided hearing impairment group than in the healthy control group (**Table 2**).

TABLE 2 | Brain regions showing group fALFF differences with *post hoc* tests analysis.

Brain regions	BA	Peak MNI Coordinates (mm) (*x*, *y*, *z*)	*t*-value
Left vs. right groups			
HG.L	38	(−55, −12, 11)	−2.25
SMG.R	48	(60, −39, 36)	−2.42
SPG.L	7	(−30, −57, 67)	2.48
IPL.R	40	(49, −47, 51)	2.72
SFG.L	6	(−13, 14, 52)	−2.67
SFG.R	8	(23, 13, 61)	2.39
Left vs. healthy controls			
IFGtri.L	45	(−52, 30, 5)	2.58
MTG.L	21	(−60, −53, 7)	2.78
Calcarine.L	17	(−4, −93,5)	2.65
Thalamus.L	/	(−8, −21,8)	2.39
Thalamus.R	/	(8, −23,12)	2.64
MOG.R	19	(32, −85,20)	2.59
SFG.R	6	(23,1,63)	2.71
Right vs. healthy controls			
ITG.R	20	(55, −14, −27)	2.31
PHG.R	20	(35, −18, −20)	2.36
Thalamus.L	/	(−5, −20,2)	2.24
Thalamus.R	/	(5, −17,20)	2.26
IFGtri.L	45	(−54,24,13)	3.26
Caudate.L	25	(−6, 19, −4)	2.43
IPL.L	40	(−35, −42, 43)	2.57

BA, Brodmann area; MNI, Montreal Neurologic Institute; HG.L, left Heschl's gyrus; SMG.R, right supramarginal gyrus; SPG.L, left superior parietal gyrus; IPL.R, right inferior parietal lobule; SFG.L, left superior frontal gyrus; SFG.R, right superior frontal gyrus; PreCG.L, left precentral gyrus; IFGtri.L, left triangular part of inferior frontal gyrus; MTG.L, left Middle temporal gyrus; Calcarine.L, left calcarine; Thalamus.L, left thalamus; Thalamus.R, right thalamus; MOG.R, right middle occipital gyrus; ITG.R, right inferior temporal gyrus; PHG.R, right parahippocampal gyrus; Caudate.L, left caudate.

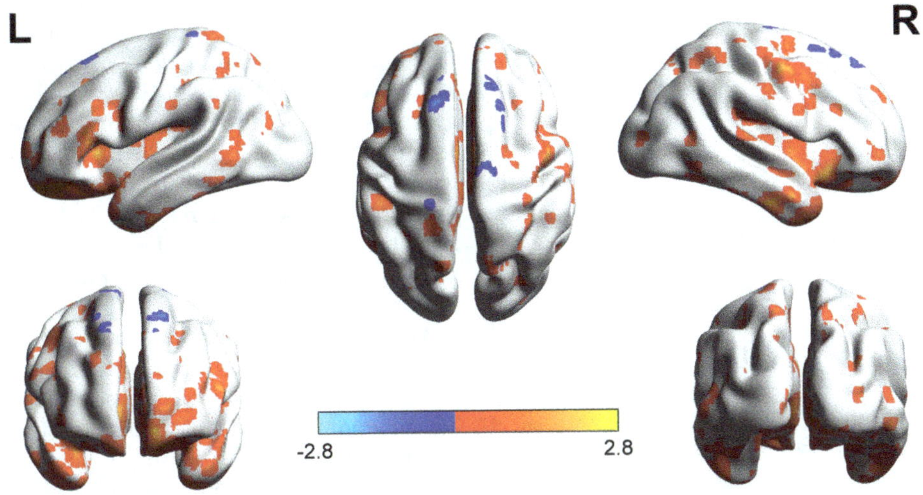

FIGURE 1 | Brain regions showed fALFF differences between left and right hearing impairment groups. The different regions with higher fALFF were observed in the left superior parietal gyrus, right inferior parietal Lobule, and right superior frontal gyrus. The regions with lower fALFF were observed mainly in the left Heschl's gyrus, right supramarginal gyrus, and left superior frontal gyrus.

TABLE 3 | Comparison of the means of the overall inter-regional connectivity between left and right hearing impairment patient groups (mean *z*-values, mean ± SD).

Brain regions	HG.L	SMG.R	SPG.L	IPL.R	SFG.L	SFG.R
Left hearing impairment	1.53 ± 0.32	1.55 ± 0.23	1.59 ± 0.34	1.72 ± 0.35	1.77 ± 0.39	1.78 ± 0.35
Right hearing impairment	1.42 ± 0.21	1.38 ± 0.21	1.44 ± 0.29	1.58 ± 0.38	1.68 ± 0.24	1.64 ± 0.39
T-values	−0.34	0.55	1.04	0.78	0.89	0.68
P-values	0.68	0.07	0.31	0.47	0.34	0.49

HG.L, left Heschl's gyrus; SMG.R, right supramarginal gyrus; SPG.L, left superior parietal gyrus; IPL.R, right inferior parietal lobule; SFG.L, left superior frontal gyrus; SFG.R, right superior frontal gyrus.

Compared with the right-sided hearing impairment group, the left-sided hearing impairment group showed significantly higher fALFF values in the left superior parietal gyrus, right inferior parietal lobule, and right superior frontal gyrus; moreover, the left-sided hearing impairment group showed significantly lower fALFF values in the left Heschl's gyrus, right supramarginal gyrus, and left superior frontal gyrus (**Figure 1** and **Table 2**).

Intergroup Comparison of Overall FC

By comparing left- and right-sided hearing impairment groups, we identified six brain regions that showed different fALFF values. However, the mean overall connectivity in these brain regions did not differ between the two groups ($P > 0.05$; **Table 3**).

Intergroup Comparison of FC Between Paired ROIs

Compared with the right-sided hearing impairment group, the left-sided hearing impairment group showed enhanced FC between the left Heschl's gyrus and right supramarginal gyrus ($P < 0.001$), left Heschl's gyrus and left superior parietal gyrus ($P < 0.001$), left superior parietal gyrus and right inferior parietal lobule ($P = 0.002$), right inferior parietal lobule and superior frontal gyrus ($P = 0.001$), and left and right superior frontal gyri ($P < 0.001$) (**Figure 2** and **Table 4**).

Correlation Analysis

In the left-sided hearing impairment group, there was a significant correlation between the FC of paired ROIs and the duration of illness, as well as between the FC of paired ROIs and PTA scores in the left Heschl's gyrus and right supramarginal gyrus (duration: $P < 0.001$, $r = -0.59$; PTA scores: $P < 0.01$, $r = -0.52$). In the right-sided hearing impairment group, there were significant correlations between the FC of paired ROIs and duration of illness in the left Heschl's gyrus and left superior parietal gyrus ($P < 0.01$, $r = -0.55$), and between the FC of ROIs and PTA scores in the right inferior parietal lobule and right superior frontal gyrus ($P = 0.02$, $r = -0.54$; **Figure 3** and **Table 5**).

DISCUSSION

Long-term unilateral hearing impairment can lead to abnormal changes in brain function, which can lead to a variety of network abnormalities in the brain involving sensory, conductive, and cognitive functions (Chen and Young, 2016; Shah et al., 2018). Awareness of abnormal changes in brain

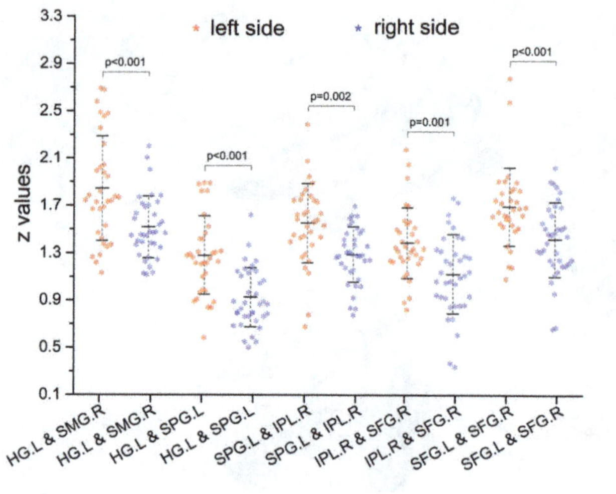

FIGURE 2 | Inter-group comparison of functional connectivity (FC) (z-values) between paired ROIs. Compared with right hearing impairment group, the paired ROIs with enhanced FC were left Heschl's gyrus and right supramarginal gyrus, left Heschl's gyrus and left superior parietal gyrus, left superior parietal gyrus and right inferior parietal lobule, right inferior parietal lobule and superior frontal gyrus, and left and right superior frontal gyrus in the left hearing impairment group.

TABLE 4 | Difference of inter-ROI functional connectivity between left and right hearing impairment patients groups.

Two brain regions	*z*-values (mean ± SD)		*t*-values	*P*-values
	Left side	Right side		
HG.L and SMG.R	1.83 ± 0.43	1.52 ± 0.26	3.84	<0.001
HG.L and SPG.L	1.29 ± 0.34	0.93 ± 0.25	4.89	<0.001
SPG.L and IPL.R	1.55 ± 0.33	1.29 ± 0.23	3.91	0.002
IPL.R and SFG.R	1.39 ± 0.29	1.13 ± 0.34	3.55	0.001
SFG.L and SFG.R	1.7 ± 0.32	1.42 ± 0.31	3.69	<0.001

HG.L, left Heschl's gyrus; SMG.R, right supramarginal gyrus; SPG.L, left superior parietal gyrus; IPL.R, right inferior parietal lobule; SFG.R, right superior frontal gyrus.

function and related functional integration will help to elucidate the neurological mechanisms by which impairment of brain function occurs in patients with long-term unilateral hearing impairment (Chen and Young, 2016). Such awareness would also be helpful for the identification areas of abnormal brain activity that could serve as clinical therapeutic targets. In this study, we used fALFF values and FC to study changes in resting brain function activity, as well as to compare changes between patients with left-sided long-term hearing impairment and those with right-sided long-term hearing impairment.

We found that the left-sided hearing impairment group showed significantly higher fALFF values in the left superior parietal gyrus, right inferior parietal lobule, and right superior frontal gyrus, compared with those in the right-sided hearing impairment group; moreover, the left-sided hearing impairment group showed significantly lower fALFF values in the left Heschl's gyrus, right supramarginal gyrus, and left superior frontal gyrus, compared with those in the right-sided hearing impairment group. Heschl's gyrus, also known as the transverse temporal gyrus, is the primary cortical structure that processes incoming auditory information (Warrier et al., 2009). A previous study has shown, using fMRI, that the transverse temporal gyrus is active during auditory processing of tone and semantic tasks (Lieu et al., 2012). Interestingly, the transverse temporal gyrus in the left hemisphere has a significantly more rapid processing rate (33 Hz), relative to that in the right hemisphere (3 Hz). This difference in processing rate is associated with the volume of the rate-related cortex in the gyrus (Zatorre and Belin, 2001).

Other brain regions that showed functional changes in patients with hearing impairments in this study have not previously been shown to play direct roles in auditory processing. The superior parietal lobule is associated with spatial orientation and receives visual and sensory inputs (Goldberg et al., 2006); the inferior parietal lobule is associated with the perception of emotions in facial stimuli and interpretation of sensory information (Peeters et al., 2009); the supramarginal gyrus forms part of the somatosensory association cortex, which interprets tactile sensory data, and is associated with the perception of space and limb location (Hartwigsen et al., 2010); the right supramarginal gyrus plays a central role in controlling empathy toward other individuals. Evidence from fMRI studies has indicated that the superior frontal gyrus is involved in self-awareness, in coordination with the actions of the sensory system (Morosan et al., 2005). The activation of the inferior parietal lobule is related to the recognition of linguistic information, while the functions of the superior frontal lobe and the middle gyrus are associated with the retention of linguistic information (Pross et al., 2015). Some studies have suggested that equivalent information about the environment can be obtained by perceptual compensation through perception of stimuli that are suitable for their own sensory patterns (Leclerc et al., 2000). Moreover, Leclerc et al. (2000) revealed that the visual area of the brain is used to perform auditory functions in individuals who are blind. Therefore, the activity observed in non-auditory areas in patients with unilateral hearing impairment in our study supports the perceptual compensation theory.

In previous studies, altered functional activity in patients with hearing impairment has been reported in the inferior frontal gyrus, superior marginal gyrus, anterior central gyrus, and posterior central gyrus (Schmithorst et al., 2014; Zhang et al., 2015). Furthermore, abnormal activation of the central anterior and posterior gyri of patients with hearing impairments is significantly higher than that in healthy controls (Bertolero et al., 2015; Chang et al., 2016; Zhang et al., 2016 Paul et al., 2017). However, in the present study, no significant differences in activation were found in the anterior and posterior gyri between patients and controls. Bushara et al. (1999) analyzed auditory and visual processing and found extensive activation in regions in the parietal lobes and inferior frontal gyrus where integration of auditory and visual information is performed. Abnormal functional activity in these regions of the brain suggests that brain reorganization might occur in patients with neurological deafness (Wang et al., 2014). Furthermore, these results indicate that the

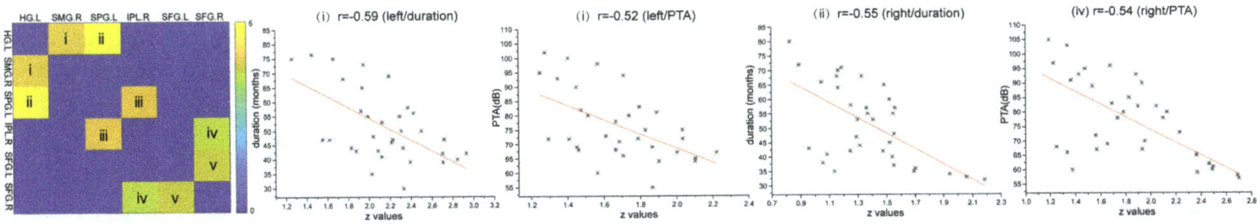

FIGURE 3 | Correlations between altered FC (z-values) of paired regions and corresponding duration and PTA scores of the patients (altered FC showed from i to v; the colorbar indicated *t*-values among bilateral comparisons in the **Table 4** which showed the degree of difference of inter-groups). In the left hearing impairment group, the FC of paired ROIs that correlated with the duration and PTA were left Heschl's gyrus and right supramarginal gyrus (i). In the right hearing impairment group, the FC of paired ROIs that correlated with the duration were the left Heschl's gyrus and superior parietal gyrus (ii), and correlated with the PTA were the right inferior parietal lobule and superior frontal gyrus (iv).

functional networks of the human brain undergo neuroplasticity under a variety of physiological conditions, in order to adapt to environmental needs and changes. Our results are inconsistent with those of previous studies. Therefore, we speculate that the mechanism of reorganization of the resting-state auditory event-related network in patients with long-term hearing impairment is complex and requires further study.

In the present study, the overall FC of each ROI was compared between the left- and right-sided hearing impairment groups. No differences were identified. The balance of overall connectivity strength in different functional regions of the brain might have been maintained because remodeling of the functional activity of the brain in these patients compensated for areas of the brain that were functionally damaged. Comparisons of FC between left- and right-sided hearing impairment groups showed that the paired regions with enhanced FC in the left-sided hearing impairment group were left Heschl's gyrus and right supramarginal gyrus, left Heschl's gyrus and left superior parietal gyrus, left superior parietal gyrus and right inferior parietal lobule, right inferior parietal lobule and right superior frontal gyrus, and left and right superior frontal gyrus. These results indicated that FC changes in these regions related to information input may contribute to remodeling of the sensory system. Furthermore, these results highlighted the role of Heschl's gyrus in processing incoming auditory information (Zhang et al., 2017b). In addition, our results indicated that the FC of the regions of the brain in the resting-state network related to auditory information was stronger in the left side than in the right side, which is consistent

TABLE 5 | Brain regions showed correlation between left and right hearing impairment groups.

Groups	Two brain regions	Correlation with	*r*-values	*P*-values
Left hearing impairment	HG.L and SMG.R	Duration	−0.59	< 0.001
	HG.L and SMG.R	PTA	−0.52	0.005
Right hearing impairment	HG.L and SPG.L	Duration	−0.55	0.002
	IPL.R and SFG.R	PTA	−0.54	0.02

HG.L, left Heschl's gyrus; SMG.R, right supramarginal; SPG.L, left superior parietal gyrus; IPL.R, right inferior parietal lobule; SFG.R, right superior frontal gyrus.

with the results of another study (Puschmann and Thiel, 2017). The functional integration network of patients with left-sided hearing impairment underwent more obvious reorganization, indicating a laterality of processing with respect to incoming auditory information in the brain; this is consistent with the findings of previous studies (Wang et al., 2016). Furthermore, we showed an asymmetry in the structure and function of the left and right hemispheres of the brain, which is consistent with the findings of a previous study that showed lateralization in the processing of auditory sensory afferent information with a dominant hemisphere effect (Burton et al., 2012).

In patients with left-sided hearing impairment, the paired ROI that showed negative correlations with both the duration of illness and PTA scores was the left Heschl's gyrus and right supramarginal gyrus. In patients with right-sided hearing impairment, the paired ROIs that showed respective negative correlations with duration and PTA scores were the left Heschl's gyrus and left superior parietal gyrus, and the right inferior parietal lobule and superior frontal gyrus. The processing of auditory information is associated with sensory transmission. Therefore, we speculate that increased sensory afferent actions may accompany increased disease severity. This may explain the close relationship between disease severity and changes in the auditory information processing in patients with hearing impairment.

This study had some limitations. First, the sample size was relatively small. Therefore, the validity of the statistical inferences is relatively low. Second, the noise of high-field magnetic resonance could not be completely eliminated with the earplugs and sponge pads that were placed on the head during the experiment; this may have been more obvious for the healthy control participants. Finally, we did not differentiate among etiologies for unilateral hearing impairment. In the future, we plan to increase our sample size, use etiological grouping, and eliminate the impact of noise from magnetic resonance, in order to confirm the findings of the present study.

In summary, this R-fMRI study provided considerable evidence for abnormal intrinsic brain activity in patients with unilateral hearing impairment. Furthermore, our data indicated differences in the mechanism of reintegration between patients with left-sided hearing impairment and those with right-sided hearing impairment. Finally, we found that the disease severity was associated with differences in functional activity in certain regions of the brain. However, further studies are needed to explore the specific underlying mechanisms by which fALFF values and functional activity are altered in patients with hearing loss.

AUTHOR CONTRIBUTIONS

XX, YL, and XH acquired and analyzed the data, drafted and revised the manuscript. PL, XH, and HQ analyzed and explained the data. JL and HY revised the manuscript for extremely important intellectual content.

ACKNOWLEDGMENTS

We thank Editage (http://editage.com/frontiers/) for their linguistic assistance during the revision of this manuscript.

REFERENCES

Andoh, J., Matsushita, R., and Zatorre, R. J. (2015). asymmetric interhemispheric transfer in the auditory network: evidence from TMS, resting-state fmri, and diffusion imaging. *J. Neurosci.* 35, 14602–14611. doi: 10.1523/JNEUROSCI.2333-15.2015

Andoh, J., and Zatorre, R. J. (2011). Inter hemispheric connectivity influences the degree of modulation of TMS-induced effects during auditory processing. *Front. Psychol.* 2:161. doi: 10.3389/fpsyg.2011.00161

Bertolero, M. A., Yeo, B. T., and D'Esposito, M. (2015). The modular and integrative functional architecture of the human brain. *Proc. Natl. Acad. Sci. U.S.A.* 112, E6798–E6807. doi: 10.1073/pnas.1510619112

Burton, H., Firszt, J. B., Holden, T., Agato, A., and Uchanski, R. M. (2012). Activation lateralization in human core, belt, and parabelt auditory fields with unilateral deafness compared to normal hearing. *Brain Res.* 1454, 33–47. doi: 10.1016/j.brainres.2012.02.066

Bushara, K. O., Weeks, R. A., and Ishii, K. (1999). Modality-specific frontaland parietal areas for auditory and visual spatial localization in humans. *Nat. Neurosci.* 2, 759–766. doi: 10.1038/11239

Chang, J. L., Pross, S. E., Findlay, A. M., Mizuiri, D., Henderson-Sabes, J., Garrett, C., et al. (2016). Spatial plasticity of the auditory cortex in single-sided deafness. *Laryngoscope* 126, 2785–2791. doi: 10.1002/lary.25961

Chen, Y.-H., and Young, Y.-H. (2016). Bilateral simultaneous sudden sensorineural hearing loss. *J. Neurol. Sci.* 362, 139–143. doi: 10.1016/j.jns.2016.01.029

Eickhoff, S. B., Stephan, K. E., Mohlberg, H., Grefkes, C., Fink, G. R., Amunts, K., et al. (2005). A new SPM toolbox for combining probabilistic cytoarchitectonic maps and functional imaging data. *Neuroimage* 25, 1325–1335. doi: 10.1016/j.neuroimage.2004.12.034

Firszt, J. B., Reeder, R. M., and Holden, L. K. (2017). Unilateral hearing loss: understanding speech recognition and localization variability-implications for cochlear implant candidacy. *Ear Hear.* 38, 159–173. doi: 10.1097/AUD.0000000000000380

Goldberg, I., Harel, M., and Malach, R. (2006). When the brain loses its self: prefrontal inactivation during sensorimotor processing. *Neuron* 50, 329–339. doi: 10.1016/j.neuron.2006.03.015

Hartwigsen, G., Baumgaertner, A., Price, C. J., Koehnke, M., Ulmer, S., and Siebner, H. R. (2010). Phonological decisions require both the left and right supramarginal gyri. *Proc. Natl. Acad. Sci. U.S.A.* 21, 16494–16499. doi: 10.1073/pnas.1008121107

Hughes, M. E., Nkyekyer, J., Innes-Brown, H., Rossell, S. L., Sly, D., Bhar, S., et al. (2018). Hearing aid use in older adults with postlingual sensorineural hearing loss: protocol for a prospective cohort study. *JMIR Res. Protoc.* 7:e174. doi: 10.2196/resprot.9916

Jing, B., Liu, C. H., Ma, X., Yan, H. G., Zhuo, Z. Z., Zhang, Y., et al. (2013). Difference in amplitude of low-frequency fluctuation between currently depressed and remitted females with major depressive disorder. *Brain Res.* 2013, 74–83. doi: 10.1016/j.brainres.2013.09.039

Kim, S., Kwon, H. J., Kang, E. J., and Kim, D. W. (2018). diffusion-tensor tractography of the auditory neural pathway : clinical usefulness in patients with unilateral sensorineural hearing loss. *Clin. Neuroradiol.* doi: 10.1007/s00062-018-0733-x [Epub ahead of print].

Kompus, K., Specht, K., Ersland, L., Juvodden, H. T., van Wageningen, H., Hugdahl, K., et al. (2012). A forced-attention dichotic listening fMRI study on 113 subjects. *Brain Lang.* 121, 240–247. doi: 10.1016/j.bandl.2012.03.004

Leaver, A. M., and Rauschecker, J. P. (2016). Functional topography of human auditory cortex. *J. Neurosci.* 36, 1416–1428. doi: 10.1523/JNEUROSCI.0226-15.2016

Leclerc, C., Saint-Amour, D., Lavoie, M. E., Lassonde, M., and Lepore, F. (2000). Brain functional reorganization in early blind humans revealed by auditory event-related potentials. *Neuroreport* 11, 545–550. doi: 10.1097/00001756-200002280-00024

Lieu, J. E., Tye-Murray, N., and Fu, Q. (2012). Longitudinal study of children with unilateral hearing loss. *Laryngoscope* 122, 2088–2095. doi: 10.1002/lary.23454

Morosan, P., Rademacher, J., Palomero-Gallagher, N., and Zilles, K. (2005). "Anatomical organization of the human auditory cortex: cytoarchitecture and transmitter receptors," in *The Auditory Cortex: A Synthesis of Human and Animal Research*, eds R. König, P. Heil, E. Budinger, and H. Scheich (Mahwah, NJ: Lawrence Erlbaum Associates Publishers), 27–50.

Paul, A., Marlin, S., Parodi, M., Rouillon, I., Guerlain, J., Pingault, V., et al. (2017). Unilateral sensorineural hearing loss: medical context and etiology. *Audiol. Neurootol.* 22, 83–88. doi: 10.1159/000474928

Peeters, R., Simone, L., Nelissen, K., Fabbri-Destro, M., Vanduffel, W., Rizzolatti, G., et al. (2009). The representation of tool use in humans and monkeys: common and uniquely human features. *J. Neurosci.* 29, 11523–11539. doi: 10.1523/JNEUROSCI.2040-09.2009

Pross, S. E., Chang, J. L., Mizuiri, D., Findlay, A. M., Nagarajan, S. S., and Cheung, S. W. (2015). Temporal cortical plasticity in single-sided deafness: a functional imaging study. *Otol. Neurotol.* 36, 1443–1449. doi: 10.1097/MAO.0000000000000821

Puschmann, S., and Thiel, C. M. (2017). Changed crossmodal functional connectivity in older adults with hearing loss. *Cortex* 86, 109–122. doi: 10.1016/j.cortex.2016.10.014

Schmithorst, V. J., Plante, E., and Holland, S. (2014). Unilateral deafness in children affects development of multi-modal modulation and default mode networks. *Front. Hum. Neurosci.* 8:164. doi: 10.3389/fnhum.2014.00164

Shah, J., Pham, G. N., Zhang, J., Pakanati, K., Raol, N., Ongkasuwan, J., et al. (2018). Evaluating diagnostic yield of computed tomography (CT) and magnetic resonance imaging (MRI) in pediatric unilateral sensorineural hearing loss. *Int. J. Pediatr. Otorhinolaryngol.* 115, 41–44. doi: 10.1016/j.ijporl.2018.09.003

Song, W., Cao, Z., Lang, C., Dai, M., Xuan, L., and Lv, K. (2017). Disrupted functional connectivity of striatal sub-regions in Bell's palsy patients. *Neuroimage Clin.* 14, 122–129. doi: 10.1016/j.nicl.2017.01.008

Ungar, O. J., Brenner-Ullman, A., Cavel, O., Oron, Y., Wasserzug, O., and Handzel, O. (2018). The association between auditory nerve neurovascular conflict and sudden unilateral sensorineural hearing loss. *Laryngoscope Investig. Otolaryngol.* 6, 384–387. doi: 10.1002/lio2.209

van de Ven, V. G., Formisano, E., Prvulovic, D., Roeder, C. H., and Linden, D. E. (2004). Functional connectivity as revealed by spatial inde pendent component analysis of fMRI measurements during rest. *Hum. Brain Mapp.* 22, 165–178. doi: 10.1002/hbm.20022

Wang, X., Fan, Y., Zhao, F., Wang, Z., Ge, J., Zhang, K., et al. (2014). Altered regional and circuit resting-state activity associated with unilateral hearing loss. *PLoS One* 9:e96126. doi: 10.1371/journal.pone.0096126

Wang, X., Xu, P., Li, P., Wang, Z., Zhao, F., Gao, Z., et al. (2016). Alterations in gray matter volume due to unilateral hearing loss. *Sci. Rep.* 6:25811. doi: 10.1038/srep25811

Warrier, C., Wong, P., Penhune, V., Zatorre, R., Parrish, T., Abrams, D., et al. (2009). Relating structure to function: heschl's Gyrus and acoustic processing. *J. Neurosci.* 29, 61–69. doi: 10.1523/JNEUROSCI.3489-08.2009

Zatorre, R. J., and Belin, P. (2001). Spectral and temporal processing in human auditory cortex. *Cereb. Cortex* 11, 946–953.

Zhang, G. Y., Yang, M., Liu, B., Huang, Z. C., Chen, H., Zhang, P. P., et al. (2015). Changes in the default mode networks of individuals with long-term unilateral sensorineural hearing loss. *Neuroscience* 285, 333–342. doi: 10.1016/j.neuroscience.2014.11.034

Zhang, G. Y., Yang, M., Liu, B., Huang, Z. C., Li, J., Chen, J. Y., et al. (2016). Changes of the directional brain networks related with brain plasticity in patients with long-term unilateral sensorineural hearing loss. *Neuroscience* 313, 149–161. doi: 10.1016/j.neuroscience.2015.11.042

Zhang, Y., Mao, Z., Feng, S., Liu, X., Zhang, J., and Yu, X. (2017a). Monaural-driven functional changes within and beyond the auditory cortical network: evidence from long-term unilateral hearing impairment. *Neuroscience* 371, 296–308. doi: 10.1016/j.neuroscience.2017.12.015

Zhang, Y., Mao, Z., Feng, S., Wang, W., Zhang, J., and Yu, X. (2017b). Convergent and divergent functional connectivity patterns in patients with long-term left-sided and right-sided deafness. *Neurosci. Lett.* 665, 74–79. doi: 10.1016/j.neulet.2017.11.050

Zou, Q. H., Zhu, C. Z., Yang, Y., Zuo, X. N., Long, X. Y., and Cao, Q. J. (2008). An improved approach to detection of amplitude of low-frequency fluctuation (ALFF) for resting-state fMRI: fractional ALFF. *J. Neurosci. Methods* 172, 137–141. doi: 10.1016/j.jneumeth.2008.04.012

13

Functional Brain Changes During Mindfulness-Based Cognitive Therapy Associated with Tinnitus Severity

*Benjamin Zimmerman[1,2], Megan Finnegan[1,2,3], Subhadeep Paul[4], Sara Schmidt[2,3], Yihsin Tai[1], Kelly Roth[1], Yuguo Chen[5] and Fatima T. Husain[1,2,3]**

[1] *Department of Speech and Hearing Science, University of Illinois at Urbana–Champaign, Champaign, IL, United States,* [2] *Beckman Institute for Advanced Science and Technology, University of Illinois at Urbana–Champaign, Champaign, IL, United States,* [3] *Neuroscience Program, University of Illinois at Urbana–Champaign, Champaign, IL, United States,* [4] *Department of Statistics, The Ohio State University, Columbus, OH, United States,* [5] *Department of Statistics, University of Illinois at Urbana–Champaign, Champaign, IL, United States*

Correspondence:
Fatima T. Husain
husainf@illinois.edu

Mindfulness-based therapies have been introduced as a treatment option to reduce the psychological severity of tinnitus, a currently incurable chronic condition. This pilot study of twelve subjects with chronic tinnitus investigates the relationship between measures of both task-based and resting state functional magnetic resonance imaging (fMRI) and measures of tinnitus severity, assessed with the Tinnitus Functional Index (TFI). MRI was measured at three time points: before, after, and at follow-up of an 8-week long mindfulness-based cognitive therapy intervention. During the task-based fMRI with affective sounds, no significant changes were observed between sessions, nor was the activation to emotionally salient compared to neutral stimuli significantly predictive of TFI. Significant results were found using resting state fMRI. There were significant decreases in functional connectivity among the default mode network, cingulo-opercular network, and amygdala across the intervention, but no differences were seen in connectivity with seeds in the dorsal attention network (DAN) or fronto-parietal network and the rest of the brain. Further, only resting state connectivity between the brain and the amygdala, DAN, and fronto-parietal network significantly predicted TFI. These results point to a mostly differentiated landscape of functional brain measures related to tinnitus severity on one hand and mindfulness-based therapy on the other. However, overlapping results of decreased amygdala connectivity with parietal areas and the negative correlation between amygdala-parietal connectivity and TFI is suggestive of a brain imaging marker of successful treatment.

Keywords: tinnitus, mindfulness-based cognitive therapy, resting state MRI, functional MRI, graph connectivity analysis

INTRODUCTION

Subjective tinnitus, the perception of sound in the absence of an external source, is a currently incurable chronic condition with a relatively large prevalence rate (12–30% of the general population) (McCormack et al., 2016). Tinnitus is a heterogeneous condition with varying perceptual qualities (e.g., pitch, loudness, type of sound) as well as varying psychological reactions to the condition. Most individuals habituate to the condition over time, but for a subset of people, the condition becomes debilitating with severe psychological effects including comorbid anxiety and depression (Bartels et al., 2008; McCormack et al., 2015).

The pursuit of better understanding and treating the condition typically falls into two overlapping lines of research. One area seeks to understand and intervene on the primary perception of the sound. The other line of research focuses more on understanding the reasons for the variability in psychological severity of the condition and pursuing ways to effectively encourage habituation and management of the perception.

Recently, mindfulness-based therapies have been introduced as a treatment option in this second category of research to reduce the psychological burden of the condition. Although the research on these treatments are still in their early days, mindfulness-based therapies have shown initial promise in modulating the severity of tinnitus (Kreuzer et al., 2012; Philippot et al., 2012; Gans et al., 2014; Roland et al., 2015; McKenna et al., 2017). These therapies teach a conception of mindfulness defined by Kabat-Zinn (1994) as 'paying attention…on purpose, in the present moment, and non-judgmentally.'

As mindfulness-based therapies have grown in popularity and have shown efficacy in a number of psychological conditions (e.g., Hofmann et al., 2010; Philippot et al., 2012; Hölzel et al., 2013; Lakhan and Schofield, 2013), there has been a growing body of literature investigating changes in functional brain activity after a period of mindfulness training. Research on the functional correlates of tinnitus has also expanded in recent years, with evidence pointing to differences in both responses to certain types of tasks as well as resting state functional activity predictive of the condition. Given the evidence for functional changes with tinnitus and functional changes due to mindfulness training, there has been growing interest in testing the hypothesis that the positive effects from mindfulness interventions on tinnitus severity are modulated through changes in brain function (Roland et al., 2015). Previous work on functional connectivity changes with tinnitus have suggested that therapies which increase connectivity with limbic regions and attention resting state networks could be effective at reducing tinnitus-related distress (Schmidt et al., 2013, 2017). Since mindfulness-based interventions have observed this pattern of connectivity change (Tang et al., 2015), there is a strong theoretical basis to expect that mindfulness-based therapies may be effective through this mechanism. In this study, it was hypothesized that mindfulness-based therapies alleviate symptoms of tinnitus by altering those functional patterns.

In addition to changes in seed-voxel connectivity, supplemental tools from network analysis are widely used to understand anatomical and functional brain connectivity patterns using data obtained from neuroimaging studies (Bassett and Bullmore, 2006; Bullmore and Sporns, 2009; Rubinov and Sporns, 2010; Meunier et al., 2010; Hutchison et al., 2013; Sporns, 2014; Zalesky et al., 2014; van den Heuvel et al., 2016; Bassett and Sporns, 2017). Various network metrics have been used to assess and differentiate between individuals in terms of cognitive abilities and disease progression in a wide range of conditions (Liu et al., 2008; Alexander-Bloch et al., 2010; Lynall et al., 2010; van den Heuvel et al., 2010, 2013; Bassett et al., 2011; Yu et al., 2011; Hutchison et al., 2013; Wang et al., 2013; Braun et al., 2015). Researchers have also observed many salient properties of brain functional networks, e.g., community (module) structure, rich club organization, network hub structure, strong local clustering, short characteristic path length, etc., which together lead to efficiency and small world property in networks. These network properties, in turn, have been associated with efficient performance of brain's tasks. A number of studies have also applied graph analysis tools to data from mindfulness or meditation studies and have found significant differences in efficiency and clustering coefficient in functional brain networks to be associated with meditation (Gard et al., 2014; van Lutterveld et al., 2017). However, these graph analysis tools have not been applied with respect to changes in tinnitus outcomes across mindfulness-based interventions.

In the current pilot study, we build upon results presented in Husain et al. (2019) showing a reduction in tinnitus severity after a mindfulness-based cognitive therapy (MBCT) intervention by analyzing the functional MRI (fMRI) data in the same subjects. We analyzed changes in brain activity during an auditory emotion task and during resting state across three sessions before, immediately after treatment, and 8 weeks after the treatment ended. The auditory emotion task was used in previous studies (Carpenter-Thompson et al., 2014) to differentiate between bothersome and mild tinnitus. As a secondary goal, we investigated whether changes in functional activity to the auditory emotion task or resting state across the sessions predicted the reductions in tinnitus severity, as assessed through the Tinnitus Functional Index (TFI: Meikle et al., 2012). Finally, we investigated how network properties change across the mindfulness intervention and if those changes reflect tinnitus severity. This study adds to the burgeoning literature on functional brain differences in effective tinnitus therapies and will deepen our knowledge of this complex and heterogeneous condition.

MATERIALS AND METHODS

Participants

Inclusion/Exclusions Criteria

Participants underwent a screening session to determine eligibility before enrolling in the study. Individuals included in the study were between the ages of 21 and 72, had a Tinnitus Handicap Inventory (THI: Newman et al., 1996) score of 28 or greater and had pure-tone thresholds less than or equal to 30 dB HL up to 2 kHz testing frequency in order to ensure that they were able to hear the MBCT instructors. The goal of recruitment was to include a broad sample of individuals with chronic, bothersome tinnitus, while excluding comorbid symptoms that may too drastically increase the heterogeneity of the tinnitus condition investigated in the study or otherwise impair the ability of the subject to participate in the study. These included transmandibular joint problems, a history of Meniere's disease, pulsatile tinnitus, drug and/or alcohol abuse in the recent past, a score greater than 25 on the Beck Anxiety Inventory (BAI: Beck et al., 1988a), a score greater than 30 on the Beck Depression Inventory (BDI: Beck et al., 1988b) or a score greater than 0 on question 9 of the BDI, which asks about suicidal ideation, neurological disorders (e.g., epilepsy), a history of or currently unmanaged post-traumatic stress disorder, unmanaged chronic health problems (e.g., hypertension, diabetes), a score of 23 or below on the Mini-Mental State Examination (MMSE: Folstein et al., 1975), or speech discrimination scores in quiet lower than 80% in the better ear.

Sample Demographics

Twenty-one participants (11 female) with problematic tinnitus were recruited from the Champaign–Urbana area via fliers, campus notifications, and newspaper advertisements. The study was approved by the University of Illinois at Urbana–Champaign Institutional Review Board (IRB Protocol Number: 16784), and all subjects gave written informed consent prior to taking part in each phase (audiological, MRI, intervention) of the study.

Of those 21 participants, 12 participants participated in the initial MRI scanning session, 10 participants remained for the post-MBCT session, and 8 participants returned for a follow-up scan 8 weeks after the conclusion of the study. Demographics for the 12 imaged participants are included in **Table 1**. **Supplementary Table 1** shows the extended demographics for the post-MBCT and follow-up sessions.

TABLE 1 | Sample demographics.

Gender	M = 5; F = 7			
	Mean	***SD***		
Age (year)	51.42	10.63		
TFI	50.92	15.57		
BDI	6.67	7.04		
BAI	10.17	8.67		
	Mean hearing thresholds at screening			
Frequency (kHz)	**Right ear mean threshold (dB HL)**	**Right ear threshold SD (dB HL)**	**Left ear mean threshold (dB HL)**	**Left ear threshold SD (dB HL)**
0.25	12.08	5.42	15.00	5.22
0.5	12.08	5.82	12.92	6.56
1	14.17	7.93	14.58	7.82
2	16.67	6.51	15.42	11.37
3	25.42	13.22	25.42	16.44
4	26.25	15.69	25.42	16.16
6	35.42	20.17	30.42	17.38
8	34.17	22.04	37.08	21.05
9	51.25	20.79	43.33	20.60
10	53.75	23.27	46.67	22.50
11.2	56.67	23.77	51.25	25.86
12.5	59.58	25.89	56.25	27.64
14	64.58	24.16	60.83	26.01
16	50.83	17.69	47.08	20.28

Mindfulness-Based Cognitive Therapy

Participants were enrolled in one of two 8-week MBCT sessions. The classes were taught by clinical psychology graduate students trained in delivery of MBCT and supervised by a licensed clinical psychologist. Classes were structured according to the MBCT curriculum developed by Segal et al. (2002) and used the student workbook developed for MBCT by Teasdale et al. (2014). Each class lasted about 2 h and involved learning about mindfulness, participating in exercises designed to illustrate principles of mindfulness, clarifying values and setting goals, and practicing techniques designed to cultivate mindfulness. After each class, home practice assignments were given according to the workbook, and participants were asked to commit to daily practice between 40 and 60 min. The classes were modified from the original curriculum to remove discussions of depression relapse prevention and include a loving-kindness meditation in the final class, but no tinnitus-specific exercises or discussions were introduced.

Behavioral Measures

Audiology

Participants received a complete audiological evaluation during an initial screening phase, as well as pre-intervention (week 0), post-intervention (week 8) and at an 8-week follow-up session. The full audiological screening and follow-up audiology assessments were reported in Husain et al. (2019).

The initial audiological screening included pure-tone audiometry (0.25–16 kHz) (Equinox 2.0 PC-based clinical audiometer) and is presented in **Table 1** with the sample demographics.

Questionnaires

Three measures of tinnitus-related handicap were given at each session including the THI, TFI and Tinnitus Primary Function Questionnaire (TPFQ: Tyler et al., 2014). TFI, which has been shown to be sensitive to changes due to previous interventions (Henry et al., 2016), was chosen to be analyzed as a covariate of interest with functional MRI changes.

In addition to the tinnitus measures, the participants were given the MMSE, BDI, BAI, Big Five Personality Test (John et al., 1991), and Five Facet Mindfulness Questionnaire (FFMQ: Baer et al., 2008). TFI, BDI, and BAI were given at each of three MRI sessions. The behavioral data for this study was previously analyzed and reported in Husain et al. (2019) and provided evidence for significant improvement in self-reported tinnitus severity. The focus of this study was to examine the change in functional MRI measures across the MBCT intervention and to analyze the relationship between brain function and tinnitus severity as the variables change over the course of the study. Since our sample was so limited in this pilot study, we chose to focus on TFI as the primary measure of tinnitus severity.

fMRI Scans

Two fMRI scans were used to acquire measures of brain function at pre-intervention, post-intervention, and follow-up sessions. First, a resting state scan was collected over approximately 10 min. During the resting state scans, participants were instructed to lay still and fixate on a cross for the duration of the scan. This task was used to analyze resting-state functional connectivity, and the change in connectivity across sessions.

The second scan was an affective sound categorization task, where participants were asked to rate sounds presented to them as pleasant, unpleasant, or neutral. Sounds were used from the International Affective Digital Sounds Database (IADS; Bradley and Lang, 2007), which include normative scores of valences (1 very unpleasant – 9 very pleasant) and arousals (1 low arousing – 9 high arousing). Only the normative valence score was used to categorize sounds into emotionally salient, including a total of 46 pleasant sounds (valence: 6.89 ± 0.25; arousal: 5.99 ± 0.27) and 46 unpleasant sounds (valence: 2.66 ± 0.38; arousal 6.95 ± 0.31), and emotionally neutral, including 46 neutral sounds (valence: 4.96 ± 0.36; arousal 4.92 ± 0.29), for analysis. At each session, a different combination of 46 sounds was played, matched for valence across sessions. Each sound in a session was played twice, totaling 92 sounds played per session. The full list and order of the sounds presented in each session is included in **Supplementary Table 2**. Sounds were delivered using Presentation software[1] on a Windows 7 machine, with an Avotec silent scan 3300 sound system[2] through sound dampening headphones.

MRI/fMRI Acquisition

MRI data were collected on a 3T Siemens MAGNETOM Prisma MRI scanner with a 20-channel Siemens head coil.

An EPI sequence was collected during the resting state scan with parameters: TR = 2000 ms, TE = 25 ms, flip angle = 90°, 38 slices, 2.5 mm × 2.5 mm × 3.0 mm, FOV = 230 mm × 230 mm, matrix size = 92 × 92, with 304 volumes.

A second EPI sequence was collected during the auditory emotion task using a sparse sampling design in order to allow enough time for the auditory stimuli to evoke a BOLD response that does not overlap with the auditory response to the scanner gradients. The sequence had parameters: TR = 9000 ms (7000 ms delay), TE = 25 ms, flip angle = 90°, 38 slices, voxel size = 2.5 mm × 2.5 mm × 3.0 mm, FOV = 230 × 230, matrix size = 92 × 92, 92 volumes.

In addition, a low-resolution T2-weighted structural image (TR = 3400 ms, TE = 65.0 ms, flip angle = 120°, 38 slices, voxel size = 1.2 mm × 1.2 mm × 3.0 mm, FOV = 230 × 230, matrix size = 192 × 192) and a high-resolution T1-weighted MPRAGE (TR = 2300 ms, TE = 2.32 ms, flip angle = 8°, 192 slices, voxel size = 0.9 mm × 0.9 mm × 0.9 mm, FOV = 230 × 230, matrix size = 256 × 256) were collected and used for co-registration.

fMRI Analysis

Two types of functional imaging analyses were conducted. First, results from the emotion task were analyzed. In the emotion task, the whole brain response to emotionally salient contrasted against emotionally neutral stimuli was analyzed for change throughout the intervention. Then, results from resting state data across the three intervention imaging sessions were analyzed. For the resting state data, the connectivity between the brain and several seed regions was analyzed for change throughout the intervention was analyzed, as well as how patterns of connectivity predicted TFI. In addition, how some graph measures of connectivity including modularity and efficiency changed across the sessions in the intervention was analyzed.

Affective Sound Categorization Task

Functional MRI data collected during the affective sound categorization task was analyzed using SPM12 software (Statistical Parametric Mapping, Welcome Trust Center for Neuroimaging[3]). Images were preprocessed in a five-step procedure including slice timing correction, realignment, coregistration, normalization, and smoothing (Gaussian kernel of 8 mm × 8 mm × 8 mm).

In the first level analysis, emotionally salient vs. neutral contrast images were generated for each subject for each session. Second level analysis analyzed sample-wide within session salient vs. neutral contrasts and contrasts between each of the session pairs using a paired t-tests. Cluster-level significance in the salient vs. neutral contrasts was assessed using a cluster-defining height threshold of p < 1e-5 and family-wise error (FWE)-corrected (p < 0.05) cluster extent defined by the SPM12 software through random field theory. Results found by reducing the height threshold to a more liberal p < 1e-4 are additionally cautiously presented.

Resting State Functional Connectivity

Functional MRI data collected during the resting state task was also analyzed using SPM12 software. Images were preprocessed using the same five-step procedure described above, but with some additional denoising steps implemented with the Functional Connectivity Toolbox (Conn)[4] (RRID:SCR_009550) for MATLAB. These denoising steps included filtering the fMRI data with a 0.008–0.08 kHz bandpass filter and regressing out the signal from the white matter and cerebrospinal fluid segmentations from SPM12.

After denoising, seed-to-voxel connectivity analysis was conducted across several seeds of interest. Certain seed locations representing the default mode network (DMN) and the dorsal attention network (DAN) were the same as those used in earlier studies in our lab for comparison (Schmidt et al., 2013). In similar fashion to the study conducted by Schmidt et al. (2013) the DAN was split into two separate networks. The DMN used 8-mm spherical seeds corresponding to the medial prefrontal cortex and posterior cingulate cortex. The DAN_1 network used 8-mm spherical seeds corresponding to the left and right posterior intraparietal sulci. The DAN_2 network used 8-mm spherical seeds corresponding to the left and right frontal eye fields. Additionally, a seed representing the bilateral amygdalae was used given the evidence for its role in tinnitus (Carpenter-Thompson et al., 2015; Zimmerman et al., 2018). This seed was generated using the left and right amygdala parcellations in the atlas provided within the Conn toolbox, from the Harvard-Oxford subcortical atlas. For each of these regions, the seeds were combined prior to the connectivity analysis.

[1] http://www.neurobs.com

[2] http://www.avotecinc.com

[3] https://www.fil.ion.ucl.ac.uk/spm/software/spm12/

[4] www.nitrc.org/projects/conn

In addition to these networks, some network connectivity was investigated in an attempt to replicate and expand on results reported by Roland et al. (2015), which investigated changes in functional connectivity in the fronto-parietal (FPN) and cingulo-opercular networks (CON). As analyzed by Roland et al. (2015), seeds for these networks were separated by hemisphere. Seeds representing the left and right FPN in the left and right prefrontal cortex and representing left and right CON in the left and right anterior insulae were taken from the canonical network atlas provided in the Conn toolbox. The seeds and their coordinates in MNI space for each connectivity analysis are provided in **Table 2**.

Cluster-level significance in seed-to-voxel connectivity was assessed using a height threshold of $p < 1\text{e-}5$, and FWE-corrected cluster extent defined by the SPM12 software through random field theory. Results found by reducing the height threshold to a more liberal $p < 1\text{e-}4$ are additionally cautiously presented.

Relationship With TFI

Generalized estimating equations (GEE) were used to estimate the extent to which TFI predicted brain function across the intervention. For both the affective sound categorization task and the resting state functional connectivity, TFI was used as a predictor at each voxel to predict the results from the first-level, within-subject contrasts in a multi-scale adaptive generalized estimating equations (MAGEE) model developed by Li et al. (2013).

MAGEE integrates the GEE approach with adaptive smoothing methods to make robust estimates of betas for each voxel. GEE models account for the within-subject correlation among the longitudinal measures through the specification of a correlation structure to estimate parameters, avoiding violations of the sphericity assumptions in analysis of variance (ANOVA) and violations of the assumption of equal observations per time point in multivariate ANOVA. GEE can thus use incomplete data under less stringent assumptions while accommodating time-varying covariates without assumptions about the structure of the covariance, improving the power of the analysis for longitudinal data (Diggle et al., 2002).

TABLE 2 | Seeds for seed-voxel connectivity analysis.

Seed	Region	MNI Coordinate
DMN	Medial prefrontal cortex	8, 59, 19
	Posterior cingulate cortex	−2, −50, 25
DAN_1	Left posterior intraparietal sulcus	−23, −70, 46
	Right posterior intraparietal sulcus	26, −62, 53
DAN_2	Left frontal eye field	−25, −11, 54
	Right frontal eye field	27, −11, 54
AMGY	Left amygdala	Harvard-Oxford atlas parcellation
	Right amygdala	Harvard-Oxford atlas parcellation
L_FPN	Left prefrontal cortex	−43, 33, 28
R_FPN	Right prefrontal cortex	41, 38, 30
L_CON	Left anterior insula	−44, 13, 1
R_CON	Right anterior insula	47, 14, 0

The multi-scale adaptive smoothing smooths over the beta estimates across a user set number of iterations (in this case 5), allowing for a balance between cluster size and peak intensities. The beta for the TFI predictor was tested against the null hypothesis that beta = 0. The MAGEE analysis outputs a map of the Wald statistic for that parameter estimate, which is compared against a chi-squared distribution with 1-degree of freedom. Cluster-level analysis was completed using the peak_nii toolbox[5]. Because of the increased power afforded by GEE, cluster-level significance was defined using a height threshold of $p < 1\text{e-}5$ and a cluster extent of 100. This height threshold and cluster extent were chosen cautiously to in order to restrict our analysis to relatively large and extended effects. However, results found by reducing the height threshold to a more liberal $p < 1\text{e-}4$ are additionally cautiously discussed. All statistical maps are presented after surface-mapping volumetric results using Connectome Workbench[6] (Marcus et al., 2011).

Graph Analysis

To obtain a whole-brain functional network from the resting state fMRI data, first, the mean region of interest (ROI) time series were obtained by averaging the fMRI time series over all voxels within an ROI. For this purpose, 90 cortical and subcortical ROIs (excluding the ones from the cerebellum and vermis regions) defined in the Automated Anatomical Labeling (AAL) atlas (Tzourio-Mazoyer et al., 2002) were chosen. Then a 90×90 pairwise correlation matrix was obtained using the time series from these 90 regions. The pairwise correlation matrix was thresholded at various target connection densities to convert it to an undirected and unweighted (binary) connection matrix. In each case, correlations whose absolute values were higher than the threshold were converted to 1 s and the remaining correlations were converted to 0 s. At low graph connection densities, only the strongest correlations are present in the graph as connections, and as the graph density increases, weaker correlations also get added to the graph. As is standard in the literature, there is no *a priori* preference for a target connection density and so graph properties at a number of such connection densities were investigated.

Static network analysis

First, a single static network for each subject was created using the resting state time series data from the whole imaging session. With these static networks, the subjects' brain networks at pre, post, and follow-up sessions were compared both at the whole network level as well as at ROI level. Since data at all three sessions were available for only eight subjects, the remaining subjects' data were excluded from this analysis. The subjects' brain networks at pre, post and follow-up sessions were analyzed in terms of three commonly employed global graph summary measures, modularity, global network efficiency, and global clustering coefficient, and also tested for association of changes in these measures with changes in TFI scores between consecutive sessions.

[5]http://www.nitrc.org/projects/peak_nii
[6]https://www.humanconnectome.org

Modularity is a quality function that measures how much the networks are modular, i.e., segregated into communities or modules as opposed to what one might expect from a random network with similar node degree patterns. The Newman–Girvan modularity is computed using the Louvain algorithm for community detection (Blondel et al., 2008). The global network efficiency is defined as the average of the inverse shortest paths between pairs of vertices in the entire network (Rubinov and Sporns, 2010). The smaller the shortest paths are between pairs of vertices in the network, the higher the global efficiency. Intuitively, shorter paths between pairs of vertices allow information to pass throughout the network more efficiently. More locally, the nodal network efficiency of node i is defined as the average of the inverse shortest paths of all nodes in the network from the node i. Finally, the local clustering coefficient for a vertex measures the ratio of pairs of neighbors of the vertex i that are themselves connected (thus forming a closed triplet or triangle), to the number of such possible connections. The global clustering coefficient is defined as the average of the local clustering coefficient across the vertices of the network. The clustering coefficient is a measure of network segregation (Rubinov and Sporns, 2010), and a large clustering coefficient indicates that an otherwise sparse network is locally clustered and dense. For the purpose of statistical testing, due to the small sample size, non-parametric tests were employed along with parametric tests. All graph analyses were carried out in the statistical analysis software R.

Beyond global summary measures, the subjects' brain network community structures between pre and post sessions were also compared by fitting the Random Effects Stochastic Block Model (Paul and Chen, 2018) with the Co-regularized Orthogonal Symmetric Non-negative Matrix Tri-Factorization (Co-OSNTF) method (Paul and Chen, 2018). The number of communities to be used with the Co-OSNTF method was obtained by taking the median of the number of communities detected in the subject networks separately using the Louvain method for community detection. The Co-OSNTF method was used to statistically test for differences in the global community structure as well as identify ROIs that have significantly different community placements between the two time sessions. Further, subjects' brain networks were compared at each ROI in terms of nodal efficiency and local clustering coefficient in an effort to identify the ROIs which exhibit differential properties.

Dynamic network analysis

Time varying networks from the ROI time series data for each subject at each session were constructed using a sliding window approach (Hutchison et al., 2013). A window size of 20 TRs (40 s) was moved by 1 TR to obtain 280 time windows. For each window, a correlation matrix is estimated from the data within that window. The absolute correlation was thresholded to obtain a sparse connection matrix with connection density of 0.10. The subjects' networks were then compared at pre and post intervention in terms of dynamic fluctuations of network efficiency, modularity and clustering coefficient.

RESULTS

Paired t-tests showed that TFI scores were significantly lower at the post-intervention compared to pre-intervention sessions [$t(9) = 4.97$, $p < 0.001$] and significantly lower at the follow-up session compared to the pre-intervention session [$t(7) = 4.67$, $p = 0.002$]. However, there was no significant difference between the post-intervention and follow-up sessions [$t(7) = 0.45$, $p = 0.66$]. **Table 3** shows the mean and standard deviations of TFI scores at each session as well as the hours of logged weekly MBCT practice for each session.

There was a large variance in hours of practice of the 8-week period of intervention and the 8-week period following the treatment. Despite a numerical decline in mean practice hours, there was not a statistically significant difference between the amount of mindfulness practice logged during the MBCT and during the 8-week period after the MBCT ended [$t(7) = 2.05$, $p = 0.08$].

Affective Sound Categorization Task

There was little evidence for changes in functional activation during the affective sound categorization task across the three sessions of the study (**Supplementary Figure 1**). There were no statistically significant changes between sessions for the salient vs. neutral contrasts.

Additionally, there was no evidence for the activation differences between salient and neutral conditions predicting TFI in the participants (**Supplementary Figure 2**).

However, results from the analysis at more liberal thresholds were also reported as possible points of follow-up for future studies, although these results should be interpreted with caution. Peak MNI coordinates and the direction of the relationship for each test are included in **Table 4**. There was only some suggestive evidence, after reducing the statistical threshold, for a change in functional activation to the salient vs. neutral contrast between the post-intervention and follow-up sessions, where a decreased activation in clusters peaking in the left inferior frontal gyrus and the right insula were observed. Patterns of functional activation to the affective sound categorization task were not significantly predicted by TFI, even after reducing the statistical threshold.

Resting State Functional Connectivity

For the resting state analysis, we assessed how the seed-to-voxel whole brain connectivity changed across the MBCT intervention. We analyzed pre-determined seeds, meant to reflect

TABLE 3 | Tinnitus Function Index and mindfulness practice.

TFI	Mean	*SD*
Pre-intervention	50.92	15.57
Post-intervention	35.40	15.80
Follow-up	35.38	21.07
Minutes of practice	**Mean**	***SD***
During MBCT	960.60	510.20
After MBCT	605.50	210.11

TABLE 4 | Results from the analysis of the affective sound categorization fMRI.

Region	Peak MNI coordinates	Beta direction
Post vs. Pre		
None		
Follow-up vs. Pre		
None		
Follow-up vs. Post		
L. inferior frontal gyrus, pars opercularis*	−52, 16, 18	−
L. insula*	−42, 14, 6	−
Prediction of TFI		
None		

$p < 1e\text{-}4$ height threshold.

TABLE 5 | Results from the analysis of the DMN.

Region	Peak MNI coordinates	Beta direction
Post vs. Pre		
L. middle temporal gyrus*	−60, −42, −4	−
Follow-up vs. Pre		
L. calcarine sulcus**	2, −92, 6	−
R. thalamus**	2, −14, 8	−
Follow-up vs. Post		
R. angular gyrus**	40, −70, 38	+
L. middle temporal gyrus*	−70, −36, 4	+
Prediction of TFI		
R. middle frontal gyrus*	36, 6, 62	+
R. putamen*	32, −4, −2	+

***$p < 1e\text{-}5$ height threshold, *$p < 1e\text{-}4$ height threshold.*

the connectivity with the DMN, DAN_1 and DAN_2, AMYG, left and right FPN, and left and right CON. Significant results are reported in the main text, but for all of the networks, the full connectivity maps for each session, the full statistical maps of all non-significant between session changes, and the non-significant statistical maps of the connectivity associated with TFI are all presented in supplement (**Supplementary Figures 3–14**).

Default Mode Network

The between-session comparisons revealed a pattern of decreased connectivity between the DMN and the right thalamus and occipital regions from pre-intervention to the follow-up session (**Figure 1A**). In contrast, there were connectivity increases between the DMN and clusters with peaks in the right angular gyrus and left superior temporal gyrus from the post-intervention session to the follow-up session (**Figure 1B**). There was some evidence that connectivity between the right middle frontal gyrus and the DMN and between the right putamen and the DMN was positively related with TFI, but there was no indication that connectivity with the DMN and these areas changed across the intervention (**Table 5**).

Amygdala

There was a significant decrease in connectivity between a cluster overlapping the left inferior parietal lobule and the amygdala from the pre-intervention session to the post-intervention session (**Figure 2**). There was also evidence for the connectivity between the amygdala and multiple areas in the brain, mostly in frontal and parietal areas, relating positively to TFI (**Figure 3A**). The combined observations of the amygdala connectivity with parietal areas is intriguing. On one hand, the connectivity between these two regions significantly and positively predicts tinnitus severity. On the other hand, the connectivity between these regions significantly decreases over the intervention, suggesting that the decreasing connectivity may reflect some of the benefits of the MBCT. **Table 6** completely summarizes the statistical tests for changes in each session and for connectivity associated with TFI.

Dorsal Attention Network

There were no changes in connectivity with either of our DAN divisions in any of the pairwise session comparisons at the

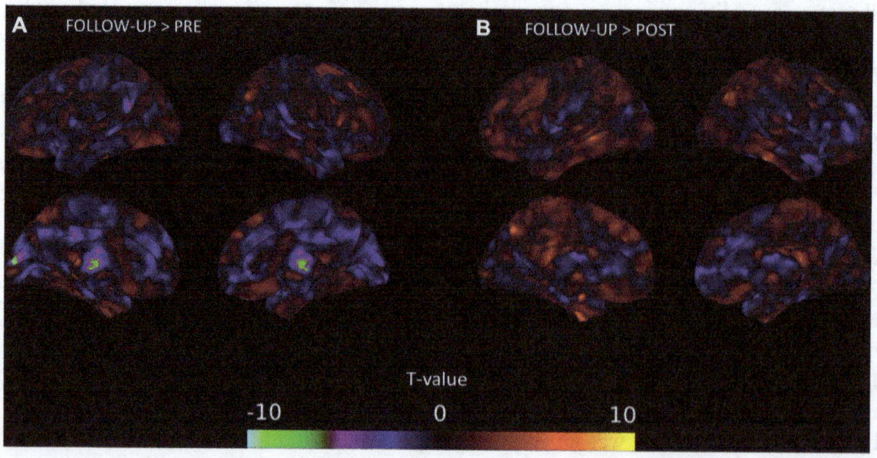

FIGURE 1 | DMN connectivity changes between time points of the mindfulness intervention. **(A)** Connectivity between the DMN and clusters in the right thalamus and left calcarine sulcus significantly decreases from the pre-intervention session to the follow-up session. **(B)** Connectivity between the DMN and a cluster in the right angular gyrus significantly increases from the post-intervention session to the follow-up session.

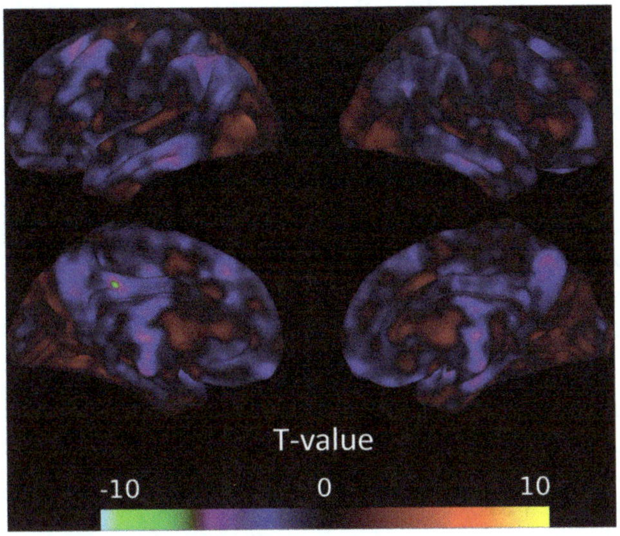

FIGURE 2 | Connectivity with the amygdala from the pre-intervention session to the post-intervention session decreases in a cluster overlapping the left inferior parietal lobule.

established threshold for significance. Even after reducing the voxel height threshold to be more liberal, no clusters emerged. Despite the lack of change in connectivity over the intervention, there were several clusters where the connectivity with DAN_1 significantly correlated with TFI (**Figure 3B**), primarily in the medial temporal lobe and cerebellum (**Table 7**).

In contrast with DAN_1, no connectivity with DAN_2 significantly predicted TFI. However, by reducing the height threshold, two suggestive clusters appeared within inferior frontal and superior occipital regions (**Table 7**).

Fronto-Parietal Network

There were no changes in connectivity with the left FPN in any of the pairwise session comparisons at the established threshold for significance, although there was some evidence for decreased connectivity between the right FPN and left caudate nucleus from pre- to post-intervention when reducing height threshold. Despite the lack of change in connectivity over the intervention, there were several clusters where the connectivity with the FPN significantly correlated with TFI (**Table 8**). These included lobule IX of the cerebellar hemisphere, the bilateral insulae, right hippocampus, right middle temporal gyrus, and the right inferior frontal gyrus (**Figures 3C,D**). In contrast, connectivity between the left FPN and the left calcarine sulcus was significantly negatively correlated with TFI (**Figure 3C**).

Cingulo-Opercular Network

The between-session comparisons revealed a pattern of decreased connectivity between the left CON and the left superior frontal gyrus from the post-intervention to the follow-up session (**Figure 4**). However, there was no indication that connectivity with the CON changed across the intervention (from the pre-intervention to the post-intervention sessions) or was predicted by TFI (**Table 9**).

Global Graph Properties

Figures 5A–C present the median modularity, global efficiency, and global clustering coefficient respectively, at pre-intervention, post-intervention and follow-up (weeks 0, 8, and 16), at various graph density thresholds or costs. From **Figure 5A** it appears that the modularity of the brain networks decreases post-intervention as compared to pre-intervention, but returns closer to the previous level at the follow-up session. There are similar trends in global efficiency and global clustering coefficient. While global efficiency increases at the post-intervention session compared to pre-intervention, the measure returns close to the previous level at the follow-up session (**Figure 5B**). This phenomenon is even more pronounced with global clustering coefficient, which is substantially lower at the post-intervention compared to pre-intervention, but almost entirely returns to the previous levels at the follow-up session (**Figure 5C**). These observations largely

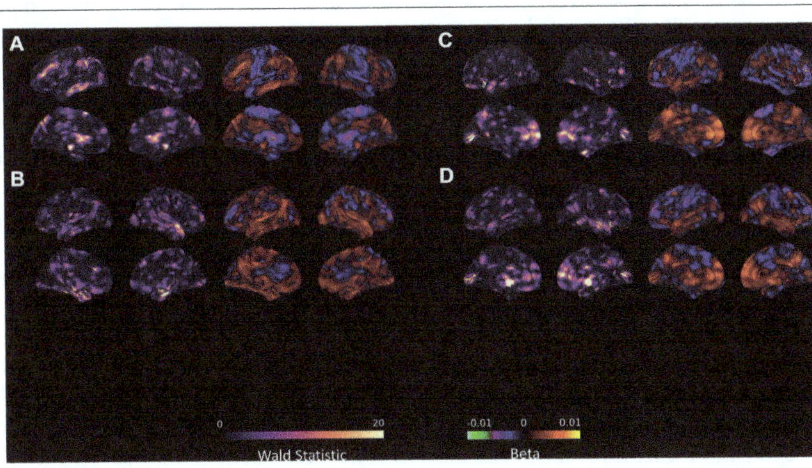

FIGURE 3 | Seed-voxel connectivity that significantly predicts TFI with the **(A)** AMYG, **(B)** DAN_1, **(C)** left FPN, and **(D)** right FPN. For each section, the left panel shows the Wald statistic, while the right panel indicates the beta value and the direction of the relationship.

TABLE 6 | Results from the analysis of the AMYG.

Region	Peak MNI coordinates	Beta direction
Post vs. Pre		
Left inferior parietal lobule**	−42, −58, 54	−
Follow-up vs. Pre		
None		
Follow-up vs. Post		
None		
Prediction of TFI		
L. precuneus**	−4, −78, 47	+
L. inferior frontal gyrus – pars triangularis**	−48, 40, 12	+
L. inferior frontal gyrus – pars triangularis**	−48, 36, 20	+
L. inferior frontal gyrus – pars triangularis*	−32, 36, 12	+
Undefined*	−26, −48, 14	−
Undefined *	−18, −42, 16	−
L. middle frontal gyrus*	−50, 22, 36	+
L. precentral gyrus*	−50, 10, 42	+
L. precentral gyrus*	−44, 12, 34	+
L. middle frontal gyrus*	−38, 20, 54	+
L. middle frontal gyrus*	−36, 30, 48	+
Undefined*	6, 0, 14	−
Undefined*	0, 6, 4	−
L. superior parietal lobule*	−32, −64, 46	+

***p < 1e-5 height threshold, *p < 1e-4 height threshold.*

hold across different brain network density or cost. Hence, at the post-intervention session, the subject networks tend to be less functionally segregated (Rubinov and Sporns, 2010) as evident with lower modularity and clustering coefficient, and more functionally integrated (Rubinov and Sporns, 2010) as evident by higher global efficiency. However, both these changes to the brain networks tend to return to pre-intervention levels by the follow-up session.

Remarkably, the distribution of TFI scores show a similar phenomenon, where the scores drop substantially at the post-intervention compared to pre-intervention, but remain stationary at the post-intervention level when measured again during the follow-up session (**Figure 5D**). The distribution of TFI scores was calculated over all subjects for whom data were available at the respective stage of data collection. Based on these observations we hypothesized that the changes in TFI scores might be related to the changes in the brain network global summary measures.

As reported in **Table 10**, the difference in TFI scores was found to be positively correlated with changes in both the measures of functional segregation (modularity and clustering coefficient) with the correlation being statistically significant [0.05 family-wise error rate (FWER), corrected for multiple comparisons] at lower graph densities of 0.05 and 0.10 (significant in all but one graph density without correction for multiple comparisons). Notably, the correlations between the change in functional segregation measures and change in TFI scores are stronger at lower graph densities. The association between the difference in TFI scores and global network efficiency was not significant at any graph density.

TABLE 7 | Results from the analysis of the DAN.

Region	Peak MNI coordinates	Beta direction
DAN_1		
Post vs. Pre		
None		
Follow-up vs. Pre		
None		
Follow-up vs. Post		
None		
Prediction of TFI		
Undefined**	16, −14, −28	+
R. parahippocampal gyrus**	22, −10, −24	+
R. parahippocampal gyrus**	26, −4, −32	+
L. lobule IV/V of cerebellar hemisphere**	−30, −36, −30	+
Undefined**	−14, −32, −34	+
L. parahippocampal gyrus**	−24, −6, −28	+
L. hippocampus**	−22, −20, −16	+
Undefined*	12, −34, −30	+
L. parahippocampal gyrus*	−20, 8, −28	+
L. inferior temporal gyrus*	−34, 8, −38	+
R. superior temporal gyrus*	46, −28, 12	+
Undefined*	34, −32, 12	+
Undefined*	22, −38, 0	+
R. hippocampus*	20, −30, −6	+
DAN_2		
Post vs. Pre		
None		
Follow-up vs. Pre		
None		
Follow-up vs. Post		
None		
Prediction of TFI		
L. superior occipital gyrus*	−14, −74, 22	+
R. inferior frontal gyrus, pars orbitalis*	41, 29, −5	+

***p < 1e-5 height threshold, *p < 1e-4 height threshold.*

Additional analysis of the global graph properties are provided in supplement, including normalizing measures of inter-session changes (**Supplementary Table 3**), analyzing a regression model of changes in TFI using global graph measures as predictors (**Supplementary Table 4**) and analyzing multiple density thresholds (**Supplementary Table 5** and **Supplementary Figure 15**). Furthermore, dynamic changes in efficiency, modularity and clustering are provided (**Supplementary Figure 17**), as well as their distribution smoothed by a kernel density estimator (**Supplementary Figure 18**).

Local Graph Properties

The subjects' networks at pre- and post-intervention were compared in terms of nodal efficiency and local clustering coefficient at each of the 90 ROIs using two-sample *t*-tests. At a connection density of 0.10, two ROIs, the right middle frontal gyrus, orbital part (Frontal_Mid_Orb_R), and the right angular gyrus (Angular_R) were found to exhibit significantly different nodal efficiency with a false discovery rate (FDR) correction of 5%

TABLE 8 | Results from the analysis of the left and right FPN.

Region	Peak MNI Coordinates	Beta direction
Left FPN		
Post vs. Pre		
None		
Follow-up vs. Pre		
None		
Follow-up vs. Post		
None		
Prediction of TFI		
L. calcarine sulcus**	0, −84, 0	−
Undefined**	−14, −86, 2	+
R. lobule IX of cerebellar hemisphere**	12, −50, −46	+
L. insula**	−29, 19, −17	+
R. hippocampus**	29, −35, 0	+
R. lobule VIII of cerebellar hemisphere*	18, −64, −38	+
L. medial frontal gyrus*	−6, 62, 4	+
R. anterior cingulate gyrus*	8, 46, 8	+
L. anterior cingulate gyrus*	−8, 36, 2	+
R. anterior cingulate gyrus*	2, 37, −1	+
L. medial frontal gyrus*	−8, 48, 6	+
Right FPN		
Post vs. Pre		
L. caudate nucleus*	−10, 12, −4	-
Follow-up vs. Pre		
None		
Follow-up vs. Post		
None		
Prediction of TFI		
Undefined**	0, −2, −10	+
Undefined**	15, −25, −37	-
R. middle temporal gyrus**	56, −6, −18	+
R. middle temporal gyrus**	52, −18, −12	+
R. insula**	33, 16, −12	+
R. inferior frontal gyrus – pars orbitalis**	34, 22, −22	+
Undefined*	26, −16, −6	+
R. lobule IX of cerebellar hemisphere*	10, −52, −40	+
L. lobule IX of cerebellar hemisphere*	−6, −52, −40	+
R. calcarine sulcus*	28, −64, 12	-
R. calcarine sulcus*	14, −80, 8	+
L. calcarine sulcus*	−8, −96, 0	+
L. calcarine sulcus*	−2, −88, 0	+
R. superior temporal pole*	46, 18, −22	+
R. medial frontal gyrus*	6, 56, 8	+
R. anterior cingulate gyrus*	6, 42, 4	+

***p < 1e-5 height threshold, *p < 1e-4 height threshold.*

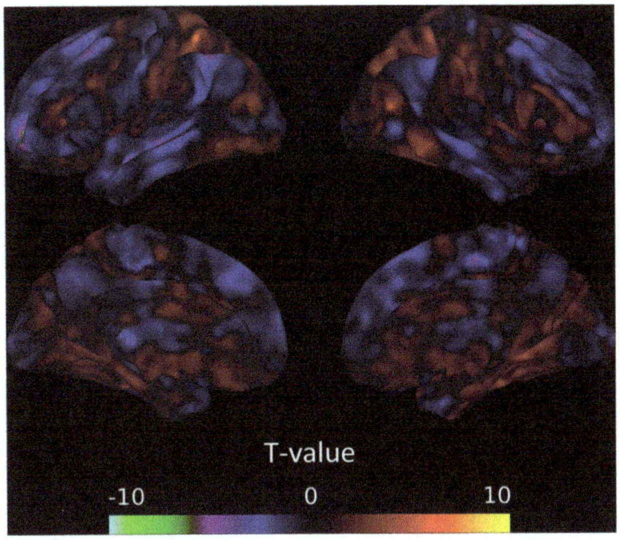

FIGURE 4 | Connectivity between the left CON and the left superior frontal gyrus decreases from the post-intervention to the follow-up session.

TABLE 9 | Results from the analysis of the left and right CON.

Region	Peak MNI coordinates	Beta direction
Left CON		
Post vs. Pre		
None		
Follow-up vs. Pre		
None		
Follow-up vs. Post		
L. superior frontal gyrus**	−32, 62, −2	−
R. lobule VI of cerebellar hemisphere*	34, −38, −38	+
Prediction of TFI		
None		
Right CON		
Post vs. Pre		
None		
Follow-up vs. Pre		
None		
Follow-up vs. Post		
R. calcarine sulcus*	18, −52, 8	+
Prediction of TFI		
None		

***p < 1e-5 height threshold, *p < 1e-4 height threshold.*

(the ROI Frontal_Mid_Orb_R was also significant at 5% FWER). One ROI, the right calcarine fissure (Calcarine_R), was found to exhibit a significantly different local clustering coefficient with an FDR correction of 5% (also significant at 5% FWER).

At a connection density of 0.20, no ROIs were found to exhibit any significantly different nodal efficiency with an FDR correction of 5%. However, two ROIs, the right medial superior frontal gyrus (Frontal_Sup_Medial_R), and the right middle occipital gyrus (Occipital_Mid_R), exhibited significantly different local clustering coefficients with an FDR correction of 5%. At pre-intervention, some ROIs were found to exhibit very low nodal efficiency, indicating a disconnect of those ROIs with the rest of the network. However, those ROIs exhibited nodal efficiency at par with other ROIs post intervention.

Next, random effects stochastic block models (RESBM) were fitted using the Co-OSNTF method (Paul and Chen, 2018) to pre- and post-intervention subject networks at 0.20

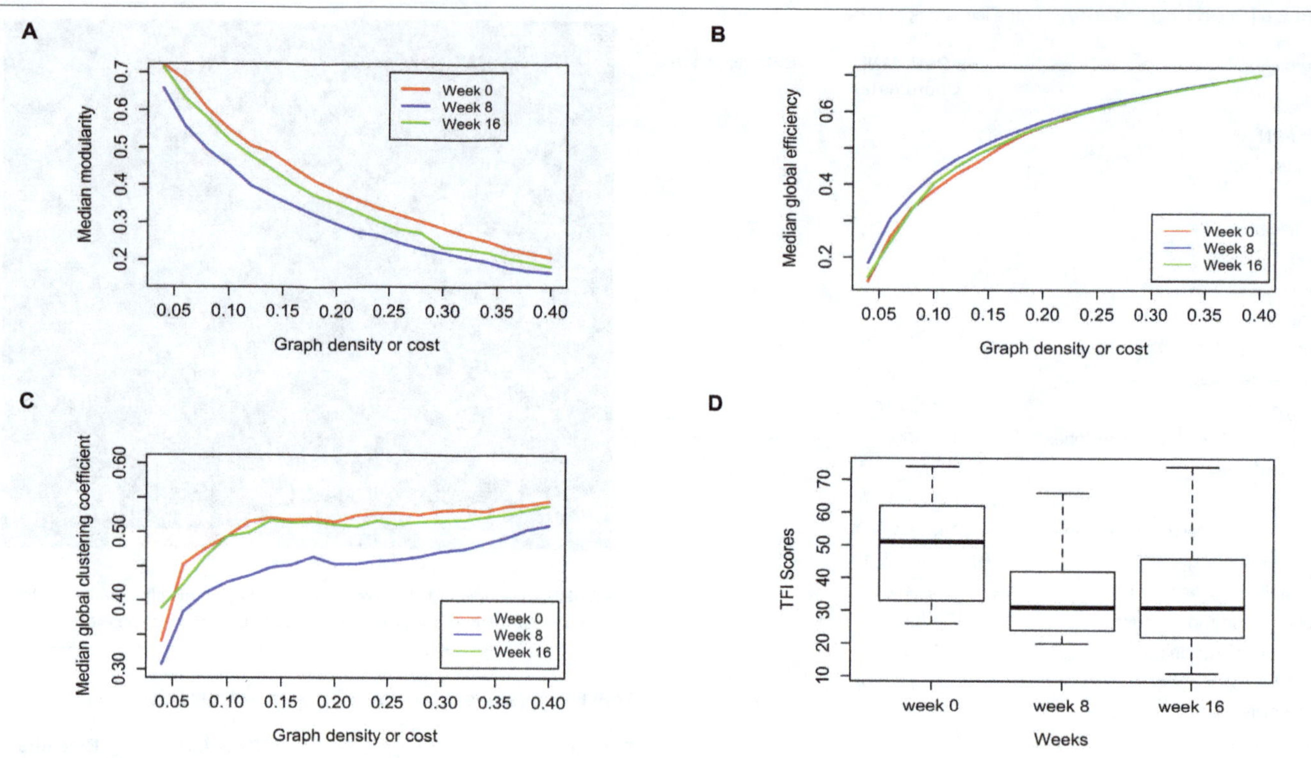

FIGURE 5 | Comparison of pre-intervention (week 0), post intervention (week 8) and follow up (week 16) session brain networks in terms of **(A)** Median modularity, **(B)** Median global efficiency, and **(C)** Median global clustering coefficient as a function of increasing network density, along with the **(D)** distribution of the TFI scores measured for subjects at those sessions.

connection densities. The median number of communities at pre-intervention brain networks was 5 and at post-intervention was 4.9 and hence 5 was selected to be the number of communities to be used with Co-OSNTF. The putative group module structures obtained from this method represent the module structures of all the 10 subjects at pre- and post-sessions and are presented in **Supplementary Figure 16.** The group module structures were found to be significantly different between pre- and post-intervention at the whole network level with $p = 0.0086$. However, no nodes were found to have significantly altered module membership at 5% FDR.

RESBM was also fitted to the pre and post-networks at 0.10 connection density with the number of communities as 6. The group module structures were found to be significantly altered between pre- and post-intervention with $p = 0.0033$. In addition, two ROIs, the left middle occipital gyrus (Occipital_Mid_L) and right inferior occipital gyrus (Occipital_Inf_R), were found to exhibit significantly altered module memberships in post-intervention as compared to pre-intervention with a 5% FDR correction (both ROIs were also significant with 5% FWER correction).

DISCUSSION

In this study, our focus was on explaining declines in tinnitus severity due to MBCT using task-based and resting-state fMRI. For the task-based fMRI, when the participants were processing affective sounds, we did not observe changes in the response of any of the brain regions at post-intervention or at follow-up. However, there were changes across the intervention in the resting state connectivity of a diverse set of regions, as well as evidence for certain patterns of functional connectivity relating to tinnitus handicap. Because we observed some overlap between changes across the intervention and a relationship to TFI, connectivity between the amygdala and parietal regions showed particular promise as an area involved in the improved tinnitus severity outcomes across the MBCT intervention. In contrast, connectivity with other ROIs that we investigated showed varying degrees of evidence for sensitivity to the intervention or as relating to TFI but lacked any overlap. This overlap is critical to interpreting the role of brain regions or connectivity benefiting from the intervention, since MBCT may induce functional brain changes that have no bearing on predicting tinnitus severity, and similarly, there may be functional patterns of brain activation that are predictive of tinnitus severity but are not influenced by the specific MBCT intervention.

Despite the sparse evidence for the resting connectivity with particular ROIs relating to the beneficial effects of the MBCT intervention (besides connectivity with the amygdala), global measures of connectivity from graph analysis did seem to have some correspondence to the decrease in tinnitus severity over the course of the intervention. Particularly, measures of functional segregation, modularity, and cross-correlation coefficient, which decreased over the MBCT intervention predicted the decreases in TFI.

Changes in RSFC During MBCT

We found evidence for changes in seed-to-voxel connectivity across the MBCT intervention in the DMN, AMYG, and left CON, but did not see evidence in the DAN or left or right FPN.

Interestingly, in both the DMN and the CON, the strongest contrasts in connectivity appeared to involve the follow-up session. In the DMN, we observed significant decreases in connectivity with the left calcarine sulcus and right thalamus from pre-intervention to the follow-up session. We also observed increased connectivity with the right angular gyrus from the post-intervention session to the follow-up. There was weaker evidence for a decrease in connectivity with the left middle temporal gyrus over the intervention, but then an increase in connectivity in the same area from the post-intervention session to the follow-up, after the intervention had ended. It is notable that the most significant changes in connectivity with the DMN occurred in contrasts with the follow-up session, suggesting that the brain may continue adapting even after the intervention. Our data suggested that there is substantial variance in practice both during and after the treatment and that our participants as a group continued their practice even after the MBCT ended.

Our work replicates other studies of mindfulness that have found decreases in connectivity between the DMN and regions involved in visual processing (Kilpatrick et al., 2011). However, we did not see any evidence of increased connectivity across the intervention with the dorsolateral prefrontal cortex, which has been identified in other studies (Brewer et al., 2011; King et al., 2016a) and has been implicated in improvement with other conditions (e.g., post-traumatic stress disorder, King et al., 2016a). It should also be noted that although researchers have observed connectivity increases *within* the DMN (e.g., Jang et al., 2011), we chose to combine seeds in the posterior cingulate cortex and medial prefrontal cortex, which limits our ability to study any within network effects.

In the CON (sometimes called the salience network), we did not observe any changes across the intervention, but did observe a decrease in connectivity between the left CON and the left dorsolateral frontal gyrus between the post-intervention and follow-up sessions. The CON has been implicated in mindfulness-based treatments primarily in its increased connectivity with self-referential regions, such as the dorsomedial prefrontal cortex, and decreased connectivity

TABLE 10 | Correlation of TFI score differences with the differences in modularity and clustering coefficient.

Graph density	Modularity (*p*-value)	Clustering coefficient (*p*-value)
0.05	0.6851 (0.0034**)	0.6597 (0.0054**)
0.10	0.6377 (0.0078**)	0.6688 (0.0046**)
0.15	0.4915 (0.0531)	0.4518 (0.0789)
0.20	0.5316 (0.0340*)	0.5355 (0.0325*)
0.25	0.5271 (0.0358*)	0.5073 (0.0448*)

**$p < 0.01$ levels ($p < 0.05$, FWER level), *$p < 0.05$.

with visual regions (Kilpatrick et al., 2011; Doll et al., 2015). Doll et al. (2015) found some trending evidence for increased connectivity between the salience network and what they refer to as the left central executive network, which included the left dorsolateral frontal gyrus, after 2 weeks of daily 20-min attention to breath training. Based on this, it seems more probable that the decrease in connectivity between post-intervention and follow-up sessions represents a return to baseline levels of connectivity after the intervention, rather than continued adaptation from the intervention. However, interpretation of any of the contrasts with the follow-up session, without significant effects at other contrasts, is very difficult, and highlights the importance of continuing this work with larger studies.

In the amygdala, we observed decreased connectivity with the left inferior parietal lobule from pre- to the post-intervention sessions. Changes in amygdala connectivity from mindfulness-based training treatments have been observed but seem to vary depending on the sample. For example, connectivity between the amygdala and anterior cingulate cortex decreased after a 3-day intensive mindfulness meditation intervention in a sample of stressed, unemployed adults (Taren et al., 2015). In a study on generalized anxiety disorder, Hölzel et al. (2013) found an increase in connectivity between the amygdala and prefrontal cortex over the course of an 8-week mindfulness-based stress reduction intervention, which correlated with the change in anxiety. King et al. (2016b) also found increased effective connectivity during an angry-faces viewing task between the left amygdala and medial frontal gyrus, dorsal anterior cingulate cortex, and lingual gyrus after a mindfulness-based exposure therapy on a sample of combat veterans with post-traumatic stress disorder. However, that study did not find significant correlations between changes in amygdala connectivity and symptom improvement.

Further research is required to determine whether connectivity changes with the amygdala are altered in a similar way across mindfulness interventions in accordance to a consistent framework or if instead changes in connectivity are highly dependent on the condition of the sample. For example, it may be possible to interpret connectivity changes across a mindfulness intervention in terms of increased cognitive control over emotional or default-mode processing, consistent across many forms of emotional dysregulation. Both research on post-traumatic stress disorder and existing research on tinnitus hypothesize that increased cognitive control over self-referential processing leads to improved outcomes (Malinowski, 2013; Husain, 2016; Schmidt et al., 2017).

Alternatively, there may be large condition specific effects. For example, in tinnitus, perhaps the emotional interpretation of primary sensory information is a critical aspect of the condition and is highlighted through changes in amygdala connectivity with the inferior parietal lobule. Conditions where the emotional interpretation of one's social position is more critical may instead be highlighted through changes in amygdala connectivity with the cingulate cortex or prefrontal cortex.

A broader review of the neural bases of both MBCT and the related mindfulness-based stress reduction (Gotink et al., 2016) revealed increased activity and gray matter volume in the prefrontal cortex, the cingular cortex, the insula and the hippocampus in both individuals with stress or anxiety and healthy participants. In contrast, the amygdala showed decreased response. A more recent systematic review of fMRI studies of mindfulness-based interventions (Young et al., 2018) did not find compelling evidence of increased response in the prefrontal cortex; rather, the authors found significant increased insular cortex activity correlated with the longitudinal interventions. Again, the authors noted the variety of findings with respect to neural bases of mindfulness-based interventions dependent on the populations and tasks.

Predicting Changes in TFI Using RSFC

One of the most striking results from this pilot study is the difference between functional connectivity that changes over a mindfulness intervention on one hand and functional connectivity that is predictive of tinnitus severity on the other. Connectivity between the FPN and broad regions of the brain predicted TFI, despite not showing any significant changes due to the intervention. Likewise, the DAN connectivity with a variety of regions, particularly limbic structures, predicted TFI, despite having no change due to MBCT. In contrast, connectivity to the DMN only weakly predicted TFI, and connectivity to the CON did not predict TFI.

We focused our analysis on resting state connectivity changes with regions that were implicated in both tinnitus and mindfulness-based treatments. Studies conducted on differences in functional connectivity in tinnitus compared to normal controls have identified changes in connectivity primarily in the DMN and networks involved in attention (Schmidt et al., 2013, 2017; Husain and Schmidt, 2014). While the results of this study largely replicate the importance of these networks in tinnitus, there were some key differences. Primarily, differences in DMN connectivity that predicted tinnitus have focused on the decreased connectivity between DMN and the precuneus (Schmidt et al., 2013, 2017), whereas this study only found weak evidence for increases in connectivity between the DMN and the right middle frontal gyrus and putamen as predictive of TFI. In addition, while the results here replicate past results (e.g., Schmidt et al., 2013) showing increased connectivity between the attention networks and limbic regions, our study additionally implicates increased connectivity between attention networks and the cerebellum, inferior frontal areas, and occipital areas in predicting TFI. Although connectivity with the DAN and FPN have similar patterns in predicting tinnitus, connectivity between the FPN and the right middle temporal gyrus additionally predicted TFI, which was an absent effect in the DAN. Connectivity with the amygdala also predicted TFI, but the effects were focused primarily to increased connectivity with frontal and parietal regions.

It should also be noted that the study here investigates how a measure of tinnitus severity, TFI, within a sample of individuals with tinnitus, predicts functional connectivity. This contrasts with most of the previous research, which focuses on differences between individuals with tinnitus vs. normal-hearing controls. It may be the case that changes in DMN connectivity strongly differentiate tinnitus patients from controls, but are far less important in predicting severity, whereas connectivity with regions involved in attention and emotion plays a far greater role in predicting severity.

Functional Correlates of Successful MBCT

Thus far, we discussed the mostly disparate results between changes in connectivity across the intervention and connectivity that predicts tinnitus severity. However, for the purpose of understanding any benefits of the intervention in terms of functional connectivity, we would like to observe changes in connectivity that also predicted TFI. This key overlap was evident in connectivity between the amygdala and parietal regions and in some of the global graph theoretical metrics of connectivity.

The cluster of amygdala connectivity with the parietal areas that changed over the intervention peaked in the left inferior parietal lobule, whereas amygdala connectivity with parietal areas that predicted TFI peaked in the left precuneus and left superior parietal lobule. Future research will be required to determine if these patterns of connectivity represent the same mechanism of some broad connectivity between the amygdala and the parietal lobe or if they represent two distinct patterns of connectivity. Interpreting the connectivity with parietal areas is further complicated by the complex functions of the parietal lobe. In fact, even within the precuneus, functions, and connections may vary widely between dorsal and ventral regions (Cavanna and Trimble, 2006; Zhang and Li, 2012). Despite these difficulties, the observation is a promising lead for future research. A large region of decreased connectivity between the amygdala and the parietal lobe appears to overlap with regions where that change predicts tinnitus severity. This overlap represents the critical result from the functional connectivity analysis, since every other measure of functional connectivity that changes over the intervention did not show any relation to tinnitus severity. With such a small sample, this may simply be due to being underpowered, but it is intriguing to speculate about the specific role of amygdala-parietal connectivity in tinnitus. On the one hand, the connectivity could be interpreted in terms of emotional regulation through the control functions of the parietal lobe. However, previous research has shown *increased* connectivity between the amygdala and cognitive control networks in response to cognitive behavioral therapy (Shou et al., 2017) and in mindfulness practice (Doll et al., 2016). Therefore, we would predict that if it was an attentional effect, the change in connectivity and the relation to tinnitus severity would be in the opposite direction from what we observed. It is possible that the reduction in connectivity observed here instead reflects a reduced need to process self-referential information related to stress. Increased connectivity between amygdala and the precuneus has been seen in response to psychosocial stress (Veer et al., 2011). In addition, Aghajani et al. (2014) observed increased amygdala-precuneus connectivity related to neuroticism and speculated that aberrant self-referential information processing reflected in this connectivity difference, may increase the propensity toward negative emotions. Despite the decreasing overall connectivity between the amygdala and parietal areas, we did observe increasing local nodal efficiency over the intervention in frontal and parietal areas as well, which may represent increased efficiency of areas involved in cognitive control. More research is clearly needed to elucidate the meaning of these findings and more finely define the spatial effects.

Besides these ROI based results, there were also global measures of connectivity that predicted the change in TFI. Specifically, decreases in measures of functional segregation (modularity and clustering coefficient) predicted decreases in TFI. Previous works have suggested meditation or mindfulness training to be associated with a decreased functional segregation and increased function integration in the brain networks (Gard et al., 2014; van Lutterveld et al., 2017). Our observations in this study are in line with those findings. While we found mindfulness training to be associated with both decreased segregation and increased integration, only the changes in the measures of segregation were found to be correlated with changes in TFI scores. Again, it is important to point out that this change in functional segregation speaks to a functional change within a sample of individuals with tinnitus and without a control it is impossible to relate to a non-tinnitus group. The relationship is particularly intriguing, since research on intervention-related plasticity typically has found modularity to positively predict behavioral outcomes across a variety of interventions (see Gallen and D'Esposito, 2019 for a review). It is possible that in the context of tinnitus or other conditions of disordered emotional processing modularity represents a different mechanism or pattern of brain function. This intriguing possibility further emphasizes the need for future research with a non-tinnitus comparison group.

Prior to this study, only one study has investigated the effects of a mindfulness-based intervention on the resting-state connectivity in tinnitus patients (Roland et al., 2015). Unlike that study, we did not observe changes to the connections between the attention networks and other regions but did note differences between DMN seeds and other regions. Interestingly, we did not see evidence that either of these patterns of connectivity overlapped with regions predicting tinnitus severity over the course of the intervention. In their study, they did not explicitly examine changes in connectivity that were predicted by tinnitus severity. The difference in the intervention effects may have been due to the difference in protocols (MBCT vs. mindfulness-based stress reduction). However, it is also probable that the small sample sizes in both studies yielded less reliable results or were underpowered to observe the effects.

Limitations and Future Directions

Despite the promise of the analysis of the study in informing future directions in research on tinnitus interventions, this pilot-study has some great limitations. First, this was an open-label study, with the participants aware of the treatment they were receiving and no control group. The lack of a control group is somewhat offset by the longitudinal nature of the study; with the baseline longitudinal data on their self-report tinnitus measures, each participant served as their own control in some regards. However, it is difficult to definitively attribute the effects to the MBCT, and the results may be due to other factors not considered here, including placebo effects.

A further major shortcoming of this study is the small sample size, further exacerbated by a high dropout rate. A small sample size is sometimes an unfortunate aspect of studies of medical conditions due to challenges in recruitment and retention. The current study did not include data from any participants that missed more than two classes, which may be too restrictive of a criterion for future research, especially if adherence to home practice is maintained. A second limitation of the small sample is the inability to model heterogenous aspects of the sample, including age. We have attempted to mitigate the small sample size by using statistical techniques that allow unequal sample sizes and focus on population-level effects (rather than within-subject effects) to improve the power of the fMRI analyses as much as possible. We also attempted to report the results in such a way that makes all of the results accessible rather than limiting the scope of the results to a single set criterion. However, due to the limited sample size, the results presented here should be taken as suggestive rather than definitive.

We plan to use findings from this pilot study to guide future research and theory building for tinnitus interventions. Mindfulness-based interventions appear to be a promising therapy for tinnitus and understanding why may open ways to enhance or substitute these effects. Randomized controlled clinical studies with larger sample sizes and control groups with and without tinnitus will help determine the answer to some of the questions that the research here brings up. First, increased power will help to make a stronger case for whether mindfulness-based therapies improve many conditions through a similar mechanism (e.g., improved attentional control over emotional processing) or whether there are unique, condition-specific effects that need to be considered while developing future interventions. Secondly, a non-tinnitus control group would be beneficial in further elucidating patterns of brain function that predict the condition of tinnitus itself and patterns of brain function that predict severity within the condition.

CONCLUSION

In this feasibility study, we measured fMRI at three time points: before, after, and at follow-up of an 8-week long MBCT intervention. In an affective sound categorization task, no significant functional activation differences were observed between sessions, nor was the activation to emotionally salient compared to neutral stimuli significantly predictive of TFI. However, we found significant changes in resting state connectivity with the DMN, cingulo-opercular network and amygdala after the intervention, and patterns of resting state connectivity with amygdala, DAN and frontoparietal network significantly predicted tinnitus-related handicap. Critically, the overlap of decreased amygdala connectivity with parietal areas and the negative correlation between amygdala-parietal connectivity and TFI is suggestive of a brain imaging marker of successful treatment of tinnitus-distress. Additionally, we found an intriguing pattern of decreased functional segregation predictive of decreased TFI over the course of the MBCT intervention. Our findings support the use of brain imaging, specifically resting state functional connectivity analyses, to provide clinicians and researchers with supplementary information to better evaluate the efficacy of interventions and to design more focused experiments in future.

ETHICS STATEMENT

This study was carried out in accordance with the recommendations of the Institutional Review Board of the University of Illinois at Urbana–Champaign, with written informed consent from all subjects. All subjects gave written informed consent in accordance with the Declaration of Helsinki. The protocol was approved by the Institutional Review Board of the University of Illinois at Urbana–Champaign.

AUTHOR CONTRIBUTIONS

FH obtained funding, directed this study, designed the research, and edited the manuscript. BZ oversaw all analysis, analyzed both resting state and task-based fMRI data, and wrote the manuscript. MF helped design the study and recruited the participants. Both MF and SS collected the MRI data and ran the initial analysis. SP and YC helped conduct graph connectivity analysis, with SP taking the lead and contributing text and figures. KR helped design the study and screened the participants. YT conducted the audiological and behavioral assessments and related data analysis. All authors contributed to manuscript revision, and read and approved the submitted version.

ACKNOWLEDGMENTS

We would like to thank Pengyu Chen, Hongtu Zhu, and Liming Zhong for their support and help in implementing the generalized estimating equation analysis. This work was conducted in part at the Biomedical Imaging Center of the Beckman Institute for Advanced Science and Technology at the University of Illinois at Urbana–Champaign (UIUC-BI-BIC).

REFERENCES

Aghajani, M., Veer, I. M., van Tol, M. J., Aleman, A., van Buchem, M. A., Veltman, D. J., et al. (2014). Neuroticism and extraversion are associated with amygdala resting-state functional connectivity. *Cogn. Affect. Behav. Neurosci.* 14, 836–848. doi: 10.3758/s13415-013-0224-0

Alexander-Bloch, A. F., Gogtay, N., Meunier, D., Birn, R., Clasen, L., Lalonde, F., et al. (2010). Disrupted modularity and local connectivity of brain functional networks in childhood-onset schizophrenia. *Front. Syst. Neurosci.* 4:147. doi: 10.3389/fnsys.2010.00147

Baer, R. A., Smith, G. T., Lykins, E., Button, D., Krietemeyer, J., and Sauer, S. (2008). Construct validity of the five facet mindfulness questionnaire in meditating and nonmeditating samples. *Assessment* 15, 329–342. doi: 10.1177/1073191107313003

Bartels, H., Middel, B. L., van der Laan, B. F. A. M., Staal, M. J., and Albers, F. W. J. (2008). The additive effect of co-occurring anxiety and depression on health status, quality of life and coping strategies in help-seeking tinnitus sufferers. *Ear Hear.* 29, 947–956. doi: 10.1097/AUD.0b013e3181888f83

Bassett, D. S., and Bullmore, E. (2006). Small-world brain networks. *Neuroscientist* 12, 512–523. doi: 10.1177/1073858406293182

Bassett, D. S., and Sporns, O. (2017). Network neuroscience. *Nat. Neurosci.* 20, 353–364. doi: 10.1038/nn.4502

Bassett, D. S., Wymbs, N. F., Porter, M. A., Mucha, P. J., Carlson, J. M., and Grafton, S. T. (2011). Dynamic reconfiguration of human brain networks during learning. *Proc. Natl. Acad. Sci.* 108, 7641–7646. doi: 10.1073/pnas.1018985108

Beck, A. T., Epstein, N., Brown, G., and Steer, R. A. (1988a). An inventory for measuring clinical anxiety: psychometric properties. *J. Consult. Clin. Psychol.* 56, 893–897. doi: 10.1037//0022-006x.56.6.893

Beck, A. T., Steer, R. A., and Carbin, M. G. (1988b). Psychometric properties of the beck depression inventory: twenty-five years of evaluation. *Clin. Psychol. Rev.* 8, 77–100. doi: 10.1016/0272-7358(88)90050-5

Blondel, V. D., Guillaume, J.-L., Lambiotte, R., and Lefebvre, E. (2008). Fast unfolding of communities in large networks. *J. Stat. Mech.* 2008:10008. doi: 10.1088/1742-5468/2008/10/P10008

Bradley, M. M., and Lang, P. J. (2007). *International Affective Digitized Sounds (IADS): Affective Ratings of Sounds and Instruction Manual.* Gainesville, Fl: University of Florida.

Braun, U., Schäfer, A., Walter, H., Erk, S., Romanczuk-Seiferth, N., Haddad, L., et al. (2015). Dynamic reconfiguration of frontal brain networks during executive cognition in humans. *Proc. Natl. Acad. Sci. U.S.A.* 112, 11678–11683. doi: 10.1073/pnas.1422487112

Brewer, J. A., Worhunsky, P. D., Gray, J. R., Tang, Y.-Y., Weber, J., and Kober, H. (2011). Meditation experience is associated with differences in default mode network activity and connectivity. *Proc. Natl. Acad. Sci. U.S.A.* 108, 20254–20259. doi: 10.1073/pnas.1112029108

Bullmore, E., and Sporns, O. (2009). Complex brain networks: graph theoretical analysis of structural and functional systems. *Nat. Rev. Neurosci.* 10, 186–198. doi: 10.1038/nrn2575

Carpenter-Thompson, J. R., Akrofi, K., Schmidt, S. A., Dolcos, F., and Husain, F. T. (2014). Alterations of the emotional processing system may underlie preserved rapid reaction time in tinnitus. *Brain Res.* 1567, 28–41. doi: 10.1016/j.brainres.2014.04.024

Carpenter-Thompson, J. R., Schmidt, S., McAuley, E., and Husain, F. T. (2015). Increased frontal response may underlie decreased tinnitus severity. *PLoS One* 10:e0144419. doi: 10.1371/journal.pone.0144419

Cavanna, A. E., and Trimble, M. R. (2006). The precuneus: a review of its functional anatomy and behavioural correlates. *Brain* 129(Pt 3), 564–583. doi: 10.1093/brain/awl004

Diggle, P. J., Heagerty, P., Liang, K.-Y., and Zeger, S. L. (2002). *Analysis of Longitudinal Data.* Oxford: Oxford University Press.

Doll, A., Hölzel, B. K., Boucard, C. C., Wohlschläger, A. M., and Sorg, C. (2015). Mindfulness is associated with intrinsic functional connectivity between default mode and salience networks. *Front. Hum. Neurosci.* 9:461. doi: 10.3389/fnhum.2015.00461

Doll, A., Hölzel, B. K., Mulej Bratec, S., Boucard, C. C., Xie, X., Wohlschläger, A. M., et al. (2016). Mindful attention to breath regulates emotions via increased amygdala-prefrontal cortex connectivity. *NeuroImage* 134, 305–313. doi: 10.1016/j.neuroimage.2016.03.041

Folstein, M. F., Folstein, S. E., and McHugh, P. R. (1975). Mini-mental state. A practical method for grading the cognitive state of patients for the clinician. *J. Psychiatr. Res.* 12, 189–198.

Gallen, C. L., and D'Esposito, M. (2019). Brain Modularity: a biomarker of intervention-related plasticity. *Trends Cogn. Sci.* 23, 293–304. doi: 10.1016/j.tics.2019.01.014

Gans, J. J., O'Sullivan, P., and Bircheff, V. (2014). Mindfulness based tinnitus stress reduction pilot study. *Mindfulness* 5, 322–333. doi: 10.1007/s12671-012-0184-4

Gard, T., Taquet, M., Dixit, R., Hölzel, B. K., de Montjoye, Y.-A., Brach, N., et al. (2014). Fluid intelligence and brain functional organization in aging yoga and meditation practitioners. *Front. Aging Neurosci.* 6:76. doi: 10.3389/fnagi.2014.00076

Gotink, R. A., Meijboom, R., Vernooij, M. W., Smits, M., and Hunink, M. G. M. (2016). 8-week Mindfulness Based Stress Reduction induces brain changes similar to traditional long-term meditation practice - a systematic review. *Brain Cogn.* 108, 32–41. doi: 10.1016/j.bandc.2016.07.001

Henry, J. A., Griest, S., Thielman, E., McMillan, G., Kaelin, C., and Carlson, K. F. (2016). Tinnitus functional index: development, validation, outcomes research, and clinical application. *Hear. Res.* 334, 58–64. doi: 10.1016/j.heares.2015.06.004

Hofmann, S. G., Sawyer, A. T., Witt, A. A., and Oh, D. (2010). The effect of mindfulness-based therapy on anxiety and depression: a meta-analytic review. *J. Consult. Clin. Psychol.* 78, 169–183. doi: 10.1037/a0018555

Hölzel, B. K., Hoge, E. A., Greve, D. N., Gard, T., Creswell, J. D., Brown, K. W., et al. (2013). Neural mechanisms of symptom improvements in generalized anxiety disorder following mindfulness training. *NeuroImage Clin.* 2, 448–458. doi: 10.1016/j.nicl.2013.03.011

Husain, F. T. (2016). Neural networks of tinnitus in humans: elucidating severity and habituation. *Hear. Res.* 334, 37–48. doi: 10.1016/j.heares.2015.09.010

Husain, F. T., and Schmidt, S. A. (2014). Using resting state functional connectivity to unravel networks of tinnitus. *Hear. Res.* 307, 153–162. doi: 10.1016/j.heares.2013.07.010

Husain, F. T., Zimmerman, B., Tai, Y., Finnegan, M. K., Kay, E., Khan, F., et al. (2019). Assessing mindfulness-based cognitive therapy intervention for tinnitus using behavioural measures and structural MRI: a pilot study. *Int. J. Audiol.* doi: 10.1080/14992027.2019.1629655 [Epub ahead of print].

Hutchison, R. M., Womelsdorf, T., Allen, E. A., Bandettini, P. A., Calhoun, V. D., Corbetta, M., et al. (2013). Dynamic functional connectivity: promise, issues, and interpretations. *NeuroImage* 80, 360–378. doi: 10.1016/j.neuroimage.2013.05.079

Jang, J. H., Jung, W. H., Kang, D.-H., Byun, M. S., Kwon, S. J., Choi, C.-H., et al. (2011). Increased default mode network connectivity associated with meditation. *Neurosci. Lett.* 487, 358–362. doi: 10.1016/j.neulet.2010.10.056

John, O. P., Donahue, E. M., and Kentle, R. L. (1991). *The Big Five Inventory—Versions 4a and 54.* Berkeley, CA: University of California.

Kabat-Zinn, J. (1994). *Wherever You Go, There You Are: Mindfulness Meditation In Everyday Life.* New York, NY: Hachette Books.

Kilpatrick, L. A., Suyenobu, B. Y., Smith, S. R., Bueller, J. A., Goodman, T., Creswell, J. D., et al. (2011). Impact of mindfulness-based stress reduction training on intrinsic brain connectivity. *NeuroImage* 56, 290–298. doi: 10.1016/j.neuroimage.2011.02.034

King, A. P., Block, S. R., Sripada, R. K., Rauch, S., Giardino, N., Favorite, T., et al. (2016a). Altered default mode network (dmn) resting state functional connectivity following a mindfulness-based exposure therapy for posttraumatic stress disorder (ptsd) in combat veterans of Afghanistan and Iraq. *Depress. Anxiety* 33, 289–299. doi: 10.1002/da.22481

King, A. P., Block, S. R., Sripada, R. K., Rauch, S. A., Porter, K. E., Favorite, T. K., et al. (2016b). A pilot study of mindfulness-based exposure therapy in OEF/OIF combat veterans with PTSD: altered medial frontal cortex and amygdala responses in social–emotional processing. *Front. Psychiatry* 7:154. doi: 10.3389/fpsyt.2016.00154

Kreuzer, P. M., Goetz, M., Holl, M., Schecklmann, M., Landgrebe, M., Staudinger, S., et al. (2012). Mindfulness-and body-psychotherapy-based group treatment of chronic tinnitus: a randomized controlled pilot study. *BMC Complement. Alternat. Med.* 12:235. doi: 10.1186/1472-6882-12-235

Lakhan, S. E., and Schofield, K. L. (2013). Mindfulness-based therapies in the treatment of somatization disorders: a systematic review and meta-analysis. *PLoS One* 8:e71834. doi: 10.1371/journal.pone.0071834

Li, Y., Gilmore, J. H., Shen, D., Styner, M., Lin, W., and Zhu, H. (2013). Multiscale adaptive generalized estimating equations for longitudinal neuroimaging data. *NeuroImage* 72, 91–105. doi: 10.1016/j.neuroimage.2013.01.034

Liu, Y., Liang, M., Zhou, Y., He, Y., Hao, Y., Song, M., et al. (2008). Disrupted small-world networks in schizophrenia. *Brain* 131(Pt 4), 945–961. doi: 10.1093/brain/awn018

Lynall, M.-E., Bassett, D. S., Kerwin, R., McKenna, P. J., Kitzbichler, M., Muller, U., et al. (2010). Functional connectivity and brain networks in schizophrenia. *J. Neurosci.* 30, 9477–9487. doi: 10.1523/JNEUROSCI.0333-10.2010

Malinowski, P. (2013). Neural mechanisms of attentional control in mindfulness meditation. *Front. Neurosci.* 7:8. doi: 10.3389/fnins.2013.00008

Marcus, D., Harwell, J., Olsen, T., Hodge, M., Glasser, M., Prior, F., et al. (2011). Informatics and data mining tools and strategies for the human connectome project. *Front. Neuroinform.* 5:4. doi: 10.3389/fninf.2011.00004

McCormack, A., Edmondson-Jones, M., Fortnum, H., Dawes, P. D., Middleton, H., Munro, K. J., et al. (2015). Investigating the association between tinnitus severity and symptoms of depression and anxiety, while controlling for neuroticism, in a large middle-aged UK population. *Int. J. Audiol.* 54, 599–604. doi: 10.3109/14992027.2015.1014577

McCormack, A., Edmondson-Jones, M., Somerset, S., and Hall, D. (2016). A systematic review of the reporting of tinnitus prevalence and severity. *Hear. Res.* 337, 70–79. doi: 10.1016/j.heares.2016.05.009

McKenna, L., Marks, E. M., Hallsworth, C. A., and Schaette, R. (2017). Mindfulness-based cognitive therapy as a treatment for chronic tinnitus: a randomized controlled trial. *Psychother. Psychosom.* 86, 351–361. doi: 10.1159/000478267

Meikle, M. B., Henry, J. A., Griest, S. E., Stewart, B. J., Abrams, H. B., McArdle, R., et al. (2012). The tinnitus functional index: development of a new clinical measure for chronic, intrusive tinnitus. *Ear Hear.* 33, 153–176. doi: 10.1097/AUD.0b013e31822f67c0

Meunier, D., Lambiotte, R., and Bullmore, E. T. (2010). Modular and hierarchically modular organization of brain networks. *Front. Neurosci.* 4:200. doi: 10.3389/fnins.2010.00200

Newman, C. W., Jacobson, G. P., and Spitzer, J. B. (1996). Development of the tinnitus handicap inventory. *Arch. Otolaryngol. Head Neck Surg.* 122, 143–148.

Paul, S., and Chen, Y. (2018). A random effects stochastic block model for joint community detection in multiple networks with applications to neuroimaging. *ArXiv*

Philippot, P., Nef, F., Clauw, L., de Romrée, M., and Segal, Z. (2012). A randomized controlled trial of mindfulness-based cognitive therapy for treating tinnitus. *Clin. Psychol. Psychother.* 19, 411–419. doi: 10.1002/cpp.756

Roland, L. T., Lenze, E. J., Hardin, F. M., Kallogjeri, D., Nicklaus, J., Wineland, A. M., et al. (2015). Effects of mindfulness based stress reduction therapy on subjective bother and neural connectivity in chronic tinnitus. *Otolaryngol. Head Neck Surg.* 152, 919–926. doi: 10.1177/0194599815571556

Rubinov, M., and Sporns, O. (2010). Complex network measures of brain connectivity: uses and interpretations. *NeuroImage* 52, 1059–1069. doi: 10.1016/j.neuroimage.2009.10.003

Schmidt, S. A., Akrofi, K., Carpenter-Thompson, J. R., and Husain, F. T. (2013). Default mode, dorsal attention and auditory resting state networks exhibit differential functional connectivity in tinnitus and hearing loss. *PLoS One* 8:e76488. doi: 10.1371/journal.pone.0076488

Schmidt, S. A., Carpenter-Thompson, J., and Husain, F. T. (2017). Connectivity of precuneus to the default mode and dorsal attention networks: a possible invariant marker of long-term tinnitus. *NeuroImage Clin.* 16, 196–204. doi: 10.1016/j.nicl.2017.07.015

Segal, Z. V., Williams, J. M. G., and Teasdale, J. D. (2002). *Mindfulness-Based Cognitive Therapy for Depression, A New Approach to Preventing Relapse*, 1st Edn. New York, NY: Guilford Publications.

Shou, H., Yang, Z., Satterthwaite, T. D., Cook, P. A., Bruce, S. E., Shinohara, R. T., et al. (2017). Cognitive behavioral therapy increases amygdala connectivity with the cognitive control network in both MDD and PTSD. *NeuroImage Clin.* 14, 464–470. doi: 10.1016/j.nicl.2017.01.030

Sporns, O. (2014). Contributions and challenges for network models in cognitive neuroscience. *Nat. Neurosci.* 17, 652–660. doi: 10.1038/nn.3690

Tang, Y.-Y., Hölzel, B. K., and Posner, M. I. (2015). The neuroscience of mindfulness meditation. *Nat. Rev. Neurosci.* 16, 213–225. doi: 10.1038/nrn3916

Taren, A. A., Gianaros, P. J., Greco, C. M., Lindsay, E. K., Fairgrieve, A., Brown, K. W., et al. (2015). Mindfulness meditation training alters stress-related amygdala resting state functional connectivity: a randomized controlled trial. *Soc. Cogn. Affect. Neurosci.* 10, 1758–1768. doi: 10.1093/scan/nsv066

Teasdale, J., Williams, M., and Segal, Z. (2014). *The Mindful Way Workbook: An 8-Week Program to Free Yourself from Depression and Emotional Distress*. New York, NY: Guilford Press.

Tyler, R., Ji, H., Perreau, A., Witt, S., Noble, W., and Coelho, C. (2014). Development and validation of the tinnitus primary function questionnaire. *Am. J. Audiol.* 23, 260–272. doi: 10.1044/2014_AJA-13-0014

Tzourio-Mazoyer, N., Landeau, B., Papathanassiou, D., Crivello, F., Etard, O., Delcroix, N., et al. (2002). Automated anatomical labeling of activations in SPM using a macroscopic anatomical parcellation of the MNI MRI single-subject brain. *NeuroImage* 15, 273–289. doi: 10.1006/nimg.2001.0978

van den Heuvel, M. P., Bullmore, E. T., and Sporns, O. (2016). Comparative connectomics. *Trends Cogn. Sci.* 20, 345–361. doi: 10.1016/j.tics.2016.03.001

van den Heuvel, M. P., Mandl, R. C. W., Stam, C. J., Kahn, R. S., and Hulshoff Pol, H. E. (2010). Aberrant frontal and temporal complex network structure in schizophrenia: a graph theoretical analysis. *J. Neurosci.* 30, 15915–15926. doi: 10.1523/JNEUROSCI.2874-10.2010

van den Heuvel, M. P., Sporns, O., Collin, G., Scheewe, T., Mandl, R. C. W., Cahn, W., et al. (2013). Abnormal rich club organization and functional brain dynamics in schizophrenia. *JAMA Psychiatry* 70, 783–792. doi: 10.1001/jamapsychiatry.2013.1328

van Lutterveld, R., van Dellen, E., Pal, P., Yang, H., Stam, C. J., and Brewer, J. (2017). Meditation is associated with increased brain network integration. *NeuroImage* 158, 18–25. doi: 10.1016/j.neuroimage.2017.06.071

Veer, I. M., Oei, N. Y., Spinhoven, P., van Buchem, M. A., Elzinga, B. M., and Rombouts, S. A. (2011). Beyond acute social stress: increased functional connectivity between amygdala and cortical midline structures. *NeuroImage* 57, 1534–1541. doi: 10.1016/j.neuroimage.2011.05.074

Wang, J., Zuo, X., Dai, Z., Xia, M., Zhao, Z., Zhao, X., et al. (2013). Disrupted functional brain connectome in individuals at risk for Alzheimer's disease. *Biol. Psychiatry* 73, 472–481. doi: 10.1016/j.biopsych.2012.03.026

Young, K. S., van der Velden, A. M., Craske, M. G., Pallesen, K. J., Fjorback, L., Roepstorff, A., et al. (2018). The impact of mindfulness-based interventions on brain activity: a systematic review of functional magnetic resonance imaging studies. *Neurosci. Biobehav. Rev.* 84, 424–433. doi: 10.1016/j.neubiorev.2017.08.003

Yu, Q., Plis, S. M., Erhardt, E. B., Allen, E. A., Sui, J., Kiehl, K. A., et al. (2011). Modular organization of functional network connectivity in healthy controls and patients with schizophrenia during the resting state. *Front. Syst. Neurosci.* 5:103. doi: 10.3389/fnsys.2011.00103

Zalesky, A., Fornito, A., Cocchi, L., Gollo, L. L., and Breakspear, M. (2014). Time-resolved resting-state brain networks. *Proc. Natl. Acad. Sci. U.S.A.* 111, 10341–10346. doi: 10.1073/pnas.1400181111

Zhang, S., and Li, C. R. (2012). Functional connectivity mapping of the human precuneus by resting state fMRI. *Neuroimage* 59, 3548–3562. doi: 10.1016/j.neuroimage.2011.11.023

Zimmerman, B. J., Abraham, I., Schmidt, S. A., Baryshnikov, Y., and Husain, F. T. (2018). Dissociating tinnitus patients from healthy controls using resting-state cyclicity analysis and clustering. *Netw. Neurosci.* 3, 67–89. doi: 10.1162/netn_a_00053

14

Neuroanatomical Alterations in Patients with Tinnitus Before and After Sound Therapy: A Voxel-Based Morphometry Study

Xuan Wei[1], Han Lv[1], Zhaodi Wang[2], Chunli Liu[2], Pengling Ren[1], Peng Zhang[1], Qian Chen[1], Yawen Liu[1], Pengfei Zhao[1], Shusheng Gong[2], Zhenghan Yang[1] and Zhenchang Wang[1]**

[1] *Department of Radiology, Beijing Friendship Hospital, Capital Medical University, Beijing, China,* [2] *Department of Otolaryngology Head and Neck Surgery, Beijing Friendship Hospital, Capital Medical University, Beijing, China*

***Correspondence:**
Han Lv
chrislvhan@126.com
Zhenchang Wang
cjr.wzhch@vip.163.com

According to previous studies, many neuroanatomical alterations have been detected in patients with tinnitus. However, few studies have reported on the morphological changes observed following sound therapy. To explore the brain anatomical alterations in patients with idiopathic tinnitus using voxel-based morphometry (VBM) analysis before and after effective 12 weeks sound therapy. The protocol was registered on ClinicalTrials.gov, ID: NCT02774122. In this study, we collected data from 27 matched healthy control (HC) individuals and 27 idiopathic tinnitus patients before and after 12 weeks of sound therapy by using adjusted narrow band sound. 3.0T MRI system and high-resolution 3D structural images were acquired with a 3D-BRAVO pulse sequence. Structural image data preprocessing was performed using the VBM8 toolbox. The Tinnitus Handicap Inventory (THI) score was acquired in the tinnitus group to assess the severity of tinnitus and tinnitus-related distress. Mann–Whitney *U* Test, Wilcoxon Signed-Ranks test, and Pearson's correlation analysis were used in the statistical analysis. We found significantly decreased gray matter (GM) volume in the left thalami, right thalami, and cochlear nucleus among the tinnitus patients before sound therapy (baseline) compared to the HC group. However, we did not find significant differences in brain regions between the 12-week treatment and HC groups. According to the results of Wilcoxon Signed-Ranks test, the 12-week sound therapy group demonstrated significant greater brain volume compared with the baseline group among these brain regions. Decreased THI score and changed GM volume were not correlated. This is a useful study for observing the characteristics of neuroanatomical changes in patients with idiopathic tinnitus before and after sound treatment. The study characterized the effect of sound therapy on brain volume. It found that sound therapy had a normalizing effect on the bilateral thalami and cochlear nucleus.

Clinical Trial Registration: www.ClinicalTrials.gov, NCT02774122.

Keywords: tinnitus, sound therapy, thalamus, voxel-based morphometry, functional magnetic resonance imaging

INTRODUCTION

Tinnitus is a phantom auditory sensation that reduces quality of life for millions worldwide (Shore et al., 2016), affecting approximately 4 to 15% of the population (Baguley et al., 2013). It has been related to listening to loud music (Axelsson and Prasher, 2000), head and neck injuries, sudden sensorineural hearing loss (Pecorari et al., 2020), ototoxic drug use (Dille et al., 2010), and other medical conditions that can affect hearing. Chronic tinnitus can trigger a range of problems, including cognitive problems, sleep disturbances (Schecklmann et al., 2015), depression (Dobie, 2003), and work disorders (Heller, 2003).

According to previous studies (Han et al., 2015; Lv et al., 2016a,b, 2018), tinnitus has been proven to be a symptom characterized by abnormal resting-state functional magnetic resonance imaging (rs-fMRI) in auditory and non-auditory brain regions (Vanneste and De Ridder, 2012) such as the posterior cingulate cortex (Vanneste et al., 2010), insula (van der Loo et al., 2011), parahippocampal region (Vanneste et al., 2011), and anterior cingulate cortex (De Ridder et al., 2011).

Structural changes in the brain have also been explored in tinnitus patients. Voxel-based morphometry (VBM) can quantitatively detect the volume of brain tissue at the voxel level and reflect the differences in the components and characteristics of brain tissue in local brain regions of different groups or individuals (Ashburner and Friston, 2000). Currently, VBM has been used to describe subtle changes in brain structure in tinnitus patients (Husain et al., 2011; Meyer et al., 2016). Studies of patients with right-sided unilateral pulsatile tinnitus have shown that compared with normal controls, patients with unilateral pulsatile tinnitus have a significantly increased gray matter (GM) volume in the bilateral superior temporal gyrus (STG) and significantly decreased volumes in the left cerebellar posterior lobe, left frontal superior orbital lobe (gyrus rectus), right middle occipital gyrus (MOG), and bilateral putamen (Liu et al., 2018).

Effective treatment for tinnitus requires a basic understanding of the functional and anatomical changes in the brain. A recent study in tinnitus patients treated with rTMS demonstrated the reversibility of structural effects after treatment (Poeppl et al., 2018). Another study analyzed the treatment effect on anatomical changes in the brain (Krick et al., 2015). The patients included were in the early stages of disease, with a disease duration of 5.1 weeks. The GM of the precuneus, medial superior frontal areas, and auditory cortex increased in acute tinnitus patients after the Heidelberg model of music therapy intervention, accompanied by significantly decreased tinnitus-related distress. Narrow band noise sound therapy is a commonly used treatment for tinnitus (Henry et al., 2002). Previous studies have demonstrated functional changes in the brain (Han et al., 2019a,b). However, we only found a few related reports on the morphological changes before and after sound therapy with an average treatment time of 1 week (Krick et al., 2015, 2017).

In this study, we applied VBM to analyze the anatomical changes in the brain in patients before and after sound therapy and to explore the morphological feature alterations after treatment. Based on previous studies on structural and functional plasticity, the bilateral thalami are considered to be a critical brain region that is closely associated with effective treatment of tinnitus. In this study, we hypothesize that the brain regions associated with tinnitus, especially the bilateral thalami, may show volume alterations after sound therapy. This study will help to gain deeper insight into the changes in the brain after treatment from a neuroanatomical perspective.

MATERIALS AND METHODS

Standard Protocol Approvals, Registrations, and Patient Consents

This research involved human participants. All authors have declared that this research was approved by the Institutional Review Board (IRB). Written informed consent was obtained from all subjects enrolled in this study. The protocol was registered on ClinicalTrials.gov, ID: NCT02774122.

Subjects

All patients and healthy volunteers were recruited in our institution. In this study, 27 patients with idiopathic tinnitus were enrolled. The tinnitus sound was described as persistent, high-pitched sound in both of the ears. The inclusion criteria were: (1) 18 to 65 years old; (2) right handedness; (3) tinnitus duration range from 6 to 48 months; (4) no significant hearing loss (hearing thresholds $\geq$ 25 dB HL at frequencies of 0.250, 0.500, 1, 2, 3, 4, 6, and 8 kHz determined by pure tone audiometry [PTA]); (5) willing to receive sound therapy for 12 weeks and return for reexamination after treatment. The exclusion criteria included: (1) other kinds of tinnitus (such as pulsatile tinnitus), Meniere's disease, sudden deafness, otosclerosis; (2) neurological signs and/or a history of neurological disease; (3) current chronic medical illness; (4) a history of head trauma; (5) a cardiovascular, pulmonary, or systemic disease; (6) claustrophobia experienced during MRI simulator session. Twenty-seven age-, gender-, education-, and handedness-matched healthy control (HC) subjects were enrolled as normal controls. None of the HCs suffered from tinnitus in the past year. Other exclusion criteria were the same as previously described. The characteristics of the subjects are presented in **Table 1**.

Sound Therapy and Clinical Evaluation

To characterize the tinnitus and prepare for treatment, all of the enrolled tinnitus patients were examined for tinnitus loudness matching (L = loudness of tinnitus), pitch matching (Tf = tinnitus frequency), minimum masking level, and residual inhibition. Narrow band sound therapy was administered to participants in the tinnitus group for 12 weeks, three times a day for 20 min at a time. For each tinnitus patient, the loudness of sound for treatment was set as L + 5 dB. The frequency was set as a 1 kHz narrow band when setting the Tf as the middle point of the delivered sound (Tf $\pm$ 0.5 kHz; for example, Tf = 4 kHz, low sound cut = 3.5 kHz, high sound cut = 4.5 kHz). Subjects who could not pitch-match their tinnitus were not included.

We also asked the patients to fill out the Tinnitus Handicap Inventory (THI) to assess the severity of tinnitus before and after

TABLE 1 | Demographic and clinical characteristics of participants.

Characteristics	Healthy controls (baseline, n = 27)	Tinnitus patients (baseline, n = 27)	Tinnitus patients (12th week, n = 27)	P value
Age (years, $\bar{x} \pm s$)	46.6 ± 9.9	46.4 ± 12.0		0.92[a]
Years of education	11.8 ± 3.0	11.4 ± 2.5		0.63[a]
Gender (male/female)	12/15	12/15		>0.99[b]
Center Frequencies	NA	4596.2 ± 1492.9	NA	NA
Tinnitus duration (months)	NA	23.4 ± 10.0		NA
THI score	NA	40.0 ± 9.5	19.0 ± 5.2	<0.001[c]
ΔTHI score	NA	21.1 ± 8.3	NA	NA

Data are presented as mean ± SD for all variables except gender. THI: Tinnitus Handicap Inventory. ΔTHI = THIpre–THIpost. NA: not applicable. [a]Two-sample t-tests. [b]Chi-square test. [c]Paired-samples t-tests.

treatment. The primary outcome of this prospective study was based on changes in THI score after treatment. A reduction of at least 16 points in the THI was considered effective treatment (Zeman et al., 2011). The HC group was not given any kind of sound during the research.

Data Acquisition

Images were acquired using a 3.0T GE Signa Excite MR scanner (General Electric Medical Systems, Milwaukee, WI, United States) equipped with an eight-channel, phased-array head coil. All imaging studies were performed at the Medical Imaging Research Center of Beijing Friendship Hospital. Parallel imaging was employed for data acquisition. High-resolution 3D structural images were acquired with a 3D-BRAVO pulse sequence with the following acquisition parameters: TR (repetition time) = 8.8 milliseconds (ms), TE (echo time) = 3.5 ms, TI (inversion time) = 450 ms, field of view (FOV) = 240 × 240 mm, matrix = 256 × 256, and slice thickness = 1 mm without a gap. In total, 196 slices of images were obtained from each subject. We acquired the MRI data of tinnitus patients at baseline and after treatment (week 12). HC individuals only underwent MRI one time.

Data Preprocessing

Image preprocessing was performed with the VBM8 toolbox in the SPM8 software package (Statistical Parametric Mapping, Wellcome Department of Cognitive Neurology, London, United Kingdom) running in MATLAB (MathWorks, Natick, MA, United States). The procedures for image preprocessing have been described in detail in our previous research (Liu et al., 2018). Briefly, image processing in this work included spatial normalization using the Montreal Neurological Institute's (MNI) 152 template and segmentation of the GM, white matter (WM), and cerebrospinal fluid (CSF). Only the GM images were analyzed in this study. Modulation was also applied to avoid volumetric deformation of the GM due to stretching and shrinking effects during the normalization procedure. The modulated GM images were smoothed with a 6 mm full width at half maximum (FWHM) isotropic Gaussian kernel. Finally, the smoothed GM images were resampled to a 3 mm × 3 mm × 3 mm voxel size for the statistical analysis. Subjects with excessive head motion (more than 1.5 mm in translation or 1.5° in rotation) were excluded from the analysis.

Statistical Analysis

Nonparametric test was used in this study. Mann–Whitney U Test and Wilcoxon Signed-Ranks test were used to extract GM volumetric changes in this study. A comparison between treated and untreated patients was performed to examine sound therapy-induced effects on structural changes. A P value of less than 0.05 was considered statistically significant [false discovery rate (FDR) corrected].

To prove our hypothesis, Pearson's correlation analyses were further conducted to investigate the relationship between changed GM volume and the clinical characteristics of tinnitus patients (disease duration at baseline, ΔTHI score [ΔTHI score = THIpre–THIpost]). $P < 0.05$ was set as the threshold to determine significance. The GM volume results were visualized with the REST Slice Viewer and BrainNet Viewer[1] (Xia et al., 2013). Pearson's correlation analysis was performed using SPSS 17 software (SPSS, Inc., Chicago, IL, United States) between the THI scores.

RESULTS

Demographics and Behaviors of Study Participants

In this study, we enrolled 54 subjects, including 27 patients with idiopathic tinnitus. In this group, we applied VBM to analyze anatomical changes in the brain before and after sound therapy. 27 HC individuals were also enrolled. Each group of subjects was age-, sex-, and education-matched (**Table 1**). THI scores were acquired before and after sound therapy. In the data preprocessing step, none of the subjects were excluded according to the head motion criteria. Significant longitudinal decreases in THI scores were observed. The results are summarized in **Table 1**.

Statistical Analysis Results

Significantly decreased GM volume was found in the left and right thalami and cochlear nucleus of the tinnitus patients prior to sound therapy (baseline) compared to participants in the HC group (**Table 2**).

As shown in **Figure 1** and **Table 2**, the statistical analysis demonstrated significant difference in GM volume in the left thalamus, right thalamus, and cochlear nucleus among the

[1]http://www.nitrc.org/projects/bnv/

TABLE 2 | Regions of significant difference with changed GM volumes in the tinnitus patients compared with the HC group according to the voxel-based morphometry analysis.

Brain Region	Number of voxels	Peak MNI (X, Y, Z)	Nonparametric tests/*P* Value		
			G1 vs. G2	G1 vs.G3	G2 vs. G3
L thalamus	44	−22, −20, 8	0.000[a]	0.001[b]	0.897[b]
R thalamus	31	18, −20, 4	0.000[a]	0.001[b]	0.622[b]
Cochlear nucleus	32	−8, −35, −40	0.012[a]	0.001[b]	0.095[b]

($P < 0\ 05$, FDR corrected). G1: Group 1 Tinnitus patients (baseline). G2: Group 2 Tinnitus patients (12th week). G3: Group 3 Healthy control. [a]Wilcoxon Signed-Ranks Test. [b]Mann–Whitney U Test. Number of voxels: The cluster sizes of the three brain regions, e.g., 44 means this cluster has 44 voxels. MNI: Montreal Neurological Institute. Peak MNI: The specific positioning of each brain region on MIN template.

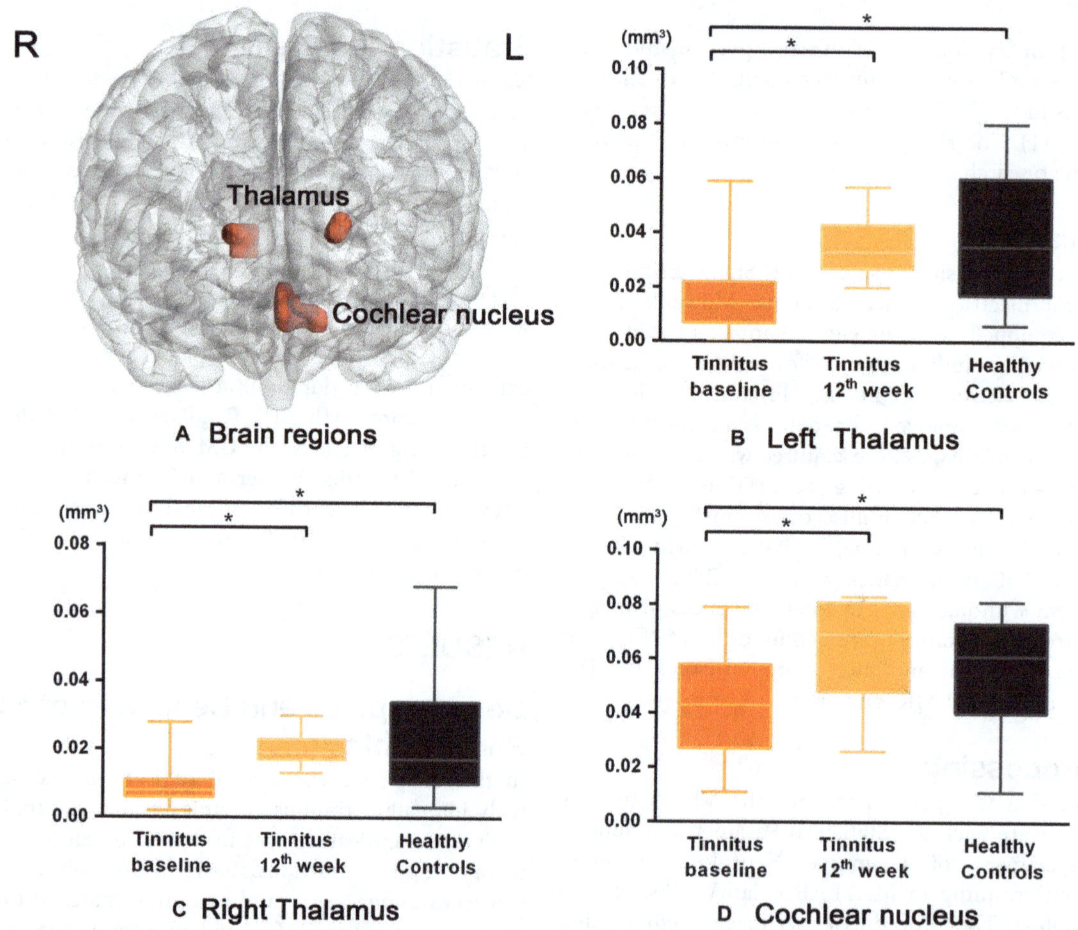

FIGURE 1 | The differences in GM volume among the baseline, after 12 weeks of sound treatment and the healthy control groups (Nonparametric tests; $P < 0.05$, corrected for false discovery rate simulations; L left, R right). **(A)** The bilateral thalamus and cochlear nucleus were the brain regions with statistical differences. Panels **(B–D)** represent the GM volume changes of each brain region in tinnitus baseline after 12 weeks of sound treatment and HC group. Wilcoxon Signed-Ranks test was used to compare tinnitus baseline with after 12 weeks treatment; Mann–Whitney *U* test was used to compare after treatment with normal people, baseline with normal people. **P* < 0.05. The results showed differences in GM volume in the left thalamus, right thalamus, and cochlear nucleus, which are shown in red. L, left; R, right; the labeled number corresponds to the number in **Table 2**. The threshold was set as $P < 0.05$ (corrected). It can be seen that the volume of gray matter increased after 12 weeks treatment compared to baseline and there was no statistically significant difference between the 12 weeks treatment and HC group.

tinnitus before sound therapy (baseline), tinnitus after sound therapy (12 weeks), and HC groups.

Compared with the baseline group, the 12-week sound therapy group demonstrated a significantly higher GM volume in all of the regions mentioned above.

Compared with the HC group, the 12-week sound therapy group demonstrated slightly lower GM volume in the bilateral thalami and slightly higher volume in the cochlear nucleus, but these differences did not reach statistical significance.

Compared with the HC group, the baseline group demonstrated a lower GM volume in the bilateral thalami and cochlear nucleus, and there was a significant difference between the two groups.

The results also showed that in the three brain regions described above, the GM volume was higher after 12 weeks of sound therapy than at baseline (**Table 3**).

Correlation

No correlation results survived the multiple comparison correction.

DISCUSSION

This is a meaningful longitudinal investigation that specifically analyzed the changes in GM volume in the bilateral thalami at baseline and after 12 weeks of sound therapy. Anatomical changes in the brain were found in patients before and after sound therapy, mainly in the left thalamus, right thalamus, and cochlear nucleus. Regarding the morphological and functional changes associated with tinnitus, most previous studies and our recent research have focused on functional aspects, including the use of rest-state and task-state fMRI with 7 Tesla MR (Berlot et al., 2020), while research on the structural aspects has been relatively limited, especially for structural changes after treatment. However, there are structural changes in tinnitus patients (Schecklmann et al., 2013) and these changes will affect structure after treatment, so it is necessary to pay more attention to the structural changes associated with tinnitus patients. Some previous studies have mentioned additional functional issues but fewer structural analyses, so the results of this study are important supplements to original research.

In this study, we found that tinnitus patients had structural changes after treatment. Although these changes may not be as significant as functional changes, the results also reflect the efficacy of sound therapy to a certain extent. One reason may be that many previous studies have focused more on functional changes, including local abnormal activities and abnormal activities of the network, than on structural changes (Han et al., 2019b). A recent study using two resting-state functional connectivity (RSFC) approaches to better understand functional network disturbances associated with tinnitus also found that there were many changes in brain function level in tinnitus patients (Leaver et al., 2016). In addition, in recent research performed before and after 12 weeks of sound therapy in tinnitus patients, our team also found that there were more changes in functional connectivity (Lv et al., 2020). A multimodal neuroimaging meta-analysis investigated the neural substrates of tinnitus by combining information from whole-brain VBM studies of GM volume of and ReHo studies of spontaneous brain activity (Cheng et al., 2020). It reported that increased volume of GM in the bilateral STG, right middle temporal gyrus (MTG), and right supramarginal gyrus and decreased GM volume in the bilateral hypothalamus, left superior frontal gyrus (SFG), and right occipital lobe were observed in tinnitus patients (Boyen et al., 2013). Although fewer structural changes have been found in previous studies, structural changes may not be as obvious as functional changes but still have important clinical significance. These brain regions could represent new neuroanatomical features of patients with tinnitus.

The tinnitus treatment options that have been subjected to randomized controlled trials (RCTs) include pharmacological interventions, sound-based interventions, psychological interventions, magnetic stimulation, electrical stimulation, manual physical therapy, relaxation therapy, complementary and alternative medicine (CAM) therapies, and so on (McFerran et al., 2019). In our study, we applied narrow band noise sound therapy. After choosing a suitable treatment method, it is particularly important to pay attention to the duration of the patient's illness and the time of treatment. These two factors have a great impact on the condition of tinnitus and the relief of the condition. A previous study with the Heidelberg model of music therapy analyzed comparisons of approximately 1 week of treatment and found that there were GM volume changes in the precuneus, medial superior frontal areas, and auditory cortex (Krick et al., 2015). Husain et al. have investigated brain structure in tinnitus patients with a minimally modified version of Mindfulness-Based Cognitive Therapy (MBCT) to treat symptoms of distress associated with tinnitus, which is a cognitive behavior therapy. All participants underwent a complete audiological evaluation during a screening phase and at subsequent pre-intervention (week 0), post-intervention (week 8), and follow-up (week 16) assessments. VBM analysis revealed clusters in bilateral SFG that exhibited significant increases in gray matter volume over the period of intervention and follow-up. Furthermore, gray matter changes in occipital and cingulate regions correlated with declines in tinnitus handicap (Husain et al., 2019). The analysis in our study was performed after 3 months of treatment with narrow band sound therapy, with a longer treatment time and a relatively better treatment effect. Therefore, the morphological changes may be different from those of previous studies, which is supported by our results, although a study reported that the overall evidence for structural abnormalities specifically related to tinnitus is poor at present (Adjamian et al., 2014). Outcomes are divergent and even contradictory across these studies, so we should listen to different opinions, which is conducive to a balanced view of our research.

In this study, it was found that patients with tinnitus had better treatment outcomes, and the brain regions with morphological changes were the bilateral thalami and cochlear nucleus. Our results showed GM volume changes in the bilateral thalami, which also illustrated the importance of the thalamus in tinnitus treatment. Previous research by our team has also found that the thalamus is a very important brain area and it plays a critical role in the perception of tinnitus (Han et al., 2019b). It is also a brain relay area that regulates sensory information flow to and from the auditory cortex (Rauschecker et al., 2010; Leaver et al., 2011). A study reported that thalamic regional expansion may signify dysfunctional auditory gating in the thalamus, where inhibition of tinnitus signals at the level of the thalamus is disrupted due to abnormal changes in the limbic system, ultimately leading to the perception of tinnitus (Tae et al., 2018). This is consistent with the results of this study. In addition to the thalamus, there are also

TABLE 3 | VBM-derived brain regions that are critical to VBM prediction, ranked by their changed in treatment time.

Brain Region	Peck MNI (X, Y, Z)	Volume in patients (baseline, *n* = 27)	Volume in patients (12th week, *n* = 27)	Volume in HC (mm^3)
L thalamus	−22, −20, 8	0.17 (0.08–0.27)	0.39 (0.33–0.51)	0.72 (0.41–0.90)
R thalamus	18, −20, 4	0.10 (0.07–0.13)	0.23 (0.20–0.28)	0.20 (0.12–0.41)
Cochlear nucleus	−8, −35, −40	0.51 (0.32–0.70)	0.83 (0.58–0.97)	0.73 (0.48–0.87)

Data are presented as quartile for all variables. The GM volume after 12 weeks treatment increased compared with the baseline GM volume, which was closer to the normal subjects.

some other important brain regions that affect tinnitus. Although they did not show morphological changes after treatment, they have functional changes and have been found in our previous research. Therefore, the results also show that structure and function do not necessarily change simultaneously, and changes between the two should be analyzed objectively.

The cochlear nucleus is referred to as a single entity but is the first relay station of the brainstem to receive auditory pulses. The cochlear nucleus is divided into the ventral cochlear nucleus (VCN) and the dorsal cochlear nucleus (DCN). The cochlear nerve further divides the ventral nucleus of the cochlea into an anteroventral cochlear nucleus (AVCN) and posteroventral cochlear nucleus (PVCN) (Mishra et al., 2018). These direct synaptic connections from one cochlear nucleus to the other could play a significant role in non-lateralized tinnitus (Levine and Oron, 2015). Our results are mostly concentrated on the left DCN. We will continue to study the role of the cochlear nucleus in tinnitus in the next experiments.

Limitations

There are several limitations in this study. First, the current sample size is small. There was no relationship between changes in GM volume and THI scores in tinnitus patients, which may be due to the small sample size in this study. Further studies should include a larger sample size, such as more than a hundred patients, which would improve the results. Of course, collecting so many subjects for treatment is also a challenge. Second, this study did not include a sham treatment group, so there may be some placebo factors that cannot be completely ruled out. Third, we only used the baseline data of HC group as control group. In the next study, we will also follow up the HCs with the same time point. Fourth, the tinnitus patients included in this study did not have significant hearing loss, which represents only a portion of patients with different types of tinnitus. Fifth, subjects who could not pitch-match their tinnitus were not included. Lastly, although many studies have used VBM to better understand tinnitus, the results may be inconsistent. There is a pressing need to standardize the use of VBM when evaluating tinnitus patients (Scott-Wittenborn et al., 2017). We should pay further attention to tinnitus heterogeneity, which could be expressed in terms of treatment response (Simoes et al., 2019). Research using machine learning may be helpful.

CONCLUSION

This study analyzed the anatomical changes in tinnitus patients before and after treatment for 3 months. The effects of sound therapy includes alterations in brain volume, especially in the bilateral thalami.

ETHICS STATEMENT

This experiment was approved by the Institutional Review Board (IRB) of Beijing Friendship Hospital, Capital Medical University, Beijing, China. Written informed consent was obtained from all subjects enrolled in this study. The protocol was registered on ClinicalTrials.gov, ID: NCT02774122. The patients/participants provided their written informed consent to participate in this study. Written informed consent was obtained from the individual(s) for the publication of any potentially identifiable images or data included in this article.

AUTHOR CONTRIBUTIONS

XW designed the experiments, performed the statistical analysis, and wrote the manuscript. PR and YL conducted the statistical analysis. PZ and PFZ contributed to the manuscript revision. HL, ZW, CL, and QC also collected the data. SG, ZY, and ZCW are guarantors of this work. HL and ZCW are the corresponding authors of this manuscript. They have full access to all the data in the study and take responsibility for the integrity of the data and the accuracy of the data analysis. All authors contributed to the article and approved the submitted version.

ACKNOWLEDGMENTS

We thank Beijing Friendship Hospital, Capital Medical University, for their support with our research. We also thank Dr. Shen Liu, from the Department of Otolaryngology Head and Neck Surgery, Beijing Friendship Hospital, Capital Medical University, for their assistance with the data collection and audiological tests.

REFERENCES

Adjamian, P., Hall, D. A., Palmer, A. R., Allan, T. W., and Langers, D. R. (2014). Neuroanatomical abnormalities in chronic tinnitus in the human brain. *Neurosci. Biobehav. Rev.* 45, 119–133. doi: 10.1016/j.neubiorev.2014.05.013

Ashburner, J., and Friston, K. J. (2000). Voxel-based morphometry–the methods. *Neuroimage* 11(6 Pt 1), 805–821. doi: 10.1006/nimg.2000.0582

Axelsson, A., and Prasher, D. (2000). Tinnitus induced by occupational and leisure noise. *Noise Health* 2, 47–54.

Baguley, D., McFerran, D., and Hall, D. (2013). Tinnitus. *Lancet* 382, 1600–1607. doi: 10.1016/S0140-6736(13)60142-7

Berlot, E., Arts, R., Smit, J., George, E., Gulban, O. F., Moerel, M., et al. (2020). A 7 Tesla fMRI investigation of human tinnitus percept in cortical and subcortical auditory areas. *Neuroimage Clin.* 25, 102166. doi: 10.1016/j.nicl.2020.102166

Boyen, K., Langers, D. R., de Kleine, E., and van Dijk, P. (2013). Gray matter in the brain: differences associated with tinnitus and hearing loss. *Hear. Res.* 295, 67–78. doi: 10.1016/j.heares.2012.02.010

Cheng, S., Xu, G., Zhou, J., Qu, Y., Li, Z., He, Z., et al. (2020). A multimodal meta-analysis of structural and functional changes in the brain of tinnitus. *Front. Hum. Neurosci.* 14:28. doi: 10.3389/fnhum.2020.00028

De Ridder, D., Vanneste, S., and Congedo, M. (2011). The distressed brain: a group blind source separation analysis on tinnitus. *PLoS One* 6:e24273. doi: 10.1371/journal.pone.0024273

Dille, M. F., Konrad-Martin, D., Gallun, F., Helt, W. J., Gordon, J. S., Reavis, K. M., et al. (2010). Tinnitus onset rates from chemotherapeutic agents and ototoxic antibiotics: results of a large prospective study. *J. Am. Acad. Audiol.* 21, 409–417. doi: 10.3766/jaaa.21.6.6

Dobie, R. A. (2003). Depression and tinnitus. *Otolaryngol. Clin. North Am.* 36, 383–388. doi: 10.1016/s0030-6665(02)00168-8

Han, L., Na, Z., Chunli, L., Yuchen, C., Pengfei, Z., Hao, W., et al. (2019a). Baseline functional connectivity features of neural network nodes can predict improvement after sound therapy through adjusted narrow band noise in tinnitus patients. *Front. Neurosci.* 13:614. doi: 10.3389/fnins.2019.00614

Han, L., Yawen, L., Hao, W., Chunli, L., Pengfei, Z., Zhengyu, Z., et al. (2019b). Effects of sound therapy on resting-state functional brain networks in patients with tinnitus: a graph-theoretical-based study. *J. Magn. Reson. Imaging* 50, 1731–1741. doi: 10.1002/jmri.26796

Han, L., Zhaohui, L., Fei, Y., Pengfei, Z., Ting, L., Cheng, D., et al. (2015). Disrupted neural activity in unilateral vascular pulsatile tinnitus patients in the early stage of disease: evidence from resting-state fMRI. *Prog. Neuropsychopharmacol. Biol. Psychiatry* 59, 91–99. doi: 10.1016/j.pnpbp.2015.01.013

Heller, A. J. (2003). Classification and epidemiology of tinnitus. *Otolaryngol. Clin. North Am.* 36, 239–248. doi: 10.1016/s0030-6665(02)00160-3

Henry, J. A., Schechter, M. A., Nagler, S. M., and Fausti, S. A. (2002). Comparison of tinnitus masking and tinnitus retraining therapy. *J. Am. Acad. Audiol.* 13, 559–581.

Husain, F. T., Medina, R. E., Davis, C. W., Szymko-Bennett, Y., Simonyan, K., Pajor, N. M., et al. (2011). Neuroanatomical changes due to hearing loss and chronic tinnitus: a combined VBM and DTI study. *Brain Res.* 1369, 74–88. doi: 10.1016/j.brainres.2010.10.095

Husain, F. T., Zimmerman, B., Tai, Y., Finnegan, M. K., Kay, E., Khan, F., et al. (2019). Assessing mindfulness-based cognitive therapy intervention for tinnitus using behavioural measures and structural MRI: a pilot study. *Int. J. Audiol.* 58, 889–901. doi: 10.1080/14992027.2019.1629655

Krick, C. M., Argstatter, H., Grapp, M., Plinkert, P. K., and Reith, W. (2017). Heidelberg neuro-music therapy enhances task-negative activity in tinnitus patients. *Front. Neurosci.* 11:384. doi: 10.3389/fnins.2017.00384

Krick, C. M., Grapp, M., Daneshvar-Talebi, J., Reith, W., Plinkert, P. K., and Bolay, H. V. (2015). Cortical reorganization in recent-onset tinnitus patients by the heidelberg model of music therapy. *Front. Neurosci.* 9:49. doi: 10.3389/fnins.2015.00049

Leaver, A. M., Renier, L., Chevillet, M. A., Morgan, S., Kim, H. J., and Rauschecker, J. P. (2011). Dysregulation of limbic and auditory networks in tinnitus. *Neuron* 69, 33–43. doi: 10.1016/j.neuron.2010.12.002

Leaver, A. M., Turesky, T. K., Seydell-Greenwald, A., Morgan, S., Kim, H. J., and Rauschecker, J. P. (2016). Intrinsic network activity in tinnitus investigated using functional MRI. *Hum. Brain Mapp.* 37, 2717–2735. doi: 10.1002/hbm.23204

Levine, R. A., and Oron, Y. (2015). Tinnitus. *Handb. Clin. Neurol.* 129, 409–431. doi: 10.1016/B978-0-444-62630-1.00023-8

Liu, Y., Lv, H., Zhao, P., Liu, Z., Chen, W., Gong, S., et al. (2018). Neuroanatomical alterations in patients with early stage of unilateral pulsatile tinnitus: a voxel-based morphometry study. *Neural Plast* 2018:4756471. doi: 10.1155/2018/4756471

Lv, H., Zhao, P., Liu, Z., Li, R., Zhang, L., Wang, P., et al. (2016a). Abnormal resting-state functional connectivity study in unilateral pulsatile tinnitus patients with single etiology: a seed-based functional connectivity study. *Eur. J. Radiol.* 85, 2023–2029. doi: 10.1016/j.ejrad.2016.09.011

Lv, H., Zhao, P., Liu, Z., Wang, G., Zeng, R., Yan, F., et al. (2016b). Frequency-dependent neural activity in patients with unilateral vascular pulsatile tinnitus. *Neural Plast* 2016:4918186. doi: 10.1155/2016/4918186

Lv, H., Zhao, P., Liu, Z., Liu, X., Ding, H., Liu, L., et al. (2018). Lateralization effects on functional connectivity of the auditory network in patients with unilateral pulsatile tinnitus as detected by functional MRI. *Prog. Neuropsychopharmacol. Biol. Psychiatry* 81, 228–235. doi: 10.1016/j.pnpbp.2017.09.020

Lv, H., Liu, C., Wang, Z., Zhao, P., Cheng, X., Yang, Z., et al. (2020). Altered functional connectivity of the thalamus in tinnitus patients is correlated with symptom alleviation after sound therapy. *Brain Imaging Behav.* doi: 10.1007/s11682-019-00218-0 [Epub ahead of print].

McFerran, D. J., Stockdale, D., Holme, R., Large, C. H., and Baguley, D. M. (2019). Why is there no cure for tinnitus? *Front. Neurosci.* 13:802. doi: 10.3389/fnins.2019.00802

Meyer, M., Neff, P., Liem, F., Kleinjung, T., Weidt, S., Langguth, B., et al. (2016). Differential tinnitus-related neuroplastic alterations of cortical thickness and surface area. *Hear. Res.* 342, 1–12. doi: 10.1016/j.heares.2016.08.016

Mishra, S., Roy, T. S., and Wadhwa, S. (2018). Morphological and morphometrical maturation of ventral cochlear nucleus in human foetus. *J. Chem. Neuroanat.* 93, 38–47. doi: 10.1016/j.jchemneu.2017.03.002

Pecorari, G., Riva, G., Bruno, G., Naqe, N., Nardo, M., Albera, A., et al. (2020). Recurrences in sudden sensorineural hearing loss: a long-term observational study. *Am. J. Audiol.* 29, 18–22. doi: 10.1044/2019_AJA-19-00061

Poeppl, T. B., Langguth, B., Lehner, A., Frodl, T., Rupprecht, R., Kreuzer, P. M., et al. (2018). Brain stimulation-induced neuroplasticity underlying therapeutic response in phantom sounds. *Hum. Brain Mapp.* 39, 554–562. doi: 10.1002/hbm.23864

Rauschecker, J. P., Leaver, A. M., and Muhlau, M. (2010). Tuning out the noise: limbic-auditory interactions in tinnitus. *Neuron* 66, 819–826. doi: 10.1016/j.neuron.2010.04.032

Schecklmann, M., Lehner, A., Poeppl, T. B., Kreuzer, P. M., Rupprecht, R., Rackl, J., et al. (2013). Auditory cortex is implicated in tinnitus distress: a voxel-based morphometry study. *Brain Struct. Funct.* 218, 1061–1070. doi: 10.1007/s00429-013-0520-z

Schecklmann, M., Pregler, M., Kreuzer, P. M., Poeppl, T. B., Lehner, A., Cronlein, T., et al. (2015). Psychophysiological associations between chronic tinnitus and sleep: a cross validation of tinnitus and insomnia questionnaires. *Biomed. Res. Int.* 2015:461090. doi: 10.1155/2015/461090

Scott-Wittenborn, N., Karadaghy, O. A., Piccirillo, J. F., and Peelle, J. E. (2017). A methodological assessment of studies that use voxel-based morphometry to study neural changes in tinnitus patients. *Hear Res.* 355, 23–32. doi: 10.1016/j.heares.2017.09.002

Shore, S. E., Roberts, L. E., and Langguth, B. (2016). Maladaptive plasticity in tinnitus–triggers, mechanisms and treatment. *Nat. Rev. Neurol.* 12, 150–160. doi: 10.1038/nrneurol.2016.12

Simoes, J., Neff, P., Schoisswohl, S., Bulla, J., Schecklmann, M., Harrison, S., et al. (2019). Toward personalized tinnitus treatment: an exploratory study based on internet crowdsensing. *Front. Public Health* 7:157. doi: 10.3389/fpubh.2019.00157

Tae, W. S., Yakunina, N., Lee, W. H., Ryu, Y. J., Ham, H. K., Pyun, S. B., et al. (2018). Changes in the regional shape and volume of subcortical nuclei in patients with tinnitus comorbid with mild hearing loss. *Neuroradiology* 60, 1203–1211. doi: 10.1007/s00234-018-2093-2

van der Loo, E., Congedo, M., Vanneste, S., Van De Heyning, P., and De Ridder, D. (2011). Insular lateralization in tinnitus distress. *Auton. Neurosci.* 165, 191–194. doi: 10.1016/j.autneu.2011.06.007

Vanneste, S., and De Ridder, D. (2012). The auditory and non-auditory brain areas involved in tinnitus. An emergent property of multiple parallel overlapping subnetworks. *Front. Syst. Neurosci.* 6:31. doi: 10.3389/fnsys.2012.00031

Vanneste, S., Heyning, P. V., and Ridder, D. D. (2011). Contralateral parahippocampal gamma-band activity determines noise-like tinnitus laterality: a region of interest analysis. *Neuroscience* 199, 481–490. doi: 10.1016/j.neuroscience.2011.07.067

Vanneste, S., Plazier, M., der Loo, E., de Heyning, P. V., Congedo, M., and De Ridder, D. (2010). The neural correlates of tinnitus-related distress. *Neuroimage* 52, 470–480. doi: 10.1016/j.neuroimage.2010.04.029

Xia, M., Wang, J., and He, Y. (2013). BrainNet viewer: a network visualization tool for human brain connectomics. *PLoS One* 8:e68910. doi: 10.1371/journal.pone.0068910

Zeman, F., Koller, M., Figueiredo, R., Aazevedo, A., Rates, M., Coelho, C., et al. (2011). Tinnitus handicap inventory for evaluating treatment effects: which changes are clinically relevant? *Otolaryngol. Head Neck Surg.* 145, 282–287. doi: 10.1177/0194599811403882

15

Abnormal Spontaneous Neural Activity of the Central Auditory System Changes the Functional Connectivity in the Tinnitus Brain: A Resting-State Functional MRI Study

Wei-Wei Cai[1,2†], Zhi-cheng Li[3†], Qin-tai Yang[3*] and Tao Zhang[1*]

[1] Department of Otolaryngology–Head and Neck Surgery, The First Affiliated Hospital of Jinan University, Guangzhou, China, [2] Department of Otolaryngology–Head and Neck Surgery, Panyu Central Hospital, Guangzhou, China, [3] Department of Otolaryngology–Head and Neck Surgery, The Third Affiliated Hospital, Sun Yat-sen University, Guangzhou, China

***Correspondence:**
Qin-tai Yang
yang.qt@163.com
Tao Zhang
tzhangt@jnu.edu.cn

† These authors have contributed equally to this work

Objective: An abnormal state of the central auditory system (CAS) likely plays a large role in the occurrence of phantom sound of tinnitus. Various tinnitus studies using resting-state functional MRI (RS-fMRI) have reported aberrant spontaneous brain activity in the non-auditory system and altered functional connectivity between the CAS and non-auditory system. This study aimed to investigate abnormal functional connections between the aberrant spontaneous activity in the CAS and the whole brain in tinnitus patients, compared to healthy controls (HC) using RS-fMRI.

Materials and Methods: RS-fMRI from 16 right-ear tinnitus patients with normal hearing (TNHs) and 15 HC individuals was collected, and the time series were extracted from different clusters of a CAS template, supplied by the Anatomy Toolbox of the Statistical Parametric Mapping software. These data were used to derive the smoothed mean amplitude of low-frequency fluctuation (smALFF) values and calculate the relationship between such values and the corresponding clinical data. In addition, clusters in the CAS identified by the smALFF maps were set as seed regions for calculating and comparing the brain-wide connectivity between TNH and HC.

Results: We identified the different clusters located in the left higher auditory cortex (HAC) and the right inferior colliculus (IC) from the smALFF maps that contained increased (HAC) and decreased (IC) activity when the TNH group was compared to the HC group, respectively. The value of increased smALFF cluster in the HAC was positively correlated with the tinnitus score, but the decreased smALFF cluster in the IC was not correlated with any clinical characters of tinnitus. The TNH group displayed increased connectivity, compared to the HC group, in brain regions that encompassed the left IC, bilateral Heschl gyrus, bilateral supplementary motor area, right insula, bilateral superior temporal gyrus, right middle temporal gyrus, left hippocampus, left amygdala, and right supramarginal gyrus.

Conclusion: Tinnitus may be linked to abnormal spontaneous activity in the HAC, which can arise from the neural plasticity induced from the increased functional connectivity between the auditory network, cerebellum, and limbic system.

Keywords: tinnitus, resting-state functional magnetic resonance imaging, amplitude of low-frequency fluctuation, auditory cortex, auditory pathway, spontaneous neural synchrony

INTRODUCTION

Tinnitus is commonly defined as the perception of sound in the absence of an external auditory source and has a prevalence ranging from 10 to 15% in the adult population (Xu et al., 2011; Heller, 2003). Many patients with tinnitus have reported symptoms that can significantly impair patients' quality of life (Langguth, 2011), such as frustration, annoyance, irritability, anxiety, depression, hearing difficulties, hyperacusis, insomnia, and concentration difficulties.

Most tinnitus accompanies obvious hearing loss, but some patients without hearing loss can also experience severe tinnitus (Savastano, 2008; Martines et al., 2010). Evidence from studies using animal models of tinnitus indicates that long-term exposure to non-traumatic noise can (Munguia et al., 2013; Lau et al., 2015; Takacs et al., 2017) induce dysfunctional brainstem projections from the cochlea that can trigger the development of abnormal neuronal baseline activity in the several levels of central auditory system (CAS).

NeuroImage techniques applying to tinnitus human studies include testing abnormally elevated spontaneous activity, investigations of brain structure, and exploring corresponding changes in non-auditory system (NAS) following tinnitus perception (Landgrebe et al., 2009; Chen et al., 2014; Geven et al., 2014; Seydell-Greenwald et al., 2014). Tinnitus is the perception of phantom sound in the absence of physical signal and is no task-based modulation of the tinnitus signal. For these reasons, tinnitus may be uniquely suited to studies using resting-state functional MRI (RS-fMRI).

Functional brain regions such as motor cortices (Biswal et al., 1995), visual cortices (Kiviniemi et al., 2004), auditory cortices (Cordes et al., 2001), and default mode network (Fox et al., 2005) that have been identified using stimulus- or task-evoked paradigms can also be identified in the resting state by examining low-frequency (0.01–0.08 Hz) fluctuations (LFFs) of the resting-state blood oxygen level dependent (BOLD) signal. These results imply that the LFFs infer neuronal activation indirectly through neurovascular coupling (Lu et al., 2007; Mantini et al., 2007; Shmuel and Leopold, 2008; Rusiniak et al., 2015; Shtark et al., 2015). These networks generally show reliable and consistent patterns of functional connectivity (FC) (Zhang et al., 2008), which is defined as the quantification of the operational interactions of multiple spatially distinct brain regions that are highly synchronous (Rogers et al., 2007). The effects of tinnitus on resting-state FC have recently been reported by using RS-fMRI and have variable results for experimental and analytical methods, partly due to heterogeneity of tinnitus subjects (Burton et al., 2012; Kim et al., 2012; Maudoux et al., 2012a,b; Wineland et al., 2012; Davies et al., 2014). These studies obtained the modulated correlation between the auditory resting-state network and the following networks: default mode, limbic, dorsal attention, and visual networks to explain the mechanism of tinnitus accompany symptoms.

The amplitude of LFFs (ALFFs), an alternative index to LFF, has been suggested as a measure of regional spontaneous neuronal activity and has been validated using a comparison between ALFF and PET imaging (Zang et al., 2007; Yuan et al., 2018). The ALFF metric has previously been used to measure intrinsic regional neural activity at the baseline state of neurological or psychiatric disorder such as attention deficit hyperactivity disorder, Parkinson disease, and depression (Rogers et al., 2007; Zang et al., 2007; Zhang et al., 2008; Skidmore et al., 2013; Huang et al., 2017; Lei et al., 2017; Li et al., 2017). In a recent tinnitus study, the ALFF has been used to reveal abnormal spontaneous neural activity in tinnitus patients (Chen et al., 2014; Lv et al., 2016) and found that aberrant ALFF brain regions (right middle temporal gyrus) in the NAS are associated with clinical tinnitus characteristics (Chen et al., 2014). However, changes in the regional spontaneous neural activity of the CAS are thought to be the first stage of sound perception in tinnitus. In fact, these changes may be the driving factor for aberrant global FC, which can induce the various disease symptoms except for phantom sound. Therefore, the mechanism of altered FC of tinnitus needs to be explored further to understand the relationship between the abnormal neural activity within the CAS and the NAS regions.

Previous RS-fMRI studies have explored aberrant FC between the CAS and the NAS to interpret various clinical dysfunctions such as anxiety and depression, which often accompany tinnitus (Burton et al., 2012; Maudoux et al., 2012a,b; Wineland et al., 2012; Davies et al., 2014). The CAS in some of these studies was isolated from the rest of the brain using independent component analyses to explore the relationship between the whole CAS and NAS (Kim et al., 2012; Maudoux et al., 2012b; Davies et al., 2014). Other studies identified the auditory cortex based on a human brain atlas and used such regions as seeds to assess abnormal FC across the whole brain (Burton et al., 2012; Wineland et al., 2012). These methods selected the whole CAS or primary auditory cortex (PAC) regardless of its active vs. inactive regions caused by tinnitus perception. While proven to be useful, the assumptions of these techniques in the processing pipeline might lead to some inaccuracies in the resulting connectivity measures and the subsequent clinical implications.

Base on prior work and theoretical consideration, we try to improve the consistency of tinnitus subjects including several factors such as unilateral tinnitus ear, the possible causes of tinnitus, and handedness to make the differences prominent between groups. The present study attempted to assess abnormal activity of the tinnitus brain and the functional connections thereof using active clusters within the CAS that were identified through a data-driven approach utilizing the ALFF metric. We hypothesized that tinnitus patients exhibit abnormal FC between various clusters of the CAS and the remainder of the brain.

MATERIALS AND METHODS

Subject Demographics

This study utilized data from two groups of subjects, tinnitus patients with normal hearing (TNHs) and healthy controls (HCs), who were recruited from various sources. The TNH group was composed of subjects recruited from outpatient clinics at The Otorhinolaryngology Department of Guangzhou Panyu Central Hospital, The First Affiliated Hospital of Jinan University, and The Third Affiliated Hospital, Sun Yat-sen University, Guangzhou, Guangdong, China, from March 2015 to May 2018. The HC group was matched in age, sex, and education to the TNH group. The TNH group comprised 16 right-handed patients between the ages of 18 and 55 years with self-reported right-ear tinnitus lasting >6 months. All tinnitus patients have occupational noise exposure or have experienced environmental noise exposure. The HC group contained 15 subjects who were recruited from the staff of Jinan University. All individuals provided written informed consent before participation in this study. This study was approved by the Research Ethics Committee of Guangzhou Panyu Central Hospital and the First Affiliated Hospital of Jinan University, Guangzhou.

Pure-tone audiometry was performed with a clinical audiometer using eight octave frequencies (0.125, 0.25, 0.5, 1, 2, 3, 4, and 8 kHz) in both the TNH and HC groups to determine audio thresholds. The audio thresholds of the TNH patients and HC are shown in **Figure 1** and **Table 1**. The severity of tinnitus was assessed by a Chinese translation of the Tinnitus Handicap Inventory (THI), a self-reported tinnitus handicap questionnaire (Meng et al., 2012). All subjects were confirmed to have a Self-Rating Depression Scale (SDS) score of <50 and a Self-Rating Anxiety Scale score of <50 (Zung, 1971, 1986).

We excluded subjects who exhibited any of the following criteria: Mènière disease; conductive deafness; alternative hearing level; cognitive or mental disorders; serious systemic diseases, such as heart failure or diabetes; epilepsy; alcoholism or use of psychiatric drugs; pregnancy; acoustic neuroma, brain stem, or inferior colliculi diseases; hyperacousia; smoking; and history of stroke, brain injury, Alzheimer's disease, or Parkinson's disease. **Table 2** summarizes the characteristics of the TNH and HC subjects in this study.

MRI Data Acquisition

Resting-state BOLD fMRI data were acquired with a 3.0 T MR scanner (MR750, GE Health Care System, United States) in the Imaging Center of the First Affiliated Hospital of Jinan University. Before the MRI, all subjects laid in the supine position on the examination bed with noise-cancelling headphones and earplugs (Mack's noise reduction ear plugs, United States) to reduce the noise level by 32 dB. To reduce head motion, a foam pad was fixed around the subjects' head for the duration of the scan. All subjects were asked to remain relaxed with their eyes closed and to avoid serious thought for approximately 20 min. In order to avoid the influence of acoustic noise produced during the MRI procedure on brain activity, the BOLD images were acquired using an echo planar-imaging sequence with the following parameters: repetition time (TR) = 2000 ms, echo time (TE) = 30 ms, slice thickness = 3 mm, flip angle = 90°, field of view = 200 × 200 mm, acquisition matrix = 64 × 64 mm, and the number of time points (volumes) = 160. Anatomical images were acquired using a 3D-fast spoiled gradient echo sequence with the following parameters: TR = 7.63 ms, TE = 3.74 ms, slice thickness = 1 mm, flip angle = 8°, field of view = 256 × 256 mm, and acquisition matrix = 256 × 256 mm. The MRI images included the whole brain.

Data Processing

All fMRI data were processed using the DPAESF (Data Processing Assistant for Resting-state fMRI) toolbox (Chao-Gan and Yu-Feng, 2010), which is embedded in the DPABI (Data Processing and Analysis for Brain Imaging) V4.3 toolbox (Yan et al., 2016), and based on Statistical Parametric Mapping SPM[1]. First, the initial 10 volumes were discarded, and slice-timing correction was performed, with all volume slices being corrected for different signal acquisition time by shifting the signal measured in each slice relative to the acquisition of the slice at the mid-point of each TR. Then, the time series of images for each subject were realigned using a six-parameter (rigid body) linear transformation with a two-pass procedure (registered to the first image and then registered to the mean of the images after the first re-alignment). After realignment, individual T1-weighted map were co-registered to the mean functional image using a 6 degree-of-freedom linear transformation without re-sampling and then segmented into gray matter, white matter, and cerebrospinal fluid (Ashburner and Friston, 2005). Finally, the transformations from individual native space to Montreal Neurological Institute (MNI) space were computed with the Diffeomorphic Anatomical Registration Through Exponentiated Lie algebra (DARTEL) tool (Ashburner, 2007). To control for head motion confounds, we utilized the Friston 24-parameter model (Friston et al., 1996) to regress out head motion effects. The Friston 24-parameter model (i.e., 6 head motion parameters, 6 head motion parameters one time point before, and the 12 corresponding squared items) was chosen based on prior work that higher-order models remove head motion effects better (Yan et al., 2013). In addition, mean FD was used to address the residual effects of motion in group analyses. Mean FD is derived from Jenkinson's relative root mean square algorithm. We used the threshold (mean FD Jenkinson, <0.2 mm) to

[1] http://www.fil.ion.ucl.ac.uk/spm

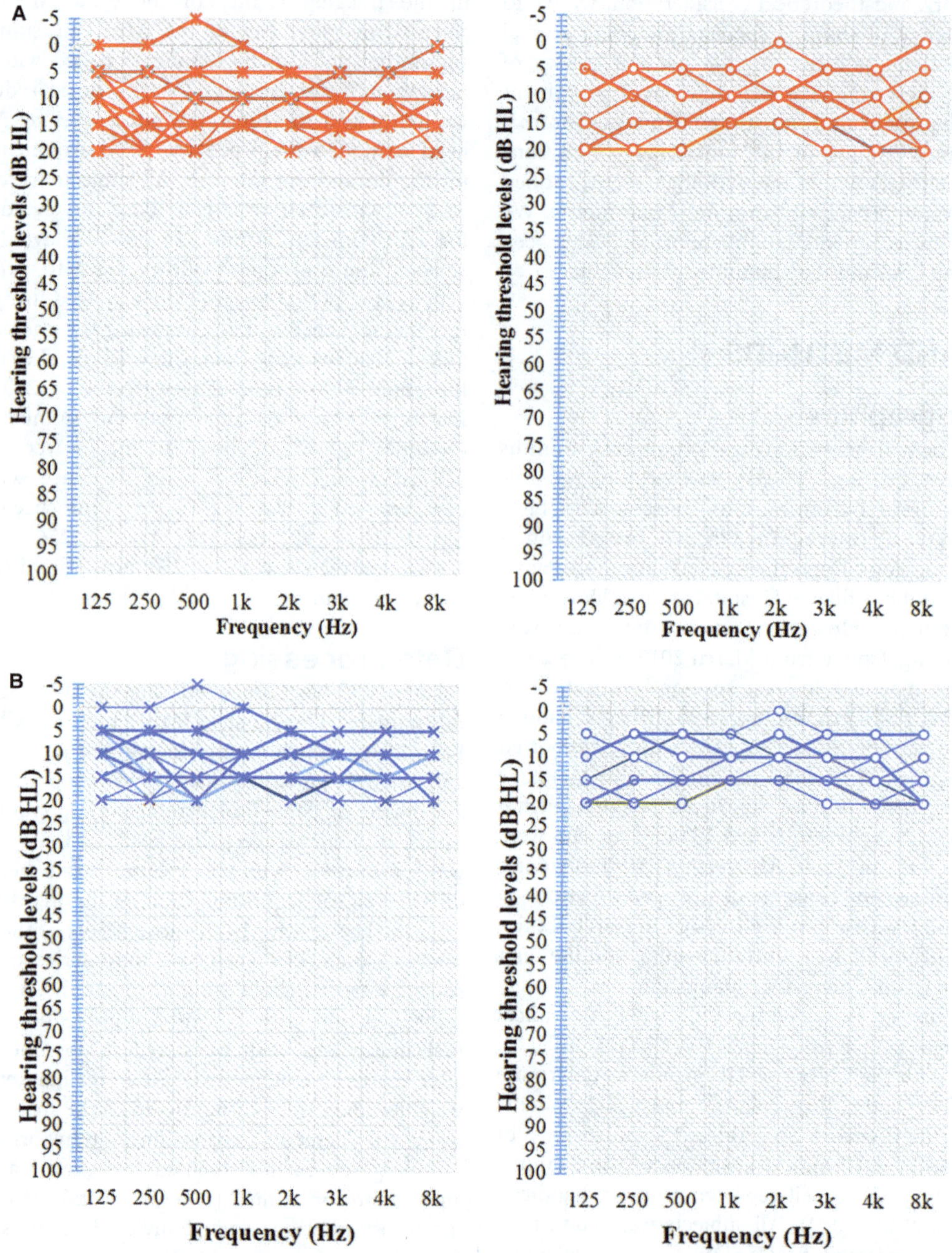

FIGURE 1 | Characteristic hearing levels of the groups. **(A)** TNH group hearing threshold (n = 16). **(B)** HC group hearing threshold (n = 15). X, left ear air conduction; O, right ear air conduction; TNH, tinnitus patients with normal hearing; HC, healthy controls. Red, hearing threshold audiogram of TNH; Blue, hearing threshold audiogram of HC.

exclude the subjects, which followed the research about the impact of head motion on RS-fMRI (Jenkinson et al., 2002). The mean FD_Jenkinson values of subjects in this study were max = 0.13, min = 0.03, and mean = 0.05 SD. None of the subjects were excluded. Global signal regression and sources of spurious variance (white matter and cerebrospinal fluid signals) were also removed from the data through linear regression to reduce respiratory and cardiac effects. In addition, linear trends were included as a regressor to account for drifts in the BOLD signal. We performed temporal filtering (0.01–0.1 Hz) on all time series except for ALFF. The ALFF results were then standardized by global mean to generate mALFF maps. Then, mALFF maps were smoothed with a Gaussian kernel [FWHM = (8 × 8 × 8) mm] to generate smoothed mean amplitude of low-frequency fluctuation (smALFF) maps. A larger smoothing kernel (8 mm) was used in this work as it has been shown to improve the reproducibility of results and more likely reflects the true effect for group comparison (Mikl et al., 2008).

TABLE 1 | Characteristic hearing levels of the participants.

	125 Hz	250 Hz	500 Hz	1 kHz	2 kHz	3 kHz	4 kHz	8 kHz
TNH (right ear, n = 16)	15.00 ± 5.477	13.75 ± 5.916	13.44 ± 5.692	11.25 ± 3.416	10.31 ± 4.270	12.50 ± 4.082	13.44 ± 4.732	14.06 ± 5.836
HC (right ear, n = 15)	15.00 ± 5.669	14.00 ± 6.036	13.33 ± 5.876	12.00 ± 3.519	10.33 ± 4.419	12.67 ± 4.169	13.67 ± 4.806	14.33 ± 5.300
P-value (df = 29)	1.000	0.908	0.960	0.947	0.989	0.911	0.895	0.894
TNH (left ear, n = 16)	10.63 ± 5.737	11.25 ± 6.191	11.56 ± 5.876	10.63 ± 5.123	10.31 ± 4.990	11.94 ± 4.090	12.19 ± 4.820	11.88 ± 5.737
HC (left ear, n = 15)	10.33 ± 5.815	11.33 ± 6.399	12.00 ± 7.270	11.00 ± 5.071	10.67 ± 4.952	12.07 ± 4.200	12.33 ± 4.952	12.00 ± 5.278
± P-value (df = 29)	0.889	0.971	0.868	0.839	0.844	0.931	0.934	0.950

TNH, tinnitus patients with normal hearing; HC, healthy controls. The auditory threshold data of TNH and HC are represented as mean ± SD.

CAS Template Setting

In order to identify the different CAS active clusters between the TNH and HC groups, the SPM anatomy toolbox v1.8[2] was used to create a template composed of the PAC and the combination of areas Te 1.0, Te1.1 (Brodmann area 41), Te1.2 (Brodmann area 42) the higher auditory cortex (HAC), and area Te3.0 (part of Brodmann area 22 and Brodmann area 42) (Morosan et al., 2001, 2005). The auditory pathway template was based on regions of interest (ROIs) reported by Muhlau et al. (2006). The ROIs are shown in **Figure 2** and were defined as the dorsal cochlear nuclei (sphere radius: 5 mm; MNI coordinates, ± 10, −38, −45), superior olivary complex (sphere radius: 5 mm; MNI coordinates, ±13, −35, −41), inferior colliculus (IC; sphere radius: 5 mm; MNI coordinates, ±6, −33, −11), and medial geniculate nucleus (sphere radius: 8 mm; MNI coordinates, ±17, −24, −2) (Muhlau et al., 2006). The SPM Marsbar toolbox was employed for ROI analysis of the HAC, PAC, and auditory pathway using the CAS template (Brett et al., 2002; **Figure 2**).

Statistical Analysis

The statistical analysis tool embedded within DPABI was used to calculate the difference between the THN and HC groups using two-sample t-tests. A permutation test was used to correct for multiple comparisons (Winkler et al., 2016), which offered the optimal balance between the family-wise error rate and test-retest reliability (Chen et al., 2018). The permutation test was two-tailed and performed with a threshold controlling family-wise error rate at $p < 0.05$ level, 5000 permutations, and no acceleration.

Comparing the smALLF maps of the TNH with HC groups within the CAS template was performed using two-sample t-tests, and the gray matter images of the TNH and HC groups were added as a covariate. To investigate the relationship between the neural activity and the clinical data of tinnitus patients, we extracted smALFF values from different clusters in smALFF maps of the TNH group and computed the Pearson's correlation coefficient with each clinical characteristic available (**Table 2**).

The different clusters of smALFF were defined as seeds to explore the different FC patterns (comparing TNH and HC); the time series of the seed voxels were used to calculate the Person correlation coefficient across the whole brain, which was defined by Whole-Brain-template of SPM8, and Whole-brain-template covers the CAS template. The FC maps using different smALLF clusters as seed regions were compared between the TNH and HC groups using two-sample t-tests.

In order to analyze the asymmetries of tinnitus brain in CAS, smALFF values of the left/right PAC and HAC were extracted from smALFF maps of all subjects to compare differences between the left and right auditory cortex in group and calculated the left/right smALFF ratio to compare difference between groups. An independent samples t-test examines the statistic differences in group and between groups. Statistical analysis was carried out using SPSS 18.0 package for Windows.

[2]www.fz-juelich.de/inm/inm-1/DE/Forschung/_docs/SPMAnatomy-Toolbox/SPMAnatomyToolbox_node.htm

TABLE 2 | Clinical characteristics of study subjects.

	TNH	HC	P-value
Gender (male/female)	6/10	5/10	0.689
Age (years)	35.33 ± 10.70	35.00 ± 10.10	0.720
Education (years)	13.50 ± 1.57	13.25 ± 1.75	0.698
SDS score	34.67 ± 7.30	35.25 ± 6.33	0.274
SAS score	35.67 ± 9.37	37.65 ± 7.23	0.240
THI score	55.33 ± 11.03	\	\
Tinnitus duration (months)	36.58 ± 18.03	\	\
Frequency range of tinnitus	5–8 kHz	\	\

SDS, Self-Rating Depression Scale; SAS, Self-Rating Anxiety Scale; THI, Tinnitus Handicap Inventory.

RESULTS

Comparison of smALFF in the CAS Between Groups

Analyses using two-sample t-tests revealed clusters with significantly different smALFF values between the TNH and HC groups. A significantly increased smALFF cluster was found in the left HAC, and a significantly decreased smALFF cluster was found in the right IC (**Figure 3**). The cluster in the HAC was 142 voxels large, and had a peak intensity of t score = 7.55 and an MNI location of peak intensity of (−57, −6, −9). The peak intensity of the active cluster was located in the left middle temporal gyrus (Automated Anatomical Labeling atlas) or Brodmann area 22.

In the TNH group, the average smALFF value of the different cluster of left HAC cluster was correlated with various clinical

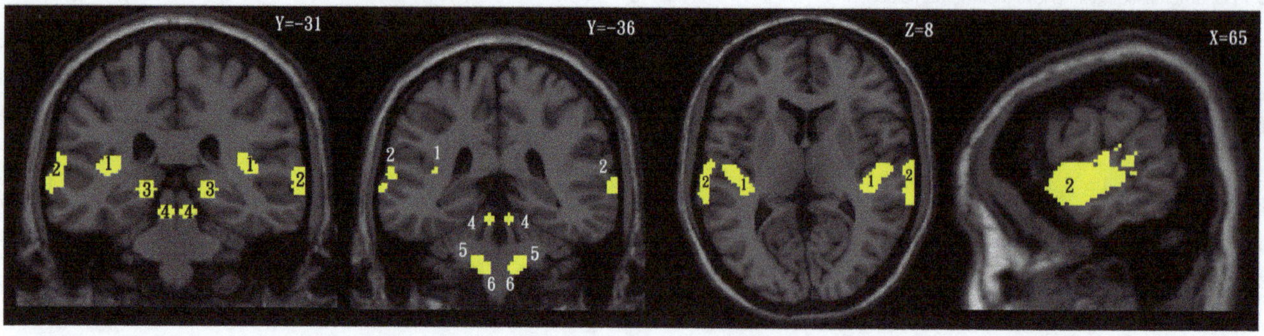

FIGURE 2 | Template of the central auditory system in the coronal (left), axial (middle), and sagittal (right) planes. 1 = primary auditory cortex, 2 = higher auditory cortex, 3 = medial geniculate nucleus, 4 = inferior colliculus, 5 = superior olivary complex, 6 = cochlear nuclei.

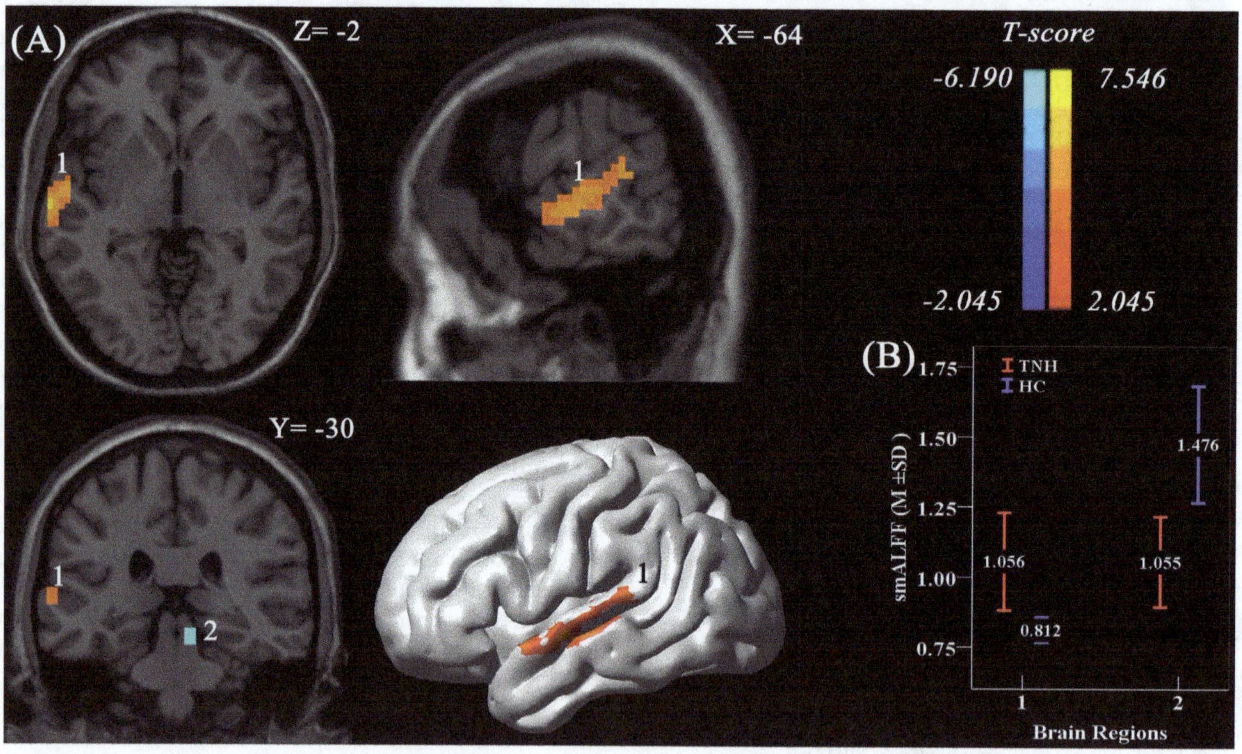

FIGURE 3 | Significant smoothed mean amplitude of low-frequency fluctuation (smALFF) differences in tinnitus patients without hearing loss, compared to healthy controls. **(A)** The differences maps at slices $Z = -2$, $X = -64$, $Y = -3{,}0$ and a 3D rendering of the left-lateral view of the brain. The permutation test was two-tailed and performed with a threshold controlling family-wise error rate at $p < 0.05$ level, 5000 permutations, and no acceleration. Blue indicates that TNH subjects had decreased smALFF compared to the HC, and the yellow indicates the opposite. Number 1 indicates that the cluster of increased smALFF value located in the left higher auditory cortex (HAC; T value's peak score: 7.55; MNI: −57, −6, −9; cluster size: 142 voxels), and number 2 indicates the cluster of decreased smALFF value located in the right inferior colliculus (T value's peak score: −6.19; MNI: 9, −30, −15; cluster size: 16 voxels). **(B)** The smoothed mean and SD of standardized ALFF at the peak voxels.

metrics, including the Duration of Tinnitus-Months (DTM) ($P < 0.01$), THI ($P < 0.01$), and SDS ($P < 0.01$) (**Figure 4**).

Brain-Wide Functional Connectivity With the CAS

When using the left HAC active cluster as the seed region for investigating brain-wide FC, we found differences in this global connectome between the TNH with HC groups (**Figure 5**). The TNH group revealed significantly increased FC between the HAC and the bilateral supplementary motor area, bilateral insula, bilateral superior temporal gyrus (STG), bilateral Heschl, left hippocampus, left amygdala, left IC, left rolandic operculum, left cerebellum (lobule 8), and right cerebellum (lobules 4, 5) (see **Figure 5** and **Table 3**). We found no regions that displayed a significant decrease in FC in the TNH group compared to

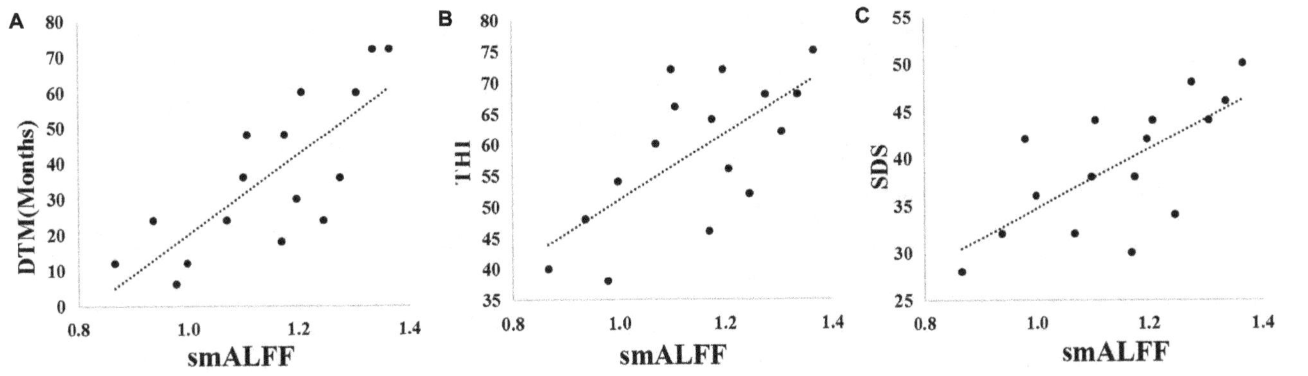

FIGURE 4 | Pearson correlations between clinical parameters [Duration of Tinnitus-Months (DTM), Tinnitus Handicap Inventory (THI) score, Self-Rating Depression Scale (SDS) score, and Self-Rating Anxiety Scale (SAS) score] and the smALFF values of the active cluster in the left HAC. **(A)** DTM-smALFF: $r = 0.778$, $p = 0.000$. **(B)** THI-smALFF: $r = 0.682$, $p = 0.004$. **(C)** SDS-smALFF: $r = 0.694$, $p = 0.003$.

the HC group. When using the right IC cluster as the seed, no active clusters survived the FC comparison between the TNH and HC groups.

Asymmetric Analysis of Auditory Cortex With smALFF in Group and Between Groups

Table 4 shows the characters of value smALFF extraction from bilaterality PAC and HAC, respectively. An independent samples *t*-test examines the statistic differences in group and between groups. Statistical analysis was carried out using SPSS 18.0 package for Windows. The asymmetric analysis results were as follows: (1) the HC group shows a higher smALFF value on the left PAC ($P = 0.048$) and right HAC ($P = 0.001$); (2) the TNH group shows no significant difference between the bilateral auditory cortex; and (3) when the asymmetry ratio (left/right auditory cortex's smALFF value) between TNH and HC was compared, there is no significant difference between TNH and HC: P (HAC) = 0.059 and P (PAC) = 0.993.

DISCUSSION

In the present study, we hypothesized that tinnitus may be the result of alterations in the spontaneous activity of the brain, and that changes in resting state CAS activity cause aberrant brain-wide FC that leads to the stress of tinnitus through plastic changes of neural behavior.

To improve the consistency of tinnitus group for making different activity in brain prominent between groups, it have been concerned several influenced factors including unilateral tinnitus, hearing level of tinnitus ear, right handedness, and the cause of tinnitus for the following reasons. (1) right ear tinnitus might have a different THI score when compared with left ear tinnitus, with the right ear having an advantage for speech sounds, and peripheral and cognitive interaction (Tai and Husain, 2018); (2) unilateral tinnitus and right handedness might help in increasing a significant difference in spontaneous activity in the tinnitus brains for the possible link between tinnitus and hemisphere dominance (Reiss and Reiss, 2001); (3) the unified cause of tinnitus may have similar mechanism. The non-traumatic noise-induced tinnitus has been found regional spontaneous neural activity in the auditory cortex and pathway (Schaette and McAlpine, 2011; Munguia et al., 2013).

In CAS, we found that smALFF maps of TNH showed hyperactivity in the left HAC (BA22) and reduced activity in the right IC (**Figure 3**) when compared with HC.

It is not sure if the increasing smALFF cluster of HAC might reflect the abnormal asymmetry or regional spontaneous neural activity of the auditory cortex caused by tinnitus. We analyzed the asymmetry of every subject with smALFF value extracted from the PAC and HAC. We found that the asymmetric feature is present in HC but not in TNH, and there is no significantly different asymmetric ratio between TNH and HC (**Table 4**). Geven et al. have a similar finding on asymmetric feature in the tinnitus and control groups (Geven et al., 2014). In previous tinnitus studies on baseline activity measurements using PET, Arnold et al. (1996) found that the left PAC had significantly more asymmetric activity in tinnitus patients and the control group also showed the same asymmetric character, which was similar to our HC group. However, the prevalence of hearing loss among the tinnitus patients in the studies makes it unclear whether the asymmetry in the left PAC reflects the abnormally spontaneous neural activity of the PAC. In a further PET study, Langguth et al. suggested that the asymmetry auditory cortical activity of tinnitus may not imply cortical hyperactivity and also have no correlation with tinnitus severity (Langguth et al., 2006). In our study, the mALFF values of the active cluster in the left HAC was found to be significantly correlated with clinical characteristics of tinnitus such as DTM, THI, and SDS (**Figure 4**). These results suggest that the activity cluster in the left HAC (BA22) might be involved in the changing baseline neural activity following tinnitus. Remarkably, the increased smALFF cluster was located in the left MTG (BA22) of TNH, the brain region links to the recognition of language and the selective attention to sound in human beings (Rinne et al., 2008).

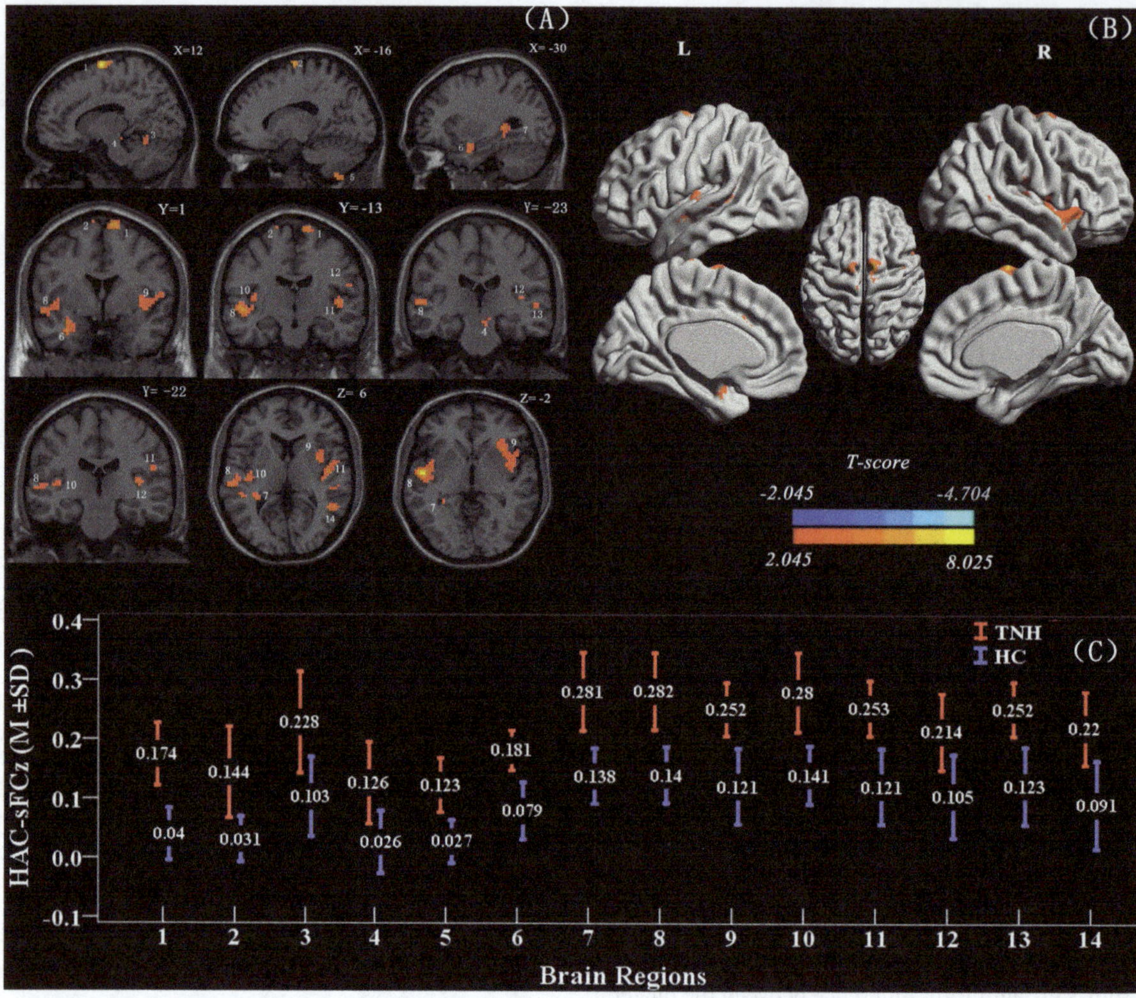

FIGURE 5 | Clusters displaying a significant difference in functional connectivity (FC) (smoothed-Z-transfer maps) between the TNH and HC groups. Results are presented as slices **(A)** and a 3D rendering **(B)**. The HAC cluster from **Figure 3** was used as the seed region to explore the functional connectivity across the whole brain. The permutation test was two-tailed and performed with a threshold controlling family-wise error rate at $p < 0.05$ level, 5000 permutations, and no acceleration. Blue indicates that TNH subjects had decreased smoothed-Z-transfer FC compared to the HC, and the yellow indicates the opposite. **(C)** The smoothed-Z transformed standardized functional connectivity at the peak voxels. Numbers (1–14) indicate the different clusters; see **Table 3** for the corresponding brain areas and the cluster characteristics.

Clinical therapy experience of tinnitus also had some pieces of evidence to support that the neural activity of HAC has a correlation with tinnitus severity. De Ridder et al. (2011) suggested that transcranial magnetic stimulation and extradural electrodes implanted over the HAC can help in tinnitus suppression. Plewnia et al. (2007) used PET to show attenuation of neural activity in the auditory cortical association area after transcranial magnetic stimulation in effectively treated patients. Emmert et al. (2017) found that tinnitus patients, who were performed neurofeedback treatment show weakened activity in the secondary auditory cortex, appeared lower relaxation index scores than pre-treatment, while no significant alteration in tinnitus loudness.

In similar RS-ALFF tinnitus research, Chen et al. found that increased spontaneous activity (measured with ALFF) in the right MTG (BA22), an auditory associated region, was correlated with tinnitus clinical characteristics, such as tinnitus duration and handicap score (Chen et al., 2014). The cause of the difference may be the tinnitus mechanism and the effect of the tinnitus side. From the study participants, all patients selected in our study had right ear tinnitus, and possible exposure factors were persistent non-invasive noise damage. As described in the previous literature, right-sided tinnitus caused by non-trauma noise exposure has a greater impact on speech recognition than left ear tinnitus and affects the severity of tinnitus symptoms (Tai and Husain, 2018). The location of abnormal activation in this study is just in the BA22 area on the left hemisphere, which have the function of recognition of language and the selective attention to sound in human beings (Rinne et al., 2008).

In animal studies, the mechanism of tinnitus following long-term exposure to non-traumatic noise might be the result of the cortical tonotopic map distortion in the PAC, which present

TABLE 3 | Characteristics of clusters displaying significantly different functional connectivity between the TNH and HC groups.

Number order of the clusters	Brain regions (AAL)	Peak intensity (T-score) (L/R)	Peak MNI coordinate	Number of voxels	Function of brain region
10, 11	Heschl (L/R)	4.56/5.23	−38, −19, 5/45, −13, 5	14/19	Auditory network
8, 13	Superior temporal gyrus (L/R)	7.50/4.51	−51, −9, −6/51, −37, 12	130/34	Auditory network
14	Middle temporal gyrus (R)	5.13	51, −51 6	28	Auditory network
4	Inferior colliculus (R)	4.16	3, −27, −15	11	Auditory network
3	Cerebellum 4,5 (L)	4.75	15, −57, −18	24	Motor planning and control
5	Cerebellum 8 (L)	6.48	−18, −63, −60	20	Motor planning and control
7	Hippocampus (L)	5.47	−30, −42, 3	55	Mood, memory, spatial navigation
6	Amygdala (L)	5.50	−30, 0, −18	27	Emotions; fear or anxiety
13	Supramarginal gyrus (R)	4.54	55, −21, 26	14	Dorsal attention network
9	Insula (R)	5.73	45, −9, 3	148	Executive control of attention
1, 2	Supplementary motor area (L/R)	6.10/8.02	−15, −6, 75 /9, −3, 75	18/53	Motor control

AAL, Automated Anatomical Labeling atlas; MNI, Montreal Neurological Institute; R, right; L, left.

decreased neural activity within the exposure frequency range and increased outside the exposure range. We did not find any difference in the PAC between TNH and HC, as we expected. Langguth et al. (2006) did not find a difference in the auditory cortices between subjects with tinnitus and controls using steady-state metabolism of PET evaluation. Chen et al. (2014) did not find different clusters in the PAC using the ALFF index. Only Shulman et al. (1995) presented hyperactivity (SPECT Tc^{99}) in the PAC of tinnitus patients without hearing evaluation (Shulman et al., 1995). In our study, the null result of the PAC might be ascribed to the fact that the tonotopic mapping area of the PAC is too small to detect the difference for limitation of low spatial resolution RS-fMRI and small size of sample in our study.

In our study, decreased smALFF values are presented in the right IC. Various research studies with noise-induced tinnitus present increases in excitation and decreases in inhibition of the CAS, which be thought to stabilize the mean activity of neurons on long time scales (Schaette and McAlpine, 2011). Most of the tinnitus subjects in our study have environmental noise exposure and low activity of the right IC, which might be induced by adaptive homeostatic plasticity to environmental noise with wideband. Smits et al. (2007) reported a similar result showing that right ear tinnitus showed sound-evoked fMRI activation in the IC and lateralized toward the right IC. Landgrebe et al. (2009) also showed increased gray matter in the right IC of tinnitus, which means that that IC has more active neurons and increased neural activity. These are not consisted with our results. There is no correlation between the clinical characteristics of tinnitus and smALFF of the right IC. The IC activity might therefore be related to maintain sound perception (Schaette and McAlpine, 2011) rather than the clinical features associated with tinnitus.

TABLE 4 | Asymmetric analysis of the auditory cortex in group and between groups (analysis with smALFF).

Items	Side	TNH (*n* = 16)	HC (*n* = 15)	*P*-value (TNH/NC)
PAC	Left	1.136 ± 0.267	1.041 ± 0.073	
PAC	Right	1.079 ± 0.161	0.990 ± 0.061	
P-value (L/R)		0.472	0.048	
HAC	Left	0.844 ± 0.120	0.707 ± 0.046	
HAC	Right	0.952 ± 0.214	0.871 ± 0.044	
P-value (L/R)		0.093	0.001	
HAC ratio (L/R)		0.926 ± 0.214	0.813 ± 0.066	0.059
PAC ratio (L/R)		1.053 ± 0.170	1.053 ± 0.069	0.993

smALFF, smoothed mean amplitude of low-frequency fluctuation; PAC, primary auditory cortex; HAC, higher auditory cortex.

In the present study, seed voxels were used to explore differences in brain-wide FC between the TNH and HC groups. When using a left HAC seed, we found increased FC with various brain regions including the bilateral supplementary motor area, bilateral STG, bilateral Heschl gyrus, bilateral insula, left amygdala, left hippocampus, right supramarginal gyrus, right cerebellum, and right inferior (**Figure 5** and **Table 3**). When using the right IC seed, we did not find any difference in brain-wide FC. Interestingly, we also found that the smALFF values of the left HAC, but not the right IC, were significantly correlated with the clinical characteristics.

Although only the HAC in the central auditory nervous system shows an increased neural baseline activity and is related to clinical indicators of tinnitus, this change is not isolated to CAS. The activity cluster in HAC has stronger FC to auditory network-related brain regions (Mantini et al., 2007) include Heschl gyri (PAC) and bilateral anterior STG and right IC which means that the alteration of neural activity in HAC drives the aberrant functional linkages throughout the auditory network. Associative auditory cortices (BA22) have close relationship with Heschl gyri (PAC), which may cause the phantom sounds (Chen et al., 2014). The results suggest that the modulation of the resting-state auditory network neural activity in HAC affects the whole CAS, and previous studies found increased FC between the ipsilateral auditory cortex and the contralateral auditory cortex and STG (Burton et al., 2012; Kim et al., 2012; Maudoux et al., 2012a). The STG is thought to play a role not only in the perception of sound but also in cognition through a pathway consisting of the amygdala and prefrontal cortex (Bigler et al., 2007; Wild et al., 2012). The IC is a necessary relay in the ascending auditory pathway, a point at which virtually all lemniscal and extra-lemniscal ascending inputs converge (Aitkin and Phillips, 1984). In the sodium salicylate-induced tinnitus animal model, the secondary auditory cortex exhibited an increased firing rate (Eggermont and Kenmochi, 1998) as well as increased FC between the auditory cortex and the IC (Rinne et al., 2008; Chen et al., 2015). In our study, the HAC exhibited FC with the IC (**Figures 3, 5**), implying that the HAC is a major hub of tinnitus without hearing loss between the auditory network and various subnetworks. We hypothesize that the right IC receives a large descending projection from the HAC (BA22) and, in effect, modulates selective auditory attention to the tinnitus phantom sound perception.

The cerebellum is mainly thought to be associated with motor control and planning (Kelly and Strick, 2003; Konoike et al., 2012; Stoodley et al., 2012), and parts of this structure, such as supplementary motor area, lobule 4, the parafloccular lobe, and the vermis, have been found to contain links to the auditory system during tinnitus in animal models (Maess et al., 2001; Brozoski et al., 2007; Bauer et al., 2013). In particular, Chen et al. have suggested that the cerebellum (lobule 4) and parafloccular lobe form a gain control mechanism that compares the afferent input from the cochlea with descending signals from the auditory network (Chen et al., 2015). Consistent with this view, our results revealed abnormal activity in the HAC of tinnitus patients and an increase in the FC between this region and cerebellum lobules 4, 5, and 8.

The amygdala and hippocampus, which play roles in emotional responses and memory (fear, anxiety, and aggression), are members of the limbic system (Blair et al., 2001; Amunts et al., 2005). The extended object-attribute model study proposed that emotional aural events involve the auditory pathways (including the auditory cortex, IC, and thalamus) as well as the limbic system (Datta et al., 2005; McLachlan and Wilson, 2010). Interestingly, the increased FC between the HAC and IC, cerebellum lobules, amygdala, and hippocampus in the TNH group illustrates the network of the extended object-attribute model (Phelps, 2004). The neurophysiological model of tinnitus proposed by Jastreboff (1990) suggests an interplay between the auditory and limbic systems, which has been supported by various RS-fMRI studies that have also found evidence for this linkage in tinnitus patients (Kim et al., 2012; Maudoux et al., 2012a). Altogether, the results of our study provide further evidence that there exists an increased FC between the auditory cortex and the amygdala in tinnitus patients.

Some limitations of the current study should be considered when interpreting these findings. First, the study sample size is small and may be an issue when considering that small differences cannot always survive after multiple comparison statistical corrections and may induce erroneously active clusters. Therefore, we tried to maximize the differences between groups while remaining consistent across our patient populations by ensuring that they all had right ear tinnitus, a history of non-traumatic noise exposure, and no hearing loss. We also matched the patient groups according to age, sex, and education level, and excluded patients with various underlying diseases, such as metabolic diseases, long-term oral drug use, or emotional disorders. We attempted to select a stringent multiple comparison correction methods, the permutation test, which has been proved reliable (Rondinoni et al., 2013), to minimize the probability of statistical error. In the future, we will enlarge the sample size and patient groups to cases with right ear, left ear, and binaural tinnitus, as well as TNH and tinnitus with hearing loss, to further explore the mechanism of tinnitus. In addition, we cannot eliminate the substantial acoustic noise produced during the fMRI procedure, which might affect baseline neural activity (Amunts et al., 2005). We tried to reduce such interference by providing the patients with ear plugs and MRI noise-cancelling headphones, and by adjusting the pulse sequence before structural scanning (Paul et al., 2009). Finally, the abnormal FC between networks in the real world effects not only the resting-state brain but also the network dynamics (Di and Biswal, 2019). It is insufficient to observe the influence of tinnitus on the FC of the brain using only RS-fMRI and the LFF feature. How tinnitus impacts working efficiency, cognitive ability, memory, etc., needs to be further researched to determine an encompassing characterization of the disease.

CONCLUSION

Tinnitus induced by no-trauma noise might be the result of abnormal spontaneous activity in the HAC and auditory pathway, which may subsequently cause plastic changes involving the increase in FC between the auditory network, cerebellum, and limbic system.

ETHICS STATEMENT

The studies involving human participants were reviewed and approved by the Research Ethics Committee of Guangzhou Panyu Central Hospital and The First Affiliated Hospital of Jinan University, Guangzhou. The patients/participants provided their written informed consent to participate in this study.

AUTHOR CONTRIBUTIONS

TZ, Q-TY, and W-WC performed the design of the investigation and collected the subjects. Z-CL and W-WC contributed to the analysis of the resting-state fMRI data and wrote the manuscript. All authors have read and approved the manuscript.

ACKNOWLEDGMENTS

Tinnitus patients were recruited from outpatient clinics at The Otorhinolaryngology Department of Panyu Central Hospital, The First Affiliated Hospital of Jinan University, and The Third Affiliated Hospital of Sun Yat-sen University, Guangzhou, China, from March 2015 to May 2018. Resting-state fMRI data acquisition and processing was performed in The First Affiliated Hospital of Jinan University. The article was written at the Panyu Central Hospital.

REFERENCES

Aitkin, L. M., and Phillips, S. C. (1984). Is the inferior colliculus an obligatory relay in the cat auditory system? *Neurosci. Lett.* 44, 259–264. doi: 10.1016/0304-3940(84)90032-6

Amunts, K., Kedo, O., Kindler, M., Pieperhoff, P., Mohlberg, H., Shah, N. J., et al. (2005). Cytoarchitectonic mapping of the human amygdala, hippocampal region and entorhinal cortex: intersubject variability and probability maps. *Anat. Embryol.* 210, 343–352. doi: 10.1007/s00429-005-0025-5

Arnold, W., Bartenstein, P., Oestreicher, E., Romer, W., and Schwaiger, M. (1996). Focal metabolic activation in the predominant left auditory cortex in patients suffering from tinnitus: a PET study with [18F]deoxyglucose. *ORL J. Otorhinolaryngol. Relat. Spec.* 58, 195–199. doi: 10.1159/000276835

Ashburner, J. (2007). A fast diffeomorphic image registration algorithm. *Neuroimage* 38, 95–113. doi: 10.1016/j.neuroimage.2007.07.007

Ashburner, J., and Friston, K. J. (2005). Unified segmentation. *Neuroimage* 26, 839–851. doi: 10.1016/j.neuroimage.2005.02.018

Bauer, C. A., Kurt, W., Sybert, L. T., and Brozoski, T. J. (2013). The cerebellum as a novel tinnitus generator. *Hear. Res.* 295, 130–139. doi: 10.1016/j.heares.2012.03.009

Bigler, E. D., Mortensen, S., Neeley, E. S., Ozonoff, S., Krasny, L., Johnson, M., et al. (2007). Superior temporal gyrus, language function, and autism. *Dev. Neuropsychol.* 31, 217–238. doi: 10.1080/87565640701190841

Biswal, B., Yetkin, F. Z., Haughton, V. M., and Hyde, J. S. (1995). Functional connectivity in the motor cortex of resting human brain using echo-planar MRI. *Magn. Reson. Med.* 34, 537–541. doi: 10.1002/mrm.1910340409

Blair, H. T., Schafe, G. E., Bauer, E. P., Rodrigues, S. M., and LeDoux, J. E. (2001). Synaptic plasticity in the lateral amygdala: a cellular hypothesis of fear conditioning. *Learn. Mem.* 8, 229–242. doi: 10.1101/lm.30901

Brett, M., Anton, J. L., Valabregue, R., and Poline, J. B. (2002). Region of interest analysis using the MarsBar toolbox for SPM 99. *Neuroimage* 16:497.

Brozoski, T. J., Ciobanu, L., and Bauer, C. A. (2007). Central neural activity in rats with tinnitus evaluated with manganese-enhanced magnetic resonance imaging (MEMRI). *Hear. Res.* 228, 168–179. doi: 10.1016/j.heares.2007.02.003

Burton, H., Wineland, A., Bhattacharya, M., Nicklaus, J., Garcia, K. S., and Piccirillo, J. F. (2012). Altered networks in bothersome tinnitus: a functional connectivity study. *BMC Neurosci.* 13:3. doi: 10.1186/1471-2202-13-3

Chao-Gan, Y., and Yu-Feng, Z. (2010). DPARSF: a MATLAB toolbox for "Pipeline" data analysis of resting-state fMRI. *Front. Syst. Neurosci.* 4:13. doi: 10.3389/fnsys.2010.00013

Chen, X., Lu, B., and Yan, C. G. (2018). Reproducibility of R-fMRI metrics on the impact of different strategies for multiple comparison correction and sample sizes. *Hum. Brain Mapp.* 39, 300–318. doi: 10.1002/hbm.23843

Chen, Y. C., Li, X., Liu, L., Wang, J., Lu, C. Q., Yang, M., et al. (2015). Tinnitus and hyperacusis involve hyperactivity and enhanced connectivity in auditory-limbic-arousal-cerebellar network. *eLife* 4:e06576. doi: 10.7554/eLife.06576

Chen, Y. C., Zhang, J., Li, X. W., Xia, W., Feng, X., Gao, B., et al. (2014). Aberrant spontaneous brain activity in chronic tinnitus patients revealed by resting-state functional MRI. *Neuroimage Clin.* 6, 222–228. doi: 10.1016/j.nicl.2014.09.011

Cordes, D., Haughton, V. M., Arfanakis, K., Carew, J. D., Turski, P. A., Moritz, C. H., et al. (2001). Frequencies contributing to functional connectivity in the cerebral cortex in "resting-state" data. *AJNR Am. J. Neuroradiol.* 22, 1326–1333.

Datta, S., Saha, S., Prutzman, S. L., Mullins, O. J., and Mavanji, V. (2005). Pontine-wave generator activation-dependent memory processing of avoidance learning involves the dorsal hippocampus in the rat. *J. Neurosci. Res.* 80, 727–737. doi: 10.1002/jnr.20501

Davies, J., Gander, P. E., Andrews, M., and Hall, D. A. (2014). Auditory network connectivity in tinnitus patients: a resting-state fMRI study. *Int. J. Audiol.* 53, 192–198. doi: 10.3109/14992027.2013.846482

De Ridder, D., Vanneste, S., Kovacs, S., Sunaert, S., Menovsky, T., van de Heyning, P., et al. (2011). Transcranial magnetic stimulation and extradural electrodes implanted on secondary auditory cortex for tinnitus suppression. *J. Neurosurg.* 114, 903–911. doi: 10.3171/2010.11.JNS10197

Di, X., and Biswal, B. B. (2019). Toward task connectomics: examining whole-brain task modulated connectivity in different task domains. *Cereb. Cortex* 29, 1572–1583. doi: 10.1093/cercor/bhy055

Eggermont, J. J., and Kenmochi, M. (1998). Salicylate and quinine selectively increase spontaneous firing rates in secondary auditory cortex. *Hear. Res.* 117, 149–160. doi: 10.1016/s0378-5955(98)00008-2

Emmert, K., Kopel, R., Koush, Y., Maire, R., Senn, P., Van De Ville, D., et al. (2017). Continuous vs. intermittent neurofeedback to regulate auditory cortex activity of tinnitus patients using real-time fMRI - A pilot study. *Neuroimage Clin.* 14, 97–104. doi: 10.1016/j.nicl.2016.12.023

Fox, M. D., Snyder, A. Z., Vincent, J. L., Corbetta, M., Van Essen, D. C., and Raichle, M. E. (2005). The human brain is intrinsically organized into dynamic, anticorrelated functional networks. *Proc. Natl. Acad. Sci. U.S.A.* 102, 9673–9678. doi: 10.1073/pnas.0504136102

Friston, K. J., Williams, S., Howard, R., Frackowiak, R. S., and Turner, R. (1996). Movement-related effects in fMRI time-series. *Magn. Reson. Med.* 35, 346–355. doi: 10.1002/mrm.1910350312

Geven, L. I., de Kleine, E., Willemsen, A. T., and van Dijk, P. (2014). Asymmetry in primary auditory cortex activity in tinnitus patients and controls. *Neuroscience* 256, 117–125. doi: 10.1016/j.neuroscience.2013.10.015

Heller, A. J. (2003). Classification and epidemiology of tinnitus. *Otolaryngol. Clin. North Am.* 36, 239–248.

Huang, M., Lu, S., Yu, L., Li, L., Zhang, P., Hu, J., et al. (2017). Altered fractional amplitude of low frequency fluctuation associated with cognitive dysfunction in first-episode drug-naive major depressive disorder patients. *BMC Psychiatry* 17:11. doi: 10.1186/s12888-016-1190-1

Jastreboff, P. J. (1990). Phantom auditory perception (tinnitus): mechanisms of generation and perception. *Neurosci. Res.* 8, 221–254. doi: 10.1016/0168-0102(90)90031-9

Jenkinson, M., Bannister, P., Brady, M., and Smith, S. (2002). Improved optimization for the robust and accurate linear registration and motion correction of brain images. *Neuroimage* 17, 825–841. doi: 10.1016/s1053-8119(02)91132-8

Kelly, R. M., and Strick, P. L. (2003). Cerebellar loops with motor cortex and prefrontal cortex of a nonhuman primate. *J. Neurosci.* 23, 8432–8444. doi: 10.1523/jneurosci.23-23-08432.2003

Kim, J. Y., Kim, Y. H., Lee, S., Seo, J. H., Song, H. J., Cho, J. H., et al. (2012). Alteration of functional connectivity in tinnitus brain revealed by resting-state fMRI? A pilot study. *Int. J. Audiol.* 51, 413–417. doi: 10.3109/14992027.2011.652677

Kiviniemi, V., Kantola, J. H., Jauhiainen, J., and Tervonen, O. (2004). Comparison of methods for detecting nondeterministic BOLD fluctuation in fMRI. *Magn. Reson. Imaging* 22, 197–203. doi: 10.1016/j.mri.2003.09.007

Konoike, N., Kotozaki, Y., Miyachi, S., Miyauchi, C. M., Yomogida, Y., Akimoto, Y., et al. (2012). Rhythm information represented in the fronto-parieto-cerebellar motor system. *Neuroimage* 63, 328–338. doi: 10.1016/j.neuroimage.2012.07.002

Landgrebe, M., Langguth, B., Rosengarth, K., Braun, S., Koch, A., Kleinjung, T., et al. (2009). Structural brain changes in tinnitus: grey matter decrease in auditory and non-auditory brain areas. *Neuroimage* 46, 213–218. doi: 10.1016/j.neuroimage.2009.01.069

Langguth, B. (2011). A review of tinnitus symptoms beyond 'ringing in the ears': a call to action. *Curr. Med. Res. Opin.* 27, 1635–1643. doi: 10.1185/03007995.2011.595781

Langguth, B., Eichhammer, P., Kreutzer, A., Maenner, P., Marienhagen, J., Kleinjung, T., et al. (2006). The impact of auditory cortex activity on characterizing and treating patients with chronic tinnitus–first results from a PET study. *Acta Otolaryngol. Suppl.* 126, 84–88. doi: 10.1080/03655230600895317

Lau, C., Zhang, J. W., McPherson, B., Pienkowski, M., and Wu, E. X. (2015). Long-term, passive exposure to non-traumatic acoustic noise induces neural adaptation in the adult rat medial geniculate body and auditory cortex. *Neuroimage.* 107, 1–9. doi: 10.1016/j.neuroimage.2014.11.048

Lei, X., Zhong, M., Liu, Y., Jin, X., Zhou, Q., Xi, C., et al. (2017). A resting-state fMRI study in borderline personality disorder combining amplitude of low frequency fluctuation, regional homogeneity and seed based functional connectivity. *J. Affect. Disord.* 218, 299–305. doi: 10.1016/j.jad.2017.04.067

Li, W., Chen, Z., Wu, M., Zhu, H., Gu, L., Zhao, Y., et al. (2017). Characterization of brain blood flow and the amplitude of low-frequency fluctuations in major depressive disorder: a multimodal meta-analysis. *J. Affect. Disord.* 210, 303–311. doi: 10.1016/j.jad.2016.12.032

Lu, H., Zuo, Y., Gu, H., Waltz, J. A., Zhan, W., Scholl, C. A., et al. (2007). Synchronized delta oscillations correlate with the resting-state functional MRI signal. *Proc. Natl. Acad. Sci. U.S.A.* 104, 18265–18269. doi: 10.1073/pnas.0705791104

Lv, H., Zhao, P., Liu, Z., Wang, G., Zeng, R., Yan, F., et al. (2016). Frequency-dependent neural activity in patients with unilateral vascular pulsatile tinnitus. *Neural Plast.* 2016:4918186. doi: 10.1155/2016/4918186

Maess, B., Koelsch, S., Gunter, T. C., and Friederici, A. D. (2001). Musical syntax is processed in Broca's area: an MEG study. *Nat. Neurosci.* 4, 540–545. doi: 10.1038/87502

Mantini, D., Perrucci, M. G., Del Gratta, C., Romani, G. L., and Corbetta, M. (2007). Electrophysiological signatures of resting state networks in the human brain. *Proc. Natl. Acad. Sci. U.S.A.* 104, 13170–13175. doi: 10.1073/pnas.0700668104

Martines, F., Bentivegna, D., Martines, E., Sciacca, V., and Martinciglio, G. (2010). Assessing audiological, pathophysiological and psychological variables in tinnitus patients with or without hearing loss. *Eur. Arch. Otorhinolaryngol.* 267, 1685–1693. doi: 10.1007/s00405-010-1302-3

Maudoux, A., Lefebvre, P., Cabay, J. E., Demertzi, A., Vanhaudenhuyse, A., Laureys, S., et al. (2012a). Auditory resting-state network connectivity in tinnitus: a functional MRI study. *PLoS One* 7:e36222. doi: 10.1371/journal.pone.0036222

Maudoux, A., Lefebvre, P., Cabay, J. E., Demertzi, A., Vanhaudenhuyse, A., Laureys, S., et al. (2012b). Connectivity graph analysis of the auditory resting state network in tinnitus. *Brain Res.* 1485, 10–21. doi: 10.1016/j.brainres.2012.05.006

McLachlan, N., and Wilson, S. (2010). The central role of recognition in auditory perception: a neurobiological model. *Psychol. Rev.* 117, 175–196. doi: 10.1037/a0018063

Meng, Z., Zheng, Y., Liu, S., Wang, K., Kong, X., Tao, Y., et al. (2012). Reliability and validity of the chinese (mandarin) tinnitus handicap inventory. *Clin. Exp. Otorhinolaryngol.* 5, 10–16. doi: 10.3342/ceo.2012.5.1.10

Mikl, M., Marecek, R., Hlustík, P., Pavlicová, M., Drastich, A., Chlebus, P., et al. (2008) Effects of spatial smoothing on fMRI group inferences. *Magn. Reson. imaging* 26, 490–503. doi: 10.1016/j.mri.2007.08.006

Morosan, P., Rademacher, J., Schleicher, A., Amunts, K., Schormann, T., and Zilles, K. (2001). Human primary auditory cortex: cytoarchitectonic subdivisions and mapping into a spatial reference system. *Neuroimage* 13, 684–701. doi: 10.1006/nimg.2000.0715

Morosan, P., Schleicher, A., Amunts, K., and Zilles, K. (2005). Multimodal architectonic mapping of human superior temporal gyrus. *Anat. Embryol.* 210, 401–406. doi: 10.1007/s00429-005-0029-1

Muhlau, M., Rauschecker, J. P., Oestreicher, E., Gaser, C., Rottinger, M., Wohlschlager, A. M., et al. (2006). Structural brain changes in tinnitus. *Cereb. Cortex* 16, 1283–1288. doi: 10.1093/cercor/bhj070

Munguia, R., Pienkowski, M., and Eggermont, J. J. (2013). Spontaneous firing rate changes in cat primary auditory cortex following long-term exposure to non-traumatic noise: tinnitus without hearing loss? *Neurosci. Lett.* 546, 46–50. doi: 10.1016/j.neulet.2013.04.048

Paul, A. K., Lobarinas, E., Simmons, R., Wack, D., Luisi, J. C., Spernyak, J., et al. (2009). Metabolic imaging of rat brain during pharmacologically-induced tinnitus. *Neuroimage* 44, 312–318. doi: 10.1016/j.neuroimage.2008.09.024

Phelps, E. A. (2004). Human emotion and memory: interactions of the amygdala and hippocampal complex. *Curr. Opin. Neurobiol.* 14, 198–202. doi: 10.1016/j.conb.2004.03.015

Plewnia, C., Reimold, M., Najib, A., Brehm, B., Reischl, G., Plontke, S. K., et al. (2007). Dose-dependent attenuation of auditory phantom perception (tinnitus) by PET-guided repetitive transcranial magnetic stimulation. *Hum. Brain Mapp.* 28, 238–246. doi: 10.1002/hbm.20270

Reiss, M., and Reiss, G. (2001). Laterality of tinnitus: relationship to functional assymetries. *Wiener klinische Wochenschrift* 113, 45–51.

Rinne, T., Balk, M. H., Koistinen, S., Autti, T., Alho, K., and Sams, M. (2008). Auditory selective attention modulates activation of human inferior colliculus. *J. Neurophysiol.* 100, 3323–3327. doi: 10.1152/jn.90607.2008

Rogers, B. P., Morgan, V. L., Newton, A. T., and Gore, J. C. (2007). Assessing functional connectivity in the human brain by fMRI. *Magn. Reson. Imaging* 25, 1347–1357. doi: 10.1016/j.mri.2007.03.007

Rondinoni, C., Amaro, E. Jr., Cendes, F., dos Santos, A. C., and Salmon, C. E. (2013). Effect of scanner acoustic background noise on strict resting-state fMRI. *Braz. J. Med. Biol.* 46, 359–367. doi: 10.1590/1414-431x20132799

Rusiniak, M., Lewandowska, M., Wolak, T., Pluta, A., Milner, R., and Skarzynski, H. (2015). The possibilities and limitations of simultaneous EEG-fMRI registration–the alpha rhythm study. *Przeglad Lekarski* 72, 616–619.

Savastano, M. (2008). Tinnitus with or without hearing loss: are its characteristics different? *Eur. Arch. Otorhinolaryngol.* 265, 1295–1300. doi: 10.1007/s00405-008-0630-z

Schaette, R., and McAlpine, D. (2011). Tinnitus with a normal audiogram: physiological evidence for hidden hearing loss and computational model. *J. Neurosci.* 31, 13452–13457. doi: 10.1523/JNEUROSCI.2156-11.2011

Seydell-Greenwald, A., Raven, E. P., Leaver, A. M., Turesky, T. K., and Rauschecker, J. P. (2014). Diffusion imaging of auditory and auditory-limbic connectivity in tinnitus: preliminary evidence and methodological challenges. *Neural Plast.* 2014:145943. doi: 10.1155/2014/145943

Shmuel, A., and Leopold, D. A. (2008). Neuronal correlates of spontaneous fluctuations in fMRI signals in monkey visual cortex: implications for functional connectivity at rest. *Hum. Brain Mapp.* 29, 751–761. doi: 10.1002/hbm.20580

Shtark, M. B., Verevkin, E. G., Kozlova, L. I., Mazhirina, K. G., Pokrovskii, M. A., Petrovskii, E. D., et al. (2015). Synergetic fMRI-EEG brain mapping in alpha-rhythm voluntary control mode. *Bull. Exp. Biol. Med.* 158, 644–649. doi: 10.1007/s10517-015-2827-7

Shulman, A., Strashun, A. M., Afriyie, M., Aronson, F., Abel, W., and Goldstein, B. (1995). SPECT imaging of brain and tinnitus-neurotologic/neurologic implications. *Int. Tinnitus J.* 1, 13–29.

Skidmore, F. M., Yang, M., Baxter, L., von Deneen, K. M., Collingwood, J., He, G., et al. (2013). Reliability analysis of the resting state can sensitively and specifically identify the presence of Parkinson disease. *Neuroimage* 75, 249–261. doi: 10.1016/j.neuroimage.2011.06.056

Smits, M., Kovacs, S., de Ridder, D., Peeters, R. R., van Hecke, P., and Sunaert, S. (2007). Lateralization of functional magnetic resonance imaging (fMRI) activation in the auditory pathway of patients with lateralized tinnitus. *Neuroradiology* 49, 669–679. doi: 10.1007/s00234-007-0231-3

Stoodley, C. J., Valera, E. M., and Schmahmann, J. D. (2012). Functional topography of the cerebellum for motor and cognitive tasks: an fMRI study. *Neuroimage* 59, 1560–1570. doi: 10.1016/j.neuroimage.2011.08.065

Tai, Y., and Husain, F. T. (2018). Right-Ear advantage for speech-in-noise recognition in patients with nonlateralized tinnitus and normal hearing sensitivity. *J. Assoc. Res. Otolaryngol.* 19, 211–221. doi: 10.1007/s10162-017-0647-3

Takacs, J. D., Forrest, T. J., and Basura, G. J. (2017). Noise exposure alters long-term neural firing rates and synchrony in primary auditory and rostral belt cortices following bimodal stimulation. *Hear. Res.* 356, 1–15. doi: 10.1016/j.heares.2017.07.004

Wild, C. J., Yusuf, A., Wilson, D. E., Peelle, J. E., Davis, M. H., and Johnsrude, I. S. (2012). Effortful listening: the processing of degraded speech depends critically on attention. *J. Neurosci.* 32, 14010–14021. doi: 10.1523/JNEUROSCI.1528-12.2012

Wineland, A. M., Burton, H., and Piccirillo, J. (2012). Functional connectivity networks in nonbothersome tinnitus. *Otolaryngol. Head Neck Surg.* 147, 900–906. doi: 10.1177/0194599812451414

Winkler, A. M., Ridgway, G. R., Douaud, G., Nichols, T. E., and Smith, S. M. (2016). Faster permutation inference in brain imaging. *Neuroimage* 141, 502–516. doi: 10.1016/j.neuroimage.2016.05.068

Xu, X., Bu, X., Zhou, L., Xing, G., Liu, C., and Wang, D. (2011). An epidemiologic study of tinnitus in a population in Jiangsu Province. *China J. Am. Acad. Audiol.* 22, 578–585. doi: 10.3766/jaaa.22.9.3

Yan, C. G., Cheung, B., Kelly, C., Colcombe, S., Craddock, R. C., Di Martino, A., et al. (2013). A comprehensive assessment of regional variation in the impact of head micromovements on functional connectomics. *Neuroimage* 76, 183–201. doi: 10.1016/j.neuroimage.2013.03.004

Yan, C. G., Wang, X. D., Zuo, X. N., and Zang, Y. F. (2016). DPABI: data processing & analysis for (Resting-State) brain imaging. *Neuroinformatics* 14, 339–351. doi: 10.1007/s12021-016-9299-4

Yuan, L. X., Wang, J. B., Zhao, N., Li, Y. Y., Ma, Y., Liu, D. Q., et al. (2018). Intra- and inter-scanner reliability of scaled subprofile model of principal component analysis on ALFF in Resting-State fMRI under eyes open and closed conditions. *Front. Neurosci.* 12:311. doi: 10.3389/fnins.2018.00311

Zang, Y. F., He, Y., Zhu, C. Z., Cao, Q. J., Sui, M. Q., Liang, M., et al. (2007). Altered baseline brain activity in children with ADHD revealed by resting-state functional MRI. *Brain Dev.* 29, 83–91. doi: 10.1016/j.braindev.2006.07.002

Zhang, D., Snyder, A. Z., Fox, M. D., Sansbury, M. W., Shimony, J. S., and Raichle, M. E. (2008). Intrinsic functional relations between human cerebral cortex and thalamus. *J. Neurophysiol.* 100, 1740–1748. doi: 10.1152/jn.90463.2008

Zung, W. W. (1971). A rating instrument for anxiety disorders. *Psychosomatics* 12, 371–379. doi: 10.1016/s0033-3182(71)71479-0

Zung, W. W. K. (1986). "Zung self-rating depression scale and depression status inventory," in *Assessment of Depression*, eds N. Sartorius and T.A. Ban (Heidelberg: Springer). doi: 10.1007/978-3-642-70486-4_21

16

Altered Resting-State EEG Microstate in Idiopathic Sudden Sensorineural Hearing Loss Patients with Tinnitus

Yuexin Cai[1,2†], Suijun Chen[1,2†], Yanhong Chen[1,2], Jiahong Li[1,2], Chang-Dong Wang[3], Fei Zhao[4,5], Cai-Ping Dang[6,7], Jianheng Liang[8], Nannan He[8], Maojin Liang[1,2] and Yiqing Zheng[1,2*]

[1] Department of Otolaryngology, Sun Yat-sen Memorial Hospital, Sun Yat-sen University, Guangzhou, China, [2] Institute of Hearing and Speech-Language Science, Sun Yat-sen University, Guangzhou, China, [3] School of Data and Computer Science, Sun Yat-sen University, Guangzhou, China, [4] Department of Speech Language Therapy and Hearing Science, Cardiff Metropolitan University, Cardiff, United Kingdom, [5] Department of Hearing and Speech Science, Xinhua College, Sun Yat-sen University, Guangzhou, China, [6] Affiliated Brain Hospital of Guangzhou Medical University, Guangzhou, China, [7] Department of Psychology, Guangzhou Medical University, Guangzhou, China, [8] College of Mathematics and Informatics, South China Agricultural University, Guangzhou, China

***Correspondence:**
Yiqing Zheng
yiqingzheng@hotmail.com

†These authors have contributed equally to this work

In order to clarify the central reorganization in acute period of hearing loss, this study explored the aberrant dynamics of electroencephalogram (EEG) microstates and the correlations with the features of idiopathic sudden sensorineural hearing loss (ISSNHL) and tinnitus. We used high-density EEG with 128 channels to investigate alterations in microstate parameters between 25 ISSNHL patients with tinnitus and 27 healthy subjects. This study also explored the associations between microstate characteristics and tinnitus features. Microstates were clustered into four categories. There was a reduced presence of microstate A in amplitude, coverage, lifespan, frequency and an increased presence of microstate B in frequency in ISSNHL patients with tinnitus. According to the syntax analysis, a reduced transition from microstate C to microstate A and an increased transition from microstate C to microstate B were found in ISSNHL subjects. In addition, the significant negative correlations were found between Tinnitus Handicap Inventory (THI) scores and frequency of microstate A as well as between THI scores and the probability of transition from microstate D to microstate A. While THI was positively correlated with the transition probability from microstate D to microstate B. To sum up, the significant differences in the characteristics of resting-state EEG microstates were found between ISSNHL subjects with tinnitus and healthy controls. This study suggests that the alterations of central neural networks occur in acute stage of hearing loss and tinnitus. And EEG microstate may be considered as a useful tool to study the whole brain network in ISSNHL patients.

Keywords: EEG, microstate, tinnitus, ISSNHL, mechanism

INTRODUCTION

Sudden sensorineural hearing loss (SSNHL) is the sudden-onset and rapidly developed hearing impairment with reduction in hearing of at least 30 dB in no less than three consecutive audiometric frequencies within 72 h (Stachler et al., 2012). The incidence of SSNHL is approximately 5 to 20 individuals per 100,000/year (Klemm et al., 2009; Stachler et al., 2012). Some studies suggest that the hearing impairment of SSNHL is usually unilateral, and less than 5% of SSNHL patients is bilateral (Oh et al., 2007; Schreiber et al., 2010). SSNHL, whose etiology and pathogenesis are mostly unclear, is usually considered as idiopathic (Chau et al., 2010). No more than one third of cases are caused by viral infection, otologic disease, trauma, cardiovascular or hematologic risk factors, neoplastic disease, and autoimmune disease (Chau et al., 2010; Lin et al., 2012). At present, the main treatment for idiopathic sudden sensorineural hearing loss (ISSNHL) is steroid therapy (Jung et al., 2016). Unfortunately, many ISSNHL patients have little improvement of their hearing function even after high-quality suitable therapy, which may lead to the poor quality of their life (Kuhn et al., 2011). The discontented state of ISSNHL treatment may be due to the unclear mechanism of ISSNHL.

Idiopathic sudden sensorineural hearing loss is often accompanied by tinnitus, vertigo, ear fullness, and so on (Koç and Sanisoğlu, 2003). Among them, tinnitus is a perceived sound without any external sound source (Kang et al., 2017). Tinnitus is a common and annoying problem in ISSNHL patients. And the incidence of tinnitus in patients with ISSNHL is 80 to 95% (Rah et al., 2015; Nogueira-Neto et al., 2016). Tinnitus not only has a high incidence in ISSNHL patients, but also has a negative impact on the life of the sufferers. For example, ISSNHL patients with tinnitus have more depressive symptoms, mental distress, and disruptive personal relationship (Chen et al., 2013). As a result, physicians should attach great importance to the treatment of ISSNHL patients with tinnitus.

To cure ISSNHL subjects with tinnitus effectively, it is necessary to explore the intrinsic mechanism of ISSNHL completely. Previous researches have showed that ISSNHL is correlated with the deviant activity of some central neural networks (Seeley et al., 2009; Musiek et al., 2013; Wang et al., 2014; Zhou and Seeley, 2014; Fan et al., 2015; Zhang et al., 2015; Golden et al., 2016; Xu et al., 2016; Micarelli et al., 2017). The development of ISSNHL is associated with several function networks, including auditory network, default mode network (DMN) and limbic network (Xu et al., 2016; Micarelli et al., 2017). A prospective case research by Fan et al. (2015) suggested that subjects with unilateral SSNHL had significant decrease in gray matter of contralateral auditory cortex. Similarly, Micarelli et al. (2017) found that ISSNHL patients had the hypometabolism in the contralateral auditory cortex by Positron emission tomography (PET). The hypothesized mechanism behind ISSNHL may be related to the unbalanced activities between excitatory and inhibitory neurons, which led to the errors about the intensity perception at cortical level (Musiek et al., 2013; Fan et al., 2015; Micarelli et al., 2017). Moreover, Wang et al. (2014) found that the deficiency of unilateral sensory input changed the activity in sensory regions and reorganized the cognitive control network. A study by Zhang et al. (2015) suggested that long-term unilateral ISSNHL patients had an abnormal change in default node network, which might influence their cognitive abilities. In addition, the insula is an important brain region to link DMN with the networks which assess sensory information and program behavioral responses (Seeley et al., 2009; Zhou and Seeley, 2014). The decreased activity of insula is related to the inhibition of activity between DMN and auditory network (Golden et al., 2016). The increase of connection between auditory network and limbic system may be associated with the generation of tinnitus in ISSNHL patients (Xu et al., 2016). Although the deviant activity of several brain functional networks had been found in ISSNHL, more studies were needed to resolve the further central mechanism behind ISSNHL. This study aimed at exploring alterations in central nervous system of ISSNHL patients with tinnitus in a novel way.

Electroencephalography (EEG) is a high temporal resolution technique for exploring electrical activity of central brain areas. It records the electrical potentials within the brain through the electrodes on the scalp (Ingber and Nunez, 2011). So far, some ways can be applied to extract useful information from multichannel EEG data. Among them, microstate analysis explores multichannel EEG recordings across the scalp and defines a set of stable microstates (Khanna et al., 2015). Therefore, it not only partly compensates for the problem of low spatial resolution in EEG, but also analyzes the aberrant dynamics of the whole brain networks. As a result, we can acquire helpful information on brain networks by microstate analysis to further explore resting-state central neural activity. In general, microstates are clustered into four categories, including microstates A, B, C, and D. (1) Microstate A is related to activation in the bilateral superior and middle temporal gyrus regions that are correlated with phonological processing. (2) Microstate B is associated with bilateral visual cortex areas. (3) Microstate C is related to a salience network, which involved the detection and orientation of both internal and external stimuli. (4) Microstate D is associated with activation in the right-lateralized dorsal and ventral regions of the frontal and parietal regions that are correlated with the central executive network (Britz et al., 2010).

At present, several studies have suggested that some central neuropsychiatric diseases have significant changes in EEG microstates, including schizophrenia, dementia, depression, and panic disorder. According to the researches about these neuropsychiatric diseases, EEG microstate analysis may be an effective way to detect the objective indicators, recognize the disease's severity, design the treatment plan and evaluate the treatment effect (Khanna et al., 2015). Additionally, EEG microstate has been used to study the neurophysiological mechanism of auditory hallucination and tinnitus. For instance, Kindler et al. (2010) found a significantly reduced presence of microstate D in hallucinating patients. Besides, Cai et al. (2018) suggested that microstate A was significantly longer and microstate D was significantly shorter in tinnitus subjects.

So far, knowledge of microstate abnormalities in ISSNHL is limited. To investigate the neurophysiological mechanism of

ISSNHL, this study explores the changes in EEG microstates between ISSNHL subjects with tinnitus and healthy subjects. Additionally, it can confirm whether EEG microstate is a useful tool to investigate ISSNHL. With the alterations of nervous activities after ISSNHL and tinnitus, the hypothesis is that the significant alterations of microstates would be found in ISSNHL patients with tinnitus at rest. The significant result can be considered as a vital electrophysiological indicator of ISSNH.

MATERIALS AND METHODS

Participants

The ISSNHL subjects with tinnitus were recruited from the Ear, Nose and Throat Clinic, Sun Yat-sen Memorial Hospital, Sun Yat-sen University, Guangzhou, China. Detailed selection criteria for inclusion and exclusion in the study were:

(1) Patients with at least 30 dB idiopathic sensorineural hearing impairment in no less than three consecutive audiometric frequencies within 72 h were recruited. In addition, ISSNHL was diagnosed by pure tone audiometry (PTA) within 72 h of conscious hearing loss or more than 72 h of conscious hearing impairment without appreciable progression of hearing damage.
(2) Patients had sought clinical help because of their hearing loss and tinnitus.
(3) Patients with acoustic neurinoma, autoimmune hearing loss, Meniere's disease, depression, or insomnia were excluded.
(4) All patients with head trauma, central nervous system disorders, middle ear surgery or pulsatile tinnitus were also excluded.

There were 25 ISSNHL patients with tinnitus (9 males and 16 females; age Mean = 46.16 years, *SD* = 13.15 years) and 27 healthy controls (10 males and 17 females; age Mean = 41.48 years, *SD* = 13.53 years). A written consent form was signed by all participants after they had been properly informed about the background and purpose of the research. Our research was approved by the Institution Review Board of the Sun Yat-sen Memorial Hospital at Sun Yat-sen University of China.

Routine Audiological Examinations

Routine audiological examinations included otoscopy and PTA. In the test of PTA, air conduction thresholds were measured at 125, 250, 500, 1000, 2000, 4000, and 8000 Hz for both ears, and bone conduction thresholds were measured between 250 and 4000 Hz in a sound-proof room. PTA was used to measure the hearing thresholds of all participants. In addition, the mean hearing threshold is defined as the average of hearing threshold at the frequencies of 0.5, 1, 2, and 4 kHz (British society of audiology recommendation, 1988; Dispenza et al., 2011; Bing et al., 2018).

Tinnitus Specific Assessments

Patients were asked to describe the laterality of tinnitus. Then, tinnitus pitch matching test was performed (Teismann et al., 2011). In the process of tinnitus pitch matching measures, the tinnitus pitch was roughly matched through the use of nine hearing frequencies, including 0.125, 0.25, 0.5, 1, 2, 3, 4, 6, and 8 kHz. Participants contrasted the perceptive tinnitus pitch and the matching pitch, and then the matching pitch was adjusted to go higher or lower according to the feedback from patients. Ultimately, an exact or closely approximate matching pitch was gained by adjusting in a half-octave step. Narrow band noise was used if no matching pure tone was obtained from subjects.

Tinnitus Handicap Inventory (THI) was used to evaluate tinnitus severity. THI assessed the perceived level of handicap in tinnitus patients, according to a 0–100 increasing handicap scale (Newman et al., 1996). Participants were required to fill in the THI prior to the experiment.

EEG Recordings

Electroencephalogram signals were recorded by a high-density EEG with 128 channels and were saved with Electrical Geodesics, Inc. (EGI, Eugene), and a NetAmps 200 amplifier. After understanding the purpose and requirements of the test, subjects were instructed to sit in a comfortable chair and remain calm. Then, participants were required to open the eyes and fixate a cross mark in front of them. A resting EEG for about 7 min was recorded. The sampling rate was set to 1000 Hz. The impedances of all electrodes were kept less than 50 kΩ and the CZ electrode was used as reference.

Preprocessing of EEG Data

The raw EEG data was preprocessed by EEGLAB 13.0.0 in the toolbox of Matlab. Firstly, the data was re-referenced against the mean reference by all electrodes. The sampling rate of the data was reduced to 500 Hz/s. A notch filter was implemented at 50 Hz and the signals were band-pass-filtered from 0.5 to 80 Hz. Gross artifacts were manually removed by visual inspection. Some artifacts originated from one or a few distinct sources or a limited volume of space were removed. In addition, some artifacts characterized by a particular temporal pattern such as exponential decay were also removed. For example, in the pretreatment of resting EEG (eye-opening state), the largest artifact comes from eye electricity. Our system has a special electrode (E127 and E126) for recording eye electricity, but the effect of eye electricity is not limited to these two electrodes, it has a great influence on the electrode of frontal region. Therefore, we use ICA algorithm to correct it. The advantages of the ICA algorithm can be viewed in the literature (Onton et al., 2006), the artifact can be separated as independent components, and the other features of the original EEG signal can be effectively retained. Other artifacts, such as eye movement, muscle artifacts and heart beats, could be also removed by independent component analysis (ICA) correction. Then, the EEG signals were reconstructed and segmented into 2 s epochs. According to the study by von Wegner et al. (2018), the invariance of the quantities implies that the tested properties are algorithm-independent, and the microstate sequences are derived from inherent features of resting state EEG. Based on the previous research (Milz et al., 2016), more than 20 artifact-free epochs were used to microstate analysis randomly.

EEG Microstate Analysis

Microstate analysis was done following the procedure described in the study by Cai et al. (2018). First of all, the global field power (GFP) was calculated by using the selected EEG epoch. Then, the clustering analysis was applied to the local maxima of the GFP. The GFP reflects the variation degree of potential across electrodes at a time point. The calculation formula is:

$$\mathrm{GFP(t)} = \sqrt{\frac{1}{K}\sum_{i=1}^{K}(V_i(t) - V_{mean}(t))^2}$$

Where, K is the number of electrodes in the EEG data. $V_i(t)$ is the potential of the i-th electrode at a certain time point. $V_{mean}(t)$ is the average value of the instantaneous potential across electrodes and the formula is $V_{mean}(t) = \frac{1}{K}\sum_{i=1}^{K} V_i(t)$. The EEG topographic maps at the local maxima of the GFP curve were taken as the local representative maps (Konig and Mellgarcia, 2009). Then, the clustering analysis was carried out to look for the stable microstates in EEG signals. All representative maps were divided into several types by the clustering analysis. It is showed that microstates can be clustered into four categories, namely microstate classes A, B, C, and D (Newman et al., 1996; Konig and Mellgarcia, 2009; Kindler et al., 2010; Teismann et al., 2011; Khanna et al., 2015; Cai et al., 2018). After obtaining the microstates of all participants, we compute the parameters of microstates, including topographical shape, amplitude, coverage, average lifespan, frequency of occurrence and transition probabilities of microstates (Cai et al., 2018). The amplitude of a microstate is the mean GFP that microstate is dominant. The coverage of a microstate is the percentage of recording time when the microstate is dominant. The average lifespan of a microstate is the average length of time when a microstate appears and remains stable. The frequency of occurrence of a microstate is the average number of times per second that a microstate occurs during a period of recording. The transition probability of a microstate means that the microstate is non-random and has the potential significance of sequence transfer.

Statistical Analysis

SPSS 19.0 software was used for all statistical analyses. t-Test was performed to explore the significant differences of the microstate parameters between two groups. We applied Pearson correlation analysis to evaluate the correlation between microstate features and the characteristics of ISSNHL and tinnitus. A p level of less than 0.05 (two-sided) was considered to be statistically significant.

RESULTS

Table 1 shows the demographic information of ISSNHL subjects with tinnitus. No significant differences were found between the ISSNHL and control groups in terms of age ($t = -1.263$, df = 50, $p = 0.212$) and gender ($x^2 = 0.006$, df = 1, $p = 0.938$). **Table 1** also shows their hearing thresholds and tinnitus features, such as tinnitus laterality, pitch and duration.

Figure 1 shows the mean microstate topographies acquired from two groups. Similar to previous studies (Lehmann et al., 2005; Britz et al., 2010), four microstate maps were found and clustered into microstates A, B, C, and D.

Independent sample t-tests for microstate parameters between the ISSNHL ($N = 25$) and control ($N = 27$) groups are given in **Table 2**. The microstate parameters included the coverage, lifespan, amplitude, and frequency of the microstates. The significant differences in microstates A and B were found by the t-test. Compared with the control group, microstates A had significant decrease in coverage ($t = 2.817$, df = 50, $p = 0.007$), lifespan ($t = 2.644$, df = 50, $p = 0.011$), amplitude ($t = 2.039$, df = 50, $p = 0.047$), and frequency ($t = 2.125$, df = 50, $p = 0.039$). And microstate B had an increased presence ($t = 3.096$, df = 50, $p = 0.03$) in frequency for the ISSNHL group compared with the control group. There was no significant difference in microstates C or D ($p > 0.05$).

As shown in **Figure 2**, there was a significant reduction in the probability of transition from microstate C to microstate A ($t = 2.978$, df = 50, $p = 0.004$) in the ISSNHL patients compared with healthy subjects. Additionally, the probability of transition from microstate C to microstate B ($t = -2.440$, df = 50, $p = 0.018$) was increased significantly. No other significant difference in the probability of transition among microstates was revealed.

The associations between alterations in microstate parameters and tinnitus characteristics were shown in **Figure 3** and **Table 3**. Significant negative correlations were revealed between THI scores and frequency of microstate A ($r = -0.417$, $p = 0.038$) as well as between THI scores and the probability of transition from microstate D to microstate A ($r = -0.447$, $p = 0.025$). While THI was significant positively associated with the transition probability from microstate D to microstate B ($r = 0.425$, $p = 0.034$). No significant correlation was revealed in the alterations of microstate characteristics with hearing threshold in ISSNHL subjects ($p > 0.05$).

DISCUSSION

As far as we know, it is the first research to explore the aberrant dynamics of EEG microstate in ISSNHL patients with tinnitus. The purpose of this research was evaluating the early stages of cortical plasticity after ISSNHL and tinnitus by using resting-state EEG microstate. There were significant differences in the temporal characteristics of the EEG microstate between ISSNHL patients and controls.

The coverage, lifespan, amplitude, and frequency of microstate A were significantly reduced in our study. Britz et al. (2010) demonstrated that microstate A was related to activation in the bilateral superior and middle temporal gyrus regions that were correlated with phonological processing. These results were similar to the finding of Fan et al. (2015), who found the decrease of contralateral auditory gray matter in unilateral

TABLE 1 | The landscape layout of ISSNHL participants with tinnitus.

Patient	Gender	Age (years)	Tinnitus duration (days)	Tinnitus laterality	Tinnitus pitch (Hz)	Hearing thresholds (dB HL) (L/R)	THI
CJH	Female	62	20	Left	125	95/19	34
CYF	Female	43	20	Left	4000	79/10	50
DL	Male	30	14	Left	8000	90/6	36
FLX	Female	61	7	Right	1000	31/81	58
HJW	Female	25	14	Right	1500	15/60	72
HDR	Female	63	7	Right	1000	53/112	78
HST	Male	42	7	Left	4000	80/25	26
LMJ	Male	54	14	Right	8000	25/110	62
LGZ	Female	58	10	Right	250	15/75	56
LJH	Male	51	20	Right	6000	47/56	26
LRH	Female	54	7	Right	6000	32/67	82
LWY	Female	49	7	Right	250	15/83	12
LSK	Male	46	25	Bilateral	2000/2000	58/63	26
LC	Male	47	2	Right	6000	19/81	12
LQ	Female	36	20	Left	125	110/9	58
MY	Male	41	7	Right	4000	38/68	4
PGJ	Male	51	20	Bilateral	4000/750	52/66	68
SWL	Male	42	10	Left	250	110/20	60
WJD	Female	57	20	Left	8000	110/22	52
WWM	Female	48	10	Right	1000	15/89	50
XWY	Female	17	14	Right	4000	8/81	16
ZMY	Female	18	10	Right	2000	20/83	48
ZYT	Female	41	8	Right	500	13/98	28
ZXH	Female	53	7	Left	6000	70/20	40
ZJH	Female	65	2	Right	4000	23/63	30

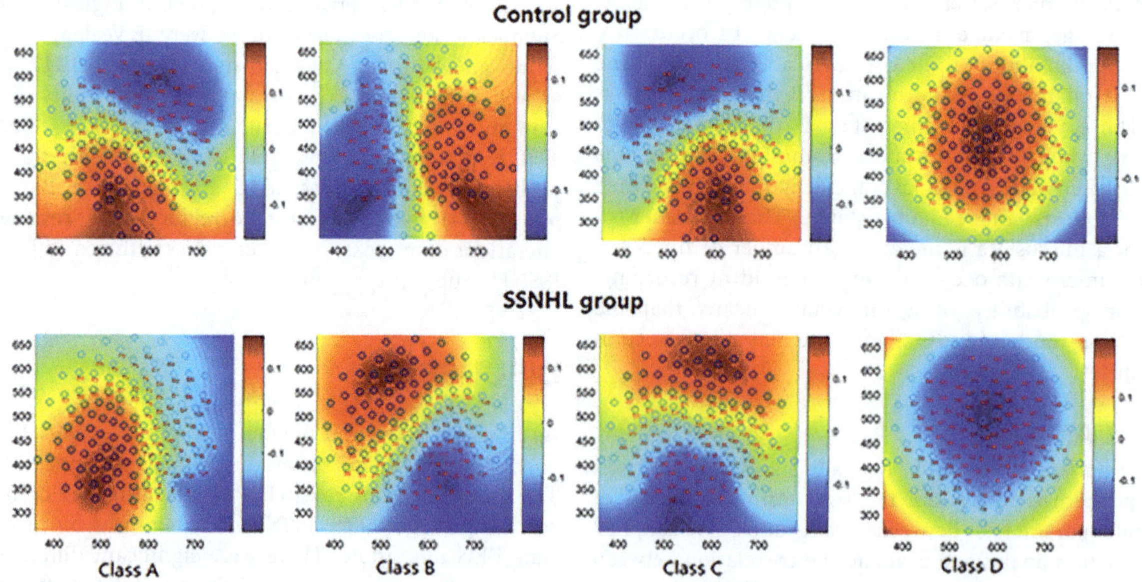

FIGURE 1 | The spatial configuration of the four microstates classes in two group. Microstate class orientations were: **(A)** right-frontal left-posterior; **(B)** left-frontal right-posterior; **(C)** anterior–posterior; **(D)** fronto-central extreme.

ISSNHL. Additionally, Micarelli et al. (2017) also showed the decrease of the metabolism in contralateral auditory cortex in ISSNHL subjects. These interesting results indicated that cortical functional alterations already existed in ISSNHL subjects during acute period and mainly occurred in the auditory network.

Increase in coverage of microstate B was also revealed in the SSNHL subjects with tinnitus. A study by Britz et al. (2010)

TABLE 2 | Comparison of the microstate analysis results in ISSNHL patients with tinnitus and control subjects.

	Class A		Class B		Class C		Class D	
	Control (Mean ± SD)	Tinnitus (Mean ± SD)	Control (Mean ± SD)	Tinnitus (Mean ± SD)	Control (Mean ± SD)	Tinnitus (Mean ± SD)	Control (Mean ± SD)	Tinnitus (Mean ± SD)
Coverage (%)	0.291 ± 0.227	0.149 ± 0.114*	0.210 ± 0.241	0.296 ± 0.201	0.322 ± 0.235	0.371 ± 0.196	0.166 ± 0.212	0.179 ± 0.199
Lifespan (ms)	251.971 ± 142.799	170.686 ± 58.921*	217.772 ± 175.857	247.793 ± 123.673	323.097 ± 315.186	307.430 ± 164.535	198.585 ± 128.154	190.289 ± 105.086
Amplitude (uV)	0.004 ± 0.081	−0.043 ± 0.087*	−0.013 ± 0.310	0.015 ± 0.056	0.002 ± 0.062	−0.006 ± 0.031	−0.009 ± 0.169	0.059 ± 0.273
Frequency	1.022 ± 0.485	0.747 ± 0.448*	0.715 ± 0.536	1.110 ± 0.360*	1.045 ± 0.354	1.189 ± 0.272	0.615 ± 0.543	0.729 ± 0.513

*Indicates the t-test was significant ($p < 0.05$).

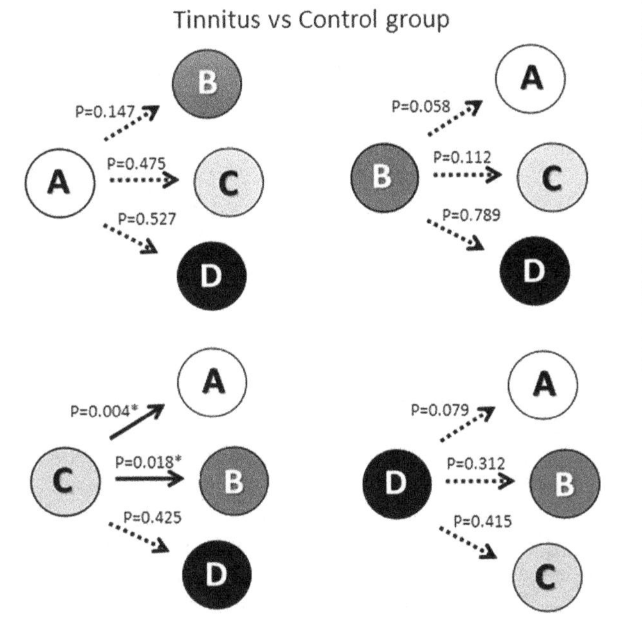

FIGURE 2 | Schematic view of the syntax pattern. * Indicates significant difference ($p < 0.05$). Solid arrow indicate significant correlation.

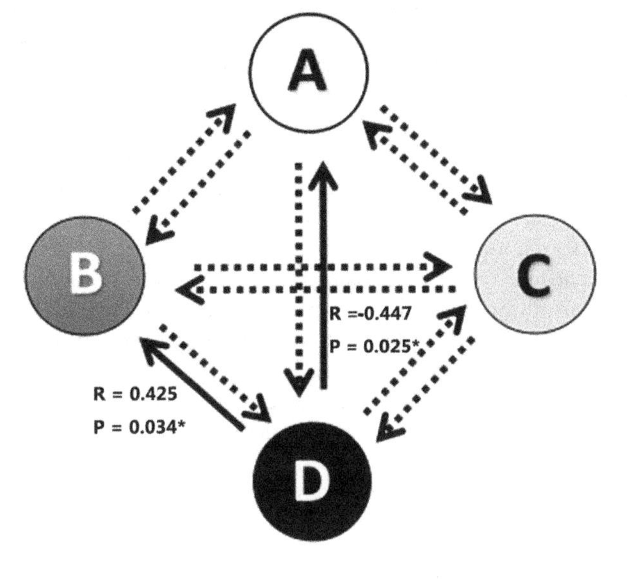

FIGURE 3 | Correlations between transitions of microstates and tinnitus subjective symptoms. * Indicates significant difference ($p < 0.05$). Solid arrow indicate significant correlation.

suggested that microstate B was associated with bilateral visual cortex areas. The increased coverage of visual network could indicate a compensatory mechanism secondary to ISSNHL. This result was similar to the finding by Campbell and Sharma (2013), who showed an alteration in cortical resource allocation with reduced activation in superior temporal gyrus and increased frontal activation in response to auditory input in hearing impairment subjects. These findings suggested that cortical

TABLE 3 | Correlations between changes of microstates and THI in ISSNHL patients with tinnitus.

THI scores	Microstate A R-value	Microstate B R-value	Microstate C R-value	Microstate D R-value
Coverage (%)	−0.358	0.197	−0.228	0.230
Lifespan (ms)	−0.235	0.137	−0.192	0.147
Amplitude (uV)	0.000	−0.411*	0.053	−0.117
Frequency	−0.417*	0.223	−0.193	0.257

*THI, Tinnitus Handicap Inventory; * Statistical significance.*

reorganization facilitated visual and auditory cross-modal recruitment for visual processing in acute period after ISSNHL.

In current study, no significant difference was found in microstate C or microstate D. Britz et al. (2010) suggested that microstate C was related to a salience network, which involved the detection and orientation of both internal and external stimuli. Microstate D was related to signals in the right-lateralized dorsal and ventral regions of the frontal and parietal cortex. These regions roughly corresponded to the central executive network (Britz et al., 2010). This result was similar to finding by Fan et al. (2015), who only found decreased auditory cortical changes in ISSNHL patients. The reason may be the short-term of duration which is not sufficient to trigger changes of cognitive functions. However, the study by Yang et al. (2014) reported not only the decreased temporal cortical activation, but also the reduced gray matter volume in non-auditory brain areas such as posterior cingulate gyrus, precuneus, and right parahippocampal gyrus. Xu et al. (2016) also showed that alterations of limbic, paralimic, and auditory networks existed in ISSNHL. The differences might be due to the heterogeneity in sample characteristics including age, gender, hearing ability, laterality of hearing loss, educational level, and research methodology (Fan et al., 2015).

According to the syntax analysis, a significant reduction in the probability of transition from microstate C to microstate A was found. The reduced transition from the salience network to the auditory network was likely due to the deficiency of auditory sensory input. In addition, the increase was significantly found in the transition probability from microstate C to microstate B. This result indicated the compensatory plasticity after hearing loss with increased activity from the salience network to the visual network. ISSNHL subjects began to rely more on the visual information to compensate for their hearing impairment (Rouger et al., 2012; Campbell and Sharma, 2014).

Another interesting finding was the negative correlations between THI scores and the frequency of microstate A as well as between THI scores and the transition probability from microstate D to microstate A. While a positive association was found between THI scores and the transition from microstate D to microstate B. These results indicated that the severity of tinnitus was related to the central plasticity after ISSNHL with alterations of auditory network and changes of cognitive function (Chen et al., 2017). The decreased transition from executive attention network to auditory network and increased to visual network indicated that generation of tinnitus in acute period may be also due to disruption of auditory and non-auditory network (Elgoyhen et al., 2015; Song et al., 2015). However, Cai et al., 2018) cannot found significant correlation between THI scores and any microstate parameters in chronical tinnitus. The reasons may be relied on the difference of the tinnitus duration and the alteration of central reorganizaiton between acute and chronic periods for tinnitus subjects. Further longitudinal study was needed to explore the central characteristics of ISSNHL and tinnitus at each stage to clarify the mechanism of the generation and maintenance of tinnitus.

All in all, the results of this study showed that there was a reduced activity in auditory network and an increased activity in visual network. In addition, the negative correlation between THI scores and frequency of microstate A was found. The findings of this study provided the theoretical basis for the treatment of ISSNHL patients with tinnitus. For example, repetitive transcranial magnetic stimulation (rTMS) is a non-invasive way that can modulate the excitability of the brain cortex (Formanek et al., 2018). And rTMS targeted on the abnormal central networks may be a strategy for the treatment of tinnitus. According to the findings of our study, we can improve the excitability of brain regions of auditory network by using rTMS, which may be beneficial for the improvement of symptoms of ISSNHL patients with tinnitus. Additionally, THI scores of acute tinnitus may reduce with the excitement of auditory network. More further studies were needed to explore the clinical effective treatment by using the findings of tinnitus associated researches.

Nonetheless, it is necessary to realize that ISSNHL is a heterogeneous disease with different hearing function, laterality and concomitant symptoms, such as tinnitus and vertigo (Fan et al., 2015). Therefore, it is hard to eliminate its heterogeneous factors completely even with the use of strict inclusion and exclusion criteria. Additionally, this study investigate aberrant dynamics of EEG microstates in ISSNHL patients with tinnitus and cannot separate the effects of acute tinnitus and ISSNHL on central nervous system respectively. Because of the perspectiveness and novelty of the study, our research has some limitations and its results need to dispose with caution. A further research with larger sample sizes and more subgroups comparisons is needed to clarify the central mechanism of ISSNHL and tinnitus in acute period.

CONCLUSION

There were several significant differences in temporal characteristics and syntax of EEG microstates between ISSNHL patients with tinnitus and the controls at rest. This study suggests that the alterations of central neural networks occur in acute stage of hearing loss and tinnitus. EEG microstate may be considered as a useful way to explore the brain network in ISSNHL patients with tinnitus.

ETHICS STATEMENT

This study was carried out in accordance with the recommendations of the Institution Review Board of the Sun Yat-sen Memorial Hospital with written informed consent from all subjects. All subjects gave written informed consent in accordance with the Declaration of Helsinki. The protocol was approved by the Institution Review Board of the Sun Yat-sen Memorial Hospital.

AUTHOR CONTRIBUTIONS

YxC and SC conceived and designed the research. YhC, JoL, and C-DW performed the experiments. JeL, NH, C-PD, and ML responsible for the data analysis. FZ, YxC, and YZ drafted the manuscript. All authors had a lot of contributions at all stages of preparing the manuscript.

ACKNOWLEDGMENTS

We want to acknowledge the proofreading from Dr. Christopher Wigham.

REFERENCES

Bing, D., Ying, J., Miao, J., Lan, L., Wang, D., Zhao, L., et al. (2018). Predicting the hearing outcome in sudden sensorineural hearing loss via machine learning models. *Clin. Otolaryngol.* 43, 868–874. doi: 10.1111/coa.13068

British society of audiology recommendation (1988). Descriptors for pure-tone audiograms. *Br. J. Audiol.* 22:123. doi: 10.3109/03005368809077807

Britz, J., Van De Ville, D., and Michel, C. M. (2010). BOLD correlates of EEG topography reveal rapid resting-state network dynamics. *Neuroimage* 52, 1162–1170. doi: 10.1016/j.neuroimage.2010.02.052

Cai, Y., Huang, D., Chen, Y., Yang, H., Wang, C., Zhao, F., et al. (2018). Deviant dynamics of resting state electroencephalogram microstate in patients with subjective tinnitus. *Front. Behav. Neurosci.* 12:122. doi: 10.3389/fnbeh.2018.00122

Campbell, J., and Sharma, A. (2013). Compensatory changes in cortical resource allocation in adults with hearing loss. *Front. Syst. Neurosci.* 7:71. doi: 10.3389/fnsys.2013.00071

Campbell, J., and Sharma, A. (2014). Cross-modal re-organization in adults with early stage hearing loss. *PLoS One* 9:e90594. doi: 10.1371/journal.pone.0090594

Chau, J. K., Lin, J. R. J., Atashband, S., Irvine, R. A., and Westerberg, B. D. (2010). Systematic review of the evidence for the etiology of adult sudden sensorineural hearing loss. *Laryngoscope* 120:1011. doi: 10.1002/lary.20873

Chen, J., Liang, J., Ou, J., and Cai, W. (2013). Mental health in adults with sudden sensorineural hearing loss: an assessment of depressive symptoms and its correlates. *J. Psychosom. Res.* 75, 72–74. doi: 10.1016/j.jpsychores.2013.03.006

Chen, Y., Wang, F., Wang, J., Bo, F., Xia, W., Gu, J., et al. (2017). Resting-state brain abnormalities in chronic subjective tinnitus: a meta-analysis. *Front. Hum. Neurosci.* 11:22. doi: 10.3389/fnhum.2017.00022

Dispenza, F., Amodio, E., De Stefano, A., Gallina, S., Marchese, D., Mathur, N., et al. (2011). Treatment of sudden sensorineural hearing loss with transtympanic injection of steroids as single therapy: a randomized clinical study. *Eur. Arch. Oto-Rhino-L* 268, 1273–1278. doi: 10.1007/s00405-011-1523-0

Elgoyhen, A. B., Langguth, B., De Ridder, D., and Vanneste, S. (2015). Tinnitus: perspectives from human neuroimaging. *Nat. Rev. Neurosci.* 16, 632–642. doi: 10.1038/nrn4003

Fan, W., Zhang, W., Li, J., Zhao, X., Mella, G., Lei, P., et al. (2015). Altered contralateral auditory cortical morphology in unilateral sudden sensorineural hearing loss. *Otol. Neurotol.* 36, 1622–1627. doi: 10.1097/MAO.0000000000000892

Formanek, M., Migalova, P., Krulova, P., Bar, M., Jancatova, D., Zakopcanova-Srovnalova, H., et al. (2018). Combined transcranial magnetic stimulation in the treatment of chronic tinnitus. *Ann. Clin. Transl. Neurol.* 5, 857–864. doi: 10.1002/acn3.587

Golden, H. L., Agustus, J. L., Nicholas, J. M., Schott, J. M., Crutch, S. J., Mancini, L., et al. (2016). Functional neuroanatomy of spatial sound processing in Alzheimer's disease. *Neurobiol. Aging* 39, 154–164. doi: 10.1016/j.neurobiolaging.2015.12.006

Ingber, L., and Nunez, P. L. (2011). Neocortical dynamics at multiple scales: EEG standing waves, statistical mechanics, and physical analogs. *Math. Biosci.* 229, 160–173. doi: 10.1016/j.mbs.2010.12.003

Jung, D. J., Park, J. H., Jang, J. H., and Lee, K. Y. (2016). The efficacy of combination therapy for idiopathic sudden sensorineural hearing loss. *Laryngoscope* 126, 1871–1876. doi: 10.1002/lary.25751

Kang, W. S., Yang, C. J., Shim, M., Song, C. I., Kim, T. S., Lim, H. W., et al. (2017). Prognostic factors for recovery from sudden sensorineural hearing loss: a retrospective study. *J. Audiol. Otol.* 21, 9–15. doi: 10.7874/jao.2017.21.1.9

Khanna, A., Pascual-Leone, A., Michel, C. M., and Farzan, F. (2015). Microstates in resting-state EEG: current status and future directions. *Neurosci. Biobehav. R* 49, 105–113. doi: 10.1016/j.neubiorev.2014.12.010

Kindler, J., Hubl, D., Strik, W. K., Dierks, T., and Koenig, T. (2010). Resting-state EEG in schizophrenia: auditory verbal hallucinations are related to shortening of specific microstates. *Clin. Neurophysiol.* 122, 1179–1182. doi: 10.1016/j.clinph.2010.10.042

Klemm, E., Deutscher, A., and Mösges, R. (2009). A present investigation of the epidemiology in idiopathic sudden sensorineural hearing loss. *Laryngo- rhino-otologie* 88:524. doi: 10.1055/s-0028-1128133

Koç, A., and Sanisoğlu, O. (2003). Sudden sensorineural hearing loss: literature survey on recent studies. *J. Otolaryngol.* 32:308. doi: 10.2310/7070.2003.11288

Konig, T., and Mellgarcia, L. (2009). "Statistical analysis of multichannel scalp field data," in *Proceedings of the EGU General Assembly Conference*, (Vienna), 169–180.

Kuhn, M., Heman-Ackah, S. E., Shaikh, J. A., and Roehm, P. C. (2011). Sudden sensorineural hearing loss: a review of diagnosis, treatment, and prognosis. *Trends Amplification* 15, 91–105. doi: 10.1177/1084713811408349

Lehmann, D., Faber, P. L., Galderisi, S., Herrmann, W. M., Kinoshita, T., Koukkou, M., et al. (2005). EEG microstate duration and syntax in acute, medication-naïve, first-episode schizophrenia: a multi-center study. *Psychiatry Res.* 138, 141–156. doi: 10.1016/j.pscychresns.2004.05.007

Lin, R. J., Krall, R., Westerberg, B. D., Chadha, N. K., and Chau, J. K. (2012). Systematic review and meta-analysis of the risk factors for sudden sensorineural hearing loss in adults. *Laryngoscope* 122, 624–635. doi: 10.1002/lary.22480

Micarelli, A., Chiaravalloti, A., Viziano, A., Danieli, R., Schillaci, O., and Alessandrini, M. (2017). Early cortical metabolic rearrangement related to clinical data in idiopathic sudden sensorineural hearing loss. *Hear. Res.* 350, 91–99. doi: 10.1016/j.heares.2017.04.011

Milz, P., Faber, P. L., Lehmann, D., Koenig, T., Kochi, K., and Pascual-Marqui, R. D. (2016). The functional significance of EEG microstates—Associations with modalities of thinking. *Neuroimage* 125, 643–656. doi: 10.1016/j.neuroimage.2015.08.023

Musiek, F., Guenette, L., and Fitzgerald, K. (2013). Lateralized auditory symptoms in central neuroaudiology disorder. *J. Am. Acad. Audiol.* 24:556. doi: 10.3766/jaaa.24.7.4

Newman, C. W., Jacobson, G. P., and Spitzer, J. B. (1996). Development of the tinnitus handicap inventory. *Arch. Otolaryngol. Head Neck Surg.* 122:143.

Nogueira-Neto, F. B., Gallardo, F. P., Suzuki, F. A. D. B., and Penido, N. D. O. (2016). Prognostic and evolutive factors of tinnitus triggered by sudden sensorineural hearing loss. *Otol. Neurotol.* 37, 627–633. doi: 10.1097/MAO.0000000000001049

Oh, J., Park, K., Lee, S. J., Shin, Y. R., and Choung, Y. (2007). Bilateral versus unilateral sudden sensorineural hearing loss. *Otolaryngol. Head Neck Surg.* 136, 87–91. doi: 10.1016/j.otohns.2006.05.015

Onton, J., Westerfield, M., Townsend, J., and Makeig, S. (2006). Imaging human EEG dynamics using independent component analysis. *Neurosci. Biobehav. Rev.* 30, 808–822. doi: 10.1016/j.neubiorev.2006.06.007

Rah, Y. C., Park, K. T., Yi, Y. J., Seok, J., Kang, S. I., and Kim, Y. H. (2015). Successful treatment of sudden sensorineural hearing loss assures improvement of accompanying tinnitus. *Laryngoscope* 125, 1433–1437. doi: 10.1002/lary.25074

Rouger, J., Lagleyre, S., Démonet, J. F., Fraysse, B., Deguine, O., and Barone, P. (2012). Evolution of crossmodal reorganization of the voice area in cochlear-implanted deaf patients. *Hum. Brain Mapp.* 33, 1929–1940. doi: 10.1002/hbm.21331

Schreiber, B. E. M., Agrup, C. P., Haskard, D. O. P., and Luxon, L. M. P. (2010). Sudden sensorineural hearing loss. *Lancet* 375, 1203–1211. doi: 10.1016/S0140-6736(09)62071-7

Seeley, W. W., Crawford, R. K., Zhou, J., Miller, B. L., and Greicius, M. D. (2009). Neurodegenerative diseases target large-scale human brain networks. *Neuron* 62, 42–52. doi: 10.1016/j.neuron.2009.03.024

Song, J. J., Vanneste, S., Schlee, W., Van de Heyning, P., and De Ridder, D. (2015). Onset-related differences in neural substrates of tinnitus-related distress: the anterior cingulate cortex in late-onset tinnitus, and the frontal cortex in early-onset tinnitus. *Brain Struct. Funct.* 220, 571–584. doi: 10.1007/s00429-013-0648-x

Stachler, R. J., Chandrasekhar, S. S., Archer, S. M., Rosenfeld, R. M., Schwartz, S. R., Barrs, D. M., et al. (2012). Clinical practice guideline: sudden hearing loss. *Otolaryngol. Head Neck Surg.* 146, S1–S35. doi: 10.1177/0194599812436449

Teismann, H., Okamoto, H., and Pantev, C. (2011). Short and intense tailor-made notched music training against tinnitus: the tinnitus frequency matters. *PLoS One* 6:e24685. doi: 10.1371/journal.pone.002468

von Wegner, F., Knaut, P., and Laufs, H. (2018). EEG microstate sequences from different clustering algorithms are information-theoretically invariant. *Front. Comput. Neurosci.* 12:70. doi: 10.3389/fncom.2018.00070

Wang, X., Fan, Y., Zhao, F., Wang, Z., Ge, J., Zhang, K., et al. (2014). Altered regional and circuit resting-state activity associated with unilateral hearing loss. *PLoS One* 9:e96126. doi: 10.1371/journal.pone.0096126

Xu, H., Fan, W., Zhao, X., Li, J., Zhang, W., Lei, P., et al. (2016). Disrupted functional brain connectome in unilateral sudden sensorineural hearing loss. *Hear. Res.* 335, 138–148. doi: 10.1016/j.heares.2016.02.016

Yang, M., Chen, H. J., Liu, B., Huang, Z. C., Feng, Y., Li, J., et al. (2014). Brain structural and functional alterations in patients with unilateral hearing loss. *Hear. Res.* 316, 37–43. doi: 10.1016/j.heares.2014.07.006

Zhang, G. Y., Yang, M., Liu, B., Huang, Z. C., Li, J., Chen, J. Y., et al. (2015). Changes of the directional brain networks related with brain plasticity in patients with long-term unilateral sensorineural hearing loss. *Neuroscience* 313, 149–161. doi: 10.1016/j.neuroscience.2015.11.042

Zhou, J., and Seeley, W. W. (2014). Network dysfunction in Alzheimer's disease and frontotemporal dementia: implications for psychiatry. *Biol. Psychiatry* 75:565. doi: 10.1016/j.biopsych.2014.01.020

17

White Matter Abnormalities of Auditory Neural Pathway in Sudden Sensorineural Hearing Loss Using Diffusion Spectrum Imaging: Different Findings From Tinnitus

Zihao Zhang[1†], Xiuqin Jia[1†], Xiaojiao Guan[2], Yi Zhang[3], Yuelei Lyu[1], Jing Yang[3] and Tao Jiang[1*]*

[1] Department of Radiology, Beijing Chaoyang Hospital, Capital Medical University, Beijing, China, [2] Department of Radiology, Beijing Shijitan Hospital, Capital Medical University, Beijing, China, [3] Department of Hyperbaric Oxygen, Beijing Chaoyang Hospital, Capital Medical University, Beijing, China

***Correspondence:**
Jing Yang
jyang2postgraduate@yeah.net
Tao Jiang
jiangt8166@hotmail.com

† These authors share first authorship

Sudden sensorineural hearing loss (SSNHL) is a complex and challenging emergency which requires evidence regarding its pathophysiological changes to guide the treatment. The aim of this study was to evaluate the white matter integrity of the auditory neural pathway in patients with unilateral SSNHL in acute stage by using diffusion spectrum imaging tractography. In the present study, 60 individuals with acute SSNHL (29 males, 50.7 ± 11.8 years) and 25 healthy controls (13 males, 45.2 ± 13.2 years) underwent diffusion spectrum imaging tractography and high resolution T1 structural examinations using a 3T magnetic resonance imaging system. The areas of the auditory neural pathway were defined as regions of interest (ROIs). The quantitative anisotropy (QA) and the generalized fractional anisotropy (GFA) were compared between the patients with unilateral SSNHL and controls in these ROIs. We further evaluated the correlation between the parameter values and hearing loss level. The mean pure tone audiometry of patients at the onset presentation was 63.2 ± 26.2 dB. The right-sided SSNHL was involved in 25 (41.7%) cases and the left-sided in 35 (58.3%) cases. The QA values in the contralateral medial geniculate body, the bilateral anterior corona radiata and the anterior limb of internal capsule were significantly reduced in SSNHL patients compared to controls. In addition, the decrease QA value of the contralateral medial geniculate body was related to the increase severity of disease, even after controlling potential confounding factors. The present study demonstrated that patients with SSNHL exhibited altered integrity of white matter in the auditory neural pathway. Furthermore, the decreased QA values in the contralateral medial geniculate body might predict the severity of this disease. In the present study, tinnitus has not been found to effect in brain area obviously.

Keywords: diffusion spectrum imaging, tractography, sudden sensorineural hearing loss, demyelination, white matter

INTRODUCTION

Sudden sensorineural hearing loss (SSNHL) is an emergency of otology. It is defined as hearing loss of at least 20 dB in two contiguous frequencies within 72 h (Editorial Committee of Chinese Journal of Otorhinolaryngology Head and Neck Surgery, and Chinese Academy of Otorhinolaryngology Head and Neck Surgery Branch, 2015). SSNHL is no longer a rare disease. Some studies have reported an annual incidence of 160 cases per 100,000 (Klemm et al., 2009). So far, the pathogenesis of the disease is unclear, and some theories have been put forward to explain this clinical problem, including the causes of infection, vascular occlusion, immune-mediated mechanisms, coagulation disorders, and breaks of labyrinthine membranes (Lin et al., 2015; Ajduk et al., 2017). The unknown etiologies lead to many empirical treatment options. Therefore, the pathophysiology of sudden hearing loss is of great significance for early targeted treatment of patients (Atay et al., 2016). However, the cause of SSNHL can be identified by conventional MR only in the presence of severe interruption of the interaxial auditory pathway, such as tumors and infarcts. In the absence of such lesions, it is difficult to determine the cause of SSNHL in conventional MR.

Conventional diffusion tensor imaging (DTI) is a sensitive and non-invasive method to evaluate white matter fiber. It can reconstruct fiber pathways to assessing the abnormalities in the central nervous system. In the past, some researches have already used DTI to study the neural changes in patients with sensorineural hearing loss (Lin et al., 2008; Wu et al., 2009; Huang et al., 2015; Tarabichi et al., 2017). But DTI cannot resolve the beginning and end point of nerve fiber or the fiber crossings in the white matter, resulting in artifacts and wrong tracts (Fernandez-Miranda et al., 2012). Diffusion spectrum imaging (DSI) (Wedeen et al., 2005; Hagmann et al., 2007; Schmahmann et al., 2007) is a modeless technique. It uses ODF (orientation distribution function) to consider the diffusion patterns in each voxel, which has been shown to better resolve the ambiguity of fiber crossing encountered in tractography. In DSI, diffusion weighted images are organized in the q-space (integral points of a cubic lattice) in the sphere and can be obtained in different directions. It proposes the probability density function (PDF) to describe the diffusion in each voxel, which specifies the three-dimensional distribution of microscopic displacements of water molecules (Wedeen et al., 2005). Through GQI (generalized q-sampling imaging) reconstruction, we can obtain the parameter of ODF, including quantitative anisotropy (QA) and generalized factional anisotropy (GFA). QA is defined as the number of anisotropic spins diffused along the fiber direction which can identify the fault structure well of cross fiber (Yeh et al., 2010). GFA reflecting the integrity of the neural fiber bundles and higher value indicates that more consistent diffusion direction of water molecules along fiber bundle (Tuch, 2004; Lo et al., 2011). Recently DSI is more and more used to study the brain nerve structure (Lin et al., 2014; Panesar et al., 2017; Yue et al., 2017). The aim of this study was to investigate the changes in the auditory neural pathway in patients with acute SSNHL by DSI tractography and measuring these DSI parameters.

MATERIALS AND METHODS

Patients

This prospective, clinical trial involved 25 healthy controls (13 males, 45.2 ± 13.2 years) and 60 patients (29 males, 50.7 ± 11.8 years) diagnosed with unilateral idiopathic SSNHL of Beijing Chaoyang Hospital, between November 2016 and July 2009. The criteria of SSNHL were the presence of a sensorineural hearing loss greater than or equal to 20 dB or exceed at least two adjacent audiometric frequencies, which developed within a few hours but no more than 2 weeks. The uniform radiological method was magnetic resonance imaging, but temporal computed tomography had also been obtained from some patients. Based on radiologic diagnosis combined with clinical information, all patients were diagnosed by clinicians. Exclusion criteria were as follows: (1) patients with abnormal anatomy, (2) otitis media, cholesteatoma and other middle ear diseases, or severe cerebral infarction and other neuromuscular or systemic diseases, (3) otological surgery history, (4) ototoxic medication history. The study was approved by the ethics committee of Beijing Chaoyang Hospital, Capital Medical University. Informed consent for the participation to the study was received from all patients.

Clinical Characteristics

The demographic data, smoking status, associated symptoms and comorbidities were recorded. The pure tone audiometry (interlacoustics; amplifon) was used to evaluate the hearing level in the sound insulation room. Hearing loss is defined as pure tone average (PTA), which follows the standards of the World Health Organization (WHO-1997).

Image Acquisition and Reconstruction

DSI data were acquired on 3T Prisma (Siemens) using a 64-channel coil. This involved a 15 min, 257-direction scan using a twice-refocused spin-echo EPI sequence and multiple q values (Wedeen et al., 2005) [echo time (TE) = 79 ms, repetition time (TR) = 7200 ms, voxel size = 2.2 × 2.2 × 2.2 mm, field of view = 220 × 220 mm, bmax = 3000 s/mm^2]. We also used high-resolution anatomical imaging as an anatomical comparison, using a 9-min T1-weighted magnetization-prepared rapid gradient echo (TE = 2.27 ms, TR = 2300 ms, 208 slices, flip angle = 8, field of view = 256 × 256 mm^2, voxel size = 1.0 × 1.0 × 1.0 mm^3). A generalized Q-sampling imaging approach (Yeh et al., 2010) were used to reconstructed DSI data. The orientation distribution functions were reconstructed to 362 discrete sampling directions with an average diffusion distance of 1.2 mm. CSF calibration uses spatial normalization to identify the position of CSF and use it as a free water diffusion to unify the amount of diffusion relative to it.

Fiber Tracking and Analysis

DSI Studio (an open-source diffusion MRI analysis tool available for free download at http://dsi-studio.labsolver.org) was used for fiber tracking. A whole brain seeding approach using multiple region of interest (ROI) masks was performed. In voxels with multiple fiber orientations, fiber tracking was initiated separately for each orientation, and fiber progression continued with a step size of 1.0 mm, minimum fiber length of 20 mm and turning angle threshold of 60. If multiple fiber orientations existed in the current progression location, the fiber orientation that was nearest to the incoming direction and formed a turning angle smaller than 60 was selected to determine the next moving direction (Fernandez-Miranda et al., 2012). To smooth each track, the next moving directional estimate of each voxel was weighted by 20% of the previous incoming direction and 80% of the nearest fiber orientation. This progression was repeated until the quantitative anisotropy of the fiber orientation dropped below a preset threshold (0.13–0.17 depending on the subject) or there was no fiber selected within the 60 angular range in the progression (Yeh et al., 2013). The ROI selected in the auditory neural pathway was shown in **Table 1**. The T1 and DSI images were spatially normalized into MNI. Then, an optical fiber tracking algorithm based on streamline is implemented by using DSI studio software, and the QA and GFA parameters of each ROI were obtained.

Statistical Analysis

Continuous variables were summarized as means (± standard deviation). For categorical variables, the percentages of patients in each category were calculated.

TABLE 1 | The selected ROI and how they were defined.

ROI	Template	MNI coordinates (x, y, z)	Volume (bilateral, cm^3)
Superior olivary nucleus	–	±13, −35, −41	5
Inferior colliculus	–	±6, −33, −11	5
Medial geniculate bodies	–	±17, −24, −2	8
Heschl	AAL	–	–
Superior temporal gyrus	AAL	–	–
Meddle temporal gyrus	AAL	–	–
Inferior tempotal gyrus	AAL	–	–
Anterior limb of internal capsule	JHU-WhiteMatter-Labels	–	–
Posterior limb of internal capsule	JHU-WhiteMatter-Labels	–	–
Anterior corona radiata	JHU-WhiteMatter-Labels	–	–
Posterior corona radiata	JHU-WhiteMatter-Labels	–	–
Lateral lemniscus	HCP842-tractography	–	–
Acoustic radiation	HCP842-tractography	–	–
Brodmann 41	Brodmann	–	–
Brodmann 42	Brodmann	–	–

Comparison of DSI parameters between patients and control group, with the usage of Student's t-test, as appropriate was to make the comparisons between subgroups of left-sided and right-sided. Results were corrected for multiple comparisons using the Bonferroni correction with a significance level of $p < 0.05/N$, where N was the number of ROIs.

Bivariate correlation and partial correlation analyses were used to identify the relationship between the DSI parameters of ROIs that exhibited significant differences and clinical severity assessment. A $P < 0.05$ was considered statistically significant. All data were analyzed by SPSS software version 19.0 of Windows (SPSS Inc. Chicago, United States).

RESULTS

Table 2 showed the patients' demographic details, clinical conditions and hearing test results at admission. In total, there were 60 patients included 29 males and 31 females, with a mean age of 50.7 ± 11.8 years. The right-sided

TABLE 2 | Characteristics of patients with unilateral sudden sensorineural hearing loss.

Clinical characteristic	Total	Left	Right
Age, Years			
Mean (SD)†	50.7 ± 11.8	50.1 ± 11.3	51.5 ± 12.7
Male sex, No. (%)	29 (48.3)	15 (42.9)	14 (56.0)
Side, NO. (%)			
Right	25 (41.7)	–	–
Left	35 (58.3)	–	–
Ever smoking, No. (%)	13 (21.7)	4 (11.4)	9 (36.0)
Length of hospital admission			
Mean (SD)	8.8 ± 4.3	8.9 ± 4.2	8.6 ± 4.5
Accompanying symptom, NO. (%)			
Tinnitus	52 (86.7)	30 (85.7)	22 (88.0)
Dizzy	21 (35.0)	16 (45.7)	5 (20.0)
Comorbidities, NO. (%)			
Cerebral ischemia	28 (47.5)	18 (51.4)	10 (41.7)
Hypertension	21 (35.0)	11 (31.4)	10 (40.0)
Type 1 or 2 diabetes	10 (16.7)	8 (22.9)	2 (8.0)
Hyperlipidemia	16 (26.7)	12 (34.3)	4 (16.0)
Severity assessment, NO. (%)			
Mild	16 (26.7)	8 (22.9)	8 (32.0)
Moderate	7 (11.7)	4 (11.4)	3 (12.0)
Moderate-severe	8 (13.3)	5 (14.3)	3 (12.0)
Severe	17 (28.3)	9 (25.7)	8 (32.0)
Extremely severe	12 (20.0)	9 (25.7)	3 (12.0)
Type			
Low-frequency hearing loss	10 (16.7)	7 (20.0)	3 (12.0)
High-frequency hearing loss	16 (26.7)	9 (25.7)	7 (28.0)
All-frequency hearing loss	33 (55.0)	19 (54.3)	14 (56.0)
Initial pta Score‡			
Mean (SD)	63.2 ± 26.2	66.1 ± 26.6	59.1 ± 25.7
Relapse, No. (%)	6 (10.0)	5 (14.3)	1 (4.0)

†Plus–minus values are means ± SD, ‡PTA means pure tone audiometry.

TABLE 3 | The QA† values obtained from the left and right sides of the subjects with SSNHL‡ and of the normal group.

Variable	Normal n = 25	Left-sided SSNHL n = 35	P§	Right-sided SSNHL n = 25	P§
Superior olivary nucleus					
Left	0.6726 ± 0.0784	0.5857 ± 0.1228	0.003	0.6597 ± 0.0889	0.589
Right	0.6584 ± 0.0910	0.5957 ± 0.1142	0.027	0.6209 ± 0.1027	0.178
Inferior colliculus					
Left	0.6531 ± 0.0800	0.6127 ± 0.1	0.100	0.6374 ± 0.0942	0.527
Right	0.6463 ± 0.0828	0.5897 ± 0.0994	0.024	0.6210 ± 0.0966	0.325
Medial geniculate bodies					
Left	0.6324 ± 0.0815	0.5721 ± 0.1042	0.019	0.5497 ± 0.0984	0.002*
Right	0.6328 ± 0.0924	0.5487 ± 0.0873	0.001*	0.5679 ± 0.1090	0.028
Lateral lemniscus					
Left	0.6531 ± 0.0816	0.6159 ± 0.0985	0.127	0.6103 ± 0.0888	0.082
Right	0.6486 ± 0.0688	0.5733 ± 0.1131	0.002*	0.6019 ± 0.0881	0.042
Anterior limb of internal capsule					
Left	0.5718 ± 0.0755	0.4957 ± 0.0741	P < 0.001*	0.4762 ± 0.0969	P < 0.001*
Right	0.5872 ± 0.0687	0.5101 ± 0.076	P < 0.001*	0.4934 ± 0.0941	P < 0.001*
Posterior limb of internal capsule					
Left	0.6947 ± 0.0635	0.6546 ± 0.1225	0.105	0.6501 ± 0.1007	0.067
Right	0.6907 ± 0.0551	0.6619 ± 0.1147	0.202	0.6580 ± 0.1175	0.213
Heschl					
Left	0.6055 ± 0.0917	0.5472 ± 0.1012	0.026	0.5492 ± 0.0822	0.027
Right	0.5793 ± 0.0764	0.4771 ± 0.1037	P < 0.001*	0.4813 ± 0.1449	0.004
Superior temporal gyrus					
Left	0.5975 ± 0.0762	0.5408 ± 0.0876	0.012	0.5337 ± 0.0851	0.008
Right	0.5942 ± 0.0732	0.5457 ± 0.087	0.027	0.5299 ± 0.0753	0.004
Meddle temporal gyrus					
Left	0.6021 ± 0.0752	0.5575 ± 0.0769	0.029	0.5421 ± 0.0764	0.007
Right	0.6065 ± 0.0721	0.5509 ± 0.0815	0.008	0.5504 ± 0.0794	0.012
Inferior temporal gyrus					
Left	0.5595 ± 0.0661	0.5104 ± 0.069	0.008	0.4937 ± 0.0778	0.002*
Right	0.5732 ± 0.0687	0.4997 ± 0.1027	0.003	0.5070 ± 0.0749	0.002*
Anterior corona radiata					
Left	0.5869 ± 0.0718	0.5218 ± 0.0743	0.001*	0.4967 ± 0.1073	0.001*
Right	0.5712 ± 0.0638	0.5154 ± 0.0661	0.002*	0.5069 ± 0.0633	0.001*
Posterior corona radiata					
Left	0.7173 ± 0.0815	0.6794 ± 0.11	0.150	0.6706 ± 0.1078	0.090
Right	0.7081 ± 0.0785	0.6668 ± 0.103	0.084	0.6660 ± 0.1086	0.124
Acoustic radiation					
Left	0.6728 ± 0.0784	0.6226 ± 0.0928	0.032	0.6156 ± 0.0916	0.022
Right	0.6617 ± 0.0827	0.6093 ± 0.0909	0.026	0.5945 ± 0.0942	0.010
Brodman 41 area	0.6350 ± 0.0790	0.5662 ± 0.1208	0.016	0.5720 ± 0.0766	0.006
Brodman 42 area	0.5483 ± 0.0793	0.4885 ± 0.0748	0.004	0.4877 ± 0.0782	0.009

*†QA means quantitative anisotropy. ‡SSNHL means sudden sensorineural hearing loss. §The left and right side of SSNHL patients was compared with normal group separately. *The asterisk denotes a significant effect under the conservative Bonferroni correction controlling the family-wise error rate among all the morphology effects hypothesis tests at 5% (adjusted threshold p = 0.05/28~0.002.*

SSNHL was involved in 25 (41.7%) cases and the left-sided in 35 (58.3%) cases. And 52 (86.7%) exhibited tinnitus, 21 (35.0%) exhibited dizzy as accompanying symptoms. Of total, 28 (47.5%) patients had cerebral ischemia and 21 (35.0%) had hypertension, which is the most common Comorbidities. Mean pure tone audiometry at the onset presentation was 63.2 ± 26.2 dB, of which 26.7% was mild, 11.7% was moderate, 13.3% was moderate-severe, 28.3% was severe and 20.0% was extremely severe. The audiogram type was low-frequency in 16.7%, high-frequency in 26.7%, and all-frequency in 55.0% cases.

DSI tractography measures of QA and GFA for each ROI of patients with SSNHL and controls were shown in **Tables 3, 4.** Compared with healthy group, the QA values of the contralateral (i.e., opposite to the lesion side) medial geniculate body, the bilateral anterior corona radiata and anterior

TABLE 4 | The GFA† values obtained from the left and right sides of the subjects with SSNHL‡ and of the normal group.

Variable	Normal *n* = 25	Left-sided SSNHL *n* = 35	*P*§	Right-sided SSNHL *n* = 25	*P*§
Superior olivary nucleus					
Left	0.0916 ± 0.0068	0.0876 ± 0.0157	0.187	0.0986 ± 0.0085	0.002*
Right	0.0906 ± 0.0077	0.0885 ± 0.0171	0.581	0.0943 ± 0.0072	0.085
Inferior colliculus					
Left	0.0941 ± 0.0055	0.0936 ± 0.0121	0.835	0.0982 ± 0.0046	0.007
Right	0.0941 ± 0.0054	0.0942 ± 0.0067	0.928	0.0966 ± 0.0060	0.132
Medial geniculate bodies					
Left	0.1002 ± 0.0096	0.0995 ± 0.0112	0.802	0.0944 ± 0.0109	0.048
Right	0.0976 ± 0.0080	0.0950 ± 0.0098	0.296	0.0950 ± 0.0111	0.355
Lateral lemniscus					
Left	0.0936 ± 0.0084	0.0945 ± 0.0067	0.653	0.0949 ± 0.0106	0.649
Right	0.0917 ± 0.0062	0.0906 ± 0.0090	0.589	0.0939 ± 0.0155	0.522
Anterior limb of internal capsule					
Left	0.0860 ± 0.0054	0.0825 ± 0.0071	0.046	0.0796 ± 0.0073	0.001*
Right	0.0883 ± 0.0042	0.0841 ± 0.0061	0.004	0.0826 ± 0.0069	0.001*
Posterior limb of internal capsule					
Left	0.1050 ± 0.0043	0.0996 ± 0.0068	P < 0.001*	0.1013 ± 0.0043	0.004
Right	0.1048 ± 0.0039	0.1006 ± 0.0054	0.001*	0.1015 ± 0.0075	0.062
Heschl					
Left	0.0898 ± 0.0103	0.0891 ± 0.0125	0.805	0.0895 ± 0.0079	0.898
Right	0.0829 ± 0.0147	0.0788 ± 0.0148	0.295	0.0804 ± 0.0221	0.637
Superior temporal gyrus					
Left	0.0938 ± 0.0045	0.0903 ± 0.0076	0.030	0.0899 ± 0.0085	0.050
Right	0.0929 ± 0.0069	0.0899 ± 0.0084	0.152	0.0888 ± 0.0063	0.032
Meddle temporal gyrus					
Left	0.0947 ± 0.0045	0.0935 ± 0.0061	0.412	0.0924 ± 0.0052	0.098
Right	0.0941 ± 0.0049	0.0907 ± 0.0068	0.039	0.0917 ± 0.0050	0.098
Inferior temporal gyrus					
Left	0.0864 ± 0.0094	0.0859 ± 0.0065	0.785	0.0857 ± 0.0080	0.779
Right	0.0890 ± 0.0070	0.0856 ± 0.0066	0.067	0.0859 ± 0.0093	0.199
Anterior corona radiata					
Left	0.0955 ± 0.0060	0.0908 ± 0.0076	0.012	0.0892 ± 0.0076	0.002*
Right	0.0940 ± 0.0048	0.0895 ± 0.0068	0.006	0.0886 ± 0.0064	0.001*
Posterior corona radiata					
Left	0.1127 ± 0.0095	0.1094 ± 0.0081	0.155	0.1106 ± 0.0098	0.456
Right	0.1120 ± 0.0104	0.1079 ± 0.0085	0.102	0.1090 ± 0.0113	0.348
Acoustic radiation					
Left	0.1033 ± 0.0071	0.1019 ± 0.0080	0.483	0.1011 ± 0.0092	0.345
Right	0.1017 ± 0.0077	0.0996 ± 0.0089	0.329	0.0995 ± 0.0095	0.363
Brodman 41 area	0.0969 ± 0.0040	0.0959 ± 0.0070	0.543	0.0958 ± 0.0070	0.534
Brodman 42 area	0.0845 ± 0.0088	0.0813 ± 0.0080	0.151	0.0811 ± 0.0078	0.153

*†GFA means generalized fractional anisotropy. ‡SSNHL means sudden sensorineural hearing loss. §The left and right side of SSNHL patients was compared with normal group separately. *The asterisk denotes a significant effect under the conservative Bonferroni correction controlling the family-wise error rate among all the morphology effects hypothesis tests at 5% (adjusted threshold p = 0.05/28̃0.002.*

limb of internal capsule were obviously reduced ($P < 0.002$) both for the left-sided and the right-sided SSNHL group (**Figure 1**). However, the GFA values of the bilateral anterior corona radiata and anterior limb of internal capsule decreased significantly only in the right-sided group ($P < 0.002$). No significant differences were identified between the left-sided SSNHL and controls. The QA and GFA values were compared between patients with or without tinnitus and dizziness by independent sample *t*-test, and found there was no difference in these areas ($p > 0.05$), as shown in the **Supplementary Table S1**.

We also further evaluated the correlation between QA values of these three brain regions and clinical severity assessment. **Table 5** showed the results of bivariate correlation analysis and partial correlation analysis. We found that the QA value of the contralateral medial geniculate body and the bilateral anterior limb of internal capsule were negatively correlated with the severity of hearing loss ($P < 0.05$).

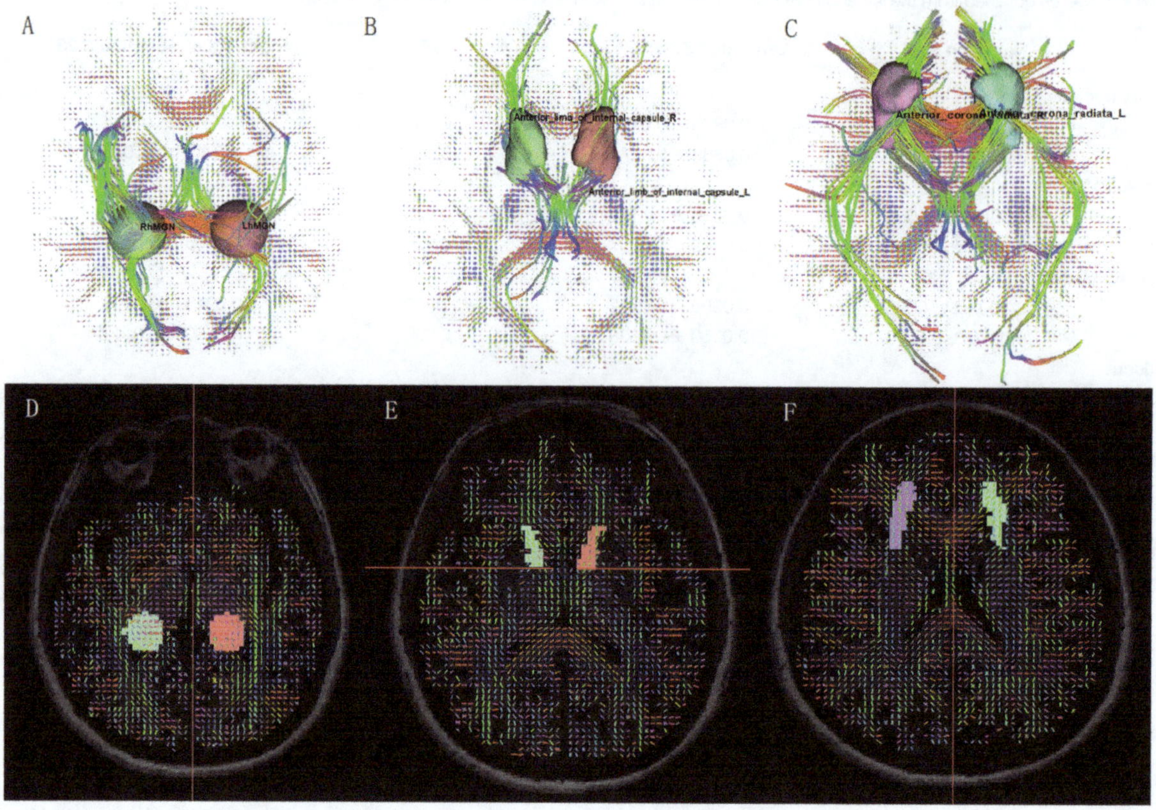

FIGURE 1 | Fiber tractography from diffusion spectrum imaging: **(A)** medial geniculate body; **(B)** anterior limb of internal capsule; **(C)** anterior corona radiata. ROI on QA map: **(D)** medial geniculate body; **(E)** anterior limb of internal capsule; **(F)** anterior corona radiata.

TABLE 5 | Results of correlation analysis between QA[†] values of selected brain areas and severity assessment of patients with sudden sensorineural hearing loss.

Variable	Left-sided SSNHL[‡]				Right-sided SSNHL			
	Bivariate correlation analysis	*P*	Partial correlation analysis*	*P*	Bivariate correlation analysis	*P*	Partial correlation analysis*	*P*
Medial geniculate bodies								
Left	–	–	–	–	−0.685	0	−0.675	0.002
Right	−0.447	0.007	−0.416	0.028	–	–	–	–
Anterior limb of internal capsule								
Left	−0.358	0.035	−0.135	0.494	−0.411	0.041	−0.380	0.120
Right	−0.350	0.039	−0.138	0.485	−0.345	0.092	−0.249	0.319
Anterior corona radiata								
Left	−0.290	0.090	−0.077	0.699	−0.250	0.228	−0.329	0.183
Right	−0.304	0.076	−0.088	0.656	−0.274	0.184	−0.243	0.332

[†]*QA means quantitative anisotropy.* [‡]*SSNHL means sudden sensorineural hearing loss.* **Partial correlation analysis controls age, gender, smoking, cerebral ischemia, hypertension, diabetes and hyperlipidemia.*

The partial correlation analysis, with controlling including age, gender, smoking, cerebral ischemia, hypertension, diabetes and hyperlipidemia, showed these relationships persisted in the contralateral medial geniculate body ($r = -0.416$, $P = 0.028$ for the left-sided group; $r = -0.675$, $P = 0.002$ for the right-sided group). The results of partial correlation analysis eliminated the influence of these possible risk factors.

DISCUSSION

To the best of our knowledge, the current study firstly applied a high angular resolution diffusion tractography technique of DSI to examine the changes of nerve fibers in the auditory neural pathway in patients with SSNHL. A major finding of this study was that compared with healthy controls, the QA values of the contralateral medial geniculate body, the bilateral anterior corona radiata and anterior limb of internal capsule in patients with sudden deafness were obviously reduced, notably in the contralateral medial geniculate body. In addition, the decrease of QA value of medial geniculate body was significantly related to the increase of disease severity, even after controlling other potential confounding factors. At present, tinnitus and dizziness have not been found to affect these areas on the auditory neural pathway.

The central auditory pathway starts from the cochlear branch of the eighth brain nerve. These synapses firstly enter the brain at the junction of pons and medulla oblongata, and transmit the encoded auditory nerve information to the cochlear nucleus of medulla oblongata. Most of the fibers project to the superior olivary nucleus on the opposite side, and a few of them project to the ipsilateral side. Then the fibers continue to go up through the lateral lemniscus. The efferent fibers project from the inferior colliculus to the medial geniculate body. Finally, the acoustic radiation from the medial geniculate body transmits the auditory information to the temporal cortex through the inner capsule (Wakana et al., 2004; Hernández-Zamora and Poblano, 2014).

The decrease of QA suggests the presence of a demyelinating process in the early stages of disease, and provides imaging verification for the pathophysiological process of the disease. It is worth noting that changes in medial geniculate body is more related to the severity of disease than that of anterior corona radiata and anterior limb of internal capsule. The more serious the disease is, the more damage of the medial geniculate body. This may be because of that the medial geniculate body is the converging site of multiple inputs from the lower auditory nuclei, which may be more sensitive to injury. Medial geniculate body has also been associated with tinnitus by inhibiting the afferent from the inferior colliculus and thalamic reticular nucleus. Thus, medial geniculate body has been used as the main target in some pharmacological experiments that enhance tonic inhibition in the treatment of auditory diseases (Richardson et al., 2012). Our finding may provide a marker for the treatment of SSNHL, which can be monitored during the treatment. On the other hand, the decrease of QA was only found in the contralateral medial geniculate body but not in the ipsilateral side. Previous studies have reported that the contralateral pathway is more important than the ipsilateral pathway in the processing of auditory stimulation (Khosla et al., 2003; Langers et al., 2005), of which 70–80% from the contralateral side and 20–30% comes from the ipsilateral side. Furthermore, the anterior limb of the internal capsule is believed to be involved in cognitive function, such as decision-making, attention, memory and so on (Nanda et al., 2017). For example, the change of QA value in this area may be related to the psychological problems such as anxiety and depression which often occur in patients with sudden hearing loss (Arslan et al., 2018). Furthermore, Husain et al. (2011) and Boyen et al. (2013) have also found similar changes of the frontal lobe which is associated with memory and higher cognitive processes in patients with hearing impaired. Consistently, the current finding of damage in the anterior limb of the internal capsule may imply the cognitive impairment in this disease.

Some previous studies have also supported the current findings. Huang et al. (2015) have found decreased FA values in regions along the auditory neural pathway using DTI in SSNHL patients, which suggests the presence of a demyelinating process in the underlying microstructures along the auditory pathway. In addition, Husain et al. (2011) also found the changes of thalamic anterior radiation, and corona radiata in patients with hearing loss, which is mainly manifested in the decrease of FA values of nerve fibers in the inner capsule. However, unlike Chang et al. (2004), Lin et al. (2008), and Wu et al. (2009) found in patients with long term sensorineural hearing loss, we did not found changes in the pathway of lateral lemniscus, olivary nucleus or subcortical inferior colliculus. This inconsistency may be due to their object of study was patients with long-term sensorineural hearing loss. Long-term hearing loss or compensatory mechanisms may lead to more extensive fiber damage (axon loss or demyelination). Other fiber expansion to the region may also lead to more disorder of white matter fiber. Consistent with Kim et al. (2009), patients in present study were in the acute stage of this disease, in which it may not occur such extensive injury or compensation in a short time. The current finding indicates that the course of disease may be related to the extent of brain nerve damage. With the prolongation of the course of disease, the range and degree of the injury will continue to progress. It suggests that early treatment may effectively control brain nerve damage and improve the prognosis of patients.

Tinnitus is the main complication of SNNHL. Previous studies have shown that the central auditory system is related to the production and maintenance of tinnitus (Noreña and Eggermont, 2003; Lanting et al., 2008), and tinnitus may also lead to changes in white matter and gray matter (Landgrebe et al., 2009; Benson et al., 2014). When compared to hearing loss patients without tinnitus, Boyen et al. (2013) have found increased gray matter volume in the primary auditory cortex in patients with tinnitus. The primary auditory cortex deals with simple auditory stimuli, such as pure tone and noise (Mirz et al., 1999). The increase of gray matter volume in primary auditory cortex may be related to continuous internal sound stimulation. In addition, Boyen et al. (2014) have further found the functional connection was significantly reduced between the inferior colliculus and the auditory cortex in patients with sensorineural hearing loss with tinnitus compared to patients without tinnitus, which suggests the thalamic dysfunction that affects the transmission of auditory information from hypothalamus to auditory cortex. However, other studies of sensorineural hearing loss have not found difference in functional connection between patients with and without tinnitus (Luan et al., 2019). Compared with normal people, Husain et al. (2011) have also found changes both in gray matter and white matter in the adjacent region of auditory cortex only in hearing loss patients with hearing loss alone and found no changes in patients with hearing loss and tinnitus, which suggests hearing loss has the greatest influence on neural tissue rather than tinnitus. Accordingly, in the present study, it was postulated that the brain area was less likely differentially affected between the two groups due to the short-term stage of patients with tinnitus that may not have a profound effect on brain regions like long-term tinnitus. Meanwhile, a small number of patients without tinnitus which limited the further clarification between the two groups in the present study. The relationship between hearing loss and tinnitus may be complex rather than simple superposition effect, which would be investigated in the further study.

Furthermore, Yeh et al. (2013) have compared FA, GFA, and QA, and found that QA is less sensitive to the partial volume effects of crossing fibers, free water, and non-diffusive materials. QA also has less noise, and the QA assisted traction imaging has better spatial resolution than the FA assisted and GFA assisted traction imaging. In this study, we also found the QA value showed significant difference between the SSNHL group and the control group, but the difference of GFA was not obvious, which supports that QA has advantage in reflecting the changes of white matter fibers. This also suggests that the demyelination of nerve fibers may be the main pathological change, while the nerve fibers are relatively intact.

There are several limitations to our study. First, our patients' data were obtained from one hospital, which may limit a generalized application of these findings. Secondly, the current study is a cross-sectional study involved in patients at acute stage. A longitudinal study is further required to clarify the white matter alteration along the course of this disease. Thirdly, the effects of concomitant symptom such as tinnitus, dizzy and psychological problems on brain structure and function needs further study.

CONCLUSION

In conclusion, the present study demonstrated that the microstructural damages in the auditory neural pathway, especially in the contralateral medial geniculate body that was related to the severity of the disease, exhibited in the acute stage of patients with SSNHL, This study provided imaging evidence for the brain changes and helped us understand the pathophysiological changes of diseases better. The QA value may be a potential biomarker of this disease, which can be used to quantitatively analyze the progress of the disease and medicinal efficacy.

ETHICS STATEMENT

The studies involving human participants were reviewed and approved by the Ethics Review Committee of the Beijing Chaoyang Hospital. The patients/participants provided their written informed consent to participate in this study.

AUTHOR CONTRIBUTIONS

ZZ and XJ contributed to research and writing. ZZ, XG, YL, and YZ contributed to study design and data collection. ZZ, XJ, and XG completed the reprocessing and data analysis. TJ and JY acted as an independent adjudicator for any discrepancies in this process and provided critical revision of the manuscript.

ACKNOWLEDGMENTS

We wish to thank the staff from the department of radiology and hyperbaric oxygen at Beijing Chaoyang Hospital.

REFERENCES

Ajduk, J., Ries, M., Trotic, R., Marinac, I., Vlatka, K., and Bedekovic, V. (2017). Hyperbaric oxygen therapy as salvage therapy for sudden sensorineural hearing loss. *J. Int. Adv. Otol.* 13, 61–64. doi: 10.5152/iao.2017.3185

Arslan, F., Aydemir, E., Kaya, Y. S., Arslan, H., and Durmaz, A. (2018). Anxiety and depression in patients with sudden one-sided hearing loss. *Ear Nose Throat J.* 97, 7–10.

Atay, G., Kayahan, B., Cinar, B. C., Sarac, S., and Sennaroglu, L. (2016). Prognostic factors in sudden sensorineural hearing loss. *Balkan Med. J.* 33, 87–93. doi: 10.5152/balkanmedj.2015.15216

Benson, R. R., Gattu, R., and Cacace, A. T. (2014). Left hemisphere fractional anisotropy increase in noise-induced tinnitus: a diffusion tensor imaging (DTI) study of white matter tracts in the brain. *Hear. Res.* 309, 8–16. doi: 10.1016/j.heares.2013.10.005

Boyen, K., De Kleine, E., Van Dijk, P., and Langers, D. R. M. (2014). Tinnitus-related dissociation between cortical and subcortical neural activity in humans with mild to moderate sensorineural hearing loss. *Hear. Res.* 312, 48–59. doi: 10.1016/j.heares.2014.03.001

Boyen, K., Langers, D. R. M., De Kleine, E., and Van Dijk, P. (2013). Gray matter in the brain: differences associated with tinnitus and hearing loss. *Hear. Res.* 295, 67–78. doi: 10.1016/j.heares.2012.02.010

Chang, Y., Lee, S., Lee, Y., Hwang, M., Bae, S., Kim, M., et al. (2004). Auditory neural pathway evaluation on sensorineural hearing loss using diffusion tensor imaging. *Neuroreport* 15, 1699–1703. doi: 10.1097/01.wnr.0000134584.10207.1a

Editorial Committee of Chinese Journal of Otorhinolaryngology Head and Neck Surgery, and Chinese Academy of Otorhinolaryngology Head and Neck Surgery Branch (2015). Guideline of diagnosis and treatment of sudden deafness (2015). *Chin. J. Otorhinolaryngol. Head Neck Surg.* 50, 443–447. doi: 10.3760/cma.j.issn.1673-0860.2015.06.002

Fernandez-Miranda, J. C., Pathak, S., Engh, J., Jarbo, K., and Friedlander, R. (2012). High-definition fiber tractography of the human brain: neuroanatomical validation and neurosurgical applications. *Neurosurgery* 71, 430–453. doi: 10.1227/NEU.0b013e3182592faa

Hagmann, P., Kurant, M., Gigandet, X., Thiran, P., Wedeen, V. J., Meuli, R., et al. (2007). Mapping human whole-brain structural networks with diffusion MRI. *PLoS One* 2:e597. doi: 10.1371/journal.pone.0000597

Hernández-Zamora, E., and Poblano, A. (2014). The auditory pathway: levels of integration of information and principal neurotransmitters. *Gac. Med. Mex.* 150, 450–460.

Huang, L., Zheng, W., Wu, C., Wei, X., Wu, X., Wang, Y., et al. (2015). Diffusion tensor imaging of the auditory neural pathway for clinical outcome of cochlear implantation in pediatric congenital sensorineural hearing loss patients. *PLoS One* 10:e140643. doi: 10.1371/journal.pone.0140643

Husain, F. T., Medina, R. E., Davis, C. W., Szymko-Bennett, Y., Simonyan, K., Pajor, N. M., et al. (2011). Neuroanatomical changes due to hearing loss and chronic tinnitus: a combined VBM and DTI study. *Brain Res.* 1369, 74–88. doi: 10.1016/j.brainres.2010.10.095

Khosla, D., Ponton, C. W., Eggermont, J. J., Kwong, B., Dort, M., and Vasama, J. (2003). Differential ear effects of profound unilateral deafness on the adult human central auditory system. *J. Assoc. Res. Otolaryngol.* 4, 235–249. doi: 10.1007/s10162-002-3014-x

Kim, D. J., Park, S., Kim, J., Lee, D. H., and Park, H. (2009). Alterations of white matter diffusion anisotropy in early deafness. *Neuroreport* 20, 1032–1036. doi: 10.1097/WNR.0b013e32832e0cdd

Klemm, E., Deutscher, A., and Mosges, R. (2009). A present investigation of the epidemiology in idiopathic sudden sensorineural hearing loss. *Laryngorhinootologie* 88, 524–527. doi: 10.1055/s-0028-1128133

Landgrebe, M., Langguth, B., Rosengarth, K., Braun, S., Koch, A., Kleinjung, T., et al. (2009). Structural brain changes in tinnitus: grey matter decrease in auditory and non-auditory brain areas. *Neuroimage* 46, 213–218. doi: 10.1016/j.neuroimage.2009.01.069

Langers, D. R. M., Dijk, P. V., and Backes, W. H. (2005). Lateralization, connectivity and plasticity in the human central auditory system. *Neuroimage* 28, 490–499. doi: 10.1016/j.neuroimage.2005.06.024

Lanting, C. P., De Kleine, E., Bartels, H., and Van Dijk, P. (2008). Functional imaging of unilateral tinnitus using fMRI. *Acta Otolaryngol.* 128, 415–421. doi: 10.1080/00016480701793743

Lin, H. C., Wang, C. H., Chou, Y. C., Shih, C. P., Chu, Y. H., Lee, J. C., et al. (2015). The correlation between lipoprotein ratios and hearing outcome in idiopathic sudden sensorineural hearing loss patients. *Clin. Otolaryngol.* 40, 355–362. doi: 10.1111/coa.12382

Lin, Y., Wang, J., Wu, C., Wai, Y., Yu, J., and Ng, S. (2008). Diffusion tensor imaging of the auditory pathway in sensorineural hearing loss: changes in radial diffusivity and diffusion anisotropy. *J. Magn. Reson. Imaging* 28, 598–603. doi: 10.1002/jmri.21464

Lin, Y. C., Shih, Y. C., Tseng, W. Y. I., Chu, Y. H., Wu, M. T., Chiu, M. J., et al. (2014). Cingulum correlates of cognitive functions in patients with mild cognitive impairment and early Alzheimer's disease: a diffusion spectrum imaging study. *Brain Topogr.* 27, 393–402. doi: 10.1007/s10548-013-0346-2

Lo, Y. C., Soong, W. T., Gau, S. F., Wu, Y. Y., Lai, M. C., Yeh, F. C., et al. (2011). The loss of asymmetry and reduced interhemispheric connectivity in adolescents with autism: a study using diffusion spectrum imaging tractography. *Psychiatry Res.* 192, 60–66. doi: 10.1016/j.pscychresns.2010.09.008

Luan, Y., Wang, C. X., Jiao, Y., Tang, T. Y., Zhang, J., and Teng, G. J. (2019). Prefrontal-temporal pathway mediates the cross-modal and cognitive reorganization in sensorineural hearing loss with or without tinnitus: a multimodal MRI study. *Front. Neurosci.* 13:222. doi: 10.3389/fnins.2019.00222

Mirz, F., Ovesen, T., Ishizu, K., Johannsen, P., Madsen, S., and Gjedde, A. (1999). Stimulus-dependent central processing of auditory stimuli: a pet study. *Scand. Audiol.* 28, 161–169. doi: 10.1080/010503999424734

Nanda, P., Banks, G. P., Pathak, Y. J., and Sheth, S. A. (2017). Connectivity-based parcellation of the anterior limb of the internal capsule. *Hum. Brain Mapp.* 38, 6107–6117. doi: 10.1002/hbm.23815

Noreña, A. J., and Eggermont, J. J. (2003). Changes in spontaneous neural activity immediately after an acoustic trauma: implications for neural correlates of tinnitus. *Hear. Res.* 183, 137–153. doi: 10.1016/s0378-5955(03)00225-9

Panesar, S. S., Yeh, F. C., Deibert, C. P., Fernandes-Cabral, D., Rowthu, V., Fernández-Miranda, J. C., et al. (2017). A diffusion spectrum imaging-based tractographic study into the anatomical subdivision and cortical connectivity of the ventral external capsule: uncinate and inferior fronto-occipital fascicles. *Neuroradiology* 59, 971–987. doi: 10.1007/s00234-017-1874-3

Richardson, B. D., Brozoski, T. J., Ling, L. L., and Caspary, D. M. (2012). Targeting inhibitory neurotransmission in tinnitus. *Brain Res.* 1485, 77–87. doi: 10.1016/j.brainres.2012.02.014

Schmahmann, J. D., Pandya, D. N., Wang, R., Dai, G., D'Arceuil, H. E., Crespigny, A. J. D., et al. (2007). Association fibre pathways of the brain: parallel observations from diffusion spectrum imaging and autoradiography. *Brain* 130, 630–653. doi: 10.1093/brain/awl359

Tarabichi, O., Kozin, E. D., Kanumuri, V. V., Barber, S., Ghosh, S., Lee, D. J., et al. (2017). Diffusion tensor imaging of central auditory pathways in patients with sensorineural hearing loss: a systematic review. *Otolaryngol. Head Neck Surg.* 158, 432–442. doi: 10.1177/0194599817739838

Tuch, D. S. (2004). Q-ball imaging. *Magn. Reson. Med.* 52, 1358–1372.

Wakana, S., Jiang, H., Nagae-Poetscher, L. M., van Zijl, P. C. M., and Mori, S. (2004). Fiber tract-based atlas of human white matter anatomy. *Radiology* 230, 77–87. doi: 10.1148/radiol.2301021640

Wedeen, V. J., Hagmann, P., Tseng, W. Y. I., Reese, T. G., and Weisskoff, R. M. (2005). Mapping complex tissue architecture with diffusion spectrum magnetic resonance imaging. *Magn. Reson. Med.* 54, 1377–1386. doi: 10.1002/mrm.20642

Wu, C. M., Ng, S. H., and Liu, T. C. (2009). Diffusion tensor imaging of the subcortical auditory tract in subjects with long-term unilateral sensorineural hearing loss. *Audiol. Neurootol.* 14, 248–253. doi: 10.1159/000191282

Yeh, F. C., Verstynen, T. D., Wang, Y., Fernández-Miranda, J. C., and Tseng, W. Y. I. (2013). Deterministic diffusion fiber tracking improved by quantitative anisotropy. *PLoS One* 8:e80713. doi: 10.1371/journal.pone.0080713

Yeh, F. C., Wedeen, V. J., and Tseng, W. Y. I. (2010). Generalized Q-sampling imaging. *IEEE Trans. Med. Imaging* 29, 1626–1635. doi: 10.1109/TMI.2010.2045126

Yue, B., Yong, W., Wei, W., and Yibao, W. (2017). The superior fronto-occipital fasciculus in the human brain revealed by diffusion spectrum imaging tractography: an anatomical reality or a methodological artifact? *Front. Neuroanat.* 11:119. doi: 10.3389/fnana.2017.00119

Neural Mechanisms of Hearing Recovery for Cochlear-Implanted Patients: An Electroencephalogram Follow-Up Study

Songjian Wang[1,2], Meng Lin[1,2], Liwei Sun[1,2], Xueqing Chen[3], Xinxing Fu[3], LiLi Yan[3], Chunlin Li[1,2] and Xu Zhang[1,2]**

[1] School of Biomedical Engineering, Capital Medical University, Beijing, China, [2] Beijing Key Laboratory of Fundamental Research on Biomechanics in Clinical Application, Capital Medical University, Beijing, China, [3] Key Laboratory of Otolaryngology Head and Neck Surgery, Beijing Tongren Hospital, Beijing Institute of Otolaryngology, Ministry of Education, Beijing, China

***Correspondence:**
Chunlin Li
lichunlin1981@163.com
Xu Zhang
zhangxu@ccmu.edu.cn

Background: Patients with severe profound hearing loss could benefit from cochlear implantation (CI). However, the neural mechanism of such benefit is still unclear. Therefore, we analyzed the electroencephalogram (EEG) and behavioral indicators of auditory function remodeling in patients with CI. Both indicators were sampled at multiple time points after implantation (1, 90, and 180 days).

Methods: First, the speech perception ability was evaluated with the recording of a list of Chinese words and sentences in 15 healthy controls (HC group) and 10 patients with CI (CI group). EEG data were collected using an oddball paradigm. Then, the characteristics of event-related potentials (ERPs) and mismatch negative (MMN) were compared between the CI group and the HC group. In addition, we analyzed the phase lag indices (PLI) in the CI group and the HC group and calculated the difference in functional connectivity between the two groups at different stages after implantation.

Results: The behavioral indicator, speech recognition ability, in CI patients improved as the implantation time increased. The MMN analysis showed that CI patients could recognize the difference between standard and deviation stimuli just like the HCs 90 days after cochlear implantation. Comparing the latencies of N1/P2/MMN between the CI group and the HC group, we found that the latency of N1/P2 in CI patients was longer, while the latency of MMN in CI users was shorter. In addition, PLI-based whole-brain functional connectivity (PLI-FC) showed that the difference between the CI group and the HC group mainly exists in electrode pairs between the bilateral auditory area and the frontal area. Furthermore, all those differences gradually decreased with the increase in implantation time.

Conclusion: The N1 amplitude, N1/P2/MMN latency, and PLI-FC in the alpha band may reflect the process of auditory function remodeling and could be an objective index for the assessment of speech perception ability and the effect of cochlear implantation.

Keywords: cochlear implant, independent component analysis, auditory function remodeling, phase lag index, functional connection, event-related potential

INTRODUCTION

Cochlear implantation (CI) is a well-established means to restore normal hearing for people with severe hearing impairment. Although the CI technology continues to advance, there remains a significant variability in speech perception performance among CI users (Paiva et al., 2016). Following CI implantation, the reacquisition of speech recognition ability is considered as the aim of CI rehabilitation (Mareike Finke et al., 2016). For CI users, behavioral measures such as the category of auditory performance score and speech intelligibility rating (SIR) score are the primary methods to evaluate speech perception ability and the effect of implantation. However, it is hard to apply these methods to people with prelingual deafness or prolonged auditory deprivation and children, since they are unable to complete the speech tests because of their poor communication and cognitive function (Mareike Finke et al., 2016). Accordingly, objective methods are needed to evaluate the effect of cochlear implantation.

Previous studies in CI users employed the electroencephalogram (EEG) to assess the status of the central auditory cortex. Event-related potentials (ERPs), also termed as long latency potentials, were previously used as indicators for auditory processing. The N1, P2, and mismatch negative (MMN) are the three widely studied components among the human auditory-evoked potentials. N1 occurs in the 60–150-ms interval after stimulus onset and is followed by the P2, a positive deflection peak at a latency around 150–250 ms (Roth et al., 1976). In addition, the MMN reflects a preattentive auditory-evoked potential (AEP) that occurs 100–300 ms following sound onset and is characterized by a front-central negativity elicited during any acoustically discriminable "deviant" sound within a regular stream of "standard" stimuli (C.W. Ponton et al., 2000; Näätänen et al., 2007; Moberly et al., 2016). N1, P2, and MMN are believed to be potential candidates in developing models of auditory information processing.

In our study, the first aim is to confirm the recovery of speech recognition and auditory perception in CI users. Previous studies suggest that ERPs can better assess the hearing recovery of patients with CI, compared with the auditory brainstem response (ABR), such that ERPs can reflect the brain activity induced by the auditory signal at the cortical level. In a seminal review on the auditory N1 wave (Roth et al., 1976), the N1 characteristic waveform detected at the central frontal electrode may originate from the auditory cortex on the dorsal surface of the temporal lobe. N1 activity is also related to the detection and discrimination of changes in the auditory environment. Besides, adult N1 would be sensitive to onset features, such as the slope and amplitude of the rise and fall of the auditory stimulus, which correlates with detection. The amplitude of N1 increases as the intensity of the standard stimulus increases, showing sensitivity to sound intensity in CI users. Previous research found that the amplitude of N1 significantly increases 1 year after CI implantation (Tremblay et al., 2014; Paiva et al., 2016). These changes may reflect the cortical reorganization of the auditory cortex and the restoration of binaural function in patients with CI.

Thus, we evaluated the change of N1 amplitude in the speech recognition experiment at different implantation stages to explore the speech recognition ability of CI users by comparing brain signals induced by standard stimuli and deviation stimuli.

The second aim is to investigate how the N1 and P2 representations changed in CI users with the increase of implantation time. Similar to N1, the P2 component also has clinical significance in evaluating the speech recognition function of CI users. P2 is thought to index some aspects of stimulus classification, reflecting processes of attentional allocation, perceptual learning, and event memory (Arnott et al., 2011; Paiva et al., 2016). It has also been suggested that its front-central prominence is related to the inhibitory process caused by irrelevant stimulation (Ferreira-Santos et al., 2012).

Accordingly, we measured the characteristic waveforms of N1 and P2 induced by standard and deviation stimuli in different implantation periods in the oddball paradigm. Besides, we compared the changes of the incubation period and amplitude at different implantation periods with the normal control group.

The third aim is to investigate MMN in CI users with the increase of implantation time. MMN is thought to represent the brain's response to a mismatch of the current stimulus representation and a trace in short- or long-term auditory memory (Naatanen et al., 2011; Moberly et al., 2016). Nina Kraus et al. (1993) studied MMN in nine postlingual adult CI users with/da/and/ta/. They found MMN in eight good CI users but not in one poor user. They suggested that MMN has the potential to be a promising objective measure for the effect of CI. Previous research found that MMN was recorded in 80–85% of good performers but in only 15–20% of poor performers. In addition, patients with higher SIR scores showed a longer duration of MMN compared with those who had lower SIR scores (Shomeshwar Singh et al., 2004). Roman's investigation showed that MMN was similar for well-performing CI users and normal hearing listeners in terms of speech perception, but abnormal or absent in poorly performing CI users (Roman et al., 2005).

As mentioned above, we used the area under MMN as the measurement of MMN, and the time point corresponding to half of the area is used as a measurement of MMN latency (Bishop and Hardiman, 2010; Moberly et al., 2016). We analyzed the changes in MMN amplitude and latency at different implantation periods and assessed the difference between CI users and healthy controls (HCs).

Fourth, we are interested in the changes in global brain functional connectivity during the recovery of CI users. A previous study found that in patients implanted with different kinds of cochlear implants, the results of behavioral tests showed consistency, but they showed differences in the functional connectivity of EEG (Maglione et al., 2017). The changes in EEG functional connectivity might better reflect the recovery of auditory function in patients with CI.

Consequently, we estimated functional connectivity using the phase lag index (PLI). By this way, we compared the difference in the EEG functional connectivity between CI users and HCs as the implantation time increased. The aim here was to find a functional connectivity measure sensitive to potential cochlear implant effects.

Overall, we measured the EEG response while patients with CI and HCs performed a speech recognition task in an oddball paradigm experiment. Using ERP analysis, we showed the time domain characteristic change in patients with CI as the implantation time increased. Using functional connectivity analysis, we demonstrated the remodeling of brain functional connectivity in patients with CI.

MATERIALS AND METHODS

Participants

Fifteen HC participants (nine males, ranging from 22 to 30 years old) and 10 postlingual deafened CI users (five males, ranging from 19 to 52 years old) took part in the experiment. Participants in both groups were right-handed and had no history of neurological or psychiatric disorders, or any cognitive impairment. The CI users wound make an appointment to activate the device about a month after recovery from cochlear surgery. At this point, we would adjust the stimulation sound at different pure-tone frequencies to ensure the effectiveness of the device in the patient. The HC participants were age-matched with CI users ($P = 0.19$, see **Table 1**). Audiometry and otoscopy were carried out for the HC participants at enrolment. Pure-tone audiometry testing was used to measure the average of the pure-tone hearing threshold (0.5, 1, 2, and 4 kHz), also known as pure-tone average (PTA). PTA lower than 20 dB is defined as normal hearing. All participants in the normal group had normal hearing. The HC participants were examined in two recording sessions that were 2 months apart. For all CI users, speech perception tests were performed before cochlear implantation, when the device was activated, and 90/180 days after the device was activated. **Tables 1, 2** show the demographic information for CI users and HC participants. The Medical Research Ethics Committee of Capital Medical University (Beijing, China) approved the study protocol in accordance with the recommendations of the Declaration of Helsinki for investigation of human participants. All participants provided written informed consent after being informed of the study details.

Speech Perception Test

Speech perception was evaluated by an audiologist who read the "Mandarin Vocabulary Adjacent Monosyllable Test Vocabulary" and "Mandarin Vocabulary Adjacent Two-syllable Test Vocabulary" to the participants by an amplifier equipment. The speech materials were presented at a comfortable level of 65 dB sound pressure level (SPL). Participants were asked to verbally repeat what they heard during the test. Eventually, the scores were calculated according to the percentage of words repeated properly. Furthermore, the speech perception tests were performed in CI users when the device was activated and 90 and 180 days after the device was activated.

TABLE 1 | Demographic information for HC subjects and CI users.

Measure	HC ($n = 15$)		CI ($n = 10$)		Statistics
	Mean	SD	Mean	SD	*P*
Age (years)	23.9	2.4	31.4	11	0.19
Gender (male)	9	n.a.	5	n.a.	0.77

HC, healthy control; CI, cochlear implant.

Stimuli and Task in the EEG/ERP Experiment

The oddball stimuli paradigm (Emmendorfer et al., 2020; Teixeira-Santos et al., 2020) with speech stimuli (350 ms duration with a 10-ms rise and fall time) was used in this study (**Figure 1**). The stimuli were delivered *via* E-Prime 2.0 (Psychology Software Tools, Inc.) and through two loudspeakers at both ears at a comfortable level of 65 dB SPL. The distance from the two loudspeakers to the participants was 100 cm. The two loudspeakers were positioned side to side and 45° to the ears. A standard stimulus/ba/was presented in 80% of the trials, together with a target stimulus/da/in 20% of the trials. There were a total of 1,000 auditory stimuli with 1,000 ms interstimulus intervals in the whole task.

EEG Data Recording and Preprocessing

During the experiment, participants were instructed to sit on a comfortable chair and watch a silent movie clip in a shielded and sound-attenuated room. They were asked to ignore the auditory stimulus category information and avoid excessive eye and body movements. They were given a short break after 500 auditory stimuli to change body position and keep alert during the test. EEG was continuously recorded by a Geodesic EEG, Inc., (EGI) system through a precabled high-density 128-channel HydroCel Geodesic Sensor Net (HCGSN-128) referenced to the vertex. The sampling rate was 500 Hz and electrode impedances were kept at or below 5 kΩ according to the recommended value for the system. The recorded signals for all the electrodes were referenced to the vertex electrode (Cz).

Electroencephalogram data were processed using EEGLAB 12.02 Toolbox[1] in MATLAB (R2013a; MathWorks, Inc.[2] and custom scripts for batch processing. First, data were down-sampled to 250 Hz and filtered from 0.5 to 40 Hz using a short non-linear infinite impulse response filter. Second, the channel location file of the EGI system was imported. The EEG data were reviewed to delete bad channels. In order to reduce highly correlated signal from nearby electrodes, we down-sampled the data to the 10–10 international electrode system, resulting in 67 electrode channels (Xu et al., 2018; Furlong et al., 2020). Third, independent component analysis (ICA) was applied to the remaining data. Independent components (ICs) representing eyeblinks and heartbeats were visually identified and then removed from all datasets. The ICA procedure was done by the Infomax algorithm in EEGLAB. Afterward, these datasets were segmented into epochs from −200 to 700 ms relative to sound onset. The prestimulus interval (−200 to 0 ms) was used for baseline subtraction. Besides, the onset of CI stimulation evokes an electrical artifact and therefore inevitably

[1] https://sccn.ucsd.edu/eeglab/
[2] https://www.mathworks.com/

TABLE 2 | Demographics of CI users.

Subject	Gender	Age (years)	Ear implanted	CI experience (days)	Implant brand	Speech processing strategy
CI1	M	33	R	180	MED-EL	FSP
CI2	M	41	R	180	MED-EL	FSP
CI3	F	24	L	180	MED-EL	FSP
CI4	F	31	R	180	MED-EL	FSP
CI5	M	43	R	180	MED-EL	FSP
CI6	F	52	L	180	MED-EL	FSP
CI7	F	21	L	180	MED-EL	FSP
CI8	M	21	L	180	MED-EL	FSP
CI9	F	29	L	180	MED-EL	FSP
CI10	M	19	L	180	MED-EL	FSP

CI, cochlear implant; FSP, fine structure processing.

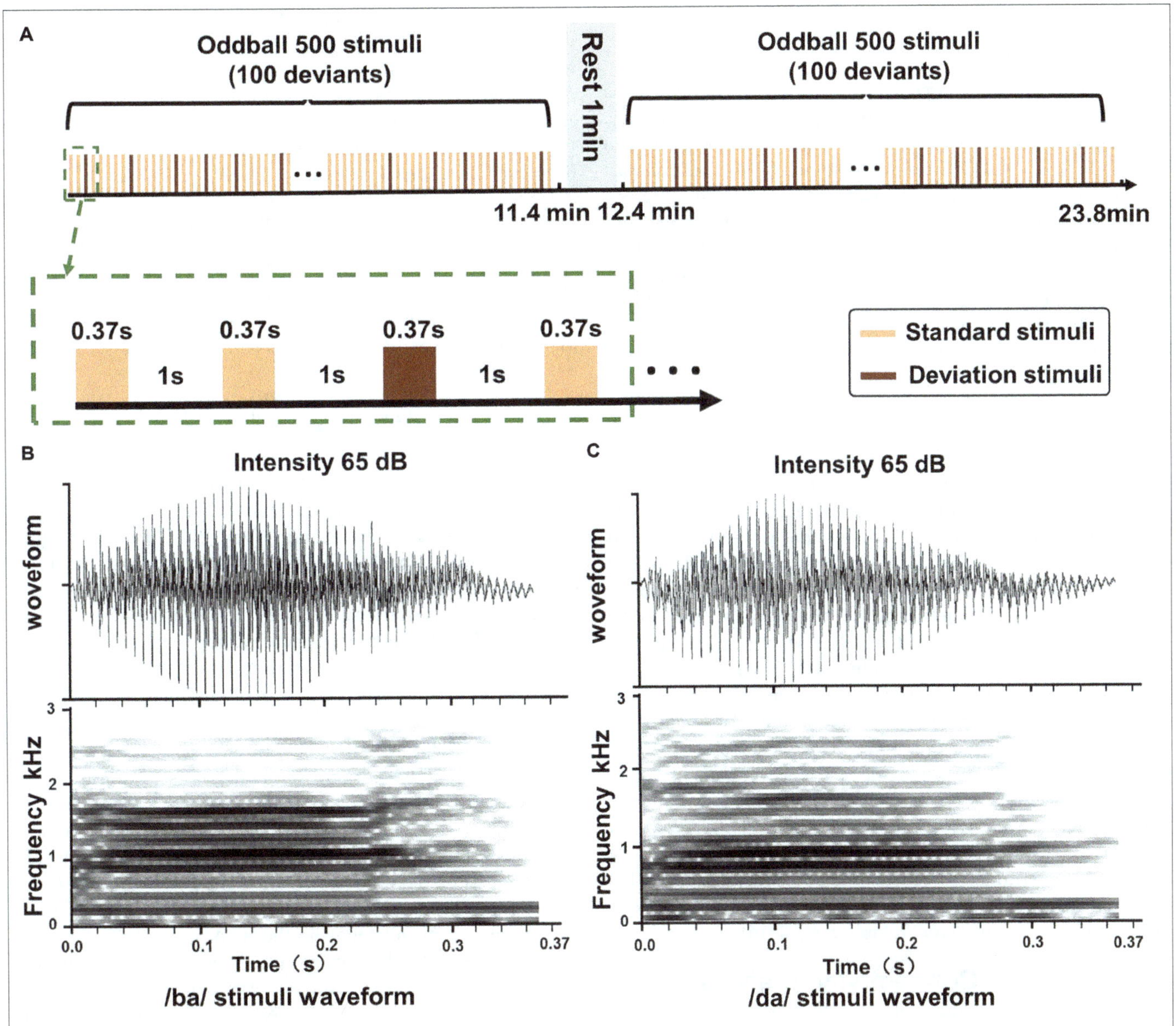

FIGURE 1 | The oddball stimuli pattern and speech stimuli. **(A)** The standard stimulus and the deviation stimulus in the oddball paradigm. **(B)** The duration and intensity of the sound/ba/stimuli. **(C)** The duration and intensity of the sound/da/stimuli.

corrupts the EEG signal. The CI artifact may largely be due to the radio frequency transmission of the signal to the receiver. Then, CI-artifact-related ICs were identified using the CI Artifact Correction (CIAC) algorithm, a plug-in in EEGLAB (Viola et al., 2009, 2011, 2012).

In our study, the CI-artifact-related ICs were selected both by CIAC and manual selection. The CI-artifact-related ICs selected by CIAC were not complete in some cases. Therefore, if the reconstruction of the individual ERPs was not reasonable after CIAC, the remaining CI-artifact-related ICs were selected manually based on the characteristics of the waveform and brain topographic maps of the ICs. The epochs contaminated by head movement were identified visually and rejected. After artifact rejection, about 700 EEG trials on average remained for standard stimuli and about 170 EEG trials on average remained for target stimuli.

ERP Analysis

Event-related potentials were calculated by averaging epochs across participants for standard and target stimuli, respectively. The largest ERPs were found in the front-central region. The ERPs at FCz, C3, and C4 were also obtained for further analysis. Measurements of N1 and P2 peak amplitude were extracted for each participant and condition. N1 peak amplitude and latency were extracted as the minimum voltage in the 60–150-ms poststimulus interval. P2 peak and latency were extracted as the maximum voltage in the 150–250-ms (Roth et al., 1976) poststimulus interval at FCz, C3, and C4. Then, we calculated the brain topographic maps of N1 and P2 within ± 5 ms of the peaks.

MMN Analysis

The difference in waveforms was also calculated between standard and target stimuli to obtain the MMN component. A valid MMN was identified when (1) a region of negativity was visibly confirmed from the differential waveform (deviant minus standard) and (2) its peak was consistent with the MMN topography (frontocentral negativity with reversals in lower temporal-posterior channels). For individuals, we performed the t test between the deviant and standard waveforms within the time window of 0–360 ms by sliding a 15-ms window with a step of 4 ms. The MMN onset was taken as the latency at which the t test (Bonferroni corrected for the number of executions) became significant. The MMN offset was taken as the latency at which the t test was no longer significant. Then, we calculated the area under the curve for the differential waveform (deviant minus standard) from the MMN onset to the MMN offset. The MMN area was used as a measurement of MMN magnitude. MMN latency was determined to be the time point that corresponded to the 50% of the area under the curve (Luck and Hillyard, 1990; Bishop and Hardiman, 2010; Moberly et al., 2016).

PLI Functional Connectivity Analysis

We analyzed PLIs in the alpha (8–13 Hz) frequency bands with time period selected at 0–450 ms. We calculated the spectral density using fast Fourier transform, extracted phase information, calculated the phase difference between electrodes, and extracted the phase difference matrix. Subsequently, we made a correlation matrix from individual PLI values using a customized code in MATLAB (Kral et al., 2017; Ueda et al., 2020).

After preprocessing, we calculated EEG data with dimensions $E \times T \times S$ (where E represents the number of electrodes, T represents the number of points in each segment, and S represents the number of segments). Each electrode pair had a PLI value at each time–frequency point. To calculate the PLI of electrode i and electrode k, we first obtain the S segment time–frequency information of the EEG signals by the short-time Fourier change

$$X(n, \omega) = \sum_{\tau=-\infty}^{\infty} x(\tau)h(n-\tau)e^{-jw\tau} \quad (1)$$

where $x(\tau)$ indicates the input EEG signal at time τ , and $h(\tau)$ indicates the length Hamming window function. The window length we chose in our research was 0.4 s with a step size of 0.4 ms. $X(n, \omega)$ is the two-dimensional function of time and frequency. At this point, we have obtained S time–frequency matrices storing phase information. We then estimated the time series of phase differences across electrodes as:

$$\Delta\phi_{i,k}(n) = \phi_i(n) - \phi_k(n) \quad (2)$$

where $\phi_i(n)$ and $\phi_k(n)$ indicate the phase value of the i electrode and the k electrode at time n (Nobukawa et al., 2019). Next, the functional connectivity was calculated as the consistency in the distribution of instantaneous phase differences $\Delta\phi_{i,k}(n)$ defined as:

$$\text{PLI} = \left| \frac{1}{S} \sum_{s=1}^{S} \text{sig}h[\Delta\phi(n_s)] \right| \quad (3)$$

where the consistency of the phase difference of S segments was examined (Zhang et al., 2018; Nobukawa et al., 2019).

The PLI ranges between 0 and 1. If the PLI is 0, the two signals are either not coupled or are coupled with a phase difference centered at approximately 0 mod π. If the PLI is 1, the two signals are perfectly phase locked at a value of $\Delta\phi$, which is different from 0 mod π. When this non-zero phase locking is strong, the PLI will be large. However, it is worth noting that the PLI does not indicate which of the two signals is leading in phase (Zhang et al., 2018).

Statistical Analysis

In each group [HC participants and CI users at three time points: as the device was activated (CI-1), 90 (CI-90), and 180 (CI-180) days after device activation], the ERP characteristics (including amplitude and latency) of the standard stimulus and deviation stimulus were tested by paired two-sample t test. One-way ANOVA analysis was performed separately on mean amplitude and mean latency on the factor group (HC, CI-1, CI-90, and CI-180). Besides, we performed the variance homogeneity test to test whether our data was variance homogeneous and $P > 0.05$ was considered homogeneous of variance. The least significant difference (LSD) method was used to correct multiple comparisons between pairs. These analyses were conducted on MMN, N1, and P2 components for both standard and target stimuli to detect any difference in amplitude and latency between HC participants and CI users at the three time points. A statistical significance level of 0.05 was considered significant, and statistical analyses were performed with SPSS 22.0.

The functional connection analysis between groups used the two-sample t test under GRETNA,[3] and $P < 0.005$ was considered a significant difference.

RESULTS

Behavioral Result

The speech recognition scores (**Figure 2**) of the HCs (95.4 ± 4.6) were significantly higher than the speech recognition scores measured in CI users (CI-1: 23.4 ± 17.3, CI-90: 42.3 ± 19.1, and CI-180: 59.6 ± 17.5). The score of the CI users gradually approximated to the HCs as the implantation time increased. The results showed that as the implantation time increased, the speech recognition level of cochlear implanters gradually increased.

ERP Components—Comparison of Standard Stimulus and Deviation Stimulus

We analyzed the FCz ERPs induced by the standard stimulus and deviation stimulus in CI users when the device was activated, 90 days after device activation, and 180 days after device activation and the HC group. The changes in the latency and amplitude of N1 and P2 induced by standard stimulation and deviation stimulation in each group were compared. The ERP characteristics of the standard and the deviation stimulus did not show a significant difference in the CI-1 group. However, the amplitude of N1 showed a significant difference ($P < 0.05$) between standard and the deviation stimulus in the CI-90 (−1.9 ± 1.2 and −3.6 ± 2.4, $t = 3.4$, $P = 0.008$) and CI-180 (−2.2 ± 1.4 and −3.5 ± 2.4, $t = 2.3$, $P = 0.046$) groups.

[3]https://www.nitrc.org/projects/gretna/

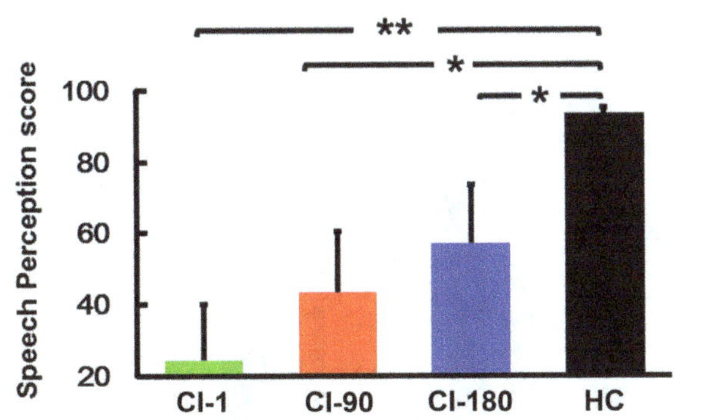

FIGURE 2 | Speech perception score within groups, where the green histogram represents when the device is activated, the red histogram represents 90 days after device activation, the blue histogram represents 180 days after device activation, and the black histogram represents healthy controls. The vertical black line means standard deviation; *$P < 0.05$ and **$P < 0.001$.

The difference was also shown in the HC group (−1.86 ± 0.9 and −3.2 ± 1.2, $t = 6.9$, $P < 0.001$) (**Figure 3**). Besides, the brain topographic maps of CI users were recovering gradually compared with the HCs.

ERP Components—Comparison Between the CI Group and the HC Group

We respectively analyzed the latency and amplitude of N1/P2 of FCz, C3, and C4 electrodes induced by standard and deviation stimuli. The results of FCz ERPs showed that the latency of N1/P2 in the CI group gradually approximated to the HC group as the implantation time increased regardless of standard stimulus or deviation stimulus (**Figure 4**). For the standard stimulus, the ANOVA analysis showed that there were significant differences in the latency of N1 ($F = 2.9$ and $P = 0.04$) and P2 ($F = 5.1$ and $P = 0.004$) among the four groups (CI-1, CI-90, CI-180, and HC). The results of N1 latency showed that CI-1 and HC were significantly different ($P = 0.01$), but CI-90 and CI-180 are not significantly different from HC. The results of P2 latency showed that CI-1 and HC and CI-90 and HC were significantly different ($P < 0.001$ and $P = 0.01$), but CI-180 is not significantly different from HC. For the deviation stimulus, the N1/P2 latency showed similar results except that CI-180 and HC were statistically different in P2 latency ($P = 0.01$). However, no similar result was found in the comparison of the amplitude of N1/P2.

Besides, for the ERPs of C3 (**Figures 5A,B**) and C4 (**Figures 5C,D**) electrodes, we did the same analysis as the FCz electrode. The results showed that the N1/P2 latency and amplitude characteristics of C3 and C4 electrodes are similar as those of the FCz electrode. The N1/P2 latency of CI users is longer than that of the HC group and approaches to the HC group regularly.

MMN—Comparison Between CI Users and HC

We analyzed the average MMN waveforms of the FCz electrodes (**Figure 6B**), and also we calculated the MMN area and latency corresponding to half of the area at the individual level. After that, we analyzed the topographic maps of the brain corresponding to the latency ±5 ms and compared the differences in the MMN area and latency between CI users and HCs in different periods by the one-way ANOVA test. It can be seen in **Figure 6** that brain topographic maps of the MMN waveform in CI users with the device activated for 180 days were closer to those of NH participants (**Figure 6A**). The statistical results of the MMM area showed that CI users and healthy subjects did not show any difference, but the latency of MMN showed significant differences ($F = 3.5$ and $P = 0.02$) (**Figure 6C**). The CI-1, CI-90, and CI-180 groups contrasted with the HC group showed significant differences ($P = 0.01$, $P = 0.017$, and $P = 0.028$). Besides, the results also showed that the MMN latency of CI users approached to the HC group with the increase of implantation time.

PLI Functional Connection

Figures 7A,B show the standard stimulus PLI for the HC group and CI group and their differences. The two-sample t test

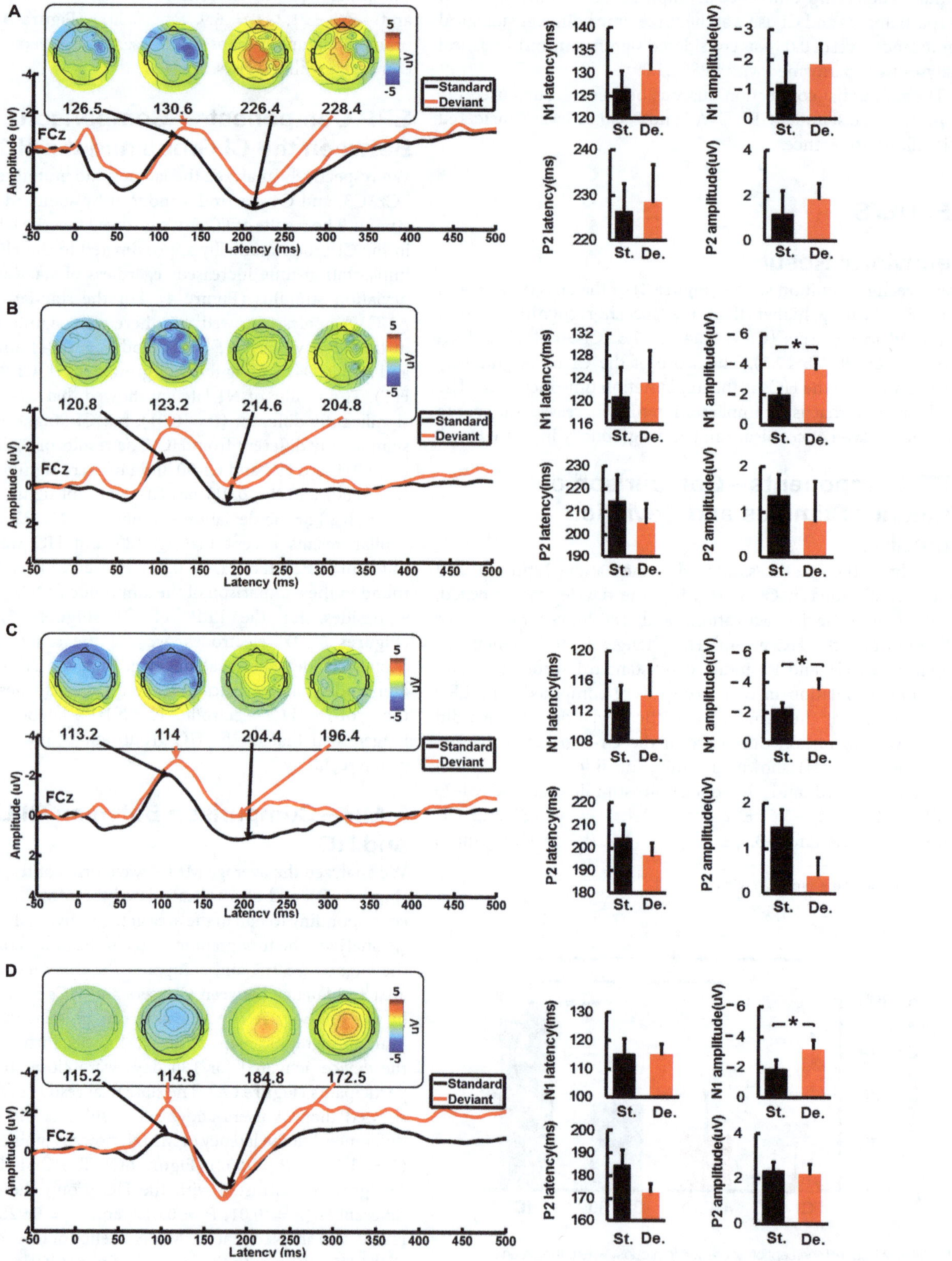

FIGURE 3 | The average waveforms of the standard stimulus and the deviation stimulus at the FCz electrode. The topographic map of the N1 and P2 feature points, and the comparison of the amplitude and the latency of the standard stimulus and the deviation stimulus for CI users and the HC group. **(A)** When the device is activated, **(B)** 90 days after device activation, **(C)** 90 days after device activation, and **(D)** healthy controls. St., standard stimulus; De., standard stimulus. The vertical black line means standard error; $^{*}P < 0.05$.

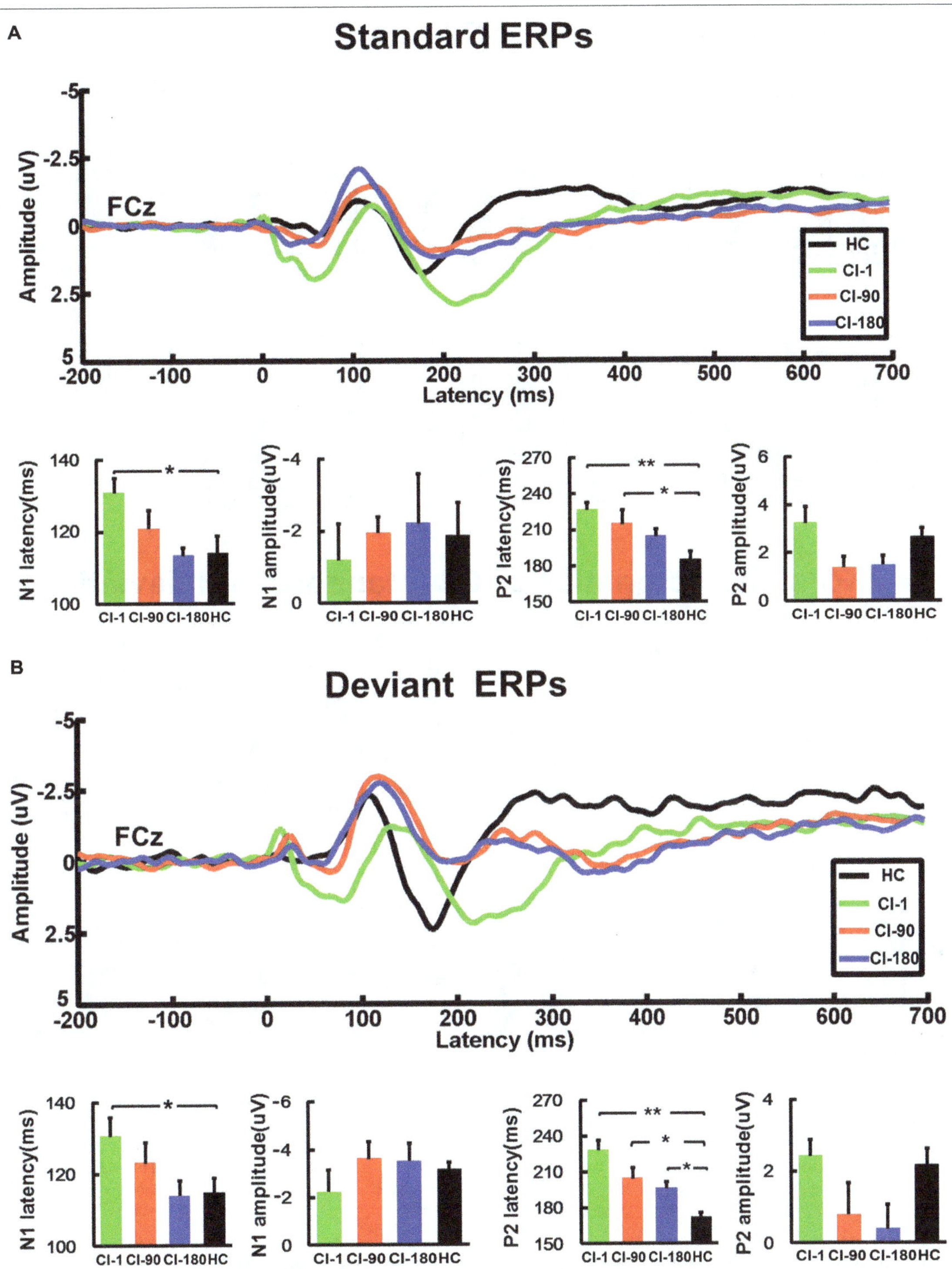

FIGURE 4 | The average standard and deviant ERP waveforms of the FCz electrode and the comparison of the amplitude and the latency of the N1/P2 for CI users and the HC group. **(A)** The standard ERPs and **(B)** the deviant ERPs. The vertical black line means standard error; $^{*}P < 0.05$ and $^{**}P < 0.001$. CI-1, when the device is activated; CI-90, 90 days after device activation; CI-180, 180 days after device activation; HC, healthy controls.

revealed the significantly reduced PLI values for the CI group (**Figure 7C**). Significantly different electrode pairs between the CI group and the HC group gradually decreased as the implantation time increases, especially for several left and right auditory areas and frontal electrode pairs. The comparison result (**Figure 7D**) of the HC and CI-1 showed the significantly different electrode pairs in AF8–T9, F2–AF3, F2–F5, FCz–T10, FC1–P9, AFz–P9, F1–T10, F3–T10, F9–F4, and FT7–T10. The comparison result of the HC

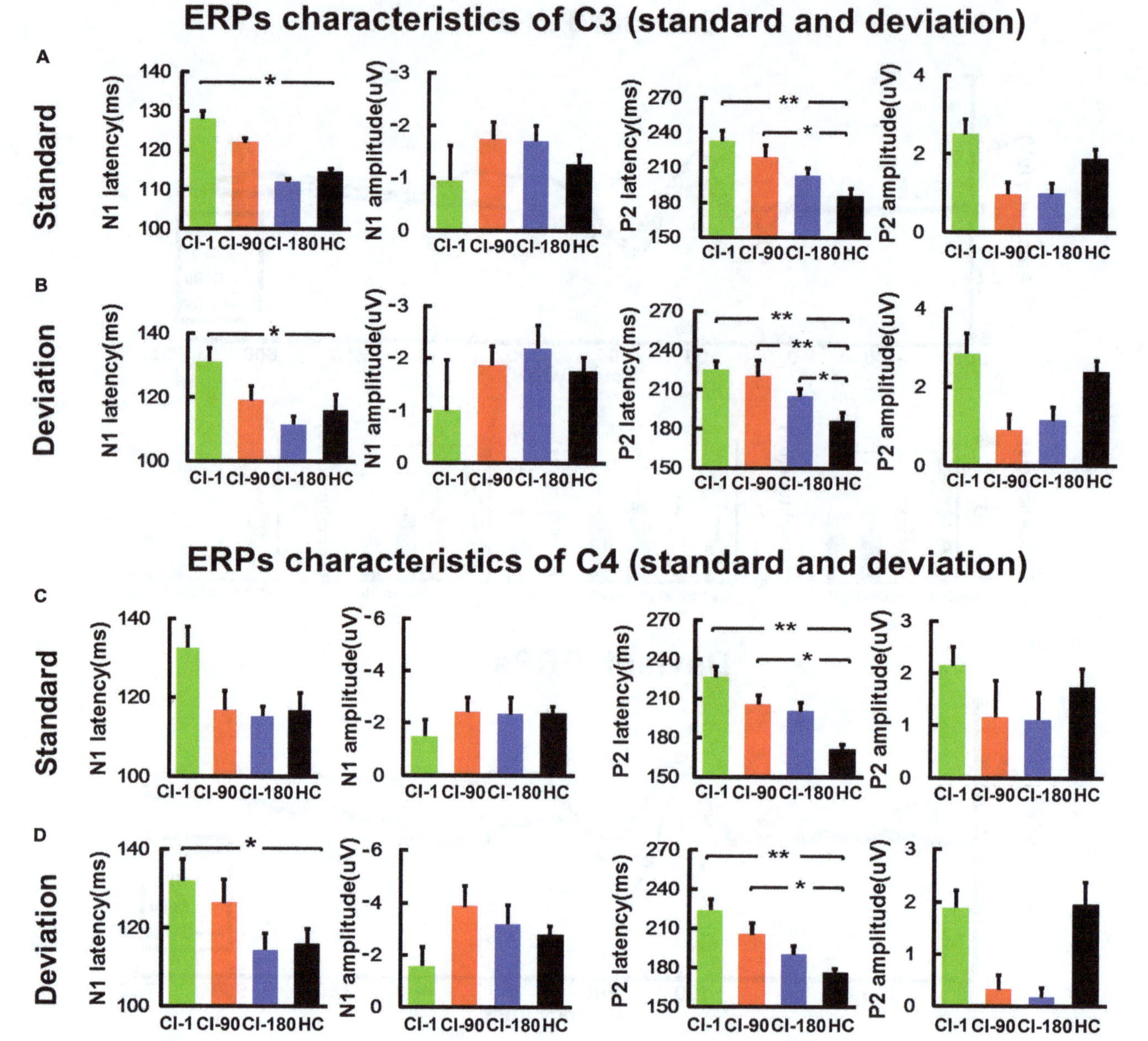

FIGURE 5 | The comparison of the amplitude and the latency of the N1/P2 for CI users and the HC group at the C3 and C4 electrodes. **(A)** The comparison of the latency and amplitude of N1 and P2 induced by the standard stimulus at the C3 electrode. **(B)** The comparison of the latency and amplitude of N1 and P2 induced by the standard stimulus at the C4 electrode. **(C)** The comparison of the latency and amplitude of N1 and P2 induced by the deviation stimulus at the C3 electrode. **(D)** The comparison of the latency and amplitude of N1 and P2 induced by the deviation stimulus at the C4 electrode. The vertical black line means standard error; **P* < 0.05 and ***P* < 0.001. CI-1, when the device is activated; CI-90, 90 days after device activation; CI-180, 180 days after device activation; HC, healthy controls.

and CI-90 showed the significantly different electrode pairs in FC1–F10, FCz–T10, FC1–FT10, F5–PO7, C1–P6, CP1–P6, and CPz–TP8. The comparison result of the HC and CI-180 showed the significantly different electrode pairs in AF8–T9, FC3–P6, FC3–PC6, C1–P6, and C3–P6.

Figures 8A,B show the deviant stimulus PLI for the HC group and CI group and their differences. Similarly, **Figure 8C** reveals the significantly reduced PLI values for the CI group. The comparison between the CI group and the HC group is also similar with the standard stimulus PLI. Significantly different electrode pairs (**Figure 8D**) between the CI group and the HC group were mainly for several left and right auditory areas and frontal electrodes. The comparison result of the HC and CI-1 showed the significantly different electrode pairs in F10–P10, FCz–T9, FC1–T9, P9–P8, and F9–CPz. The comparison result of the HC and CI-90 showed the significantly different electrode pairs in Fp2–FC3, Fz–FC3, F1–PO7, AF7–O1, and FC5–FT10. The comparison result of the HC and CI-180 showed the significantly different electrode pairs in Fp2–FC3, F3–Fz, FC3–Fz, and T9–PO4.

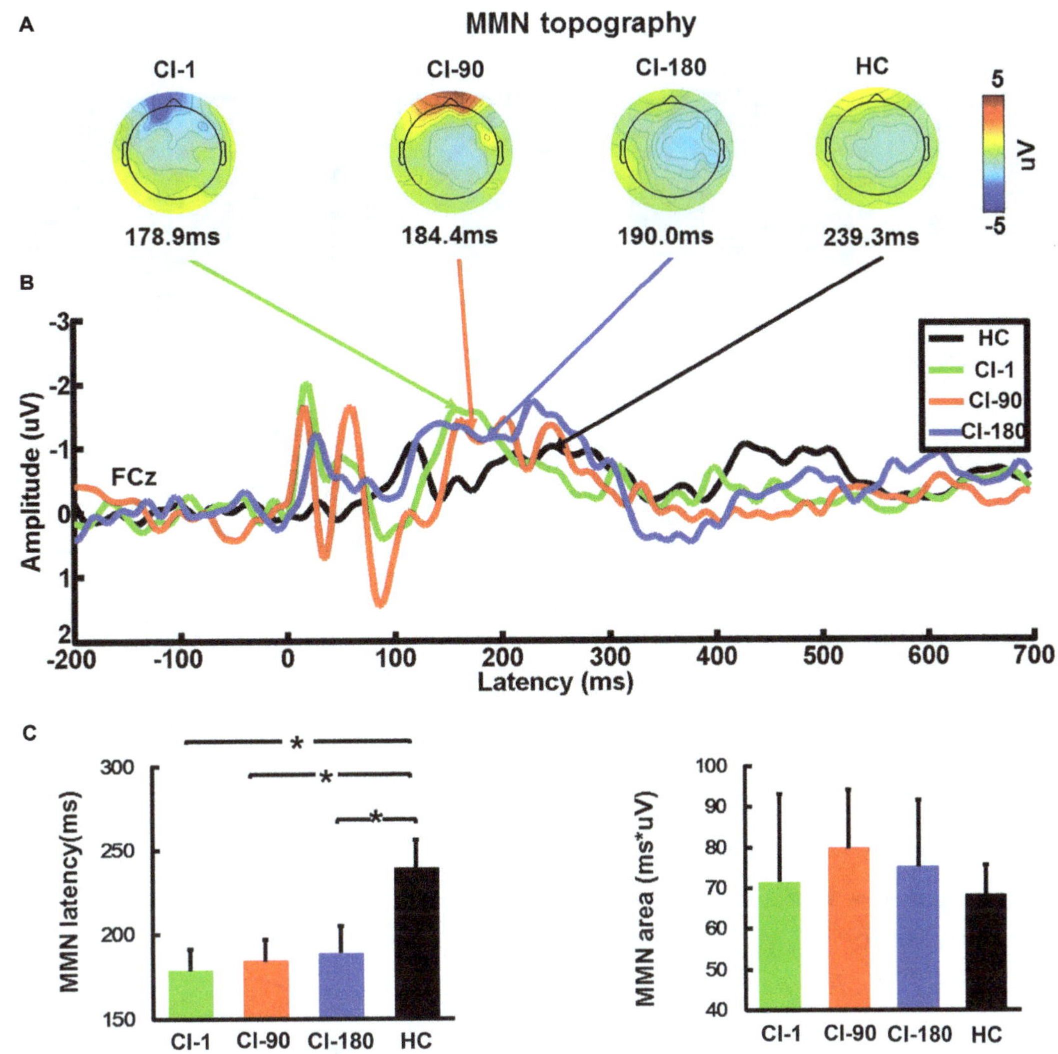

FIGURE 6 | The average waveform of the FCz electrode MMN, the topographic map, and the comparison of the area and the latency of the MMN for CI users and HC. **(A)** The topographic map of MMN (latency ± 10 ms), **(B)** the average waveform of MMN at different implantation periods in the CI group and the HC group, and **(C)** the comparison of the area and the latency of the MMN for CI users and HC. The vertical black line means standard error; $^{*}P < 0.05$. CI-1, when the device is activated; CI-90, 90 days after device activation; CI-180, 180 days after device activation; HC, healthy controls.

DISCUSSION

The present study examined the characteristics of ERPs/MMN and brain topographic maps in CI users after the CI-related artifacts were removed with ICA. Besides, we compared the difference in the EEG functional connection between CI patients and HCs. The ERP/MMN components and functional connection analysis used in this study may reflect some phases of auditory perception processes generated from auditory thalamocortical and corticocortical pathways such as primary and association cortices (Eggermont and Ponton, 2002; Ponton et al., 2002).

Removal of CI-Related Artifacts

Artifact removal in the EEG recordings of CI users is of great significance in the study of auditory cortex functions. In agreement with previous studies, our results show that CI-related artifacts can be successfully reduced with ICA (Debener et al., 2008). Functional imaging methods such as functional MRI and PET are limited in their ability to study changes of neuronal function in CI users because of their safety and invasiveness, respectively (Anne Lise Giraud, 2009). Therefore, artifact removal with ICA enables the study of auditory cortex function to be more specific, and it may be of great clinical importance to use ERPs as an objective index of auditory cortical changes in CI users.

In our experiment, we first evaluated the speech recognition ability of CI users using the speech score scale and found that the implantation of cochlear implants can significantly improve the speech recognition ability of patients. However, for people who cannot be evaluated through behavioral assessments (such as people with prelingual deafness), we should find indicators

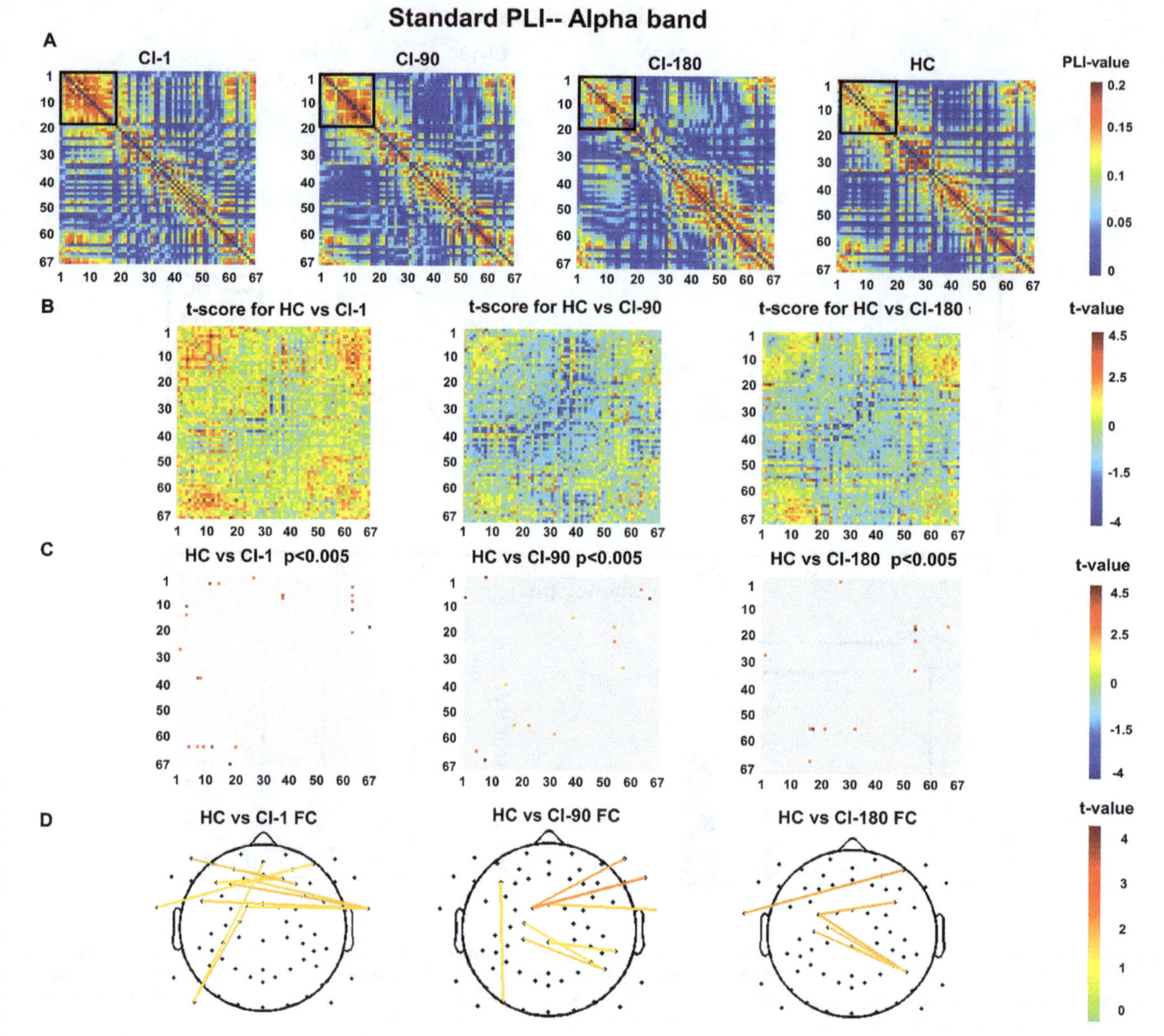

FIGURE 7 | The standard stimulus function connection analysis **(A)** presents the values of the standard stimulus phase lag index (PLI) for 67 electrode pairs in the CI group and the HC group. **(B)** The *t* scores for differences between the HC and the CI groups and **(C)** adjusted for the false discovery rate $P < 0.005$. **(D)** The *t* scores adjusted for $P < 0.005$ and differential functional connection across the topography. The black box indicates the electrode pair area with the main difference. FC, functional connection.

to evaluate the effect of cochlear implants through the non-invasive scalp EEG test.

From this experiment, we found that several ERP indicators changed regularly during the recovery process of CI users and gradually approximated to the HC group as the implantation time increased.

Characteristics of ERP Components

First, we found that the amplitude of N1 induced by the standard stimulus and the deviation stimulus was significantly different ($P < 0.05$; **Figure 3D**), which reflected the ability to recognize speech in the HC group. When the cochlear implant was implanted, there was no difference in the N1 amplitude induced by the standard stimulus and the deviation stimulus for CI users (**Figure 3A**), but after 90 days of adaptation, the N1 amplitude began to show a difference (**Figure 3B**), which also existed at 180 days (**Figure 3C**). The difference indicated that after 90 days of cochlear implantation, the speech recognition ability of CI users had improved. Here, we refer to the recovery of hearing abilities with CIs as a habilitation process, pointing out that the brain learns new strategies to adapt to the electrical input and thereby improves hearing. The improvement in speech perception was accompanied by an increase in their neural responses in the auditory cortex to complex tones. In fact, in

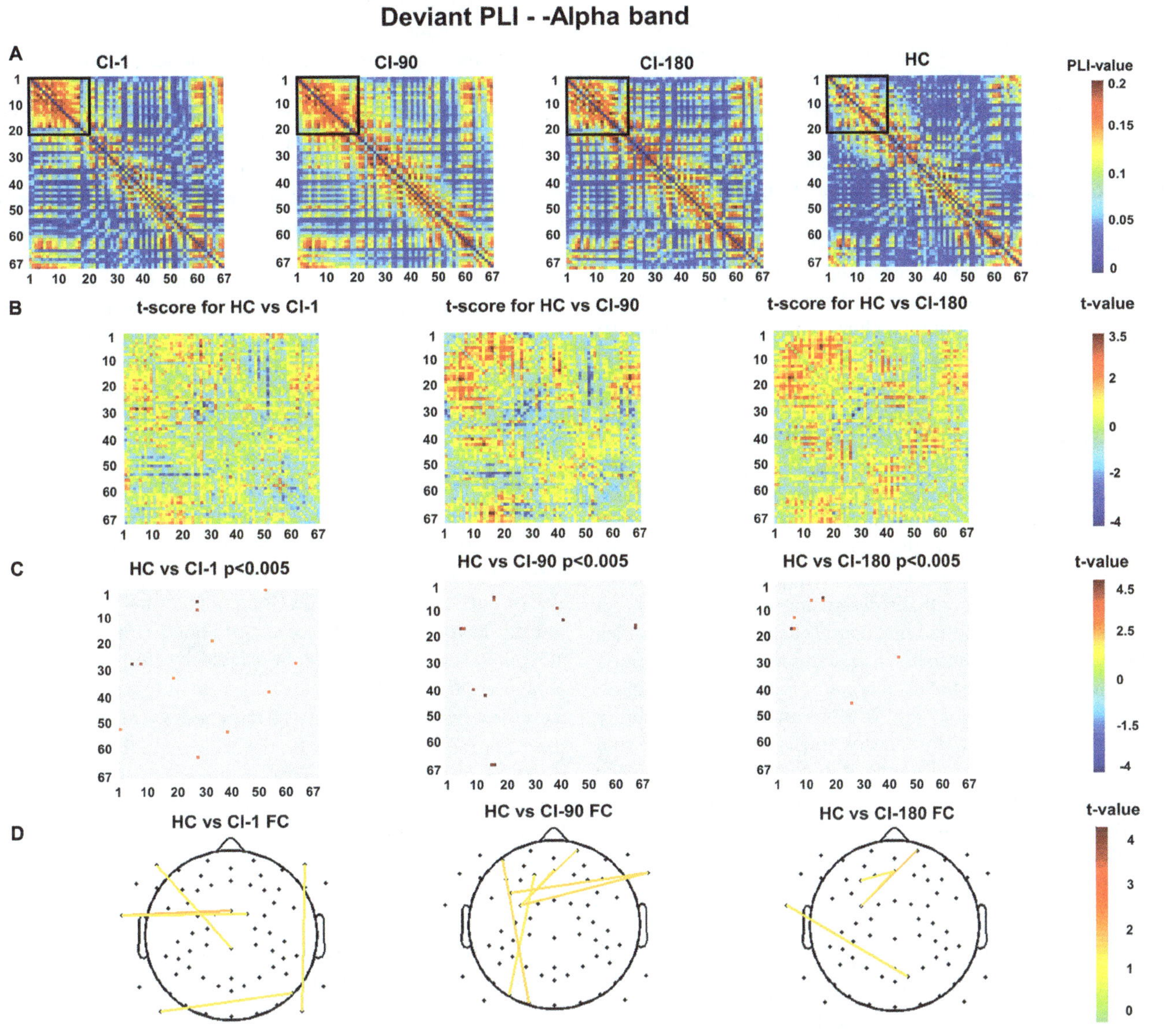

FIGURE 8 | The deviant stimulus function connection analysis **(A)** presents the values of the deviant stimulus phase lag index (PLI) for 67 electrode pairs in the CI group and the HC group. **(B)** The *t* scores for differences between the HC and the CI groups and **(C)** adjusted for the false discovery rate $P < 0.005$. **(D)** The *t* scores adjusted for $P < 0.005$ and differential functional connection across the topography. The black box indicates the electrode pair area with the main difference. FC, functional connection.

HC participants, the target stimuli often elicit larger N1 than the standard stimuli (Näätänen and Picton, 1987), which is also consistent with our results. Previous studies showed that this N1 effect is caused by the habituation, refractoriness, or adaptation of neural populations, which is more sensitive to the change in stimuli properties (Horvath et al., 2008). The change of N1 in CI users may be caused by the enhancive neural synchrony owing to the reorganization of auditory cortical neurons. This reflects the gradual restoration of auditory nerve activity in CI users and makes it easy to increase the neural activity when processing target stimuli. Similarly, Sandmann et al. (2015) found that improvement in frequency discrimination and speech recognition was most pronounced over the first 8 weeks of CI experience. Also, they found a larger activation in the contralateral than in the ipsilateral auditory cortex, confirming the view that in CI users auditory information is predominantly processed in the contralateral auditory cortex, at least in the first year after implantation.

Second, we found that the N1/P2 latency of the standard stimulus and the deviation stimulus in the CI group was greater than that in the HC group. This indicates that CI patients are more sluggish than the HC group in processing target sounds (Han et al., 2016). More recent data suggest that the generators of N1 activity are located in the posterior face of the superior temporal sulcus (Picton et al., 1999). Contrary to the N1, the neural substrates of the P2 component are less well understood, and multiple sources have been implicated in its generation. These include the auditory output of the mesencephalic reticular activating system, the planum temporale, and Brodmann's area 22 (Godey et al., 2001; Yvert et al., 2005). Besides, the latency of N1/P2 gradually decreases with the increase of implantation time, and it approaches the HC group. This also reflects the recovery effect of cochlear implantation. There was another study that conducted longitudinal research in cochlear implant users. Pantev et al. (2006) found that the increase of evoked brain activity over several months after implantation is the result of neural plasticity in the human auditory system, and within 180 days after implantation, CI patients may benefit most from postimplantation training. They also found that larger P1 and N1 amplitudes corresponded to a stronger perception in their MEG study.

Characteristics of MMN Components

Third, our research found that the latency of the MMN of CI users was shorter than that of the HC group and there was a statistical difference ($P < 0.05$) in the stage of CI (CI-1, CI-90, and CI-180). However, the change of the latency of the MMN of CI users was gradually increasing, and the difference with the HC group was gradually decreasing (**Figure 4C**). Direct electrical stimulation of functional neural elements in the cochlea bypasses acoustic and mechanical transmission delays through the auditory periphery, which can account for a minor reduction in peak latencies (Don, 1995). MMN can reflect the ability of auditory perception and memory and is an important tool for auditory perception and memory in cognitive neuroscience research (Moberly et al., 2016). There are two major hypotheses about the generation of MMN: the adjustment mechanism and the adaptation mechanism. According to some studies, MMN depends on a memory trace created by the preceding stimuli. To be specific, the standard stimuli evoke neural responses that create a neural memory trace, and the MMN will be generated if the target stimuli arrive while the memory trace is still available (Zhang et al., 2011). Some studies have shown that standard and target stimuli can be different in terms of acoustic characteristics (intensity, frequency, duration, etc.) for MMN (Opitz et al., 2002; Doeller et al., 2003). Another mechanism recently put forward showed that MMN is generated from a much simpler local neuronal adaptation in the auditory cortex (Jääskeläinen et al., 2004). Here, we should pay attention to whether the duration of sound deprivation will affect the MMN response, as longer duration of sound deprivation might lose the auditory memory. A recent longitudinal study showed that within days after the initial switch-on of the implant, postlingually deaf CI users improved significantly in their hearing discrimination ability, and this relatively quick adaptation seems to take place even in individuals who experienced a long period of hearing deprivation (Sandmann et al., 2015; Stropahl et al., 2017). We supposed that the sound memory of the CI users will also be reconstructed with the improvement of speech recognition ability and this difference should be studied in future research. In our results, the MMN latency could be increased close to that in NH participants, which indicated the adaptation fits well with the increasing use of CI (Kelly et al., 2005; Alemi and Lehmann, 2019).

PLI Functional Connectivity

Fourth, previous studies demonstrated that low-frequency EEG oscillations entrain to temporal modulations of sensory input. Different spatiotemporal characteristics of delta EEG encoding suggest that they potentially reflect different aspects of auditory motion processing (Bednar and Lalor, 2018). We analyzed the value of PLI in the alpha (8–13 Hz) band of CI users and HCs and calculated the difference in functional connection between CI users and HCs at different stages of implantation. Through statistical comparison, we found that the functional connection of the HCs was stronger than that of the CI users. Significant differences of electrode pairs mainly appear in the left and right auditory area and frontal electrodes, and the electrode pair gradually decreases as the implantation time increases. This result allows us to recognize the process of remodeling the auditory function of CI patients after CI more intuitively.

Limitations

There are also some limitations to this study. First, the sample size should be increased and different types of speech stimuli should be used, since there is some variability in a small sample size of participants. In the PLI function connection analysis, we did not have the result of correction, but set the threshold of P at < 0.005, which may also be caused by the small amount of data. Second, the ERP components were only studied in CI users with the device activated for 180 days because of the limitation of time. For more information on the change of ERP characteristics, the time should be prolonged to 1–2 years or more after the CI device is activated. The third limitation we should consider is the generality of our EEG indicators. The principle of cochlear implants is that the CI increases auditory sensitivity by direct electrical activation of auditory nerve fibers, enabling phonemic awareness, discrimination, and identification, ultimately yielding speech understanding (Hossain et al., 2012). However, the various styles of cochlear implants with different manufacturers and algorithms (spectral peak, continuous interleaved sampler, advanced confined encoding, etc.) and the duration and intensity of stimuli might affect the results of data analysis. In this study, our task adopted the classic oddball paradigm, and the brands of cochlear implants are the same.

Besides, the applicability of multichannel EEG recordings might be more limited than a single-channel EEG acquisition, a faster and more comfortable technique, in a clinical setting (Mc Laughlin et al., 2013), but it allows the use of an ICA-based approach to attenuate the CI-related artifacts, providing a good solution for attenuating artifacts. Furthermore, multichannel EEG recordings could provide spatial information about the ERP with the brain topographic maps, which might be a better objective measure of CI performance together with the characteristics of an ERP waveform in the time domain.

Conclusion

The behavioral performance revealed by speech perception scores showed a significant improvement with the increasing use of

CI. The recovery of speech recognition ability can be evaluated by comparing the N1 amplitude of the standard stimulus and the deviation stimulus. In addition, the N1/P2/MMN latency characteristics and the PLI index in the alpha band can be used as the reference index for the remodeling of brain functional connectivity in CI patients and could be the objective index for the assessment of speech perception and the effects of cochlear implantation.

ETHICS STATEMENT

The studies involving human participants were reviewed and approved by the Medical Research Ethics Committee of Capital Medical University (Beijing, China). The patients/participants provided their written informed consent to participate in this study.

AUTHOR CONTRIBUTIONS

SW contributed to the study conception, design, data analysis and interpretation, statistical analyses, and manuscript writing. CL contributed to the conception, design, data acquisition and interpretation, and manuscript writing. ML and LS contributed to the conception, design, data acquisition and interpretation, and manuscript writing. XZ contributed to the conception, design, data acquisition and interpretation, and manuscript writing. All authors read and approved the final manuscript.

REFERENCES

Alemi, R., and Lehmann, A. (2019). Middle latency responses to optimized chirps in adult cochlear implant users. *J. Am. Acad. Audiol.* 30, 396–405. doi: 10.3766/jaaa.18014

Anne Lise Giraud, C. J. P. (2009). Functional plasticity of language-related brain areas after cochlear implantation. *Brain* 124, 1307–1316. doi: 10.1093/brain/124.7.1307

Arnott, S. R., Bardouille, T., Ross, B., and Alain, C. (2011). Neural generators underlying concurrent sound segregation. *Brain Res.* 1387, 116–124. doi: 10.1016/j.brainres.2011.02.062

Bednar, A., and Lalor, E. C. (2018). Neural tracking of auditory motion is reflected by delta phase and alpha power of EEG. *Neuroimage* 181, 683–691. doi: 10.1016/j.neuroimage.2018.07.054

Bishop, D. V., and Hardiman, M. J. (2010). Measurement of mismatch negativity in individuals: a study using single-trial analysis. *Psychophysiology* 47, 697–705. doi: 10.1111/j.1469-8986.2009.00970.x

Debener, S., Hine, J., Bleeck, S., and Eyles, J. (2008). Source localization of auditory evoked potentials after cochlear implantation. *Psychophysiology* 45, 20–24. doi: 10.1111/j.1469-8986.2007.00610.x

Doeller, C. F., Opitz, B., Mecklinger, A., Krick, C., Reith, W., and Schröger, E. (2003). Prefrontal cortex involvement in preattentive auditory deviance detection. *NeuroImage* 20, 1270–1282. doi: 10.1016/s1053-8119(03)00389-6

Don, C. W. P. M. (1995). The mismatch negativity in cochlear implant users. *Ear Hear.* 16, 131–147. doi: 10.1097/00003446-199502000-00010

Eggermont, J. J., and Ponton, C. W. (2002). The neurophysiology of auditory perception: from single units to evoked potentials. *Audiol. Neurootol.* 7, 71–99. doi: 10.1159/000057656

Emmendorfer, A. K., Correia, J. M., Jansma, B. M., Kotz, S. A., and Bonte, M. (2020). ERP mismatch response to phonological and temporal regularities in speech. *Sci. Rep.* 10:9917. doi: 10.1038/s41598-020-66824-x

Ferreira-Santos, F., Silveira, C., Almeida, P. R., Palha, A., Barbosa, F., and Marques-Teixeira, J. (2012). The auditory P200 is both increased and reduced in schizophrenia? A meta-analytic dissociation of the effect for standard and target stimuli in the oddball task. *Clin. Neurophysiol.* 123, 1300–1308. doi: 10.1016/j.clinph.2011.11.036

Finke, M., Billinger, M., and Büchner, A. (2016). Toward automated cochlear implant fitting procedures based on event-related potentials. *Ear Hear.* 38, 118–127. doi: 10.1097/AUD.0000000000000377

Furlong, S., Cohen, J. R., Hopfinger, J., Snyder, J., Robertson, M. M., and Sheridan, M. A. (2020). Resting-state EEG connectivity in young children with ADHD. *J. Clin. Child Adolesc. Psychol.* [Epub ahead of print]. doi: 10.1080/15374416.2020.1796680

Godey, B., Schwartz, D., de Graaf, J., Chauvel, P., and Liégeois-Chauvel, C. (2001). Neuromagnetic source localization of auditory evoked fields and intracerebral evoked potentials: a comparison of data in the same patients. *Clin. Neurophysiol.* 112, 1850–1859. doi: 10.1016/S1388-2457(01)00636-8

Han, J. H., Zhang, F., Kadis, D. S., Houston, L. M., Samy, R. N., Smith, M. L., et al. (2016). Auditory cortical activity to different voice onset times in cochlear implant users. *Clin. Neurophysiol.* 127, 1603–1617. doi: 10.1016/j.clinph.2015.10.049

Horvath, J., Czigler, I., Jacobsen, T., Maess, B., Schroger, E., and Winkler, I. (2008). MMN or no MMN: no magnitude of deviance effect on the MMN amplitude. *Psychophysiology* 45, 60–69. doi: 10.1111/j.1469-8986.2007.00599.x

Hossain, M. D., Raghunandhan, S., Kameswaran, M., and Ranjith, R. (2012). A clinical study of cortical auditory evoked potentials in cochlear implantees. *Indian J. Otolaryngol. Head Neck Surg.* 65, 587–593. doi: 10.1007/s12070-012-0563-0

Jääskeläinen, I. P., Ahveninen, J., Bonmassar, G., Dale, A. M., Ilmoniemi, R. J., Levänen, S., et al. (2004). Human posterior auditory cortex gates novel sounds to consciousness. *PNAS* 101, 6809–6814. doi: 10.1073/pnas.0303760101

Kelly, A. S., Purdy, S. C., and Thorne, P. R. (2005). Electrophysiological and speech perception measures of auditory processing in experienced adult cochlear implant users. *Clin. Neurophysiol.* 116, 1235–1246. doi: 10.1016/j.clinph.2005.02.011

Kral, A., Yusuf, P. A., and Land, R. (2017). Higher-order auditory areas in congenital deafness: top-down interactions and corticocortical decoupling. *Hear. Res.* 343, 50–63. doi: 10.1016/j.heares.2016.08.017

Kraus, N., Micco, A. G., Koch, D. B., McGee, T., Carrell, T., Sharma, A., et al. (1993). The mismatch negativity cortical evoked potential elicited by speech in cochlear-implant users. *Hear. Res.* 65, 118–124. doi: 10.1016/0378-5955(93)90206-G

Luck, S. J., and Hillyard, S. A. (1990). Electrophysiological evidence for parallel and serial processing during visual search. *Percept. Psychophys.* 48, 603–617. doi: 10.3758/BF03211606

Maglione, A. G., Cartocci, G., Modica, E., Rossi, D., Colosimo, A., Di Flumeri, G., et al. (2017). Evaluation of different cochlear implants in unilateral hearing patients during word listening tasks: a brain connectivity study. *IEEE* 17, 2470–2473. doi: 10.1109/EMBC.2017.8037357

Mc Laughlin, M., Lopez Valdes, A., Reilly, R. B., and Zeng, F. G. (2013). Cochlear implant artifact attenuation in late auditory evoked potentials: a single channel approach. *Hear. Res.* 302, 84–95. doi: 10.1016/j.heares.2013.05.006

Moberly, A. C., Bhat, J., and Shahin, A. J. (2016). Acoustic cue weighting by adults with cochlear implants: a mismatch negativity study. *Ear Hear.* 37, 465–472. doi: 10.1097/AUD.0000000000000257

Naatanen, R., Kujala, T., and Winkler, I. (2011). Auditory processing that leads to conscious perception: a unique window to central auditory processing opened by the mismatch negativity and related responses. *Psychophysiology* 48, 4–22. doi: 10.1111/j.1469-8986.2010.01114.x

Näätänen, R., Paavilainen, P., Rinne, T., and Alho, K. (2007). The mismatch negativity (MMN) in basic research of central auditory processing: a review. *Clin. Neurophysiol.* 118, 2544–2590. doi: 10.1016/j.clinph.2007.04.026

Näätänen, R., and Picton, T. (1987). The N1 wave of the human electric and magnetic response to sound: a review and an analysis of the component structure. *Psychophysiology* 24, 375–425. doi: 10.1111/j.1469-8986.1987.tb00311.x

Nobukawa, S., Kikuchi, M., and Takahashi, T. (2019). Changes in functional connectivity dynamics with aging: a dynamical phase synchronization approach. *Neuroimage* 188, 357–368. doi: 10.1016/j.neuroimage.2018.12.008

Opitz, B., Rinne, T., Mecklinger, A., von Cramon, D. Y., and Schroger, E. (2002). Differential contribution of frontal and temporal cortices to auditory change detection: fMRI and ERP results. *Neuroimage* 15, 167–174. doi: 10.1006/nimg.2001.0970

Paiva, T. O., Almeida, P. R., Ferreira-Santos, F., Vieira, J. B., Silveira, C., Chaves, P. L., et al. (2016). Similar sound intensity dependence of the N1 and P2 components of the auditory ERP: averaged and single trial evidence. *Clin. Neurophysiol.* 127, 499–508. doi: 10.1016/j.clinph.2015.06.016

Pantev, C., Dinnesen, A., Ross, B., Wollbrink, A., and Knief, A. (2006). Dynamics of auditory plasticity after cochlear implantation: a longitudinal study. *Cereb. Cortex* 16, 31–36. doi: 10.1093/cercor/bhi081

Picton, T. W., Alain, C., Woods, D. L., John, M. S., Scherg, M., Valdes-Sosa, P., et al. (1999). Intracerebral sources of human auditory-evoked potentials. *Audiol. Neurootol.* 4, 64–79. doi: 10.1159/000013823

Ponton, C., Eggermont, J. J., Khosla, D., Kwog, B., and Don, M. (2002). Maturation of human central auditory system activity:separating auditory evoked potentials by dipole source modeling. *Clin. Neurophysiol.* 113, 107–420. doi: 10.1016/S1388-2457(01)00733-7

Ponton, C. W., Eggermont, J. J., Don, M., Waring, M. D., Kwong, B., Cunningham, J., et al. (2000). Maturation of the mismatch negativity: effects of profound deafness and cochlear implant use. *Audiol. Neurootol.* 5, 167–185. doi: 10.1159/000013878

Roman, S., Canevet, G., Marquis, P., Triglia, J. M., and Liegeois-Chauvel, C. (2005). Relationship between auditory perception skills and mismatch negativity recorded in free field in cochlear-implant users. *Hear. Res.* 201, 10–20. doi: 10.1016/j.heares.2004.08.021

Roth, W. T., Ford, J. M., Stephen, J. L., and Kopell, B. S. (1976). Effects of stimulus probability and task-televance on event-related potentials. *Psychophysiology* 13:317. doi: 10.1111/j.1469-8986.1976.tb03082.x

Sandmann, P., Plotz, K., Hauthal, N., de Vos, M., Schonfeld, R., and Debener, S. (2015). Rapid bilateral improvement in auditory cortex activity in postlingually deafened adults following cochlear implantation. *Clin. Neurophysiol.* 126, 594–607. doi: 10.1016/j.clinph.2014.06.029

Singh, S., Liasis, A., Rajput, K., Towell, A., and Luxon, L. (2004). Event-related potentials in pediatric cochlear implant patients. *Ear Hear.* 25, 598–610. doi: 10.1097/00003446-200412000-00008

Stropahl, M., Chen, L.-C., and Debener, S. (2017). Cortical reorganization in postlingually deaf cochlear implant users: intra-modal and cross-modal considerations. *Hear. Res.* 343, 128–137. doi: 10.1016/j.heares.2016.07.005

Teixeira-Santos, A. C., Pinal, D., Pereira, D. R., Leite, J., Carvalho, S., and Sampaio, A. (2020). Probing the relationship between late endogenous ERP components with fluid intelligence in healthy older adults. *Sci. Rep.* 10:11167. doi: 10.1038/s41598-020-67924-4

Tremblay, K. L., Ross, B., Inoue, K., McClannahan, K., and Collet, G. (2014). Is the auditory evoked P2 response a biomarker of learning? *Front. Syst. Neurosci.* 8:28. doi: 10.3389/fnsys.2014.00028

Ueda, R., Takeichi, H., Kaga, Y., Oguri, M., Saito, Y., Nakagawa, E., et al. (2020). Atypical gamma functional connectivity pattern during light sleep in children with attention deficit hyperactivity disorder. *Brain Dev.* 42, 129–139. doi: 10.1016/j.braindev.2019.11.001

Viola, F. C., De Vos, M., Hine, J., Sandmann, P., Bleeck, S., Eyles, J., et al. (2012). Semi-automatic attenuation of cochlear implant artifacts for the evaluation of late auditory evoked potentials. *Hear. Res.* 284, 6–15. doi: 10.1016/j.heares.2011.12.010

Viola, F. C., Thorne, J., Edmonds, B., Schneider, T., Eichele, T., and Debener, S. (2009). Semi-automatic identification of independent components representing EEG artifact. *Clin. Neurophysiol.* 120, 868–877. doi: 10.1016/j.clinph.2009.01.015

Viola, F. C., Thorne, J. D., Bleeck, S., Eyles, J., and Debener, S. (2011). Uncovering auditory evoked potentials from cochlear implant users with independent component analysis. *Psychophysiology* 48, 1470–1480. doi: 10.1111/j.1469-8986.2011.01224.x

Xu, L., Wang, C. D., Liang, M. J., Cai, Y. X., and Zheng, Y. Q. (2018). Brain network regional synchrony analysis in deafness. *Biomed. Res. Int.* 2018:6547848. doi: 10.1155/2018/6547848

Yvert, B., Fischer, C., Bertrand, O., and Pernier, J. (2005). Localization of human supratemporal auditory areas from intracerebral auditory evoked potentials using distributed source models. *Neuroimage* 28, 140–153. doi: 10.1016/j.neuroimage.2005.05.056

Zhang, F., Hammer, T., Banks, H.-L., Benson, C., Xiang, J., and Fu, Q.-J. (2011). Mismatch negativity and adaptation measures of the late auditory evoked potential in cochlear implant users. *Hear. Res.* 275, 17–29. doi: 10.1016/j.heares.2010.11.007

Zhang, J., Dong, X., Wang, L., Zhao, L., Weng, Z., Zhang, T., et al. (2018). Gender differences in global functional connectivity during facial emotion processing: a visual MMN study. *Front. Behav. Neurosci.* 12:220. doi: 10.3389/fnbeh.2018.00220

19

Baseline Functional Connectivity Features of Neural Network Nodes can Predict Improvement After Sound Therapy Through Adjusted Narrow Band Noise in Tinnitus Patients

Lv Han[1], Zeng Na[2], Liu Chunli[3,4], Chen Yuchen[5], Zhao Pengfei[1], Wang Hao[1], Cheng Xu[1], Zhang Peng[1], Wang Zheng[1], Yang Zhenghan[1], Gong Shusheng[3] and Wang Zhenchang[1]**

[1] Department of Radiology, Beijing Friendship Hospital, Capital Medical University, Beijing, China, [2] National Clinical Research Center for Digestive Diseases, Beijing Friendship Hospital, Capital Medical University, Beijing, China, [3] Department of Otolaryngology Head and Neck Surgery, Beijing Friendship Hospital, Capital Medical University, Beijing, China, [4] Department of Otolaryngology, Affiliated Hospital of Chengde Medical College, Chengde, China, [5] Department of Radiology, Nanjing First Hospital, Nanjing Medical University, Nanjing, China

***Correspondence:**
Lv Han
chrislvhan@126.com
Wang Zhenchang
cjr.wzhch@vip.163.com

Previous resting-state functional magnetic resonance imaging (fMRI) studies have shown neural connectivity alterations after the treatment of tinnitus. We aim to study the value of the baseline functional connectivity features of neural network nodes to predict outcomes of sound therapy through adjusted narrow band noise. The fMRI data of 27 untreated tinnitus patients and 27 matched healthy controls were analyzed. We calculated the graph-theoretical metric degree centrality (DC) to characterize the functional connectivity of the neural network nodes. Therapeutic outcomes are determined by the changes in the Tinnitus Handicap Inventory (THI) score after a 12-week intervention. The connectivity of 10 brain nodes in tinnitus patients was significantly increased at baseline. The functional connectivity of right insula, inferior parietal lobule (IPL), bilateral thalami, and left middle temporal gyrus was significantly modified with the sound therapy, and such changes correlated with THI changes in tinnitus patients. Receiver operating characteristic curve analyses revealed that the measurements from the five brain regions were effective at classifying improvement after therapy. After age, gender, and education correction, the adjusted area under the curve (AUC) values for the bilateral thalami were the highest (left, 0.745; right, 0.708). Our study further supported the involvement of the fronto-parietal-cingulate network in tinnitus and found that the connectivity of the thalamus at baseline is an object neuroimaging-based indicator to predict clinical outcome of sound therapy through adjusted narrow band noise.

Keywords: tinnitus, sound therapy, functional magnetic resonance imaging, functional connectivity, degree centrality, neural biomarker, graph theory

INTRODUCTION

Tinnitus, the perception of sound without any external stimuli, is highly prevalent, affecting 10 to 25% of the general population (Baguley et al., 2013; Bauer, 2018). Without effective treatment, patients with persistent tinnitus experience substantial distress that significantly affects their quality of life, even leading to suicide. New and effective therapeutic approaches are desperately needed.

Current therapeutic approaches include tinnitus retraining therapy (Scherer et al., 2014; Kim et al., 2016), counseling, cognitive behavior therapy (Conrad et al., 2015; Weise et al., 2016), transcranial magnetic stimulation (Kreuzer et al., 2017; Formanek et al., 2018), hearing aids (Searchfield et al., 2010), pharmacological treatments (von Boetticher, 2011), and several innovative sound-based treatments (e.g., Heidelberg Neuro-Music Therapy) (Krick et al., 2015, 2017a,b), Cochleural Alternating Acoustic Beam Therapy (CAABT) (Liu et al., 2018), and Tailor-Made Notched Music Training (TMNMT) (Okamoto et al., 2010; Kim et al., 2017; Lee et al., 2017). Sound therapy is considered as a cost-effective management for tinnitus (Tunkel et al., 2014; Walker et al., 2016; Makar et al., 2017) and is one of the most commonly used first-line therapy interventions for decades (Henry et al., 2002). An adjusted narrow band noise was commonly used in sound therapy. For tinnitus patients, sound therapy may not totally eliminate the symptoms, but it could help patients become familiar with tinnitus and offer relief from tinnitus-related distress, subsequently improving their quality of life (Hobson et al., 2007, 2012; Newman and Sandridge, 2012; Hoare et al., 2014; Aytac et al., 2017; Mahboubi et al., 2017). Determining the factors that can predict the treatment efficacy of sound therapy will help to deliver cost-effectiveness therapy in tinnitus patients.

For patients with tinnitus, the functional connectivity differs from that of control individuals (Husain, 2016). Effective treatments for tinnitus have been shown to correlate with alterations in brain activities. Brain regions in the posterior cingulate cortex (PCC)/precuneus (Krick et al., 2017a), rostral and pregenual anterior cingulate cortices (rACC/pgACC), auditory cortex, parahippocampus (Kim et al., 2016), and inferior frontal gyrus (Roland et al., 2015) were reported to have significantly altered functional activity after therapy. However, very few studies have investigated the value of a non-invasive test, i.e., neuroimaging to predict clinical outcome, especially with sound therapy through adjusted narrow band noise. If a set of parameters is determined through such study, it would be valuable to guide patient selection and to deliver personalized therapeutic strategies.

Among numerous neural network measures, degree centrality (DC) is regarded as a reliable graph-theoretical-based analytic method with moderate to high test–retest reliability for the measurement of functional connectivity features of neural network nodes (Zuo and Xing, 2014). In graph theory, the DC of a node is defined as the number of functional connections to other nodes in the brain atlas (Bullmore and Sporns, 2009; Tomasi and Volkow, 2010). Thus, DC value could reflect functional connectivity features. Nodes with a higher DC are considered more important in the brain network, i.e., neural network hubs. Thus, DC results could indicate the highly connected regions of the brain and quantify the importance of each node in the brain network (Lv et al., 2018). DC features simplicity in understanding and performance. It has been successfully used to measure altered functional connectivity in idiopathic tinnitus (Chen et al., 2016), pulsatile tinnitus (Lv et al., 2015), schizophrenia (Zhuo et al., 2014), and Alzheimer's disease (Dai et al., 2015). Alteration of DC in brain regions is closely correlated with symptom severity. In addition, DC at baseline could also provide objective neuroimaging-based indicators to predict response to treatment, such as in obsessive–compulsive disorder (Gottlich et al., 2015) and major depressive disorder (Shen et al., 2015). These results suggested the potential use of neuroimaging-based network features to predict response to treatment in tinnitus.

We hypothesized that functional connectivity features of the brain nodes determined by DC can predict the response of sound therapy through adjusted narrow band noise. In this study, we will analyze the functional connectivity of the neural network nodes within a standardized brain atlas (Power et al., 2011). We will compare the baseline and post-treatment functional brain network architectures in the cohort of patients with tinnitus. Furthermore, multiple regression analyses were applied to explore the potential of baseline functional connectivity features of neural network hubs to classify improvement status for patients.

MATERIALS AND METHODS

Standard Protocol Approvals, Registrations, and Patient Consents

This experiment was approved by the Institutional Review Board (IRB) of Beijing Friendship Hospital, Capital Medical University, Beijing, China. Written informed consent was obtained from all subjects enrolled in this study. The protocol was registered on ClinicalTrials.gov, ID: NCT02774122.

Participants

A total of 29 patients with untreated persistent tinnitus were recruited in this study. Twenty-eight age-, sex-, and education-level-matched healthy controls were also enrolled. The inclusion criteria for patients were as follows: aged 18 to 65 years and suffered from idiopathic tinnitus for more than 6 months persistently. Tinnitus was present as a hissing sound without any rhythm. Based on audiogram results, we excluded subjects with hearing loss, which was defined as more than 25 dB hearing loss at frequencies ranging from 250 to 8 kHz in puretone audiometry examination (PTA). Other exclusion criteria were hyperacusis on physical examination, otosclerosis, sudden deafness, Ménière's disease, stroke, trauma, brain tumor, and other neurological diseases. The hearing thresholds of normal controls were also examined by PTA. Importantly, subject with hearing loss was one of the exclusion criteria. Other exclusion criteria for healthy controls were the same as above.

We asked patients to fill in the Tinnitus Handicap Inventory (THI) to assess the severity of disease at baseline

(Newman et al., 1996). Tinnitus patients were treated by sound therapy through adjusted narrow band noise for 12 weeks, 20 min each time for three times per day. The intervention sound was matched with the clinical examination results, including loudness, and pitch matching. Specifically, the initial volume of noise sound was set as 5 dB over the loudness of tinnitus. For the frequency of the intervention sound, we first determined the tinnitus frequency (Tf) according to the results of tinnitus pitch matching. We then set an adjusted narrow band noise 1 kHz narrow band, Tf frequency. It would be necessary to adjust treated sound parameters based on examination every 2 weeks if the tinnitus sound is changed following treatment. We also asked the patients to fill out the THI again at the end of treatment. A reduction of at least 16 points in THI was considered effective (Zeman et al., 2011). Two of the patients were excluded due to lack of response to treatment according to this criterion.

MRI Data Acquisition

For both tinnitus patients and healthy controls, MRI data acquisition was performed at baseline. All of the subjects were scanned using a 3.0 T GE (General Electric) scanner with an eight-channel head coil. Resting-state functional magnetic resonance imaging (fMRI) data were obtained with the following parameters (echo planar imaging sequence): TR/TE = 2,000/35 ms; field of view (FOV) = 240 × 240 mm; flip angle = 90°; matrix = 64 × 64; 28 slices; 4-mm slice thickness; 1-mm gap; and 200 time points in total. Additionally, high-resolution structural images were obtained with the following parameters: TR/TE/TI = 8.8/3.5/450 ms; FOV = 240 × 240 mm; flip angle = 15°; matrix = 256 × 256; 196 slices; and 1 mm thickness without gap.

Image Preprocessing

Image preprocessing was performed using SPM 8[1] and the Graph-theoretical Network Analysis Toolkit v2.0.0 (GRETNA[2]) in MATLAB (Wang et al., 2015). Our procedures included discarding the first 10 time points, slice timing, realigning, correcting head motion, spatial normalization to the MNI (Montreal Neurological Institute) space with resampled images (3 mm × 3 mm × 3 mm), detrending, and bandpass filtering (0.01–0.08 Hz). Nuisance variables including signals of white matter and ventricular and friston 24 head motion parameters (Yan et al., 2013) were regressed out. For the quality control, one of the enrolled healthy controls was excluded according to the exclusion criteria (spatial movement in any direction more than 2.0 mm or degrees). Notably, we did not perform smoothing in the image preprocessing procedure to prevent the possible introduction of artifactual correlations in the next DC calculation step (Zuo et al., 2012; Lv et al., 2018).

Degree Centrality Calculation and Network Construction

Qualified images were subjected to further brain network construction and DC calculation using the GRETNA toolbox (Wang et al., 2015). A total of 264 defined brain nodes covering the whole brain were set as invested regions of interest (ROIs), as described in a widely used standardized brain atlas (Power et al., 2011). There were two main approaches when calculating DC: binary graph and weighted graph. The binary graph of DC is calculated as the number of functional connections. The weighted graph is computed as the sum of weights over every functional connection, providing a more precise centrality characterization of brain networks (Cole et al., 2010). Weighted networks generate more reliable numerical results compared to binarized networks (Wang et al., 2011). Thus, we adopted a weighted graph to calculate DC in this study. Specifically, the functional connectivity among ROIs was measured by computing the Pearson correlation coefficients (r) among the time series of every possible pair nodes. After calculation, all of the resulting DC maps were spatially smoothed (a Gaussian kernel with a full-width at half maximum = 6 mm). Finally, the DC maps were z-transformed (z-values of DC) to allow for averaging and between-subject comparisons.

Statistical Analysis

Sample Characteristics and Degree Centrality Differences Among Groups at Baseline

The demographic data of the patients and healthy controls were compared using SPSS 12.0 software (SPSS, Inc., Chicago, IL, United States) through two-sample t-tests, paired two-sample t-tests, and a Fisher's exact test. The results were considered significant with $P < 0.05$. Longitudinal changes in THI scores were calculated as: $\Delta THI = THI_{pre} - THI_{post}$. The ΔTHI would represent the therapeutic effect of treatment. Imaging data were analyzed in the SPM. Differences in the z-values of DC between tinnitus patients and healthy controls were analyzed by a two-sample t-test (false discovery rate (FDR) corrected for multiple comparisons, $P < 0.05$). The results were visualized with the REST Slice Viewer and BrainNet Viewer[3] (Song et al., 2011; Xia et al., 2013).

Degree Centrality Differences at Baseline

After DC calculation and network construction, we produced a continuously weighted network (264 × 264 matrix) for each subject. To reveal the differences of DC between tinnitus patients and healthy controls at baseline, we used a two-sample t-test. The results were FDR corrected with $P < 0.05$.

Correlation Between Degree Centrality Maps and Tinnitus Handicap Inventory Score

According to a one-sample Kolmogorov–Smirnov test, the THI score at baseline and the ΔTHI values were both normally distributed. To identify brain nodes that were significantly related to the outcome of treatment for tinnitus patients, we conducted a correlation analysis between the z-values of DC and baseline THI as well as ΔTHI. Age and gender were added as covariates during the calculations.

Adjusted Receiver Operating Characteristic Curve

To further examine whether the DC at baseline might be sufficiently sensitive and specific to serve as a potential neural

[1]http://www.fil.ion.ucl.ac.uk/spm

[2]http://www.nitrc.org/projects/gretna/

[3]http://www.nitrc.org/projects/bnv/

biomarker for predicting improvement after intervention, we employed adjusted receiver operating characteristic (ROC) curves (Janes et al., 2009). We added age, gender, and education as covariates to recalculate ROC results. Analytic strategies were performed for each node whose baseline DC was significantly correlated with the clinical response of treatment in tinnitus patients.

Additionally, according to the standard defined by Zeman et al. (2011), a reduction of at least 40 points in THI represents relative better effects of the therapy. Thus, we set THI = 40 as a cutoff value to identify brain regions that predict improvements after treatment with high specificity and sensitivity.

RESULTS

Demographics and Clinical Characteristics

A total of 27 tinnitus patients and 27 healthy controls completed the study (**Table 1**). For tinnitus patients, THI scores longitudinally decreased significantly. ΔTHI were also calculated.

Functional Connectivity Differences Between Patients and Healthy Controls at Baseline

We calculated the DC of the 264 defined brain nodes within the whole brain. As shown in **Table 2**, when compared to healthy controls, the anterior cingulate cortex (ACC), right insula, bilateral superior frontal gyrus (SFG), right middle frontal gyrus (MFG), right inferior parietal lobule (IPL), bilateral thalami, and right middle temporal gyrus [two separate brain regions: the anterior part overlapped within the default mode network (DMN) and the posterior part overlapped with the associate auditory cortex (AAC)] showed increased DC in tinnitus patients. No node with decreased DC was found. These results suggest that an objective neuroimaging-based indicator can differentiate tinnitus from healthy controls.

Correlation Between Degree Centrality Maps and Tinnitus Handicap Inventory Score

Positive correlations between THI at baseline and DC values were found in the right insula ($r = 0.415$, $p = 0.031$). As shown in

TABLE 1 | Summarized demographic and clinical characteristics of the enrolled subjects.

	Tinnitus patients (baseline, $n = 27$)	Tinnitus patients (12th week, $n = 27$)	Healthy controls (baseline, $n = 27$)	Healthy controls (12th week, $n = 27$)	*P*-value
Age (years)	23–62 (37.5 ± 10.6)		25–59 (38.4 ± 11.3)		0.78[a]
Gender (male/female)	12/15		12/15		> 0.99[b]
Education (years)	6–16 (11.4 ± 3.0)		6–19 (12.3 ± 3.6)		0.33[a]
Handedness	27 right-handed		27 right-handed		> 0.99[a]
Tinnitus duration (months)	6–48 (25.0 ± 13.4)		NA		NA
THI score	40–90 (66.6 ± 13.9)	12–50 (30.4 ± 11.1)	NA		< 0.01[c]
ΔTHI score	24–52 (36.2 ± 8.8)		NA		NA

Data are presented as min–max ranges (mean ± SD) for all variables except gender. THI: Tinnitus Handicap Inventory. $\Delta THI = THI_{pre} - THI_{post}$. NA: not applicable. [a]*Two-sample t-tests.* [b]*Chi-square test.* [c]*Paired-sample t-tests.*

TABLE 2 | Brain nodes with significant differences in DC values in tinnitus patients relative to healthy controls at baseline.

Brain region	Peak MNI, mm *x*	*y*	*z*	DC value of tinnitus patients	DC value of healthy controls	*T*
Anterior cingulate cortex	−3	26	44	73.75 ± 3.21.25	57.42 ± 7.22.45	2.75
R insula	37	32	−2	70.87 ± 0.20.96	54.27 ± 4.18.42	3.09
L superior frontal gyrus	−20	45	39	73.75 ± 3.21.25	57.42 ± 7.22.45	2.75
R superior frontal gyrus	26	50	27	73.75 ± 3.22.17	57.50 ± 7.15.56	3.12
R middle frontal gyrus	43	49	−2	65.73 ± 5.24.29	48.06 ± 8.15.05	3.21
R inferior parietal lobule	49	−42	45	69.96 ± 9.23.02	52.69 ± 2.22.68	2.78
L thalamus	−15	4	8	84.88 ± 4.25.69	61.31 ± 1.21.43	3.66
R thalamus	9	−4	6	82.12 ± 2.27.21	61.84 ± 1.27.48	2.73
R middle temporal gyrus (anterior part, DMN)	65	−24	−19	74.87 ± 4.21.47	58.78 ± 8.21.19	2.77
L middle temporal gyrus (posterior part, SAC)	−56	−50	10	84.42 ± 4.25.85	66.14 ± 6.23.97	2.69

For the DC values, data are presented as the mean ± SD. DC, degree centrality (note that the DC value was z-transformed); R, right; L, left; MNI, Montreal Neurological Institute; DMN, default mode network. SAC, secondary auditory cortex. Peak T scores and location of node maxima in MNI coordinates are listed. The significance threshold was set as $P < 0.05$ corrected for multiple comparisons using FDR.

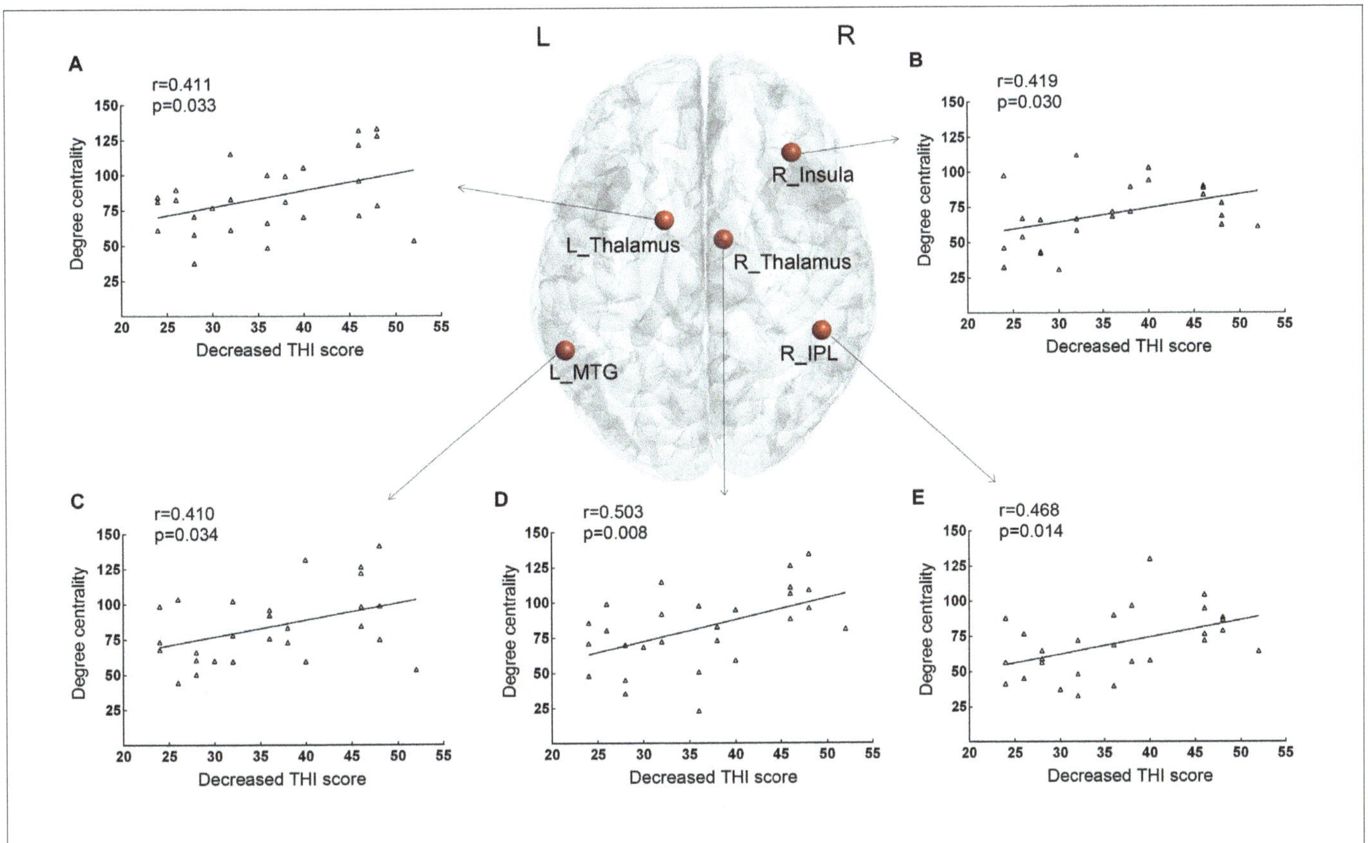

FIGURE 1 | Brain nodes with baseline DC values that were significantly correlated with decreased THI scores after 12 weeks of sound therapy through adjusted narrow band noise. **(A)** Results of the left thalamus. **(B)** Results of the right insula. **(C)** Results of the left middle temporal gyrus. **(D)** Results of the right thalamus. **(E)** Results of the right inferior parietal lobule. L, left; R, right; DC, degree centrality; THI, tinnitus handicap inventory; MTG, middle temporal gyrus; IPL, inferior parietal lobule. X-axis, Decreased THI score; Y-axis, number of Degree Centrality.

Figure 1, for correlative analysis of DC values and therapeutic effect, significant positive correlations between increased z-values of DC and ΔTHI were found in the right insula (r = 0.419, p = 0.030), right IPL (r = 0.468, p = 0.014), bilateral thalamus (left: r = 0.411, p = 0.033; right: r = 0.503, p = 0.008, respectively), and posterior part of the left MTG (SAC; r = 0.410, p = 0.034) after age and gender correction. There were no additional significant correlations reported in this study.

Sensitivity and Specificity of Baseline Degree Centrality in Predicting Treatment Effect

According to the standard, a reduction of at least 40 points represents better effects of the therapy (Zeman et al., 2011). We further tested whether the DC had predictive value for treatment effectiveness of the intervention. The ROC analyses revealed that these five brain regions performed well in classifying better effects of therapy after 12 weeks of treatment. As shown in **Figure 2**, after age, gender, and education correction, the adjusted area under the curve (AUC) values of the nodes were recalculated. The functional connectivity features of other brain nodes were as follows: right insula, AUC = 0.704, sensitivity = 77.8%, specificity = 88.9%, cutoff value = 69.0; right IPL, AUC = 0.701, sensitivity = 70.4%, specificity = 96.3%, cutoff value = 72.3; left thalamus, AUC = 0.745, sensitivity = 51.9%, specificity = 81.5%, cutoff value = 91.0; right thalamus, AUC = 0.708, sensitivity = 77.8%, specificity = 92.6%, cutoff value = 88.3; and posterior part of left MTG (SAC), AUC = 0.682, sensitivity = 51.9%, specificity = 74.1%, cutoff value = 82.5. We noted that the AUC of bilateral thalami had the highest values (left, 0.745; right, 0.708). The observed AUC values and bias are listed in **Table 3**. We also added unadjusted AUC values of each node to illustrate the impact of covariates on ROC values in tinnitus research.

DISCUSSION

This study demonstrated the potential of using a neuroimaging biomarker in predicting the therapeutic improvement of tinnitus patients. To our knowledge, this is the first study to evaluate the predictive value of the graph-theoretical metric parameters for the outcomes of sound therapy through adjusted narrow band noise.

Based on a widely used standardized brain atlas consisting of 264 brain nodes, we first identified 10 brain nodes with significant differences in their DC values between tinnitus patients and healthy controls. These brain nodes were widely distributed within the whole brain and were mainly located in

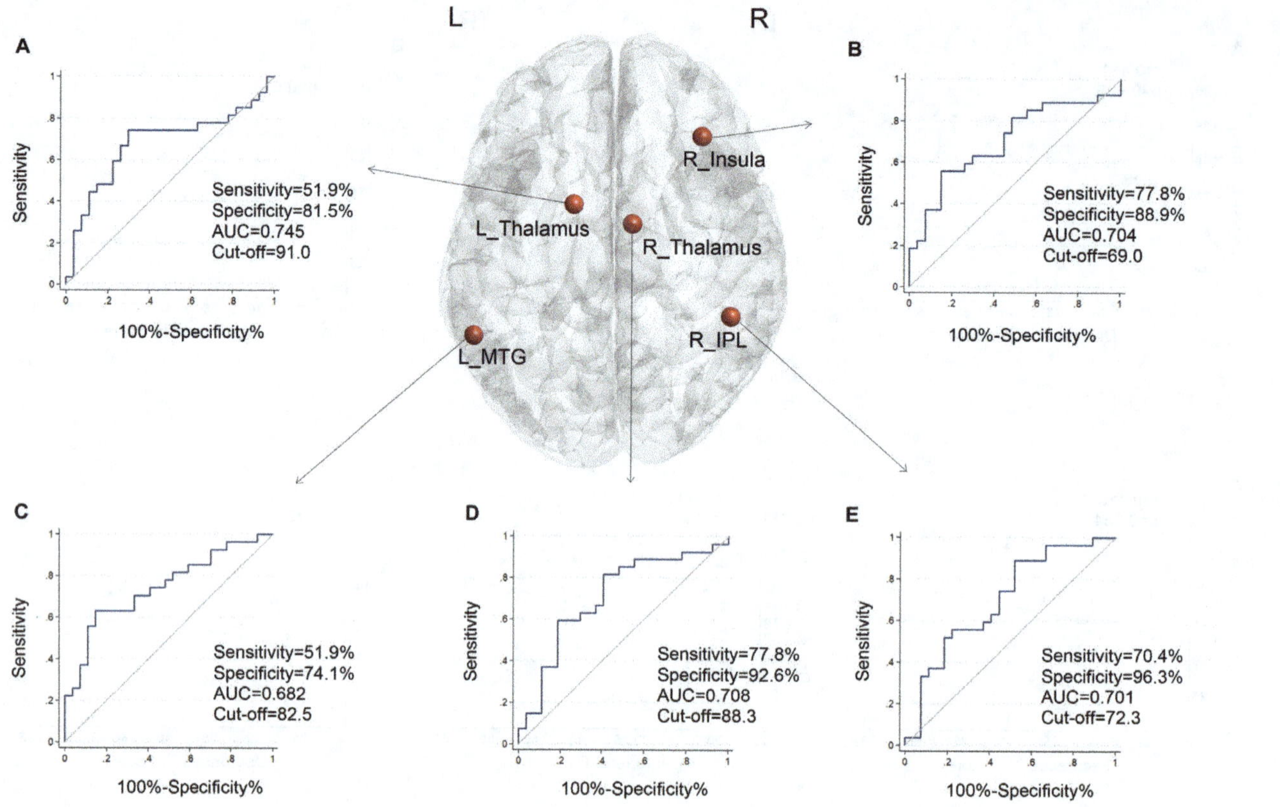

FIGURE 2 | The adjusted ROC curves and AUC values of the five nodes when classifying improvements in tinnitus patients after treatment, with age, gender, and education as corrections. **(A)** Results of the left thalamus. **(B)** Results of the right insula. **(C)** Results of the left middle temporal gyrus. **(D)** Results of the right thalamus. **(E)** Results of the right inferior parietal lobule. X-axis, 100%-Specificity%; Y-axis, Sensitivity.

the frontal lobe (left SFG, right SFG and MFG), parietal lobe (right IPL), and ACC. These brain regions largely overlap with the emotional processing areas, which are core structures within the fronto-parietal-cingulate network (Golm et al., 2013; Husain, 2016). Additionally, the thalamus, identified as an important brain node within the thalamocortical pathway in mediating auditory–limbic interactions, had a significantly increased DC in tinnitus patients compared to healthy controls at baseline. After retrospective data analysis, we identified five nodes with significant correlations between their DC values at baseline and decreased THI scores after treatment. Importantly, the DC of these five nodes had different predictive value for better treatment responses. Among which, the left thalamus was one of two brain regions with the highest AUC values, while the other brain region is the right IPL. However, after age, gender, and education correction, the adjusted AUC values for the bilateral thalami were the highest (left, 0.745; right, 0.708). According to our results, the DC value of the thalamus is an objective neuroimaging-based indicator to predict better response to treatment. An improved understanding of neural correlates of tinnitus after therapy should motivate the development of innovative neural-based means for assessing the efficacy of sound therapy through adjusted narrow band noise.

TABLE 3 | The adjusted AUC values and bias of the brain nodes.

	AUC (unadjusted; adjusted)	Bias	Bootstrap standard error	95% confidence interval (unadjusted; adjusted)
R insula	0.713			0.574, 0.828
	0.704	0.00819	0.07431	0.539, 0.831
R inferior parietal lobule	0.716			0.577, 0.830
	0.701	−0.00043	0.08184	0.524, 0.844
L thalamus	0.752			0.615, 0.859
	0.745	0.00027	0.07514	0.575, 0.868
R thalamus	0.704			0.564, 0.820
	0.708	0.00740	0.07941	0.535, 0.846
L middle temporal gyrus (posterior part, SAC)	0.700			0.560, 0.817
	0.682	−0.00336	0.08011	0.528, 0.835

95% confidence interval: bias-corrected confidence interval. R, right; L, left; SAC, secondary auditory cortex.

Methodological Considerations

When analyzing functional connectivity features of the neural network, there are several methods that can be applied. Seed-based functional connectivity is one of the most commonly used methods. The coupling of time series between brain areas indicates that they are involved in the same underlying functional process, and thus can be interpreted as functionally connected (Lv et al., 2018). The computation is relatively simple, and the results are easily understood. The modest to high test–retest reliability across connections (Shehzad et al., 2009) further facilitates its application. However, one of the major disadvantages of seed analysis is its dependence on the selection of ROIs in conducting ROI-wise analysis. When the selected seed changes, it may limit the reproducibility of the results. Thus, it would be more precise if selected brain nodes are defined prior to data analysis and set as a standard atlas.

To overcome the problems mentioned above, we first applied the DC analytic method. Featuring high test–retest reliability (Zuo et al., 2012), the DC values reflect the entirety of functional connections between one node to other nodes in the brain atlas, rather than identifying each connection (Bullmore and Sporns, 2009; Tomasi and Volkow, 2010). Thus, the results of DC are quantified values that characterize the importance of a node (Lv et al., 2018). For the definition of nodes, we applied a widely used standardized brain atlas, which included 264 defined nodes (Power et al., 2011). Thus, neural activity could be measured among those 264 predefined nodes within a graph theoretic framework without selection bias. These methodological considerations increased the validity of results and minimized possible confounding factors in this study.

Results of correlation analysis were also needed to be discussed. We performed correlative analysis with both baseline THI score at baseline and the ΔTHI. However, for the results, we only found positive correlations between the DC values and THI score at baseline in the right insula, but there were five brain nodes whose DC values were positively correlated with the ΔTHI, including the right insula. It indicated that correlations between brain activity and THI score or ΔTHI score may be different. One reason may be the different focused aspect when we do statistical analysis. One focused on the cross-sectional aspect and the other focused on the longitudinal changes. As a result, results may be different and not necessarily overlapped. Similar phenomena also exist in a previous study on patients with obsessive–compulsive disorder (Gottlich et al., 2015). Thus, it is reasonable to presume that results may be different and not be necessarily overlapped. For another reason, it may indicate that the DC value is more appropriate for prediction of treatment effect longitudinally rather than assessment of disease severity. It would be also one of the advantages that we apply DC as a predictive biomarker in this study.

The Involvement of the Fronto-Parietal-Cingulate Network in Tinnitus

The fronto-parietal-cingulate network has been implicated in tinnitus (Golm et al., 2013; Husain and Schmidt, 2014; Husain, 2016). Brain regions related to the fronto-parietal-limbic network may include the anterior and PCC, insula, frontal brain areas (SFG, MFG, especially dorsal lateral prefrontal cortex), amygdala, parahippocampal gyrus (limbic), and precuneus. These brain regions are closely correlated with emotional processing. This network is more active in patients with highly distressing tinnitus and high THI scores and is also a specific distress network in tinnitus (Golm et al., 2013). In another study, increased functional connectivity was detected between the frontoparietal regions and other parts of the brain (Maudoux et al., 2012). In the current study, we also found increased functional connectivity of several regions within the fronto-parietal-cingulate network, which was reflected by increased DC values. As a result, our study provided additional evidence that FC of this network was mainly increased in the perception of tinnitus. The functional alterations of the fronto-parietal-cingulate network as well as anatomical changes were involved in the perception of tinnitus. Gray matter volume changes in the thalamic level were considered to be critical findings of tinnitus (Muhlau et al., 2006). According to recent studies, correlations of tinnitus distress with cortical thickness and cortical surface area in bilateral cingulate cortex were also reported (Meyer et al., 2016). Morphological changes were also detected in frontal areas after treatment (Krick et al., 2015) and were interpreted as tinnitus-specific gray matter alterations, which was closely correlated with emotional changes of tinnitus. Additionally, the THI score of the patients was 66.6 ± 13.9 at baseline, representing a relatively high distress state. Thus, it is reasonable that core structures of the fronto-parietal-limbic network with significantly increased functional connectivity could be identified. Our study further supports the involvement of this neural network in tinnitus processing.

The THI score also significantly decreased after treatment in this study, representing alleviation of symptoms. However, we did not identify correlations between decreased THI scores and the DC values of most regions of the fronto-parietal-limbic network at baseline, except for the right insula. The nature of THI may be one reason. In fact, THI is a moderately accurate test for assessing psychiatric disorder of tinnitus patients (AUC = 0.792, according to previous study) (Salviati et al., 2013). As one of the most widespread validated questionnaires in the tinnitus research field (Newman et al., 1996), it is commonly applied to quantify tinnitus severity rather than tinnitus-related distress (Langguth et al., 2007). For the evaluation of distress, both the Global Severity Index (GSI) of Symptomatic Check List-90-Revised (SCL-90-R) and Stress-related Vulnerability Scale (VRS) have higher sensitivity and specificity (Salviati et al., 2013). Thus, a decrease in the THI score may not be specific to relief from tinnitus-related distress. It would be helpful to acquire GSI or VRS scores to specifically investigate the activity of the fronto-parietal-limbic network.

For the right insula, we identified positive correlations between the DC value and baseline THI as well as a decreased THI score. It may represent that functional connectivity of the right insula would be an indication for severe patients and may also indicate that high functional connectivity of the right insula have potential predictive value for effective treatment. The insula is one of the major hubs that modulate tinnitus-related distress (Husain, 2016). As a core structure of the salience network, many studies have indicated the important role of the insula in emotional processing, as reviewed by De Ridder et al. (2014). When it is active, an external auditory stimulus is perceived by the subject (Sadaghiani et al., 2009). For tinnitus patients, an elevated response of functional activity was found in the right insula and bilateral parahippocampus when processing affective stimuli (Carpenter-Thompson et al., 2014). The insula and ACC are more active in chronic tinnitus compared to recent-onset tinnitus (Vanneste et al., 2011). Greater functional connectivity was also detected in both the right anterior insula and left inferior frontal gyrus in a tinnitus group compared with healthy controls (Burton et al., 2012). Abnormal regional neural activity and functional interactions between the right insula and DMN and auditory network were also reported in patients with persistent pulsatile tinnitus (Lv et al., 2017). Anatomical changes were also reported in the insula, according to a voxel-based morphometry study with a large sample (Schecklmann et al., 2013). Those studies indicated the importance of the insula in tinnitus mediation. In this study, we found that the insula DC value performed well in classifying improvements of the tinnitus patients after treatment. Our study provided additional evidence for this core structure in the salience network in tinnitus.

Auditory–Limbic Interaction Pathway Through the Thalamus

The thalamus is the subcortical auditory processing region. The medial geniculate nucleus in the thalamus, accompanied by the primary and secondary sites in the superior temporal gyrus, forms a typical auditory perception pathway. Further, thalamic function plays a critical role in the perception of tinnitus and in regulating the flow of signal among the auditory network and limbic network. One hypothesis concerning tinnitus perception is that the thalamic reticular nucleus mediates information between the limbic and auditory cortex. Under normal circumstances, the unwanted signal is inhibited in the thalamus, and thus the propagation of tinnitus is reduced. In chronic tinnitus, cortico-thalamic activity is increased and prevents inhibition of the tinnitus signal (Rauschecker et al., 2010; Zhang, 2013). Thus, changes in the cortico-thalamic feedback loop result in increased alteration of functional connection of the thalamus (Leaver et al., 2011). In our study, we mainly enrolled patients with moderate to severe tinnitus. Those patients were also featured by relatively higher DC value of the bilateral thalamus. Although we did not find a positive correlation between DC value and THI score at baseline, increased FC of the bilateral thalamus could also further support this theory.

In a different model, the thalamus also plays a major role in the development of tinnitus. As analyzed by magneto-encephalography (MEG), the thalamo-cortical loop has normal rhythms in the normal state relating to sleep and consciousness (Llinas and Ribary, 1993). When there is reduced functional input to the thalamus or protracted functioning of the thalamus, the rhythms of the thalamus change to a large-scale but slow-rate oscillatory coherent activity, reducing lateral inhibition and disinhibiting high-frequency gamma waves (Llinas et al., 1999). To compare the results, the relationship between fMRI and MEG was preliminarily analyzed (Houck et al., 2017). The spatial patterns of the two kinds of analysis were similar but not identical. Interestingly, the functional connectivity results may be inversed in the two kinds of studies. Thus, theoretically, the thalamus would be identified with increased FC in fMRI analysis, as demonstrated by increased DC in our study. As a result, for both of the models, it was reasonable that thalamus plays a critical role in mediating tinnitus perception. Besides, similar to a previous study, our results may further indicate the inverse relationship of FC revealed by MEG and fMRI analyses.

To further validate the proposed tinnitus models, one previous study specifically analyzed the functional connectivity features of the thalamus in tinnitus patients (Zhang et al., 2015). Both increased and decreased FC were detected between the left and right thalamus and brain regions in the cerebral cortex. Different from the results of this study, we only identified increased functional connectivity (indicated by higher DC values) in the bilateral thalamus relative to healthy controls. There are two possible reasons. Firstly, similar to the introduction and methodological considerations mentioned above, DC calculates the sum of weights over every functional connection (Cole et al., 2010), while functional connectivity measures the connection between several brain regions. Thus, the connectivity feature of each brain node revealed by DC values will be averaged. There might be decreased FC between the left or right thalamus and other brain nodes, but this effect may be covered up by increased FC values in this study. This circumstance may also explain why the sensitivity and specificity of the DC values of both the left and the right thalamus were only moderate to high in predicting the therapeutic effect. This is also one limitation of the DC analytic method. However, we should also pay special attention to the accuracy of traditional ROC. As suggested by Holly Janes, covariates, e.g., age and gender, are factors that should be incorporated into ROC analysis (Janes et al., 2009). Thus, in this study, we added age, gender, and education as covariates to recalculate the ROC results. After correction, the adjusted AUC values for the bilateral thalami were the highest (left, 0.745; right, 0.708). These results further highlighted the importance of the thalamo-cortical pathway in processing tinnitus information.

Secondly, a previous study (Zhang et al., 2015) identified disconnection of the FC of the right thalamus and left STG, especially in patients with extended disease duration (~10 years). Additionally, decreased FC was negatively correlated with tinnitus duration, possibly indicating habituation of tinnitus. In our study, the disease duration of enrolled tinnitus patients was less than 48 months. As a result, the disconnection effect may not be obvious in patients in the early stage of disease, resulting in a relatively high DC value at baseline. Sound therapy also has habituation effects on tinnitus. In our research, higher DC values in the bilateral thalamus are considered to be potential biomarkers for predicting the effect of sound therapy through adjusted narrow band noise. Thus, in light of the previous study, we hypothesize that DC of the thalamus decreases after treatment. As this is a core structure that mediates information between the limbic and auditory cortex, it is critical to test our hypothesis by analyzing the functional connectivity features of the thalamus in patients with longer disease duration, as well as the alteration of DC value of bilateral thalamus after sound therapy in further studies.

Limitations

There are several limitations of this study. Firstly, we excluded two patients who did not respond to treatment in this study. However, only two subjects would not be enough to do statistical analysis in an fMRI study. It is important to analyze brain functional activity in these kinds of patients in order to provide more information about the neural mechanism of sound therapy and help to improve treatment strategy in further studies. Secondly, tinnitus patients enrolled in the current study did not show any degree of hearing loss, which is not representative for most tinnitus patients. Thirdly, it would be much more helpful to enroll a tinnitus group with sham treatment in order to exclude the placebo effect of tinnitus treatment. Last but not least, we applied adjusted narrow band noise (1 kHz narrow band, Tf $\pm$ 0.5 kHz) for the treatments of patients, but it indicated that we were providing more energy in high frequencies where critical bands are narrower. It would be better if octave bands or similar bands were applied so that critical bandwidth was considered in further studies.

CONCLUSION

Our study further supports the involvement of the fronto-parietal-cingulate network in mediating tinnitus and suggests that the DC value of the thalamus at baseline is an objective neuroimaging-based indicator for predicting effectiveness of sound therapy through adjusted narrow band noise. This preliminary analysis has important implications in motivating innovative neuroimaging-based approaches for predicting the efficacy of treatment, thus guiding earlier personalized therapeutic strategies for tinnitus patients. Further studies analyzing functional connectivity of the thalamus are still needed to further validate the predictive effect of its DC value at baseline.

ETHICS STATEMENT

This study was carried out in accordance with the recommendations of LH of guidelines, the Institutional Review Board (IRB) of Beijing Friendship Hospital, Capital Medical University with written informed consent from all subjects. All subjects gave written informed consent in accordance with the Declaration of Helsinki. The protocol was approved by the Institutional Review Board (IRB) of Beijing Friendship Hospital, Capital Medical University.

AUTHOR CONTRIBUTIONS

LH designed the experiments, collected the data, performed the statistical analysis, and wrote the manuscript. ZN conducted the statistical analysis. LC and ZoP contributed to the discussion and manuscript revision. LC, WH, CX, WZheng, and ZgP collected the data. WZhenchang, YZ, and GS are guarantors of this work. LH and WZhenchang are the corresponding authors of this manuscript, who have full access to all the data in the study and take responsibility for the integrity of the data and the accuracy of the data analysis.

ACKNOWLEDGMENTS

We thank Dr. Liu Shen and Dr. Wang Zhaodi from the Department of Otolaryngology – Head and Neck Surgery, Beijing Friendship Hospital, Capital Medical University, for their assistance with the data collection and audiological tests. We would like to especially thank Dr. Fang Ba from the University of Alberta, Canada, for her elaborate assistance with the edit of the whole manuscript.

REFERENCES

Aytac, I., Baysal, E., Gulsen, S., Tumuklu, K., Durucu, C., Mumbuc, L. S., et al. (2017). Masking treatment and its effect on tinnitus parameters. *Int. Tinnitus J.* 21, 83–89. doi: 10.5935/0946-5448.20170017

Baguley, D., McFerran, D., and Hall, D. (2013). Tinnitus. *Lancet* 382, 1600–1607. doi: 10.1016/S0140-6736(13)60142-7

Bauer, C. A. (2018). Tinnitus. *N. Engl. J. Med.* 378, 1224–1231.

Bullmore, E., and Sporns, O. (2009). Complex brain networks: graph theoretical analysis of structural and functional systems. *Nat. Rev. Neurosci.* 10, 186–198. doi: 10.1038/nrn2575

Burton, H., Wineland, A., Bhattacharya, M., Nicklaus, J., Garcia, K. S., and Piccirillo, J. F. (2012). Altered networks in bothersome tinnitus: a functional connectivity study. *BMC Neurosci.* 13:3. doi: 10.1186/1471-2202-13-3

Carpenter-Thompson, J. R., Akrofi, K., Schmidt, S. A., Dolcos, F., and Husain, F. T. (2014). Alterations of the emotional processing system may underlie preserved rapid reaction time in tinnitus. *Brain Res.* 1567, 28–41. doi: 10.1016/j.brainres.2014.04.024

Chen, Y. C., Feng, Y., Xu, J. J., Mao, C. N., Xia, W., Ren, J., et al. (2016). Disrupted brain functional network architecture in chronic tinnitus patients. *Front. Aging Neurosci.* 8:174. doi: 10.3389/fnagi.2016.00174

Cole, M. W., Pathak, S., and Schneider, W. (2010). Identifying the brain's most globally connected regions. *Neuroimage* 49, 3132–3148. doi: 10.1016/j.neuroimage.2009.11.001

Conrad, I., Kleinstauber, M., Jasper, K., Hiller, W., Andersson, G., and Weise, C. (2015). The changeability and predictive value of dysfunctional cognitions in cognitive behavior therapy for chronic tinnitus. *Int. J. Behav. Med.* 22, 239–250. doi: 10.1007/s12529-014-9425-3

Dai, Z., Yan, C., Li, K., Wang, Z., Wang, J., Cao, M., et al. (2015). Identifying and mapping connectivity patterns of brain network hubs in Alzheimer's disease. *Cereb. Cortex* 25, 3723–3742. doi: 10.1093/cercor/bhu246

De Ridder, D., Vanneste, S., Weisz, N., Londero, A., Schlee, W., Elgoyhen, A. B., et al. (2014). An integrative model of auditory phantom perception: tinnitus as a unified percept of interacting separable subnetworks. *Neurosci. Biobehav. Rev.* 44, 16–32. doi: 10.1016/j.neubiorev.2013.03.021

Formanek, M., Migalova, P., Krulova, P., Bar, M., Jancatova, D., Zakopcanova-Srovnalova, H., et al. (2018). Combined transcranial magnetic stimulation in the treatment of chronic tinnitus. *Ann. Clin. Transl. Neurol.* 5, 857–864. doi: 10.1002/acn3.587

Golm, D., Schmidt-Samoa, C., Dechent, P., and Kroner-Herwig, B. (2013). Neural correlates of tinnitus related distress: an fMRI-study. *Hear. Res.* 295, 87–99. doi: 10.1016/j.heares.2012.03.003

Gottlich, M., Kramer, U. M., Kordon, A., Hohagen, F., and Zurowski, B. (2015). Resting-state connectivity of the amygdala predicts response to cognitive behavioral therapy in obsessive compulsive disorder. *Biol. Psychol.* 111, 100–109. doi: 10.1016/j.biopsycho.2015.09.004

Henry, J. A., Schechter, M. A., Nagler, S. M., and Fausti, S. A. (2002). Comparison of tinnitus masking and tinnitus retraining therapy. *J. Am. Acad. Audiol.* 13, 559–581.

Hoare, D. J., Searchfield, G. D., El, R. A., and Henry, J. A. (2014). Sound therapy for tinnitus management: practicable options. *J. Am. Acad. Audiol.* 25, 62–75. doi: 10.3766/jaaa.25.1.5

Hobson, J., Chisholm, E., and El, R. A. (2012). Sound therapy (masking) in the management of tinnitus in adults. *Cochrane Database Syst. Rev.* 11:CD006371. doi: 10.1002/14651858.CD006371.pub3

Hobson, J., Chisholm, E., and Loveland, M. (2007). *Sound Therapy (masking) in the Management of Tinnitus in Adults.* Hoboken, NJ: John Wiley & Sons. Ltd.

Houck, J. M., Cetin, M. S., Mayer, A. R., Bustillo, J. R., Stephen, J., Aine, C., et al. (2017). Magnetoencephalographic and functional MRI connectomics in schizophrenia via intra- and inter-network connectivity. *Neuroimage* 145(Pt A), 96–106. doi: 10.1016/j.neuroimage.2016.10.011

Husain, F. T. (2016). Neural networks of tinnitus in humans: elucidating severity and habituation. *Hear. Res.* 334, 37–48. doi: 10.1016/j.heares.2015.09.010

Husain, F. T., and Schmidt, S. A. (2014). Using resting state functional connectivity to unravel networks of tinnitus. *Hear. Res.* 307, 153–162. doi: 10.1016/j.heares.2013.07.010

Janes, H., Longton, G., and Pepe, M. (2009). Accommodating covariates in ROC analysis. *Stat. J.* 9, 17–39. doi: 10.1177/1536867x0900900102

Kim, S. H., Jang, J. H., Lee, S. Y., Han, J. J., Koo, J. W., Vanneste, S., et al. (2016). Neural substrates predicting short-term improvement of tinnitus loudness and distress after modified tinnitus retraining therapy. *Sci. Rep.* 6:29140. doi: 10.1038/srep29140

Kim, S. Y., Chang, M. Y., Hong, M., Yoo, S. G., Oh, D., and Park, M. K. (2017). Tinnitus therapy using tailor-made notched music delivered via a smartphone application and Ginko combined treatment: a pilot study. *Auris Nasus Larynx* 44, 528–533. doi: 10.1016/j.anl.2016.11.003

Kreuzer, P. M., Poeppl, T. B., Rupprecht, R., Vielsmeier, V., Lehner, A., Langguth, B., et al. (2017). Individualized repetitive transcranial magnetic stimulation treatment in chronic tinnitus? *Front. Neurol.* 8:126. doi: 10.3389/fneur.2017.00126

Krick, C. M., Argstatter, H., Grapp, M., Plinkert, P. K., and Reith, W. (2017a). Heidelberg neuro-music therapy enhances task-negative activity in tinnitus patients. *Front. Neurosci.* 11:384. doi: 10.3389/fnins.2017.00384

Krick, C. M., Argstatter, H., Grapp, M., Plinkert, P. K., and Reith, W. (2017b). Heidelberg neuro-music therapy restores attention-related activity in the angular gyrus in chronic tinnitus patients. *Front. Neurosci.* 11:418. doi: 10.3389/fnins.2017.00418

Krick, C. M., Grapp, M., Daneshvar-Talebi, J., Reith, W., Plinkert, P. K., and Bolay, H. V. (2015). Cortical reorganization in recent-onset tinnitus patients by the heidelberg model of music therapy. *Front. Neurosci.* 9:49. doi: 10.3389/fnins.2015.00049

Langguth, B., Goodey, R., Azevedo, A., Bjorne, A., Cacace, A., Crocetti, A., et al. (2007). Consensus for tinnitus patient assessment and treatment outcome measurement: tinnitus research initiative meeting, regensburg, July 2006. *Prog. Brain Res.* 166, 525–536. doi: 10.1016/s0079-6123(07)66050-6

Leaver, A. M., Renier, L., Chevillet, M. A., Morgan, S., Kim, H. J., and Rauschecker, J. P. (2011). Dysregulation of limbic and auditory networks in tinnitus. *Neuron* 69, 33–43. doi: 10.1016/j.neuron.2010.12.002

Lee, H. Y., Choi, M. S., Chang, D. S., and Cho, C. S. (2017). Combined bifrontal transcranial direct current stimulation and tailor-made notched music training in chronic tinnitus. *J. Audiol. Otol.* 21, 22–27. doi: 10.7874/jao.2017.21.1.22

Liu, C., Lv, H., Jiang, T., Xie, J., He, L., Wang, G., et al. (2018). The cochleural alternating acoustic beam therapy (CAABT): a pre-clinical trial. *Am. J. Otolaryngol.* 39, 401–409. doi: 10.1016/j.amjoto.2018.04.002

Llinas, R., and Ribary, U. (1993). Coherent 40-Hz oscillation characterizes dream state in humans. *Proc. Natl. Acad. Sci. U.S.A.* 90, 2078–2081. doi: 10.1073/pnas.90.5.2078

Llinas, R. R., Ribary, U., Jeanmonod, D., Kronberg, E., and Mitra, P. P. (1999). Thalamocortical dysrhythmia: a neurological and neuropsychiatric syndrome characterized by magnetoencephalography. *Proc. Natl. Acad. Sci. U.S.A.* 96, 15222–15227. doi: 10.1073/pnas.96.26.15222

Lv, H., Wang, Z., Tong, E., Williams, L. M., Zaharchuk, G., Zeineh, M., et al. (2018). Resting-state functional MRI: everything that nonexperts have always wanted to know. *AJNR Am. J. Neuroradiol.* 39, 1390–1399. doi: 10.3174/ajnr.A5527

Lv, H., Zhao, P., Liu, Z., Li, R., Zhang, L., Wang, P., et al. (2017). Abnormal regional activity and functional connectivity in resting-state brain networks associated with etiology confirmed unilateral pulsatile tinnitus in the early stage of disease. *Hear. Res.* 346, 55–61. doi: 10.1016/j.heares.2017.02.004

Lv, H., Zhao, P., Liu, Z., Yan, F., Li, T., Dong, C., et al. (2015). Resting-state functional connectivity density mapping of etiology confirmed unilateral pulsatile tinnitus patients: altered functional hubs in the early stage of disease. *Neuroscience* 310, 27–37. doi: 10.1016/j.neuroscience.2015.09.032

Mahboubi, H., Haidar, Y. M., Kiumehr, S., Ziai, K., and Djalilian, H. R. (2017). Customized versus noncustomized sound therapy for treatment of tinnitus: a randomized crossover clinical trial. *Ann. Otol. Rhinol. Laryngol.* 126, 681–687. doi: 10.1177/0003489417725093

Makar, S. K., Mukundan, G., and Gore, G. (2017). Treatment of tinnitus: a scoping review. *Int. Tinnitus J.* 21, 144–156. doi: 10.5935/0946-5448.20170027

Maudoux, A., Lefebvre, P., Cabay, J. E., Demertzi, A., Vanhaudenhuyse, A., Laureys, S., et al. (2012). Connectivity graph analysis of the auditory resting state network in tinnitus. *Brain Res.* 1485, 10–21. doi: 10.1016/j.brainres.2012.05.006

Meyer, M., Neff, P., Liem, F., Kleinjung, T., Weidt, S., Langguth, B., et al. (2016). Differential tinnitus-related neuroplastic alterations of cortical thickness and surface area. *Hear. Res.* 342, 1–12. doi: 10.1016/j.heares.2016.08.016

Muhlau, M., Rauschecker, J. P., Oestreicher, E., Gaser, C., Rottinger, M., Wohlschlager, A. M., et al. (2006). Structural brain changes in tinnitus. *Cereb. Cortex* 16, 1283–1288. doi: 10.1093/cercor/bhj070

Newman, C. W., Jacobson, G. P., and Spitzer, J. B. (1996). Development of the tinnitus handicap inventory. *Arch. Otolaryngol. Head Neck Surg.* 122, 143–148.

Newman, C. W., and Sandridge, S. A. (2012). A comparison of benefit and economic value between two sound therapy tinnitus management options. *J. Am. Acad. Audiol.* 23, 126–138. doi: 10.3766/jaaa.23.2.7

Okamoto, H., Stracke, H., Stoll, W., and Pantev, C. (2010). Listening to tailor-made notched music reduces tinnitus loudness and tinnitus-related auditory cortex activity. *Proc. Natl. Acad. Sci. U.S.A.* 107, 1207–1210. doi: 10.1073/pnas.0911268107

Power, J. D., Cohen, A. L., Nelson, S. M., Wig, G. S., Barnes, K. A., Church, J. A., et al. (2011). Functional network organization of the human brain. *Neuron* 72, 665–678.

Rauschecker, J. P., Leaver, A. M., and Muhlau, M. (2010). Tuning out the noise: limbic–auditory interactions in tinnitus. *Neuron* 66, 819–826. doi: 10.1016/j.neuron.2010.04.032

Roland, L. T., Lenze, E. J., Hardin, F. M., Kallogjeri, D., Nicklaus, J., Wineland, A. M., et al. (2015). Effects of mindfulness based stress reduction therapy on subjective bother and neural connectivity in chronic tinnitus. *Otolaryngol. Head Neck Surg.* 152, 919–926. doi: 10.1177/0194599815571556

Sadaghiani, S., Hesselmann, G., and Kleinschmidt, A. (2009). Distributed and antagonistic contributions of ongoing activity fluctuations to auditory stimulus detection. *J. Neurosci.* 29, 13410–13417. doi: 10.1523/JNEUROSCI.2592-09.2009

Salviati, M., Macri, F., Terlizzi, S., Melcore, C., Provenzano, A., Capparelli, E., et al. (2013). The tinnitus handicap inventory as a screening test for psychiatric comorbidity in patients with tinnitus. *Psychosomatics* 54, 248–256. doi: 10.1016/j.psym.2012.05.007

Schecklmann, M., Lehner, A., Poeppl, T. B., Kreuzer, P. M., Rupprecht, R., Rackl, J., et al. (2013). Auditory cortex is implicated in tinnitus distress: a voxel-based morphometry study. *Brain Struct. Funct.* 218, 1061–1070. doi: 10.1007/s00429-013-0520-z

Scherer, R. W., Formby, C., Gold, S., Erdman, S., Rodhe, C., Carlson, M., et al. (2014). The tinnitus retraining therapy trial (TRTT): study protocol for a randomized controlled trial. *Trials* 15:396. doi: 10.1186/1745-6215-15-396

Searchfield, G. D., Kaur, M., and Martin, W. H. (2010). Hearing aids as an adjunct to counseling: tinnitus patients who choose amplification do better than those that don't. *Int. J. Audiol.* 49, 574–579. doi: 10.3109/14992021003777267

Shehzad, Z., Kelly, A. M., Reiss, P. T., Gee, D. G., Gotimer, K., Uddin, L. Q., et al. (2009). The resting brain: unconstrained yet reliable. *Cereb. Cortex* 19, 2209–2229. doi: 10.1093/cercor/bhn256

Shen, Y., Yao, J., Jiang, X., Zhang, L., Xu, L., Feng, R., et al. (2015). Sub-hubs of baseline functional brain networks are related to early improvement following two-week pharmacological therapy for major depressive disorder. *Hum. Brain Mapp.* 36, 2915–2927. doi: 10.1002/hbm.22817

Song, X. W., Dong, Z. Y., Long, X. Y., Li, S. F., Zuo, X. N., Zhu, C. Z., et al. (2011). REST: a toolkit for resting-state functional magnetic resonance imaging data processing. *PLoS One* 6:e25031. doi: 10.1371/journal.pone.0025031

Tomasi, D., and Volkow, N. D. (2010). Functional connectivity density mapping. *Proc. Natl. Acad. Sci. U.S.A.* 107, 9885–9890. doi: 10.1073/pnas.1001414107

Tunkel, D. E., Bauer, C. A., Sun, G. H., Rosenfeld, R. M., Chandrasekhar, S. S., Cunningham, E. J., et al. (2014). Clinical practice guideline: tinnitus. *Otolaryngol. Head Neck Surg.* 151(2 Suppl.), S1–S40.

Vanneste, S., van de Heyning, P., and De Ridder, D. (2011). The neural network of phantom sound changes over time: a comparison between recent-onset and chronic tinnitus patients. *Eur. J. Neurosci.* 34, 718–731. doi: 10.1111/j.1460-9568.2011.07793.x

von Boetticher, A. (2011). Ginkgo biloba extract in the treatment of tinnitus: a systematic review. *Neuropsychiatr. Dis. Treat.* 7, 441–447. doi: 10.2147/NDT.S22793

Walker, D. D., Cifu, A. S., and Gluth, M. B. (2016). Tinnitus. *JAMA* 315, 2221–2222.

Wang, J., Wang, X., Xia, M., Liao, X., Evans, A., and He, Y. (2015). GRETNA: a graph theoretical network analysis toolbox for imaging connectomics. *Front. Hum. Neurosci.* 9:386. doi: 10.3389/fnhum.2015.00386

Wang, J. H., Zuo, X. N., Gohel, S., Milham, M. P., Biswal, B. B., and He, Y. (2011). Graph theoretical analysis of functional brain networks: test–retest evaluation on short- and long-term resting-state functional MRI data. *PLoS One* 6:e21976. doi: 10.1371/journal.pone.0021976

Weise, C., Kleinstauber, M., and Andersson, G. (2016). Internet-delivered cognitive–behavior therapy for tinnitus: a randomized controlled trial. *Psychosom. Med.* 78, 501–510. doi: 10.1097/PSY.0000000000000310

Xia, M., Wang, J., and He, Y. (2013). BrainNet viewer: a network visualization tool for human brain connectomics. *PLoS One* 8:e68910. doi: 10.1371/journal.pone.0068910

Yan, C. G., Cheung, B., Kelly, C., Colcombe, S., Craddock, R. C., Di Martino, A., et al. (2013). A comprehensive assessment of regional variation in the impact of head micromovements on functional connectomics. *Neuroimage* 76, 183–201. doi: 10.1016/j.neuroimage.2013.03.004

Zeman, F., Koller, M., Figueiredo, R., Aazevedo, A., Rates, M., Coelho, C., et al. (2011). Tinnitus handicap inventory for evaluating treatment effects: which changes are clinically relevant? *Otolaryngol. Head Neck Surg.* 145, 282–287. doi: 10.1177/0194599811403882

Zhang, J. (2013). Auditory cortex stimulation to suppress tinnitus: mechanisms and strategies. *Hear. Res.* 295, 38–57. doi: 10.1016/j.heares.2012.05.007

Zhang, J., Chen, Y. C., Feng, X., Yang, M., Liu, B., Qian, C., et al. (2015). Impairments of thalamic resting-state functional connectivity in patients with chronic tinnitus. *Eur. J. Radiol.* 84, 1277–1284. doi: 10.1016/j.ejrad.2015.04.006

Zhuo, C., Zhu, J., Qin, W., Qu, H., Ma, X., Tian, H., et al. (2014). Functional connectivity density alterations in schizophrenia. *Front. Behav. Neurosci.* 8:404. doi: 10.3389/fnbeh.2014.00404

Zuo, X. N., Ehmke, R., Mennes, M., Imperati, D., Castellanos, F. X., Sporns, O., et al. (2012). Network centrality in the human functional connectome. *Cereb. Cortex* 22, 1862–1875. doi: 10.1093/cercor/bhr269

Zuo, X. N., and Xing, X. X. (2014). Test–retest reliabilities of resting-state FMRI measurements in human brain functional connectomics: a systems neuroscience perspective. *Neurosci. Biobehav. Rev.* 45C, 100–118. doi: 10.1016/j.neubiorev.2014.05.009

20

Aberrant Functional and Causal Connectivity in Acute Tinnitus with Sensorineural Hearing Loss

Yuexin Cai[1,2†], Mingwei Xie[3†], Yun Su[3], Zhaopeng Tong[1,2], Xiaoyan Wu[3], Wenchao Xu[1,2], Jiahong Li[1,2], Fei Zhao[4,5], Caiping Dang[6,7], Guisheng Chen[1,2], Liping Lan[1,2], Jun Shen[3] and Yiqing Zheng[1,2]**

[1] Department of Otolaryngology, Sun Yat-sen Memorial Hospital, Sun Yat-sen University, Guangzhou, China, [2] Institute of Hearing and Speech-Language Science, Sun Yat-sen University, Guangzhou, China, [3] Department of Radiology, Sun Yat-sen Memorial Hospital, Sun Yat-sen University, Guangzhou, China, [4] Department of Speech and Language Therapy and Hearing Science, Cardiff Metropolitan University, Cardiff, United Kingdom, [5] Department of Hearing and Speech Science, Xinhua College, Sun Yat-sen University, Guangzhou, China, [6] Affiliated Brain Hospital of Guangzhou Medical University, Guangzhou, China, [7] Department of Psychology, Guangzhou Medical University, Guangzhou, China

Correspondence:
Jun Shen
shenjun@mail.sysu.edu.cn
Yiqing Zheng
zhengyiq@mail.sysu.edu.cn

† These authors have contributed equally to this work

Purpose: The neural bases in acute tinnitus remains largely undetected. The objective of this study was to identify the alteration of the brain network involved in patients with acute tinnitus and hearing loss.

Methods: Acute tinnitus patients (n = 24) with hearing loss and age-, sex-, education-matched healthy controls (n = 21) participated in the current study and underwent resting-state functional magnetic resonance imaging (fMRI) scanning. Regional homogeneity and amplitude of low-frequency fluctuation were used to investigate the local spontaneous neural activity and functional connectivity (FC), and Granger causality analysis (GCA) was used to analyze the undirected and directed connectivity of brain regions.

Results: Compared with healthy subjects, acute tinnitus patients had a general reduction in FC between auditory and non-auditory brain regions. Based on FC analysis, the superior temporal gyrus (STG) revealed reduced undirected connectivity with non-auditory brain regions including the amygdala (AMYG), nucleus accumbens (NAc), the cerebellum, and postcentral gyrus (PoCG). Using the GCA algorithm, increased effective connectivity from the right AMYG to the right STG, and reduced connectivity from the right PoCG to the left NAc was observed in acute tinnitus patients with hearing loss. The pure-tone threshold was positively correlated with FC between the AMYG and STG, and negatively correlated with FC between the left NAc and the right PoCG. In addition, a negative association between the GCA value from the right PoCG to the left NAc and the THI scores was observed.

Conclusion: Acute tinnitus patients have aberrant FC strength and causal connectivity in both the auditory and non-auditory cortex, especially in the STG, AMYG, and NAc. The current findings will provide a new perspective for understanding the neuropathophysiological mechanism in acute tinnitus.

Keywords: acute tinnitus, hearing loss, functional magnetic resonance imaging (fMRI), functional connectivity, causal connectivity

INTRODUCTION

Tinnitus is defined as the perception of a phantom sound in the absence of an internal or external sound source (Chen et al., 2017c; Cai et al., 2018; Vanneste et al., 2019). The prevalence of tinnitus reaches about 10–15% of the adult population. Of these, about 10–20% of patients are affected severely and sought medical therapy (Cai et al., 2017; Yang et al., 2018). At present, the clinical treatment for tinnitus includes counseling, sound therapy, cognitive behavioral therapy, etc., however, no identified treatments have been effective and unequivocal to all types of tinnitus (Chen et al., 2017b; Tsai et al., 2018). One of the most important reasons is that the mechanism of tinnitus remains unclear. Nowadays, it is widely accepted that tinnitus in not only caused by peripheral cochlear impairment, but also the aberrant activity in the central nervous system (Chen et al., 2017b; Cai et al., 2018). A large number of neuroimaging studies have reported that abnormality of central activities are involved in both auditory and non-auditory brain regions for chronic tinnitus (Chen et al., 2017c; Vanneste et al., 2019).

In auditory cortices, several studies revealed that this brain region, including the middle temporal gyrus (MTG) and superior temporal gyrus (STG), predominantly had hyperactivity in patients with chronic tinnitus (Chen et al., 2017c; Han et al., 2018). Middle temporal gyrus has been proven to be a key region of the default mode network (DMN), whose activity might depend on people's attention or goal-directed behavior (Raichle et al., 2001; Mantini et al., 2007). The perception of a phantom auditory sensation from tinnitus might lead to its hyperfunction. In addition, the hyperactivity of STG has been considered to reflect the auditory phantom phenomenon (Smits et al., 2007). In non-auditory brain regions, especially the limbic system, altered neural activity has been regarded as neural decompensation for the tinnitus auditory phantom. Equivalent to the descending pain inhibitory system, a similar "noise canceling" system mainly consisting of the nucleus accumbens (NAc) and the ventromedial prefrontal cortex (vmPFC) has been evidenced and found in studies using both anatomical and functional magnetic resonance imaging (fMRI). Rauschecker et al. (2015) showed disrupted core areas of these regions, which consequently, might cause the occurrence or/and persistence of tinnitus (Rauschecker et al., 2015). In addition, Song et al. (2015) demonstrated that the neural activity of rostral anterior cingulate cortex (ACC) and the connectivity between primary auditory cortex and ACC had a significantly negative correlation with the tinnitus awareness grade. As a result, the authors suggested that rostral ACC is likely to become another core area of the noise canceling system in response to the perception of tinnitus (Song et al., 2015).

Furthermore, many pathophysiological models have also been developed to explain the mechanism of chronic tinnitus, including central gain, neural synchrony, frontostriatal gating, noise canceling deficits, and global workspace (Vanneste et al., 2011; Hashmi et al., 2013; Elgoyhen et al., 2015; Rauschecker et al., 2015; Wallhäusser-Franke et al., 2017; Cai et al., 2018; Zhou et al., 2019). However, few studies have investigated central neural processing during an acute period, thus, the mechanism of acute tinnitus remains unclear. It is therefore crucial to clarify the alteration of the brain network of acute tinnitus to prevent its development from acute to chronic tinnitus. The abnormalities in the auditory and non-auditory brain regions found in patients with chronic tinnitus could provide important clues for further research of acute tinnitus.

A recent study by Zhou et al. (2019) investigated the alterations of brain function using resting-state functional magnetic resonance imaging (rs-fMRI) in 28 patients with unilateral acute tinnitus and hearing loss. Abnormal neural activity and altered connectivity in both the auditory and non-auditory cortex were found. The disrupted cortex regions included increased activity in the right temporal gyrus and decreased in the cerebellar vermis, the right calcarine cortex, the right precuneus, the right supramarginal gyrus (SMG), as well as the right middle frontal gyrus (MFG) in acute tinnitus, which associated with the DMN, attention network, visual network, and executive control network (Zhou et al., 2019). In a recent electroencephalography (EEG) study, reduced activity in the left frontal cortex, decreased connectivity between the temporal gyrus and the SMG, as well as the central cingulate gyrus and frontal gyrus in a comparison between 25 acute tinnitus subjects and 27 healthy controls, was shown (Cai et al., 2019). These studies support the aberrant central changes in brain activity in tinnitus during the acute period, however, the findings from these studies are inconsistent and the causal connectivity in neural networks in acute tinnitus remains largely undetected.

Tinnitus is usually associated with sensorineural hearing loss (HL). Sensorineural hearing loss has been identified as the most relevant factor to trigger tinnitus. About 75% of unilateral tinnitus and over 80% of bilateral tinnitus patients have a HL in the standard audiogram detection with thresholds exceeding 20 dB (Wallhäusser-Franke et al., 2017). Studies on acute tinnitus are usually concerned with tinnitus following idiopathic sudden sensorineural hearing loss (ISSNHL). Idiopathic sudden sensorineural hearing loss with tinnitus is a good candidate for the investigation of the pathophysiological mechanism of acute tinnitus (Mühlmeier et al., 2016; Wallhäusser-Franke et al., 2017).

Resting-state fMRI has been widely used to detect intrinsic neuro-pathophysiological mechanisms in terms of aberrant neural activity and brain functional connectivity (FC) changes in various neurological related disorders, such as chronic tinnitus, Alzheimer's disease, and Parkinson (Chen et al., 2018b,c,d). Resting-state fMRI measurement is based on the low-frequency (0.01–0.1 Hz) fluctuations in blood-oxygenation-level dependent (BOLD) signals, and thus regional homogeneity (ReHo) can be applied to demonstrate abnormal neural coherence across the whole brain, by quantifying the local synchronization within adjacent voxels during resting state (Zang et al., 2004). With regards to this measurement, amplitude of low-frequency fluctuation (ALFF) is widely regarded as an effective approach that measures intrinsic neural response at the sing-voxel level to reflect the intensity of regional neuronal spontaneous activity (Biswal et al., 1995). Moreover, fractional ALFF (fALFF) is a better approach to detect the resting-state regional spontaneous neural activity in comparison to ALFF analysis, due to the reduction of physiological noise (Zou et al., 2008).

Functional connectivity is an effective method to explore the synchronization of functional activities in different brain regions as well as the correlations between them, while Granger causality analysis (GCA) is explicitly used to examine the functional relationship in a directed manner (Friston et al., 2013), emphasizing the causality between brain regions. The purpose of this study is therefore, to investigate the aberrant functional and causal connectivity of central neural regions in patients with acute tinnitus, by combining FC and GCA analysis. It is hypothesized that alterations of the central neural network can reveal the central neural mechanisms associated with the characteristics of acute tinnitus.

MATERIALS AND METHODS

Participants

In this study, 28 right-handed ISSNHL patients with tinnitus, and 23 age- and gender-matched healthy subjects were recruited from the Ear, Nose, and Throat clinic, Sun Yat-sen Memorial hospital, Guangzhou, China, through recruitment advertisements. The selection criteria for ISSNHL subjects with tinnitus were as follows:

- Patients had no less than 30 dB sensorineural hearing impairment associated with tinnitus in more than three consecutive audiometric frequencies that had onset within 3 days.
- The duration of patients' relevant symptom was less than 1 month.
- Patients had sought clinical help due to hearing impairment and tinnitus.
- Subjects with middle ear surgery, pulsatile tinnitus, Ménière's disease, autoimmune hearing loss, acoustic neurinoma, central nervous system disorders, head trauma, depression, insomnia or magnetic resonance imaging (MRI) contraindications were excluded.
- Subjects with a head motion greater than 2.0 mm translation in any plane or a 2.0° rotation in any direction during MRI scanning were excluded.

The hearing thresholds of all participants were determined by pure tone audiometry (PTA) examination. Subjects were asked to sit in an acoustically shielded room for the test. Air conduction thresholds at 0.125, 0.25, 0.5, 1, 2, 4, and 8 kHz were measured on both ears. Bone conduction thresholds at 0.25, 0.5, 1, 2, and 4 kHz were also determined. Mean hearing threshold was calculated from hearing thresholds at 0.5, 1, 2, and 4 kHz (Audiology, 1988; Cai et al., 2019).

All patients were asked to describe the duration and laterality of tinnitus. Afterward, a tinnitus pitch matching test was performed (Teismann et al., 2011), in which the tinnitus pitch match was determined using the frequencies 0.125, 0.25, 0.5, 1, 2, 3, 4, 6, and 8 kHz. In the process of the test, participants were asked to contrast the perceptive tinnitus pitch and the matching pitch, and the matching pitch was adjusted according to the feedback from the subjects. Ultimately, a more precise or approximate matching pitch was obtained by adjusting the frequency in half-octave steps. If no matching pure tone was gained from subjects, narrow band noise was applied.

Moreover, the tinnitus handicap inventory (THI; Newman et al., 1996), was used to assess the severity of tinnitus and related distress after the tinnitus specific assessment. The duration of education of all subjects were also collected.

Data was collected before patients received any therapeutic intervention, within 30 days, however, four ISSNHL patients with tinnitus and two healthy volunteers were excluded because of excessive head motion during MRI scanning. Therefore, 24 ISSNHL patients with tinnitus (10 males and 14 females; age mean = 43.57 years, SD = 15.42 years) and 21 healthy subjects (12 males and 9 females; age mean = 44.48 years, SD = 17.05 years) were finally included for the data analysis. Among the patients, eight subjects have tinnitus in the right ear, 10 subjects in the left ear, and six subjects in bilateral ears. All participants were informed of the background and purpose of the study and they signed a written consent form. This study was approved by the Ethics Committee of Sun Yat-sen Memorial Hospital, and written informed consent was obtained from each participant.

MRI Acquisition

Magnetic resonance imaging was performed on a 3.0 T MRI scanner (Ingenia, Philips Medical Systems, Netherlands) with an 8-channel receiver array head coil. Head motion and scanner noise were reduced using foam padding and earplugs. The subjects were required to lie quietly with their eyes closed but not to fall asleep, to avoid thinking of anything in particular, and to avoid head motion during the scan. Functional images were obtained axially using a gradient echo-planar imaging sequence as follows: repetition time (TR) = 2000 ms, echo time (TE) = 30 ms, slices = 33, thickness = 3.5 mm, gap = 0.7 mm, field of view (FOV) = 224 mm × 224 mm, acquisition matrix = 64 × 64, and flip angle (FA) = 90°. The voxel size was 3.5 mm × 3.5 mm × 3.5 mm, and 240 functional volumes were obtained. High resolution T1-weighted, 3D anatomical images were collected followed by the resting scan for normalization with the following parameters: TR/TE = 7/3.2 ms, slices = 192, thickness = 1 mm, gap = 0 mm, FA = 7°, acquisition matrix = 256 × 256, and FOV = 256 mm × 256 mm. The fMRI sequence lasted 8 min and 8 s, and the structural sequence lasted 6 min and 20 s. All scans were acquired with parallel imaging using the sensitivity encoding (SENSE) technique, SENSE factor = 2.

Data Preprocessing

Resting-State fMRI data were preprocessed using Data Processing & Analysis for Brain Imaging (DPABI; Yan et al., 2016), which is based on Statistical Parametric Mapping (SPM12)[1] and the MATLAB R2013a platform. The first 10 volumes were discarded, and the remaining 230 consecutive volumes were corrected for the slice time delay. The realignment was performed to evaluate the degree of head motion and any subjects with a head motion greater than 2.0 mm translation in any plane, or a 2.0° rotation in any direction were excluded. Four sudden deafness with tinnitus,

[1] http://www.fil.ion.ucl.ac.uk/spm

patients and two healthy volunteers were excluded because of excessive head motion during scanning. The 3D anatomical image was co-registered to the functional space, and segmented into white matter, gray matter, and cerebrospinal fluid. According to the segmental information, the realigned functional images were normalized to the standard Montreal Neurological Institute (MNI) template (resampling voxel size = 3 mm × 3 mm × 3 mm). In the calculations, we also regressed out nuisance covariates, including head motion profiles (Friston 24-parameter model; Friston et al., 1995), the linear trend signal, white matter signal, and the cerebrospinal fluid signal.

Regional Homogeneity Analysis

Temporal bandpass filtering (0.01–0.1 Hz) was performed to reduce the effect of high-frequency before the ReHo calculation. For each participant, ReHo map was generated by Kendall's coefficient of concordance (KCC), which was used to measure the local synchronization of a given voxel with its 26 nearest neighbors. The ReHo value of each voxel was standardized by partitioning the primal value using the global mean ReHo value. The normalized data were then smoothed with an isotropic Gaussian kernel [full width at half maximum (FWHM) = 4 mm] for further statistical analysis.

Fractional Amplitude of Low-Frequency Fluctuations Analysis

To increase the signal-to-noise ratio of the preprocessed image, spatial smoothing (FWHM = 4 mm) was conducted before the fALFF calculation. The time courses were then converted to the frequency domain with Fast Fourier Transform and the power spectrum for each voxel was evaluated. Finally, the fALFF map was generated by the ratio of the square root of the power spectrum at the low-frequency band (0.01–0.1 Hz) to the entire detectable frequency band.

Seed-Based Functional Connectivity Analysis

Twenty (10 left, 10 right) 5-mm-radius spherical regions of interest (ROIs), several prominent brain areas identified in the tinnitus literature, were defined as the seed ROIs for seed-based FC analysis (De Ridder et al., 2011, 2014a,b; Rauschecker et al., 2015; Song et al., 2015; Hullfish et al., 2019): the bilateral auditory cortices, NAc, AMYG, parahippocampal gyrus (PHG), pregenual anterior cingulate cortices (pACC), subgenual ACC, and the ventromedial prefrontal cortices (PFC). The specific MNI coordinates of the seed ROIs are shown in **Table 1**. For each ROI, we analyzed FC between the seed region and the whole brain at the voxel level using Pearson's correlation analysis, and a FC map was acquired. The FC map was standardized to a z score map using Fisher r to z transfer, and a zFC map was obtained for each subject.

Granger Causality Analysis

The ROI-wise GCA was performed using the REST-GCA in the REST toolbox[2] to detect the effective connectivity between each pair of brain regions, which presented significant group-difference in the seed-based FC analysis. For each pair, we extracted time series of the brain regions (x, y). Signed path coefficients were then calculated as a GCA value, including $x \rightarrow y$ and $y \rightarrow x$, according to Zang et al. (2012) the extended vector AR model for each subject.

[2]http://www.restfmri.net/forum/

TABLE 1 | Seed regions of interest, center coordinates in MNI space.

Regions of interest	L/R	Center-of mass coordinates		
		x	*y*	*z*
Auditory cortices				
M-TG	L	−57	−18	−15
	R	58	−17	−15
STG	L	−62	−23	12
	R	63	−24	12
	L	−46	−29	10
	R	47	−29	10
	L	−56	−25	5
	R	56	−22	3
Limbic system				
NAc	L	−10	12	−13
	R	13	11	−13
AMYG	L	−24	−6	−18
	R	24	−6	−18
PHG	L	−26	−36	−10
	R	26	−36	−10
Pregenual ACC	L	−4	38	4
	R	4	38	4
Subgenual ACC	L	−4	26	−10
	R	4	26	−10
Ventromedial PFC	L	−3	44	−8
	R	3	44	−8

Coordinates are described in MNI coordinates. MNI, Montreal Neurological Institute; MTG, middle temporal gyrus; STG, superior temporal gyrus; NAc, nucleus accumbens; AMYG, amygdala; PHG, paraHippocampal gyrus; ACC, anterior cingulate cortices; PFC, prefrontal cortices; L, left hemisphere; R, right hemisphere.

Statistical Analysis

Two-sample t-tests were used to test group differences in demographic and clinical data, such as the age, the PTA, the duration, and the THI. The χ^2-test was used to compare the between-group difference of gender and education (statistical significance set at $p < 0.05$).

For the ReHo map, fALFF map, and seed-based zFC map, we used two-sample t-tests to detect the difference between the ISSNHL patients and healthy controls, and threshold-free cluster enhancement (TFCE) with family-wise error (FWE) correction ($p < 0.05$) was used for multiple comparisons (Chen et al., 2018a). Furthermore, two-sample t-tests were used for the GCA value to determine the differences between the two groups. The significance level was set at $p < 0.05$.

Pearson's correlation was applied to investigate the association between the clinical characteristics and the altered FC/GCA in acute tinnitus subjects ($p < 0.05$, uncorrected for zFC; $p < 0.0063$, Bonferroni correction for GCA).

RESULTS

Demographic Information

Except for PTA ($p < 0.05$), there was no significant between-group differences in demographic and other clinical information ($p > 0.05$). The specific information of patients and the healthy subjects is shown in **Table 2**.

ReHo Analysis and fALFF Analysis

There was no significant difference in the ReHo value and the fALFF value between ISSNHL patients and the healthy controls in any brain region ($p > 0.05$, TFCE with FWE correction).

Functional Connectivity Analysis

In contrast to the healthy controls, ISSNHL subjects demonstrated prominent decreased FC between the left STG and the right CER4_5 and the left precentral gyrus. In addition, the reduced FC was also observed between the right STG and the right CERCRU2_R, AMYG, postcentral gyrus (PoCG), the left CER8, CER6, MOG, ITG, and the PCL ($p < 0.05$, TFCE with FWE correction; **Table 3** and **Figure 1**). Moreover, in the limbic system, we also detected decreased FC between the left NAc and the right PoCG and the homolateral SFG in ISSNHL patients with tinnitus compared to the healthy subjects. Instead of the NAc, the AMYG, and PHG had similar inhibitions of the FC to other brain regions. Compared with the healthy subjects, the left AMYG had decreased FC to the right STG. The FC also decreased between the left PHG and the right SMA ($p < 0.05$, TFCE with FWE correction; **Table 4** and **Figure 2**).

Granger Causality Analysis

According to our seed-based FC analysis results, 16 pairs of brain regions with significant group-differences were selected for the GCA analysis between each pair. In contrast to the healthy controls, patients with ISSNHL demonstrated a significantly increased GCA value from the right AMYG to the right STG ($p < 0.05$; **Figure 3**). In contrast, a reduced GCA value from the right PoCG to the left NAc was observed in ISSNHL patients ($p < 0.05$; **Figure 3**).

Correlation Analysis

Figure 4 shows that the PTA was positively correlated with the FC between the right STG and the AMYG ($r = 0.436$, $p = 0.033$). Moreover, the Pearson's correlation analyses revealed the negative correlation between the PTA and the FC between the left NAc and the right PoCG ($r = -0.461$, $p = 0.023$). In addition, a negative association between the GCA value from the right PoCG to the left NAc and the THI was observed ($r = -0.595$, $p < 0.002$; **Figure 3**).

DISCUSSION

This is the first study to use both FC and GCA approaches to explore intrinsic dysfunctional network connectivity related to acute tinnitus. These results highlight the general hypo-connectivity between auditory and non-auditory regions. Based on FC analysis, we found significant decreased connectivity between the STG and several non-auditory regions, including the AMYG, NAc, the cerebellum, and the somatosensory cortex. Using the GCA algorithm, significant increased effective connectivity from the right AMYG to the right STG, and reduced connectivity from the right PoCG to the left NAc was observed in acute tinnitus patients with hearing loss. Moreover, these abnormalities of connectivity were correlated to the intensity of hearing loss and tinnitus distress. Our study clearly demonstrates interregional changes in neural function in acute tinnitus with hearing loss.

Functional Connectivity and Spontaneous Brain Activation in the STG in Acute Tinnitus With Hearing Loss

The present study showed reduced connections between the STG and associative areas that constitute an emerging feature of brain architecture. Our finding demonstrates that the STG is the main cortical hub in the brain network that is affected by acute tinnitus with hearing loss, which is in line with the hypothesis that the dysconnectivity pattern of the STG is involved in tinnitus perception (Chen et al., 2017a; Qu et al., 2019; Berlot et al., 2020). The STG is regarded as a critical region which receives the neuronal projection from auditory pathway (Binder, 2017) and has been reported to be associated with cognitive functions including memory, auditory cognition and semantics (Jackson et al., 2018). Several neurophysiological models related to STG have been raised as being involved in the acute stage of tinnitus and hearing loss (Fan et al., 2015; Micarelli et al., 2017). In addition, hearing loss may lead to a hypofunction of the auditory cortex which consequently presents a decreased FC between the STG and associative regions. However, a recent study found no significant spontaneous neural activity in the STG and associative areas in ISSNL subjects, which may be due to the short duration of the tinnitus. This finding is in contrast to some previous studies, for example, a PET study reported the decreased FDG uPTAke in the STG, MTG and MFG regions in ISSNHL subjects. The various neuroimaging methods employed, and the tinnitus sample's heterogeneity may have contributed to the inconsistent results. These results indicated that the short duration of tinnitus accompanying hearing loss, may not necessarily evoke the compensatory enhancement of spontaneous activity, but disrupted FC occurred before the altered local neural changes took place.

Our study also found that non-auditory associative regions reduced connectivity with the STG, which included the cerebellum, PreCG, and the PoCG. The cerebellum is considered as an important hub in detecting auditory afferent and sound processing (Zhou et al., 2019), as well as plays a critical role in a gating control mechanism (Micarelli et al., 2017). Our finding is in line with this previous study, which shows a reduction of cerebellum activity in acute tinnitus. Maudoux et al. also found disrupted connectivity between the auditory cortex and the cerebellum (Maudoux et al., 2012). Therefore, the disrupted connectivity between the cerebellum and STG may induce a reduced capability of contrasting and integrating afferent signals

TABLE 2 | Demographic and clinical characteristics of sudden deafness with tinnitus patients and healthy controls.

	Patients (*n* = 24)	Controls (*n* = 21)	*p* value
Age (year)	43.57 ± 15.42	44.48 ± 17.05	0.868[a]
Gender (male; female)	10:14	12:9	0.300[b]
Education levels (years)	12.54 ± 3.50	12.61 ± 4.13	0.293[a]
Tinnitus laterality (right/left/bilateral)	8/10/6	N/A	N/A
PTA of right ear	36.96 ± 28.98	15.57 ± 4.52	0.002[a]
PTA of left ear	38.08 ± 25.99	14.52 ± 4.43	<0.001[a]
Average PTA	36.27 ± 13.84	15.05 ± 4.20	<0.001[a]
Duration (days)	9.95 ± 7.08	N/A	N/A
THI	36.25 ± 21.75	N/A	N/A

Values are represented as Mean ± SD. [a]Two-sample t-tests. [b]χ^2-test. PTA, pure tone audiometry; THI, tinnitus handicap inventory; N/A, non-applicable.

TABLE 3 | Regions showing significant differences of auditory-FC between ISSNHL patients and healthy controls.

Seed region	Brain regions	Peak MNI coordinates *x, y, z* (mm)	Peak *T* value	Voxels
STG.L (-62, −23, 12)	CER4_5.R	18, −42, −26	−4.83	82
STG.R (63, −24, 12)	CERCRU2.R	3, −78, −39	−4.29	45
	CER6.R	−15, −57, −25	−4.89	45
STG.L (-56, −25, 5)	PreCG.L	−18, −18, 69	−5.59	233
STG.R (56, −22, 3)	CER8.L	−30, −51, −57	−5.15	52
	CER6.L	−12, −66, −24	−4.64	41
	MOG.L	−39, −89, −7	−4.18	267
	ITG.L	−36, 15, −41	−4.27	309
	PCL.L	−9, −27, 72	−4.74	457
	CERCRU2.R	6, −84, −42	−4.36	89
	AMYG.R	24, −3, −15	−4.97	160
	PoCG.R	60, −21, 45	−5.68	188

MNI, Montreal Neurological Institute; STG, superior temporal gyrus; PoCG, postcentral gyrus; MOG, middle occipital gyrus; ITG, inferior temporal gyrus; PCL, paracentral lobule; AMYG, amygdala; CERCRU2, cerebellum_Crus2; CER4_5, cerebellum_4_5; CER6, cerebellum_6; CER8, cerebellum_8; L, left hemisphere; R, right hemisphere. A corrected threshold of $p < 0.05$ was determined by threshold-free cluster enhancement (TFCE) with family-wise error (FWE) correction.

from the auditory cortex, triggering a phantom sound during acute hearing loss.

The PreCG is the anatomical location of the primary motor cortex, which is responsible for controlling voluntary motor movement of the body and involved in the executive functioning of response inhibition. This was consistent with a resting state PET study that patients with SSNHL presented Glucose uPTAke reduced in PreCG and suggested PreCG as a vital region in auditory associated events related to word recognition and phonological processing (Micarelli et al., 2017). The disconnection between PreCG and STG may lead to auditory processing functional decline during the acute stage of tinnitus and hearing loss.

Functional Connectivity and Correlation Analysis in Limbic System in Acute Tinnitus With Hearing Loss

Tinnitus is often associated with emotional distress and anxiety, these complications may be associated with maladaptive functional connections to the limbic structure, such as the AMYG, hippocampus and the NAc (Hashmi et al., 2013; Lanting et al., 2014; Chen et al., 2017a,c). In this study, reduced undirected connectivity between the AMYG and STG but an increased connectivity between the GCA from the AMYG to the STG was found. The AMYG is a vital part of the subcortical limbic structure, which receives and sends auditory information to the auditory cortex to relay emotional attributes (Yan, 2003; Keuroghlian and Knudsen, 2007; Qu et al., 2019; Xu et al., 2019). Furthermore, the AMYG not only receives information from auditory cortex, but also receives directed projection from subcortical areas of the ascending auditory pathway (Pannese et al., 2016). Therefore, after the acute stage of peripheral auditory deafferentation, the dysfunctional neural synchrony of inter-regions would induce declined connectivity between the AMYG and STG. However, enhanced influence from the AMYG to the STG reflect a central reorganization in the acute period of tinnitus and hearing loss. The AMYG is thought to decode the affective value to the sound perception that is pre-processed, especially in the auditory cortex (Kumar et al., 2012). This is consistent with the findings from previous neuroimaging studies showing that the abnormalities in the AMYG could account for tinnitus and induce chronic depression in tinnitus patients (Micarelli et al., 2017). Activation of the AMYG can augment the central neural plasticity in the auditory cortex (Froemke and Martins, 2011), which could be interpreted as an attempt in conflict monitoring

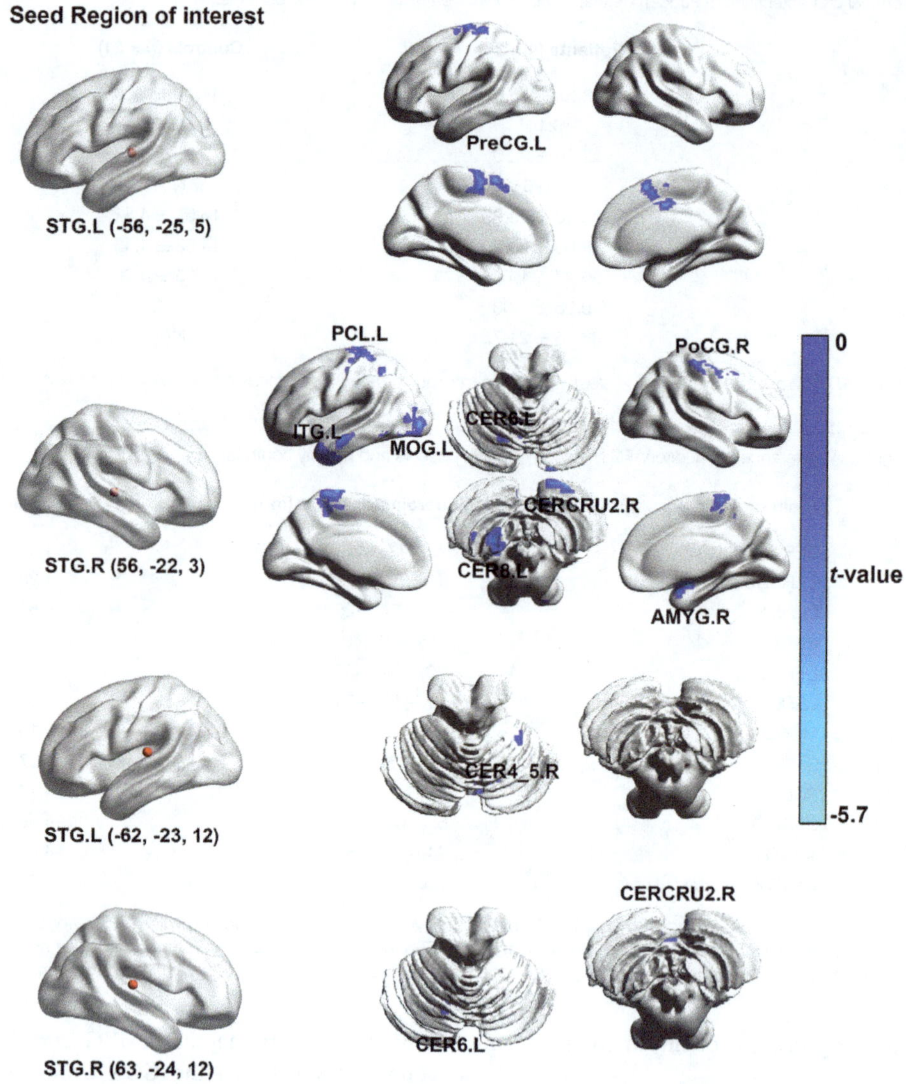

FIGURE 1 | The brain regions with significant difference in the auditory-FC between ISSNHL patients and healthy controls. Left brain diagram shows the seed region of interesting of auditory system, right brain diagram presents the regions with significant group-difference. FC, functional connectivity; STG, superior temporal gyrus; PoCG, postcentral gyrus; MOG, middle occipital gyrus; ITG, inferior temporal gyrus; PCL, paracentral lobule; AMYG, amygdala; CERCRU2, cerebellum_Crus2; CER4_5, cerebellum_4_5; CER6, cerebellum_6; CER8, cerebellum_8; L, left hemisphere; R, right hemisphere. The color bar represents the *t*-value.

TABLE 4 | Regions showing significant differences of limbic-FC between ISSNHL patients and healthy controls.

Seed region	Brain regions	Peak MNI coordinates x, y, z (mm)	Peak *T* value	Voxels
NAc.L	PoCG.R	39, −30, 45	−4.78	53
	SFG.R	15, −9, 63	−4.70	28
AMYG.L	STG.R	57, −21, 0	−4.57	33
PHG.L	SMA.R	6, 0, 48	−4.95	57

MNI, Montreal Neurological Institute; STG, superior temporal gyrus; PoCG, postcentral gyrus; NAc, nucleus accumbens; SFG, superior frontal gyrus; AMYG, amygdala; PHG, paraHippocampal gyrus; SMA, supplementary motor area; L, left hemisphere; R, right hemisphere. A corrected threshold of $p < 0.05$ was determined by threshold-free cluster enhancement (TFCE) with family-wise error (FWE) correction.

and in informative trace integration coming from sensory error detection, such as those represented by an unexpected auditory input impairment. This heightened influence from the AMYG to the STG might be interpreted as a dysfunctional inhibitory response, directing attention to a phantom sound perception, which may be the possible reason of induced tinnitus.

An interesting finding is the positive correlation between the PTA and FC of the AMYG and STG, which highlight the theories

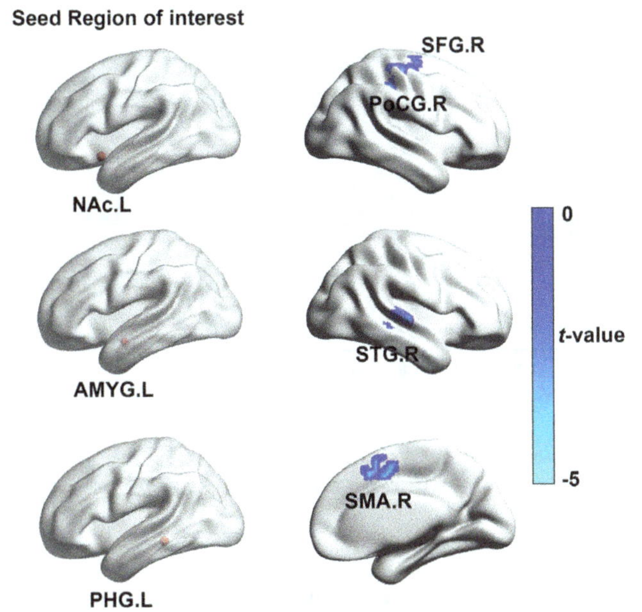

FIGURE 2 | The brain regions show significant difference of the limbic-FC between ISSNHL patients and healthy controls. Left brain diagram shows the seed region of interesting of limbic system, right brain graph presents the regions with significant group-difference. FC, functional connectivity; STG, superior temporal gyrus; PoCG, postcentral gyrus; NAc, nucleus accumbens; SFG, Superior frontal gyrus; AMYG, amygdala; PHG, paraHippocampal gyrus; SMA, supplementary motor area; L, left hemisphere; R, right hemisphere. The color bar represents the *t*-value.

of the compensatory effect of the emotional limbic network. These theories indicate that more intensive hearing loss may be concurrent with more emotional flow from the limbic system to the auditory cortex. However, no significant correlation was observed between the THI scores and the increased influence from the AMYG to the STG, which may be due to the fact that most of the tinnitus subjects presented with lower scores in the THI tests.

Moreover, reduced FC between the PoCG to the NAc and effective connectivity from the PoCG to the NAc was found for ISSNHL with tinnitus. The NAc and associated paralimbic areas play an important role in long-term habituation of continuous unpleasant sounds as well as engaging in the emotional and reward circuit (Hashmi et al., 2013; Lanting et al., 2014). Furthermore, the PoCG belongs to the vital part of somatosensory system. The balance of auditory and somatosensory integration would be altered after loss of auditory input (Froemke and Martins, 2011), which is in line with our finding of a reduced FC between the STG and PoCG in the acute stage of tinnitus and hearing loss. Therefore, besides peripheral auditory system damage, such somatosensory dysfunction may be involved in tinnitus (Job et al., 2012). Previous studies have demonstrated that tinnitus and pain shared a common neuropathological pattern, which suggests a role of the autonomous sympathetic system in tinnitus (Job et al., 2004, 2012). The auditory information was directed *via* the somatosensory system to the NAc for evaluation of the sound's emotional content. The NAc was also the core region of the noise canceling system (Song et al., 2015). This system leads to the filtering out of unwanted sounds, which then do not reach conscious perception in the auditory cortex. In addition, the FC between the PoCG and NAc was negatively correlated with PTA and also had negative correlations between THI scores and effective connectivity from the PoCG to NAc, indicating that the disruption of information flow from the somatosensory system to the NAc may comprise the noise canceling system after intensive peripheral auditory deafferentation. Consequently the abnormal sound may be passed on to the cortex, causing the conscious perception of tinnitus in ISSNHL patients.

In addition, the NAc is the vital region of brain rewarding circuitry, which plays an important role in discerning and reacting to rewarding and aversive stimuli. As a result, it regulates

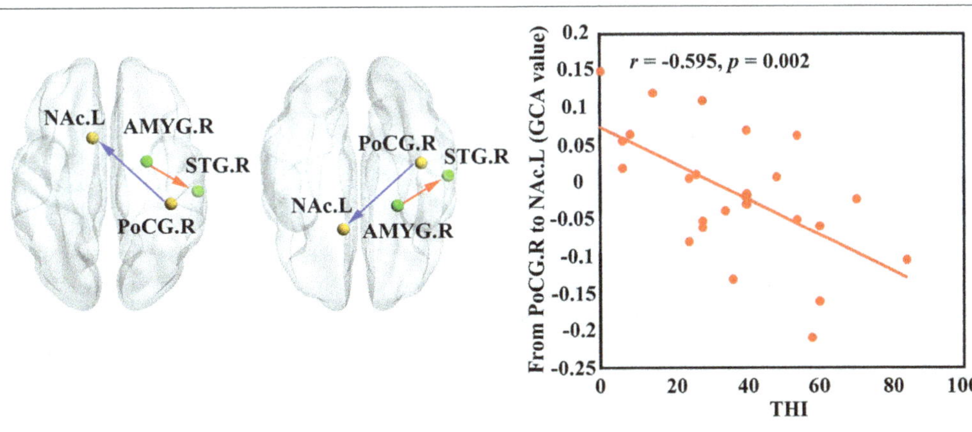

FIGURE 3 | Increased GCA value from AMYG.R to STG.R (in red) and decreased GCA value from PoCG.R to NAc.L (in blue) were found in the ISSNHL patients. The correlations between abnormal GCA value and THI in the ISSNHL patients. The red dots represent each ISSNHL patient. FC, functional connectivity; GCA, granger causality analysis; THI, tinnitus handicap inventory; STG, superior temporal gyrus; AMYG, amygdala; NAc, nucleus accumbens; PoCG, postcentral gyrus; left hemisphere; R, right hemisphere.

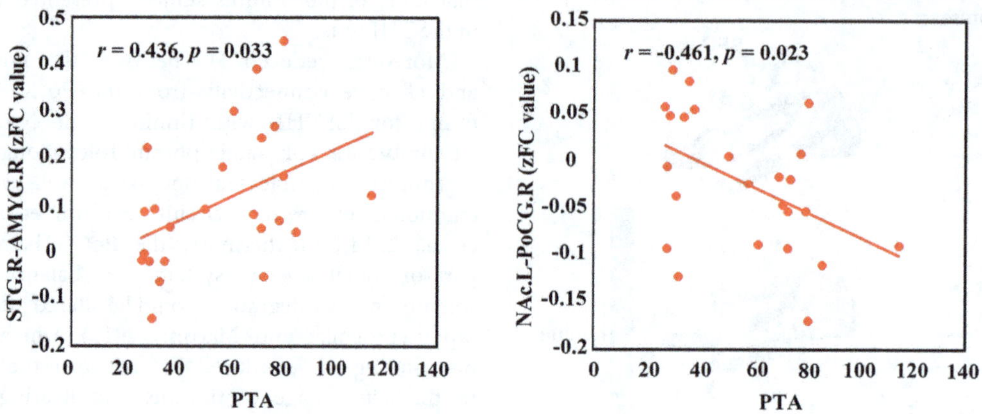

FIGURE 4 | The correlations between the FC with significant group-difference and PTA in the ISSNHL patients. The red dots represent each ISSNHL patient. FC, functional connectivity; PTA, pure tone audiometry; STG, superior temporal gyrus; AMYG, amygdala; NAc, nucleus accumbens; PoCG, postcentral gyrus; left hemisphere; R, right hemisphere.

emotional and cognitive behavior (Russo and Nestler, 2013). In the brain reward circuitry, the ventral tegmental area with dopaminergic neurons projected to the NAc is thought to "gate" the flow of rewarding information from limbic afferents to basal ganglia outputs. In numerous studies of depression, the NAc contributes neural substrate with the inability to experience pleasure and engage in rewarding activities (Pizzagalli et al., 2009; Russo and Nestler, 2013). Therefore, in association with the reduced connectivity between the PoCG and NAc, the current results indicate that the rewarding pathway dysfunction may underlie a pathophysiology of tinnitus associated depression.

LIMITATION

It should be noted that this study has several limitations. This is a cross-sectional study with a limited sample size. In addition, acute tinnitus patients have high heterogeneity in terms of laterality, hearing loss, and related symptoms. It is difficult to eliminate the heterogeneous factors completely even when using strict inclusion and exclusion criteria. Therefore, we should interpret the current results with caution. More extensive and longitudinal investigation with a larger sample size and more subgroups is needed to explore the changes of the directed and undirected FC in a follow-up study of patients with acute tinnitus. Moreover, even though we attempted to diminish the MRI noise by providing earplugs, the subjects could not be completely prevented from hearing noise during the MRI scan, which may influence the neural activity to a certain degree during resting state measurement. This confounding factor should be taken into consideration for all resting-state fMRI studies.

CONCLUSION

In this study, we found an aberrant functional network within auditory and non-auditory regions revealed by FC and GCA presented in acute tinnitus with hearing loss. Acute tinnitus patients showed reduced FC between the STG and cerebellum, limbic system, and the somatosensory cortex. Increased effective connectivity from the right AMYG to the right STG and reduced connectivity from the right PoCG to the left NAc were observed in a causal connectivity analysis. A correlation analysis showed functional changes in multiple neural regions between the auditory and limbic areas associated with the gradual increase in the degree of hearing loss during the acute stage of tinnitus. Alteration in brain functional network architecture will contribute to a better understanding of the neuropathophysiological mechanism in acute tinnitus.

ETHICS STATEMENT

The studies involving human participants were reviewed and approved by The Ethics Committee of Sun Yat-sen Memorial Hospital. The patients/participants provided their written informed consent to participate in this study.

AUTHOR CONTRIBUTIONS

YC and MX conceived and designed the study. XW, ZT, and YS performed the experiments. WX, JL, FZ, and CD analyzed the data. GC and LL drafted the manuscript. JS and YZ contributed to the discussion and manuscript revision. All authors had contributions on preparing this manuscript.

ACKNOWLEDGMENTS

We would like to acknowledge two reviewers for their helpful comments and suggestions.

REFERENCES

Audiology, B. S. O. (1988). Descriptors for pure-tone audiograms. *Br. J. Audiol.* 22:43.

Berlot, E., Arts, R., Smit, J., George, E., Gulban, O. F., Moerel, M., et al. (2020). A 7 Tesla fMRI investigation of human tinnitus percept in cortical and subcortical auditory areas. *Neuroimage* 25:102166. doi: 10.1016/j.nicl.2020.102166

Binder, J. R. (2017). Current controversies on Wernicke's area and its role in language. *Curr. Neurol. Neurosci. Rep.* 17:58.

Biswal, B., Yetkin, F. Z., Haughton, V. M., and Hyde, J. S. (1995). Functional connectivity in the motor cortex of resting human brain using echo-planar MRI. *Magn. Reson. Med.* 34, 537–541. doi: 10.1002/mrm.1910340409

Cai, Y., Huang, D., Chen, Y., Yang, H., Wang, C.-D., Zhao, F., et al. (2018). Deviant dynamics of resting state electroencephalogram microstate in patients with subjective tinnitus. *Front. Behav. Neurosci.* 12:122. doi: 10.3389/fnbeh.2018.00122

Cai, Y., Li, J., Chen, Y., Chen, W., Dang, C., Zhao, F., et al. (2019). Inhibition of brain area and functional connectivity in idiopathic sudden sensorineural hearing loss with tinnitus based on resting-state EEG. *Front. Neurosci.* 13:851. doi: 10.3389/fnins.2019.00851

Cai, Y., Zhou, Q., Yang, H., Jiang, J., Zhao, F., Huang, X., et al. (2017). Logistic regression analysis of factors influencing the effectiveness of intensive sound masking therapy in patients with tinnitus. *BMJ Open* 7:e018050. doi: 10.1136/bmjopen-2017-018050

Chen, X., Lu, B., and Yan, C. G. (2018a). Reproducibility of R-fMRI metrics on the impact of different strategies for multiple comparison correction and sample sizes. *Hum. Brain Mapp.* 39, 300–318. doi: 10.1002/hbm.23843

Chen, Y.-C., Chen, H., Bo, F., Xu, J.-J., Deng, Y., Lv, H., et al. (2018b). Tinnitus distress is associated with enhanced resting-state functional connectivity within the default mode network. *Neuropsychiatr. Dis. Treat.* 14:1919. doi: 10.2147/ndt.s164619

Chen, Y.-C., Liu, S., Lv, H., Bo, F., Feng, Y., Chen, H., et al. (2018c). Abnormal resting-state functional connectivity of the anterior cingulate cortex in unilateral chronic tinnitus patients. *Front. Neurosci.* 12:9. doi: 10.3389/fnins.2018.00009

Chen, Y.-C., Zhang, H., Kong, Y., Lv, H., Cai, Y., Chen, H., et al. (2018d). Alterations of the default mode network and cognitive impairment in patients with unilateral chronic tinnitus. *Quant. Imaging Med. Surg.* 8:1020. doi: 10.21037/qims.2018.11.04

Chen, Y.-C., Bo, F., Xia, W., Liu, S., Wang, P., Su, W., et al. (2017a). Amygdala functional disconnection with the prefrontal-cingulate-temporal circuit in chronic tinnitus patients with depressive mood. *Progr. in Neuro Psychopharmacol. Biol. Psychiatry* 79, 249–257. doi: 10.1016/j.pnpbp.2017.07.001

Chen, Y.-C., Wang, F., Wang, J., Bo, F., Xia, W., Gu, J.-P., et al. (2017b). Resting-state brain abnormalities in chronic subjective tinnitus: a meta-analysis. *Front. Hum. Neurosci.* 11:22. doi: 10.3389/fnhum.2017.00022

Chen, Y. C., Xia, W., Chen, H., Feng, Y., Xu, J. J., Gu, J. P., et al. (2017c). Tinnitus distress is linked to enhanced resting-state functional connectivity from the limbic system to the auditory cortex. *Hum. Brain Mapp.* 38, 2384–2397. doi: 10.1002/hbm.23525

De Ridder, D., Elgoyhen, A. B., Romo, R., and Langguth, B. (2011). Phantom percepts: tinnitus and pain as persisting aversive memory networks. *Proc. Natl. Acad. Sci. U.S.A.* 108, 8075–8080. doi: 10.1073/pnas.1018466108

De Ridder, D., Vanneste, S., and Freeman, W. (2014a). The Bayesian brain: phantom percepts resolve sensory uncertainty. *Neurosci. Biobehav. Rev.* 44, 4–15. doi: 10.1016/j.neubiorev.2012.04.001

De Ridder, D., Vanneste, S., Weisz, N., Londero, A., Schlee, W., Elgoyhen, A. B., et al. (2014b). An integrative model of auditory phantom perception: tinnitus as a unified percept of interacting separable subnetworks. *Neurosci. Biobehav. Rev.* 44, 16–32. doi: 10.1016/j.neubiorev.2013.03.021

Elgoyhen, A. B., Langguth, B., De Ridder, D., and Vanneste, S. (2015). Tinnitus: perspectives from human neuroimaging. *Nat. Rev. Neurosci.* 16, 632–642. doi: 10.1038/nrn4003

Fan, W., Zhang, W., Li, J., Zhao, X., Mella, G., Lei, P., et al. (2015). Altered contralateral auditory cortical morphology in unilateral sudden sensorineural hearing loss. *Otol. Neurotol.* 36:1622. doi: 10.1097/mao.0000000000000892

Friston, K., Moran, R., and Seth, A. K. (2013). Analysing connectivity with Granger causality and dynamic causal modelling. *Curr. Opin. Neurobiol.* 23, 172–178. doi: 10.1016/j.conb.2012.11.010

Friston, K. J., Ashburner, J., Frith, C. D., Poline, J. B., Heather, J. D., and Frackowiak, R. S. (1995). Spatial registration and normalization of images. *Hum. Brain Mapp.* 3, 165–189. doi: 10.1002/hbm.460030303

Froemke, R. C., and Martins, A. R. O. (2011). Spectrotemporal dynamics of auditory cortical synaptic receptive field plasticity. *Hear. Res.* 279, 149–161. doi: 10.1016/j.heares.2011.03.005

Han, Q., Zhang, Y., Liu, D., Wang, Y., Feng, Y., Yin, X., et al. (2018). Disrupted local neural activity and functional connectivity in subjective tinnitus patients: evidence from resting-state fMRI study. *Neuroradiology* 60, 1193–1201. doi: 10.1007/s00234-018-2087-0

Hashmi, J. A., Baliki, M. N., Huang, L., Baria, A. T., Torbey, S., Hermann, K. M., et al. (2013). Shape shifting pain: chronification of back pain shifts brain representation from nociceptive to emotional circuits. *Brain* 136, 2751–2768. doi: 10.1093/brain/awt211

Hullfish, J., Abenes, I., Yoo, H. B., De Ridder, D., and Vanneste, S. (2019). Frontostriatal network dysfunction as a domain-general mechanism underlying phantom perception. *Hum. Brain Mapp.* 40, 2241–2251. doi: 10.1002/hbm.24521

Jackson, R. L., Bajada, C. J., Rice, G. E., Cloutman, L. L., and Ralph, M. A. L. (2018). An emergent functional parcellation of the temporal cortex. *Neuroimage* 170, 385–399. doi: 10.1016/j.neuroimage.2017.04.024

Job, A., Cian, C., Esquivié, D., Leifflen, D., Trousselard, M., Charles, C., et al. (2004). Moderate variations of mood/emotional states related to alterations in cochlear otoacoustic emissions and tinnitus onset in young normal hearing subjects exposed to gun impulse noise. *Hear. Res.* 193, 31–38. doi: 10.1016/j.heares.2004.02.010

Job, A., Pons, Y., Lamalle, L., Jaillard, A., Buck, K., Segebarth, C., et al. (2012). Abnormal cortical sensorimotor activity during "Target" sound detection in subjects with acute acoustic trauma sequelae: an fMRI study. *Brain Behav.* 2, 187–199. doi: 10.1002/brb3.21

Keuroghlian, A. S., and Knudsen, E. I. (2007). Adaptive auditory plasticity in developing and adult animals. *Progr. Neurobiol.* 82, 109–121. doi: 10.1016/j.pneurobio.2007.03.005

Kumar, S., von Kriegstein, K., Friston, K., and Griffiths, T. D. (2012). Features versus feelings: dissociable representations of the acoustic features and valence of aversive sounds. *J. Neurosci.* 32, 14184–14192. doi: 10.1523/jneurosci.1759-12.2012

Lanting, C. P., de Kleine, E., Langers, D. R., and van Dijk, P. (2014). Unilateral tinnitus: changes in connectivity and response lateralization measured with fMRI. *PLoS One* 9:e110704. doi: 10.1371/journal.pone.0110704

Mantini, D., Perrucci, M. G., Del Gratta, C., Romani, G. L., and Corbetta, M. (2007). Electrophysiological signatures of resting state networks in the human brain. *Proc. Natl. Acad. Sci. U.S.A.* 104, 13170–13175. doi: 10.1073/pnas.0700668104

Maudoux, A., Lefebvre, P., Cabay, J.-E., Demertzi, A., Vanhaudenhuyse, A., Laureys, S., et al. (2012). Auditory resting-state network connectivity in tinnitus: a functional MRI study. *PLoS One* 7:e36222. doi: 10.1371/journal.pone.0036222

Micarelli, A., Chiaravalloti, A., Viziano, A., Danieli, R., Schillaci, O., and Alessandrini, M. (2017). Early cortical metabolic rearrangement related to clinical data in idiopathic sudden sensorineural hearing loss. *Hear. Res.* 350, 91–99. doi: 10.1016/j.heares.2017.04.011

Mühlmeier, G., Baguley, D., Cox, T., Suckfüll, M., and Meyer, T. (2016). Characteristics and spontaneous recovery of tinnitus related to idiopathic sudden sensorineural hearing loss. *Otol. Neurotol.* 37:634. doi: 10.1097/mao.0000000000001081

Newman, C. W., Jacobson, G. P., and Spitzer, J. B. (1996). Development of the tinnitus handicap inventory. *Arch. Otolaryngol. Head Neck Surg.* 122, 143–148.

Pannese, A., Grandjean, D., and Fruhholz, S. (2016). Amygdala and auditory cortex exhibit distinct sensitivity to relevant acoustic features of auditory emotions. *Cortex* 85, 116–125. doi: 10.1016/j.cortex.2016.10.013

Pizzagalli, D. A., Holmes, A. J., Dillon, D. G., Goetz, E. L., Birk, J. L., Bogdan, R., et al. (2009). Reduced caudate and nucleus accumbens response to rewards in unmedicated individuals with major depressive disorder. *Am. J. Psychiatry* 166, 702–710. doi: 10.1176/appi.ajp.2008.08081201

Qu, T., Qi, Y., Yu, S., Du, Z., Wei, W., Cai, A., et al. (2019). Dynamic Changes of Functional Neuronal Activities Between the Auditory Pathway and Limbic Systems Contribute to Noise-Induced Tinnitus with a Normal Audiogram. *Neuroscience* 408, 31–45. doi: 10.1016/j.neuroscience.2019.03.054

Raichle, M. E., MacLeod, A. M., Snyder, A. Z., Powers, W. J., Gusnard, D. A., and Shulman, G. L. (2001). A default mode of brain function. *Proc. Natl. Acad. Sci. U.S.A.* 98, 676–682. doi: 10.1073/pnas.98.2.676

Rauschecker, J. P., May, E. S., Maudoux, A., and Ploner, M. (2015). Frontostriatal gating of tinnitus and chronic pain. *Trends Cogn. Sci.* 19, 567–578. doi: 10.1016/j.tics.2015.08.002

Russo, S. J., and Nestler, E. J. (2013). The brain reward circuitry in mood disorders. *Nat. Rev. Neurosci.* 14, 609–625. doi: 10.1038/nrn3381

Smits, M., Kovacs, S., de Ridder, D., Peeters, R. R., van Hecke, P., and Sunaert, S. (2007). Lateralization of functional magnetic resonance imaging (fMRI) activation in the auditory pathway of patients with lateralized tinnitus. *Neuroradiology* 49, 669–679. doi: 10.1007/s00234-007-0231-233

Song, J. J., Vanneste, S., and De Ridder, D. (2015). Dysfunctional noise cancelling of the rostral anterior cingulate cortex in tinnitus patients. *PLoS One* 10:e0123538. doi: 10.1371/journal.pone.0123538

Teismann, H., Okamoto, H., and Pantev, C. (2011). Short and intense tailor-made notched music training against tinnitus: the tinnitus frequency matters. *PLoS One* 6:e24685. doi: 10.1371/journal.pone.0024685

Tsai, M.-C., Cai, Y.-X., Wang, C.-D., Zheng, Y.-Q., Ou, J.-L., and Chen, Y.-H. (2018). Tinnitus abnormal brain region detection based on dynamic causal modeling and exponential ranking. *Biomed Res. Int.* 2018:8656975.

Vanneste, S., Alsalman, O., and De Ridder, D. (2019). Top-down and bottom-up regulated auditory phantom perception. *J. Neurosci.* 39, 364–378. doi: 10.1523/jneurosci.0966-18.2018

Vanneste, S., Van de Heyning, P., and De Ridder, D. (2011). The neural network of phantom sound changes over time: a comparison between recent-onset and chronic tinnitus patients. *Eur. J. Neurosci.* 34, 718–731. doi: 10.1111/j.1460-9568.2011.07793.x

Wallhäusser-Franke, E., D'Amelio, R., Glauner, A., Delb, W., Servais, J. J., Hörmann, K., et al. (2017). Transition from acute to chronic tinnitus: predictors for the development of chronic distressing tinnitus. *Front. Neurol.* 8:605. doi: 10.3389/fneur.2017.00605

Xu, J.-J., Cui, J., Feng, Y., Yong, W., Chen, H., Chen, Y.-C., et al. (2019). Chronic tinnitus exhibits bidirectional functional dysconnectivity in frontostriatal circuit. *Front. Neurosci.* 13:1299. doi: 10.3389/fnins.2019.01299

Yan, C.-G., Wang, X.-D., Zuo, X.-N., and Zang, Y.-F. (2016). DPABI: data processing & analysis for (resting-state) brain imaging. *Neuroinformatics* 14, 339–351. doi: 10.1007/s12021-016-9299-4

Yan, J. (2003). Canadian Association of Neuroscience Review: development and plasticity of the auditory cortex. *Can. J. Neurol. Sci.* 30, 189–200. doi: 10.1017/s0317167100002572

Yang, H., Cai, Y., Guo, H., Xiong, H., Sun, Y., Huang, X., et al. (2018). Prevalence and factors associated with tinnitus: data from adult residents in Guangdong province. *South of China. Int. J. Audiol.* 57, 898–905. doi: 10.1080/14992027.2018.1506169

Zang, Y., Jiang, T., Lu, Y., He, Y., and Tian, L. (2004). Regional homogeneity approach to fMRI data analysis. *Neuroimage* 22, 394–400. doi: 10.1016/j.neuroimage.2003.12.030

Zang, Z.-X., Yan, C.-G., Dong, Z.-Y., Huang, J., and Zang, Y.-F. (2012). Granger causality analysis implementation on MATLAB: a graphic user interface toolkit for fMRI data processing. *J. Neurosci. Methods* 203, 418–426. doi: 10.1016/j.jneumeth.2011.10.006

Zhou, G.-P., Shi, X.-Y., Wei, H.-L., Qu, L.-J., Yu, Y.-S., Zhou, Q.-Q., et al. (2019). Disrupted intraregional brain activity and functional connectivity in unilateral acute tinnitus patients with hearing loss. *Front. Neurosci.* 13:1010. doi: 10.3389/fnins.2019.01010

Zou, Q. H., Zhu, C. Z., Yang, Y., Zuo, X. N., Long, X. Y., Cao, Q. J., et al. (2008). An improved approach to detection of amplitude of low-frequency fluctuation (ALFF) for resting-state fMRI: fractional ALFF. *J. Neurosci. Methods* 172, 137–141. doi: 10.1016/j.jneumeth.2008.04.012

21

Altered Spatial and Temporal Brain Connectivity in the Salience Network of Sensorineural Hearing Loss and Tinnitus

*Xiao-Min Xu[1], Yun Jiao[1], Tian-Yu Tang[1], Chun-Qiang Lu[1], Jian Zhang[1], Richard Salvi[2] and Gao-Jun Teng[1]**

[1] Jiangsu Key Laboratory of Molecular and Functional Imaging, Department of Radiology, Zhongda Hospital, Medical School of Southeast University, Nanjing, China, [2] Center for Hearing and Deafness, University at Buffalo, Buffalo, NY, United States

***Correspondence:**
Gao-Jun Teng
gjteng@seu.edu.cn*

Sensorineural hearing loss (SNHL), sometimes accompanied with tinnitus, is associated with dysfunctions within and outside the classical auditory pathway. The salience network, which is anchored in bilateral anterior insula and dorsal anterior cingulate cortex, has been implicated in sensory integration. Partial auditory deprivation could alter the characteristics of the salience network and other related brain areas, thereby contributing to hearing impairments-induced neuropsychiatric symptoms. To test this hypothesis, we performed fMRI scanning and neuropsychological tests on 32 subjects with long-term bilateral hearing impairment and 30 well-matched Controls. Non-directional functional connectivity and directional Granger causality analysis were used to identify aberrant spatial and temporal patterns of connections targeting bilateral anterior insula and dorsal anterior cingulate cortex. We found that the left anterior insula showed decreased connectivity with right precentral gyrus and superior frontal gyrus. The connections between the dorsal anterior cingulate cortex and middle frontal gyrus, superior parietal gyrus and supplementary motor area (SMA) were also reduced. Relative to Controls, SNHL patients showed abnormal effective connectivity of the salience network, including inferior temporal gyrus, cerebellum lobule VI, lobule VIII, precentral gyrus, middle frontal gyrus and SMA. Furthermore, correlation analysis demonstrated that some of these atypical connectivity measures were correlated with performance of neuropsychiatric tests. These findings suggest that the inefficient modulation of the salience network might contribute to the neural basis of SNHL and tinnitus, as well as associated cognition and emotion deficits.

Keywords: sensorineural hearing loss, tinnitus, functional connectivity, effective connectivity, salience network, non-auditory symptom

INTRODUCTION

Sensorineural hearing loss (SNHL), which accounts for about 90% of all cases of hearing loss, results largely from the degeneration of cochlear sensory hair cells and their afferent auditory neurons (Charizopoulou et al., 2011; Li et al., 2017). SNHL is often accompanied by tinnitus (ringing in the ear), hyperacusis (loudness intolerance), impaired speech perception and poor temporal processing (Manohar et al., 2017; Paul et al., 2017). Since the sensory hair cells and auditory nerve fibers do not regenerate, the auditory deficits associated with SNHL are largely irreversible and can only be partially ameliorated with hearing aids or cochlear implants (Gordon et al., 2013). The auditory cortex, like other sensory cortices, forms parallel connections with other brain networks each with its own unique function(s) (Menon, 2011; Sepulcre, 2014). There is growing awareness that the lack of sensory input from the peripheral auditory system can disrupt neural circuits within and outside the classically defined auditory pathway, disruptions that could affect higher order cognitive, emotional, motivational, and attentional processes.

The salience network (SN), with major hubs in the dorsal anterior cingulate cortex (dACC) and anterior insula (AI), connects with subcortical and limbic structures (Seeley et al., 2007). It is well positioned to integrate internal and external stimuli, including those from the auditory pathway (Heywood et al., 2017). In patients experiencing auditory hallucinations, activity within the SN was perturbed and increased activation was present in the AI, suggesting greater relevance and attention to the internally generated auditory percepts (Sommer et al., 2008; Lefebvre et al., 2016). The AI is also activated in tasks designed to detect temporal disparities between auditory and visual stimuli (Bushara et al., 2001). Activity in the AI and dACC increased as auditory/visual information became more ambiguous and the task more difficult, suggesting that these structures might be of importance in sensory integration and cognition (Lamichhane et al., 2016). As the integrity of the SN was the basis of normal network functioning, white-matter damage in the SN could predict worse default mode network (DMN) function (Bonnelle et al., 2012; Luo et al., 2014; Sidlauskaite et al., 2016; Wu et al., 2016; Chang et al., 2017). As SNHL makes auditory processing more difficult, it deprives the SN of important auditory information needed for sensory integration, directing attention, decision making, and performing motivationally relevant tasks. Therefore, it should come as no surprise to learn that SNHL is associated with cognitive impairment, anxiety, depression and impaired executive function (Husain et al., 2011; Kronenberger et al., 2013; Basner et al., 2014). However, the potential mechanisms underlying SNHL-related neuropsychiatric symptoms and the relationships with the SN need to be further explored.

Functional connectivity (FC) is used to characterize the statistical dependence between the functional activity in two or more brain regions without making predictions about the causal nature of the interactions (Leavitt et al., 2012; Seth et al., 2015; Chen et al., 2017). By examining the time-lagged in the relationships between two or more brain regions, effective connectivity (EC) revealed by Granger causality analysis (GCA) tries to predict the direction of information flow in the network. These two powerful techniques can be used to identify the magnitude and direction of functional connections between different brain regions in a variety of neurological and psychiatric disorders (Demirci et al., 2009; Anderson et al., 2011; De Pisapia et al., 2012; Feng et al., 2016; Jiang et al., 2018). In the current study, we employed both FC and GCA to determine if SNHL disrupted non-directional and directional connectivity patterns using three major nodes in the SN as regions of interest (ROIs).

We hypothesized that SNHL would disrupt the normal flow of neural activity within the SN and other parallel brain regions in the central nervous system. To determine if the disturbances in the SN were associated with a particular phenotype, we correlated the changes in FC and EC with performance on a series of cognition, depression, and anxiety tests.

MATERIALS AND METHODS

Subjects

The study was conducted with two groups of subjects (**Table 1**); one group of 32 subjects had long term bilateral SNHL and the second group of 30 subjects, which formed the Control group, had clinically normal hearing. The SNHL sample included 22 males and 10 females with a mean age of 54.5 years ± 9.3 (*SD*), a mean body mass index (BMI) of 23.8 (± 3.3 *SD*), and a mean education level of 11.0 years (± 3.0 *SD*). The etiologies of long term bilateral SNHL were: unknown (n = 28), ototoxic drugs (n = 2) and chronic middle ear infection (n = 2). The Control group consisted of 14 males and 16 females with a mean age of 53.6 years (± 8.0 *SD*), a mean BMI of 23.2 (± 2.5 *SD*) and mean education level of 11.8 years (± 3.6 *SD*). Subjects were recruited into the study through clinical referrals though the outpatient clinics in Zhongda Hospital in Nanjing or through newspaper advertisements. All above procedures were approved by the Ethics Committee of Zhongda Hospital, Southeast University in Nanjing, China (2016ZDSYLL031.0). Every participant signed an informed consent form prior to participating in the study.

Only right-handed subjects between the ages of 20–65 years were included in the study. All subjects first underwent audiological testing to determine if they met the criteria for normal hearing (≤20 dB HL, octave interval from 0.25 to 8 kHz) for the Control group. The criteria for inclusion in

TABLE 1 | Demographic and clinical characteristics of long-term bilateral SNHL and Control groups. Mean data (±*SD*) and *p*-values (*$p < 0.05$; ***$p < 0.001$) shown for SNHL and Control group.

Characteristic	SNHL group (n = 32)	Control group (n = 30)	*p*-value
Age (years)	54.5 ± 9.3	53.6 ± 8.0	0.698
Gender (male:female)	22:10	14:16	0.122
BMI	23.8 ± 3.3	23.2 ± 2.5	0.397
Education level (years)	11.0 ± 3.0	11.8 ± 3.6	0.348
Hearing loss durations (years)	8.0 ± 8.9	–	–
Framewise displacement	0.217 ± 0.097	0.227 ± 0.148	0.187
MMSE	29.6 ± 0.8	29.8 ± 0.6	0.315
SDMT	34.3 ± 12.5	41.5 ± 10.1	0.015*
AVLT-5 min	6.0 ± 2.7	6.8 ± 2.0	0.189
AVLT-20 min	5.9 ± 2.8	6.8 ± 1.8	0.140
SAS	36.1 ± 7.4	30.5 ± 3.7	0.001***
HAMD	6.1 ± 4.0	3.9 ± 3.2	0.024*

Mean data (±SD) and p-values ($p < 0.05$; ***$p < 0.001$) shown for SNHL and Control group. SNHL, sensorineural hearing loss; BMI, body mass index; MMSE, mini-mental state examination; SDMT, symbol digit modalities test; AVLT, auditory verbal learning test; SAS, self-rating anxiety scale; HAMD, hamilton depression scale.*

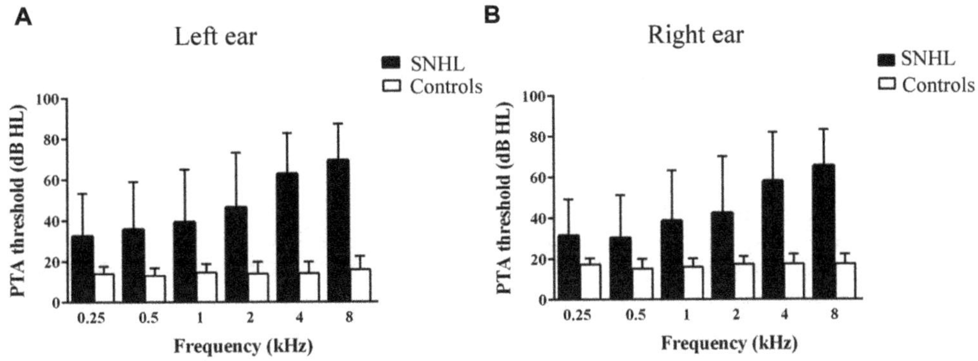

FIGURE 1 | Hearing thresholds at 0.25, 0.5, 1, 2, 4, and 8 kHz. **(B)** Mean right-ear audiogram of SNHL group and Control group. **(A)** Mean left-ear audiogram of SNHL group and Control group.

SNHL were: (1) hearing loss duration> 1 year, (2) post-lingual hearing loss, (3) hearing thresholds ≥30 dB HL in both ears. Exclusion criteria included: abnormal visual acuity, Meniere's diseases, acoustic neuroma, pulsatile tinnitus, drug or alcohol addiction, severe heart diseases, pregnancy, breast feeding, or MRI contraindications. Additionally, people were removed from this study if they had a history of depression or other psychiatric illness, Alzheimer's disease, stroke, or head trauma.

Audiological Tests

A clinical audiologist performed pure tone audiometry (PTA) using a GSI-61 audiometer in the ENT department of Zhongda Hospital. Air conduction thresholds in the left and right ear were assessed at 0.25, 0.5, 1, 2, 4, and 8 kHz using standard clinical procedures (**Figure 1**). Impedance testing was conducted to rule out middle ear dysfunction test and conductive hearing loss.

Neuropsychological Evaluation

Before MRI scanning, subjects underwent several cognitive and mental tests. The Mini-Mental State Examination (MMSE) is of high validation (Tombaugh and McIntyre, 1992) and can be easily performed to assess global cognition (Magni et al., 1996). Subjects with MMSE scores <26 were removed from our study. The Auditory Verbal Learning Test (AVLT) is a powerful tool for assessing episodic memory which consists of immediate and 20-min delayed recall, as well as recognition of 12 words (Brugnolo et al., 2014). It has been widely used for assessing cognition in dementia and pre-dementia conditions (Estevez-Gonzalez et al., 2003). The Symbol Digit Modalities Test (SDMT) was used to assess attention, processing speed and executive function (Benedict et al., 2017; Jaywant et al., 2018). The Self-Rating Anxiety Scale (SAS) contains 20 questions; 15 questions assess increasing anxiety levels and five questions assess decreasing anxiety levels (Yang et al., 2015). The Hamilton Depression Scale (HAMD) is considered as "gold standard" to capture core depressive symptoms in clinical research (Hamilton, 1967).

MRI Scanning Protocol

MRI data were collected at the Radiology Department of Zhongda Hospital using a 3.0 T MRI system (Siemens, Erlangen, Germany) with an 8-channel receiver array head coil. Structural images were acquired with a T1-weighted 3D spoiled gradient-echo sequence: sections = 176, repetition time (TR) = 1900 ms, echo time (TE) = 2.48 ms, slices = 176, section thickness = 1.0 mm, flip angle (FA) = 90°, FOV = 256 × 256 mm^2, acquisition matrix = 256 × 256. The fMRI data were obtained axially using a gradient-echo-planar (EPI) imaging sequence with the following parameters: 36 slices, TR/TE = 2000/25 ms, section thickness = 4.0 mm, FA = 90°, FOV = 240 × 240 mm^2, acquisition matrix = 64 × 64. The fMRI data were acquired over a period of 8 min and 6 s and images were acquired in an interleaved order. Subjects wore earplugs and earphones to attenuate scanner noise (approximately 32 dB) and a head cushion was used to reduce head motion. Subjects were instructed to keep their eyes closed, remain awake, lie quietly, and avoid specific thoughts.

Data Processing

Our data processing and analysis procedure have been described in detail in earlier publications (Cui et al., 2014, 2015). Briefly, functional data analyses were preprocessed using Data Processing Assistant for Resting-State software[1] and SPM 12 toolbox[2]. The first 10 time points were discarded to allow for signal equilibrium and the remaining 230 consecutive volumes were used for subsequent analysis. Afterward, slice timing correction and realignment were performed. Structural and functional images were then coregistered to Montreal Neurological Institute (MNI) space, and data were resampled to 3 mm^3. Six motion parameters, 6 temporal derivatives, 12 corresponding squared items were regressed using the Friston-24 parameter model to minimize the effect of head motion (Yan et al., 2013). The mean framewise displacement (FD) was computed from each time point for every subjects (Power et al., 2012; Van Dijk et al., 2012), and subjects with FD of >0.5 were excluded from the analysis. None of our

[1] http://rfmri.org/DPARSF
[2] http://www.fil.ion.ucl.ac.uk/spm

subjects were removed because of excessive head motion and there was no significant difference in FD between SNHL and Control group (**Table 1**). Finally, data were smoothed with an isotropic Gaussian kernel (FWHM = 6.0 mm) and filtering from 0.01 to 0.08 Hz.

Functional Connectivity

Functional connectivity was performed using REST software[3]. We used three primary nodes in the SN as ROIs (**Figure 2**) from the functional imaging in neuropsychiatric disorders lab at Stanford University[4] (Shirer et al., 2012). The time-series of each region was averaged and correlated with every other voxel within the gray-matter mask. The FC correlation maps were converted using the Fisher r-to-z transform. Two-sample *t*-test was performed to explore the difference between SNHL patients and Controls. The statistical maps were thresholded at $p < 0.001$ at voxel level and $p < 0.05$ by Gaussian Random Fields (GRF) correction with age, gender and FD corrected. Significant clusters were mapped onto the surface of brain using BrainNet Viewer software[5].

Effective Connectivity

Effective connectivity was also analyzed by REST-GCA using the REST software and the same ROIs as described above. GCA is a statistical tool to depict the directionality flow of information in time series analysis (Stokes and Purdon, 2017). If the temporal progression of brain activity in one region allows the prediction of future time series activity in another brain area, it is assumed that the first brain region causally influences the second area (Granger, 1969). In present study, the time series from the left AI, right AI, and bilateral dACC were defined as the three seed time series, x, while the time series of all voxels in the brain were identified as the time series, y. $Fx \rightarrow y$ and $Fy \rightarrow x$ were calculated voxel by voxel as the linear direct influence from the time series x to y and from y to x, respectively. We transformed the residual-based F to a normally distributed F', then converted the normally distributed *F*-values to standardized *Z*-scores ($Z_{x\rightarrow y}$ and $Z_{y\rightarrow x}$). Two Granger causality maps, ($Z_{x\rightarrow y}$ and $Z_{y\rightarrow x}$), were generated for each subject. Since we selected three seeds, six Granger causality maps were generated (left AI, $Z_{x\rightarrow y}$ and $Z_{y\rightarrow x}$, right AI with $Z_{x\rightarrow y}$ and $Z_{y\rightarrow x}$, and dorsal ACC, $Z_{x\rightarrow y}$ and $Z_{y\rightarrow x}$) for both the SNHL and Control groups. The GCA threshold was set at $p < 0.01$ at the voxel level and $p < 0.05$ corrected by GRF correction in two-sample *t*-tests with age, gender and FD corrected.

Correlation Analysis

We also evaluated the relationships among the clinical variables and the functional MRI data. First, the clusters of significance in FC and GCA were extracted. Then, the mean *z*-values of the abnormal connectivity region masks (i.e., significant differences between the long term bilateral SNHL and Control groups) were calculated and used to perform a Person correlation analysis between the mean *z*-values of FC and each of the clinical variables (e.g., SDMT score, SAS scores, hearing ability, etc.,) using SPSS software (Version 18.0; Chicago, IL, United States). The significant *p*-value was set at $p < 0.05$, corrected for multiple comparison.

[3]http://www.restfmri.net

[4]http://findlab.stanford.edu/functional_ROIs.html

[5]http://www.nitrc.org/projects/bnv/

RESULTS

Clinical Data and Neuropsychological Findings

Table 1 summarizes the demographic features, cognition and emotion status of the SNHL group and Control group. The two groups did not differ in terms of age, BMI, or education level. Consistent with our hypothesis, the SNHL group had significantly lower SDMT scores ($p < 0.05$), suggestive of poorer executive control or cognition among subjects with SNHL. The SAS scores ($p < 0.001$) and HAMD scores ($p < 0.05$) in the SNHL group were higher than those in the Control group suggesting greater anxiety and/or depression in subjects with long-term SNHL.

Hearing Characteristic

All subjects in the control group had thresholds ≤20 dB HL at all frequencies in both ears (Yang et al., 2014) and normal middle ear function (Gwer et al., 2013); and subjects with SNHL had bilateral hearing thresholds ≥30 dB HL for more than 1 year (**Figures 1A,B**). Most SNHL patients had moderate to severe, sloping high frequency hearing loss although a few had profound hearing loss in one or more ears.

Functional Connectivity

The left AI, right AI, and dACC were used as three nodes in our ROI analysis. We compared FC matrices in the SNHL and Control groups. SNHL did not lead to an increase FC between any of our three ROIs and other brain regions. Instead, we observed significant decreases in FC in the SNHL group compared to the Control group (**Figures 3A,B** and **Table 2**, $p < 0.001$, GRF corrected). The left AI showed decreased FC with the right precentral gyrus (PreCG) and superior frontal gyrus (SFG). Moreover, the dACC showed weakened connections with the right medial frontal gyrus (MFG) and

TABLE 2 | Regions of decreased functional connectivity in the SNHL group compared to the control group with the seed ROIs in the left AI, right AI, and dACC.

Seed region	Brain region	BA	MNI coordinate x,y,z (mm)	Peak *t*-score	Cluster size
Left AI	R precentral gyrus	6	18,−27,69	−4.4713	180
	R superior frontal gyrus	6	27,6,60	−4.9222	98
dACC	R medial frontal gyrus	11	12,39, −24	−4.0982	158
	R superior parietal gyrus	19	18, −84,45	−4.1949	154
	L supplementary motor area	6	−3,0,66	−4.5348	161

BA, Brodmann area; MNI, Montreal Neurological Institute coordinates (MNI); AI, anterior insula; dACC, dorsal anterior cingulate cortex; L, left; R, right.

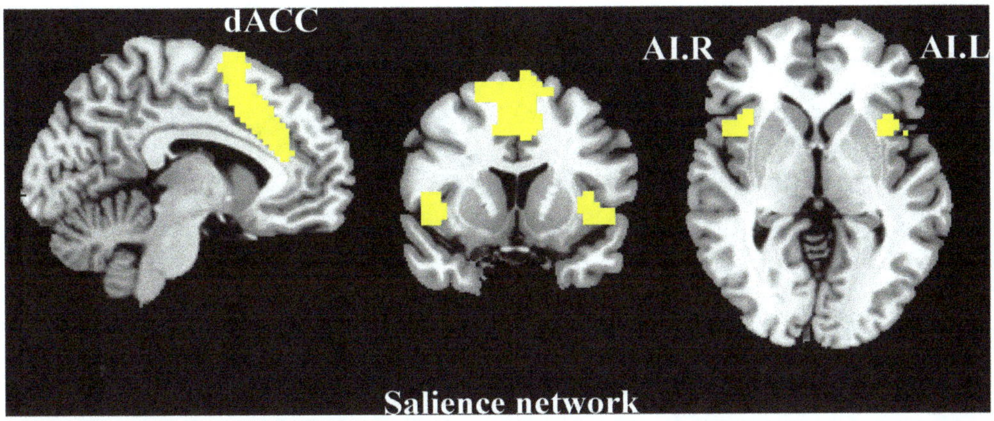

FIGURE 2 | Schematic showing three ROIs, the dorsal anterior cingulate cortex (dACC), left anterior insula (AI), and right anterior insula (AI), as nodes in the salience network.

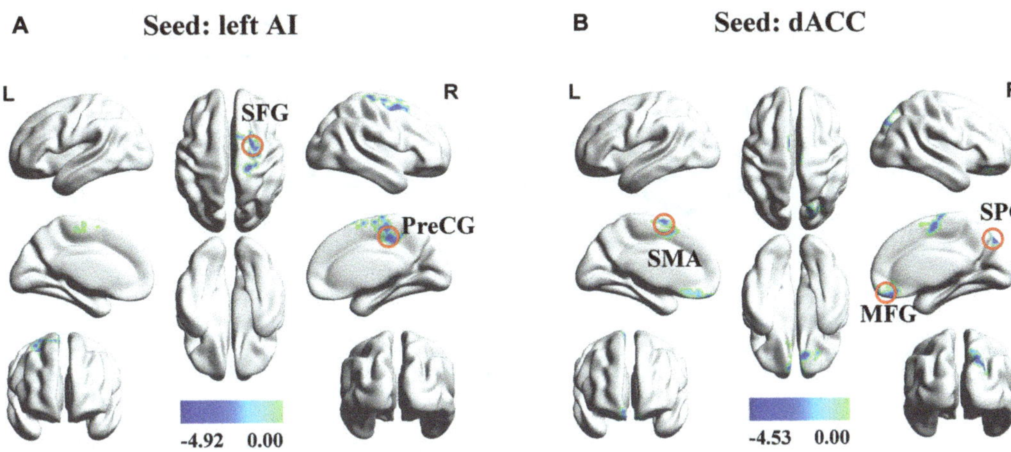

FIGURE 3 | Significant differences in functional connectivity between SNHL and Control group with ROIs in the left AI, right AI, and dACC. **(A)** Reduced functional connectivity using the left AI as the seed. **(B)** Reduced functional connectivity using the dACC as the seed. Heat maps shows *z*-values; threshold set at $p < 0.001$ at the voxel level and $p < 0.05$ after Gaussian Random field correction. AI, anterior insula; dACC, dorsal anterior cingulate cortex; SFG, superior frontal gyrus; PreCG, precentral gyrus; SMA, supplementary motor area; MFG, superior frontal gyrus; SPG, superior parietal gyrus; L, left; R, right.

superior parietal gyrus (SPG), as well as the left supplementary motor area (SMA).

Effective Connectivity

In addition to assessing the magnitude of FC, GCA attempts to identify the directionality or presumed causality of information flow in a network (Goebel et al., 2003). We used GCA to determine if SNHL disrupted FC and its directionality in our three ROIs. Compared to Controls, the SNHL group demonstrated decreased outflow GCA values from the left AI to the left cerebellum lobule VI, right MFG and right PreCG (**Figure 4A**). The inflow from right inferior temporal gyrus (ITG) to the left AI was also decreased (**Figure 4B**). Meanwhile, the outflow from the right AI to bilateral MFG was reduced in SNHL subjects (**Figure 4C**). Significant changes in directional connectivity were also evaluated using the dACC as the ROI. We observed decreased outflow from the dACC to the left PreCG and right SMA, but increased inflow from right cerebellum lobule VIII (**Figures 4D,E** and **Table 3**).

Correlation Analysis

Our neuropsychological data indicated that SNHL was associated with decreased executive function (SDMT scores), increased anxiety (SAS scores) and depression scores (HAMD scores) as noted in **Table 1**. To determine if these neuropsychological deficits were associated with the FC and EC changes, we correlated the SDMT, SAS, and HAMD scores with the changes in FC and EC for each of the three ROIs using voxel-wise methods. The SDMT performance showed positive correlations with dACC-left SMA FC ($r = 0.487$, $p = 0.005$, **Figure 5A**) and left AI-right SFG FC ($r = 0.491$, $p = 0.004$, **Figure 5B**). The connectivity between dACC and right SPG was negatively correlated with HAMD scores ($r = -0.498$, $p = 0.004$, **Figure 5C**). In addition, higher SAS scores were correlated with lower GCA

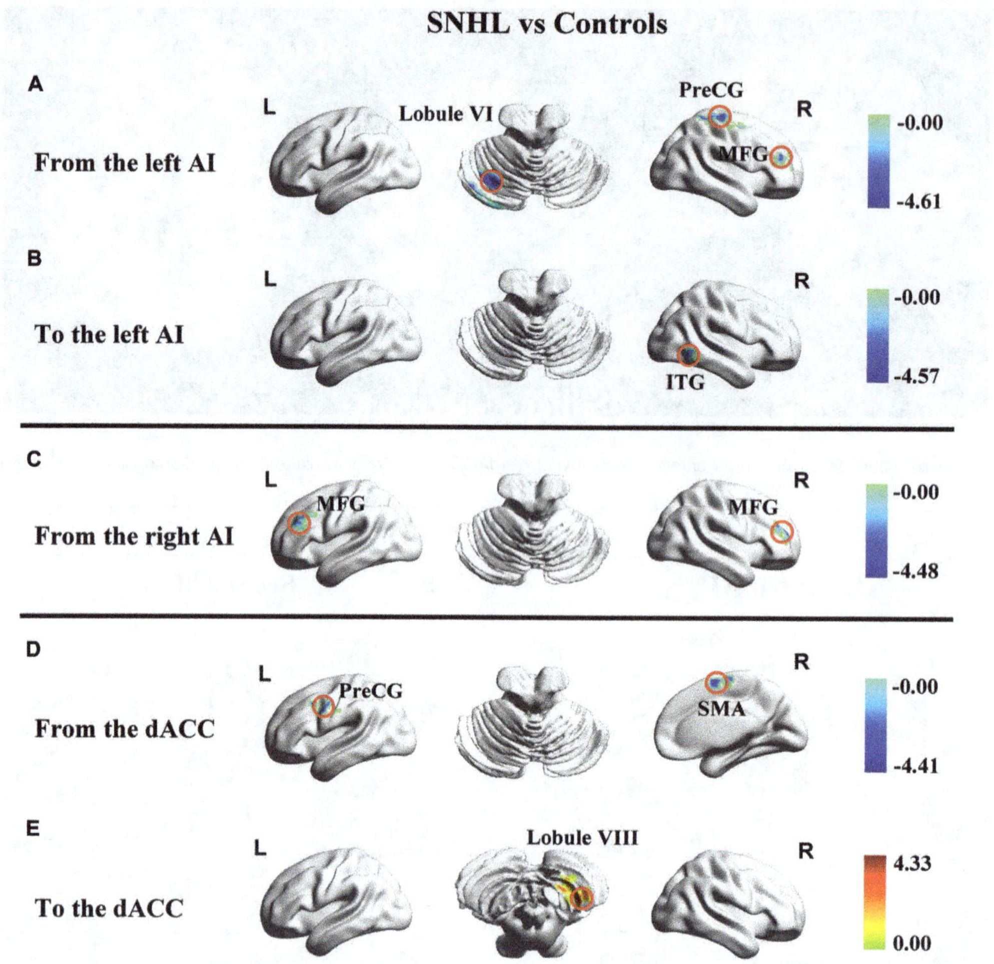

FIGURE 4 | Changes in effective connectivity in the SNHL group compared to the control group using three key nodes in the salience network as ROIs (left AI, right AI, and dACC). **(A)** Decreased outflow effective connectivity from the left AI to left cerebellum lobule VI and right PreCG, MFG, and ITG highlighted by blue color; **(B)** Decreased inflow effective causal connectivity from right ITG to dACC highlighted by blue color; **(C)** Decreased outflow effective connectivity from the right AI to left and right MFG highlighted by blue color; **(D)** Decreased outflow effective connectivity from the dACC to the left PreCG and right SMA highlighted by blue color; **(E)** Increased inflow effective causal connectivity from the right cerebellum lobule VIII to the dACC highlighted by red color. Heat maps shows *z*-values; threshold set at $p < 0.01$ at the voxel level and $p < 0.05$ after Gaussian random field correction. SNHL, sensorineural hearing loss; AI, anterior insula; dACC, dorsal anterior cingulate cortex; PreCG, precentral gyrus; MFG, middle frontal gyrus; ITG, interior temporal gyrus; SMA, supplementary motor area.

values from left AI to left cerebellum lobule VI ($r = -0.534$, $p = 0.002$, **Figure 5D**).

DISCUSSION

To date, little research has focused on the spatial and temporal brain connectivity patterns in subjects with long-term bilateral SNHL. This is the first study combing non-directional FC and directional EC to uncover the abnormalities of intrinsic organization in brain regions using three key nodes of the SN as ROIs since the SN is found to play an crucial role in auditory processing (Li et al., 2015). Widely decreased connections were observed in the SNHL group. Significant alterations of EC appeared in multiple areas emanating from and to bilateral AI or dorsal ACC. In addition, some alterations in FC and EC were correlated with clinical measurements. Our results provide emerging evidence of changed functional architecture in the SNHL brain, providing new insight into the role of the SN and associated brain regions in deafness.

When processing speech, greater activation occurred in the AI as word recognition scores declined suggesting greater salience or attention in difficult listening situations (Harris et al., 2009). In order for effective aural communication to occur, a listener must selectively attend to the relevant acoustic signal in a noisy environment in order to from a coherent auditory stream, a task normal listeners perform effortlessly (Lee et al., 2008). The involvement of the SN has been implicated in tinnitus, as increased activity in the SN and enhanced insula-auditory cortex couplings might be associated with tinnitus percept and continuous awareness (Vanneste et al., 2013). Listeners with SNHL have great difficulty

TABLE 3 | Changes in effective connectivity in the SNHL group compared to the control group using three key nodes in the salience network as ROIs (left AI, right AI, and dACC).

Brain region	BA	MNI coordinate x,y,z (mm)	Peak *t*-score	Cluster size
Casual outflow from left AI to the rest of brain (X to Y)				
L cerebellum lobule VI	19	−24, −69, −21	−4.6058	89
R middle frontal gyrus	45	45,42,18	−3.9075	140
R precentral gyrus	6	30, −21,63	−4.498	131
Casual inflow to the left AI from the rest of brain (Y to X)				
R inferior temporal gyrus	37	60, −51, −21	−4.569	80
Casual outflow from right AI to the rest of brain (X to Y)				
L middle frontal gyrus	46	−42,42,27	−3.8855	88
R middle frontal gyrus	46	33,51,18	−4.4832	141
Casual outflow from dACC to the rest of brain (X to Y)				
L precentral gyrus	6	−45,0,33	−4.2246	93
R supplementary motor area	6	3,0,60	−4.4094	97
Casual outflow to dACC from the rest of brain (Y to X)				
R cerebellum lobule VIII	-	30, −51, −51	4.3345	56

BA, Brodmann area; MNI, Montreal Neurological Institute coordinates (MNI); AI, anterior insula; dACC, dorsal anterior cingulate cortex; L, left; R, right.

filtering out irrelevant acoustic information resulting in impaired auditory processing, diminished attention and an inability to use memory and cognition to fill in missing information in an auditory stream. Interestingly, we observed weakened non-directional and directional AI-PreCG connections in SNHL subjects. Although the PreCG is part of the posterior frontal lobe and traditionally functions as the primary motor cortex, evidence has indicated its role in auditory-associated events. Zhang et al. (2015) found decreased thalamic connectivity to the PreCG in tinnitus patients and the connections between the thalamus and insula have already been demonstrated in healthy adults (Namkung et al., 2017), so that decreased AI-PreCG connectivity in the SNHL group seems reasonable. However, there were some inconsistent findings, likely due to the various kinds of hearing impairments and disease durations. [^{18}F]fluorodeoxyglucose (FDG)-PET, a quiet and reliable auditory imaging technique, demonstrated increased FDG uptake in the insula and PreCG within 72 h of onset of sudden SNHL. Glucose consumption in the PreCG was positively correlated with the speech discrimination scores (Micarelli et al., 2017). Compared to hearing non-dyslexics subjects, congenital deafness and dyslexic adults showed greater activation in the PreCG using a rhyme judgment task (MacSweeney et al., 2009). Taken together, these results suggest that the PreCG might participate in word recognition and phonological processing. Further experiments with these specific tasks in long-term SNHL could reveal the potential mechanism of the PreCG after partial hearing deprivation.

We found reduced AI-SFG FC and EC from AI to MFG in current study. Voxel-based morphometry (VBM) analysis (Husain et al., 2011) delineated gray matter changes in the SFG and MFG suggesting decreased use of executive control network (ECN) in chronic hearing loss patients, which supports our correlation between AI-SFG and SDMT scores (a symbol substitution test that examines an individual's cognitive ability, including executive control and switching attention, which also requires oculomotor scanning and visuomotor coordination (Forn et al., 2009; Pascoe et al., 2018). Conversely, metabolic PET studies found increased FDG uptake in SFG and MFG in sudden hearing loss (Micarelli et al., 2017), indicative of enhanced neural activity in ECN regions. The increased metabolic activity might reflect enhanced conflict monitoring caused by the unexpected auditory input impairment and/or an emotional response in acute hearing loss period (Chen et al., 2013), while our aberrant ECN function was not immediate but occurred over time. Moreover, our connectivity results suggest abnormal interactions between the SN and the ECN (which includes dorsolateral prefrontal cortex) and casual flows from SN to ECN in SNHL. It has been reported that the SN plays a critical role in switching between the ECN and DMN, allocating information toward ECN and DMN (Sridharan et al., 2008). The SN has positive connectivity with the ECN and they can be co-activated during cognition tasks (Greicius et al., 2003). Here, hearing impairments altered inter-connectivity between SN and ECN, which could insights on cognitive control in SNHL.

It is important to note that the cerebellum is affected by SNHL. Emerging evidence shows that the cerebellum is not only associated with motor function, but also cognition processing and emotion control (Schmahmann and Caplan, 2006; Moreno-Rius, 2018). The cerebellum is considered to have a much border role in sensory and perceptual processing (Baumann et al., 2015). Except the primary auditory cortex, parts of the cerebellum are activated during various auditory tasks (Petacchi et al., 2005). Human and animal studies have also found activation in various regions of the cerebellum in its participation in hearing impairments, including tinnitus, hyperacusis and hearing loss (Stoodley and Schmahmann, 2009; Chen et al., 2015). Manganese-enhanced magnetic resonance imaging demonstrated increased spontaneous activity in portions of the cerebellum in rat with tinnitus, suggesting that it might serve as a tinnitus generator (Brozoski et al., 2007). Neuroimaging in unilateral hearing loss revealed enhanced and weakened connectivity between cerebellar networks and other systems (Zhang et al., 2018). In the present study, we observed weakened EC from left AI to left cerebellum lobule VI; this was negatively correlated with anxiety status revealed by SAS scores. Interestingly, lobule VI is considered part of the neural circuit of anxiety and fear (Lange et al., 2015).

EEG beta power of dACC was associated with a hyper-responsiveness state to non-noxious auditory stimuli in tinnitus and positively correlated with scores on tinnitus questionnaires (Song et al., 2014), which might contribute to presistent vigilance in tinnitus. In cochlear implant users, the dACC can be activated by sound stimuli and is engaged dual-stream auditory processing (Song et al., 2015), supporting its involvement in hearing impairments. The dACC showed decreased connections with the SPG and dACC-SPG FC was negatively correlated with HAMD scores. Contemporary views of brain function have emphasized the role of SPG in depression (Yang et al., 2017), tinnitus and hearing loss (Siedentopf et al., 2007), which correspond well to our correlation analysis. In our study,

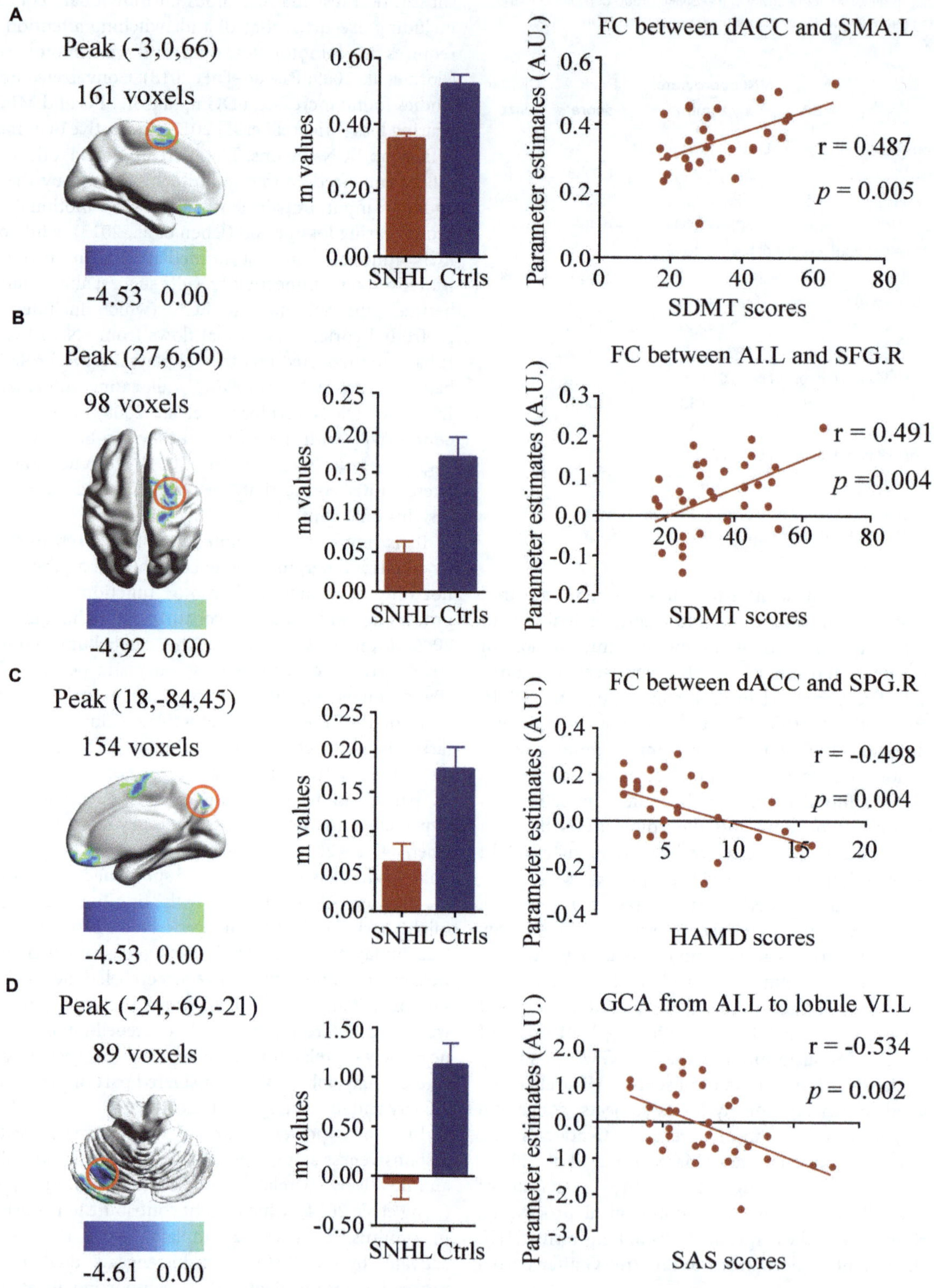

FIGURE 5 | Relationships between fMRI and clinical neuropsychiatric scales. **(A)** Positive correlation between the SDMT scores and functional connectivity of dACC and left SMA ($r = 0.487$, $p = 0.005$); **(B)** Positive correlation between the SDMT scores and functional connectivity of left AI and right SFG ($r = 0.491$, $p = 0.004$); **(C)** Negative correlation between the HAMD scores and functional connectivity of left dACC and right SPG ($r = -0.498$, $p = 0.004$); **(D)** Negative correlation between the SAS scores and the decreased effective connectivity from the left AI to the left cerebellum lobule VI($r = -0.534$, $p = 0.002$). SNHL, sensorineural hearing loss; Ctrls, controls; AI, anterior insula; dACC, dorsal anterior cingulate cortex; SMA, supplementary motor area; SFG, superior frontal gyrus; SPG, superior parietal gyrus; SDMT, symbol digit modalities test; HAMD, hamilton depression scale; SAS; self-anxiety scale.

the outflow from dACC to PreCG was disrupted in subjects with SNHL. FC and independent component analysis (ICA) have suggested a robust relationship between the PreCG and dACC (Chen et al., 2018). White et al. (2010) found a weakened relationship between the PreCG and dACC in schizophrenia similar to our causal finding from the dACC and PreCG. We also observed the participation of SMA (falling with SFG) which is involved in motor action (Cona et al., 2017). Existing research shows that the dACC not only provides supplemental function to the SMA, but also resides at a higher level than the SMA (Hatanaka et al., 2003) in motor control, consistent with our correlation between dACC-SMA FC and SDMT performance. PET and fMRI studies found recruitment of the SMA in the perception of speech (Adank, 2012) and addressed the candidate role of SMA in auditory processing and auditory imagery (Lima et al., 2016). Moreover, the directed FC from the dACC to SMA is another aspect of a contribution from the frontal executive network (Asemi et al., 2015), and involvement of sensory process in executive control (Funahashi, 2001). Our data show that auditory deprivation results in abnormal directed and unidirectional connectivity from the dACC to SMA. However, further research is needed to elucidate the role of the SMA auditory processing pathway and disclose its role in SNHL-induced non-auditory symptoms.

Limitation

There were several limitations in our preliminary study. First, this cross-sectional research does not provide direct evidence of causal relationships of functional MRI and hearing loss distress. Follow-up work using a longitudinal, within-subjects design are needed to confirm these findings. Second, the related approach should be expanded to sub-regions of bilateral AI and dACC, as well as other brain areas involved in ECN and emotional function. Third, further study using a larger sample size could be used to identify differences in the SN between SNHL subjects with tinnitus and without tinnitus. Finally, despite the fact that hearing protection was used by the subjects, scan noise from the MRI would influence spontaneous neural activity in the brain.

CONCLUSION

To conclude, we identified disrupted functional and EC in the SN in long-term SNHL patients. In addition, cognitive impairments, depression and anxiety correlated with alterations in non-directional and directional connections. The imbalances between the SN and other brain regions could potentially disclose the neuropathological mechanism underlying hearing impairments and associated reorganization of complex networks.

AUTHOR CONTRIBUTIONS

X-MX, collected the fMRI data, performed the analysis, and wrote the manuscript. JZ helped with data collecting. YJ and T-YT contributed to fMRI data analysis and discussion. C-QL helped with data processing. RS revised this manuscript. G-JT designed the MRI experiment and manuscript revision.

ACKNOWLEDGMENTS

We thank Xu Feng and Jing Zhao, Department of Otolaryngology, affiliated Zhongda Hospital of Southeast University, for her assistance with the data collection and audiological tests.

REFERENCES

Adank, P. (2012). The neural bases of difficult speech comprehension and speech production: two activation likelihood estimation (ALE) meta-analyses. *Brain Lang.* 122, 42–54. doi: 10.1016/j.bandl.2012.04.014

Anderson, J. S., Nielsen, J. A., Froehlich, A. L., DuBray, M. B., Druzgal, T. J., Cariello, A. N., et al. (2011). Functional connectivity magnetic resonance imaging classification of autism. *Brain* 134(Pt 12), 3742–3754. doi: 10.1093/brain/awr263

Asemi, A., Ramaseshan, K., Burgess, A., Diwadkar, V. A., and Bressler, S. L. (2015). Dorsal anterior cingulate cortex modulates supplementary motor area in coordinated unimanual motor behavior. *Front. Hum. Neurosci.* 9:309. doi: 10.3389/fnhum.2015.00309

Basner, M., Babisch, W., Davis, A., Brink, M., Clark, C., Janssen, S., et al. (2014). Auditory and non-auditory effects of noise on health. *Lancet* 383, 1325–1332. doi: 10.1016/S0140-6736(13)61613-X

Baumann, O., Borra, R. J., Bower, J. M., Cullen, K. E., Habas, C., Ivry, R. B., et al. (2015). Consensus paper: the role of the cerebellum in perceptual processes. *Cerebellum* 14, 197–220. doi: 10.1007/s12311-014-0627-7

Benedict, R. H., DeLuca, J., Phillips, G., LaRocca, N., Hudson, L. D., Rudick, R., et al. (2017). Validity of the symbol digit modalities test as a cognition performance outcome measure for multiple sclerosis. *Mult. Scler.* 23, 721–733. doi: 10.1177/1352458517690821

Bonnelle, V., Ham, T. E., Leech, R., Kinnunen, K. M., Mehta, M. A., Greenwood, R. J., et al. (2012). Salience network integrity predicts default mode network function after traumatic brain injury. *Proc. Natl. Acad. Sci. U.S.A.* 109, 4690–4695. doi: 10.1073/pnas.1113455109

Brozoski, T. J., Ciobanu, L., and Bauer, C. A. (2007). Central neural activity in rats with tinnitus evaluated with manganese-enhanced magnetic resonance imaging (MEMRI). *Hear. Res.* 228, 168–179. doi: 10.1016/j.heares.2007.02.003

Brugnolo, A., Morbelli, S., Arnaldi, D., De Carli, F., Accardo, J., Bossert, I., et al. (2014). Metabolic correlates of Rey auditory verbal learning test in elderly subjects with memory complaints. *J. Alzheimers Dis.* 39, 103–113. doi: 10.3233/JAD-121684

Bushara, K. O., Grafman, J., and Hallett, M. (2001). Neural correlates of auditory-visual stimulus onset asynchrony detection. *J. Neurosci.* 21, 300–304. doi: 10.1523/JNEUROSCI.21-01-00300.2001

Chang, Y. T., Lu, C. H., Wu, M. K., Hsu, S. W., Huang, C. W., Chang, W. N., et al. (2017). Salience network and depressive severities in parkinson's disease with mild cognitive impairment: a structural covariance network analysis. *Front. Aging Neurosci.* 9:417. doi: 10.3389/fnagi.2017.00417

Charizopoulou, N., Lelli, A., Schraders, M., Ray, K., Hildebrand, M. S., Ramesh, A., et al. (2011). Gipc3 mutations associated with audiogenic seizures and sensorineural hearing loss in mouse and human. *Nat. Commun.* 2:201. doi: 10.1038/ncomms1200

Chen, H. J., Zhang, L., Ke, J., Qi, R., Xu, Q., Zhong, Y., et al. (2018). Altered resting-state dorsal anterior cingulate cortex functional connectivity in patients with post-traumatic stress disorder. *Aust. N. Z. J. Psychiatry* 53, 68–79. doi: 10.1177/0004867418812674

Chen, J., Liang, J., Ou, J., and Cai, W. (2013). Mental health in adults with sudden sensorineural hearing loss: an assessment of depressive symptoms and its correlates. *J. Psychosom. Res.* 75, 72–74. doi: 10.1016/j.jpsychores.2013.03.006

Chen, Y. C., Li, X., Liu, L., Wang, J., Lu, C. Q., Yang, M., et al. (2015). Tinnitus and hyperacusis involve hyperactivity and enhanced connectivity in auditory-limbic-arousal-cerebellar network. *eLife* 4:e06576. doi: 10.7554/eLife.06576

Chen, Y. C., Xia, W. Q., Chen, H. Y., Feng, Y., Xu, J. J., Gu, J. P., et al. (2017). Tinnitus distress is linked to enhanced resting-state functional connectivity from the limbic system to the auditory cortex. *Hum. Brain Mapp.* 38, 2384–2397. doi: 10.1002/hbm.23525

Cona, G., Marino, G., and Semenza, C. (2017). TMS of supplementary motor area (SMA) facilitates mental rotation performance: evidence for sequence processing in SMA. *Neuroimage* 146, 770–777. doi: 10.1016/j.neuroimage.2016.10.032

Cui, Y., Jiao, Y., Chen, H. J., Ding, J., Luo, B., Peng, C. Y., et al. (2015). Aberrant functional connectivity of default-mode network in type 2 diabetes patients. *Eur. Radiol.* 25, 3238–3246. doi: 10.1007/s00330-015-3746-8

Cui, Y., Jiao, Y., Chen, Y. C., Wang, K., Gao, B., Wen, S., et al. (2014). Altered spontaneous brain activity in type 2 diabetes: a resting-state functional MRI study. *Diabetes* 63, 749–760. doi: 10.2337/db13-0519

De Pisapia, N., Turatto, M., Lin, P., Jovicich, J., and Caramazza, A. (2012). Unconscious priming instructions modulate activity in default and executive networks of the human brain. *Cereb. Cortex* 22, 639–649. doi: 10.1093/cercor/bhr146

Demirci, O., Stevens, M. C., Andreasen, N. C., Michael, A., Liu, J., White, T., et al. (2009). Investigation of relationships between fMRI brain networks in the spectral domain using ICA and granger causality reveals distinct differences between schizophrenia patients and healthy controls. *Neuroimage* 46, 419–431. doi: 10.1016/j.neuroimage.2009.02.014

Estevez-Gonzalez, A., Kulisevsky, J., Boltes, A., Otermin, P., and Garcia-Sanchez, C. (2003). Rey verbal learning test is a useful tool for differential diagnosis in the preclinical phase of Alzheimer's disease: comparison with mild cognitive impairment and normal aging. *Int. J. Geriatr. Psychiatry* 18, 1021–1028. doi: 10.1002/gps.1010

Feng, Z., Xu, S., Huang, M., Shi, Y., Xiong, B., and Yang, H. (2016). Disrupted causal connectivity anchored on the anterior cingulate cortex in first-episode medication-naive major depressive disorder. *Prog. Neuropsychopharmacol. Biol. Psychiatry* 64, 124–130. doi: 10.1016/j.pnpbp.2015.07.008

Forn, C., Belloch, V., Bustamante, J. C., Garbin, G., Parcet-Ibars, M. A., Sanjuan, A., et al. (2009). A symbol digit modalities test version suitable for functional MRI studies. *Neurosci. Lett.* 456, 11–14. doi: 10.1016/j.neulet.2009.03.081

Funahashi, S. (2001). Neuronal mechanisms of executive control by the prefrontal cortex. *Neurosci. Res.* 39, 147–165. doi: 10.1016/S0168-0102(00)00224-8

Goebel, R., Roebroeck, A., Kim, D. S., and Formisano, E. (2003). Investigating directed cortical interactions in time-resolved fMRI data using vector autoregressive modeling and granger causality mapping. *Magn. Reson. Imaging* 21, 1251–1261. doi: 10.1016/j.mri.2003.08.026

Gordon, K. A., Wong, D. D., and Papsin, B. C. (2013). Bilateral input protects the cortex from unilaterally-driven reorganization in children who are deaf. *Brain* 136(Pt 5), 1609–1625. doi: 10.1093/brain/awt052

Granger, C. W. J. (1969). Investigating causal relations by econometric models and cross-spectral methods. *Econometrica* 37, 424–438. doi: 10.2307/1912791

Greicius, M. D., Krasnow, B., Reiss, A. L., and Menon, V. (2003). Functional connectivity in the resting brain: a network analysis of the default mode hypothesis. *Proc. Natl. Acad. Sci. U.S.A.* 100, 253–258. doi: 10.1073/pnas.0135058100

Gwer, S., Chengo, E., Newton, C. R. J. C., and Kirkham, F. J. (2013). Unexpected relationship between tympanometry and mortality in children with nontraumatic coma. *Pediatrics* 132, E713–E717. doi: 10.1542/peds.2012-3264

Hamilton, M. (1967). Development of a rating scale for primary depressive illness. *Br. J. Soc. Clin. Psychol.* 6, 278–296. doi: 10.1111/j.2044-8260.1967.tb00530.x

Harris, K. C., Dubno, J. R., Keren, N. I., Ahlstrom, J. B., and Eckert, M. A. (2009). Speech recognition in younger and older adults: a dependency on low-level auditory cortex. *J. Neurosci.* 29, 6078–6087. doi: 10.1523/JNEUROSCI.0412-09.2009

Hatanaka, N., Tokuno, H., Hamada, I., Inase, M., Ito, Y., Imanishi, M., et al. (2003). Thalamocortical and intracortical connections of monkey cingulate motor areas. *J. Comp. Neurol.* 462, 121–138. doi: 10.1002/cne.10720

Heywood, R., Gao, Q., Nyunt, M. S. Z., Feng, L., Chong, M. S., Lim, W. S., et al. (2017). Hearing loss and risk of mild cognitive impairment and dementia: findings from the singapore longitudinal ageing study. *Dement. Geriatr. Cogn. Disord.* 43, 259–268. doi: 10.1159/000464281

Husain, F. T., Medina, R. E., Davis, C. W., Szymko-Bennett, Y., Simonyan, K., Pajor, N. M., et al. (2011). Neuroanatomical changes due to hearing loss and chronic tinnitus: a combined VBM and DTI study. *Brain Res.* 1369, 74–88. doi: 10.1016/j.brainres.2010.10.095

Jaywant, A., Barredo, J., Ahern, D. C., and Resnik, L. (2018). Neuropsychological assessment without upper limb involvement: a systematic review of oral versions of the trail making test and symbol-digit modalities test. *Neuropsychol. Rehabil.* 28, 1055–1077. doi: 10.1080/09602011.2016.1240699

Jiang, Y., Duan, M., Chen, X., Zhang, X., Gong, J., Dong, D., et al. (2018). Aberrant prefrontal-thalamic-cerebellar circuit in schizophrenia and depression: evidence from a possible causal connectivity. *Int. J. Neural Syst.* 16:1850032. doi: 10.1142/S0129065718500326

Kronenberger, W. G., Pisoni, D. B., Henning, S. C., and Colson, B. G. (2013). Executive functioning skills in long-term users of cochlear implants: a case control study. *J. Pediatr. Psychol.* 38, 902–914. doi: 10.1093/jpepsy/jst034

Lamichhane, B., Adhikari, B. M., and Dhamala, M. (2016). The activity in the anterior insulae is modulated by perceptual decision-making difficulty. *Neuroscience* 327, 79–94. doi: 10.1016/j.neuroscience.2016.04.016

Lange, I., Kasanova, Z., Goossens, L., Leibold, N., De Zeeuw, C. I., van Amelsvoort, T., et al. (2015). The anatomy of fear learning in the cerebellum: a systematic meta-analysis. *Neurosci. Biobehav. Rev.* 59, 83–91. doi: 10.1016/j.neubiorev.2015.09.019

Leavitt, V. M., Wylie, G., Genova, H. M., Chiaravalloti, N. D., and DeLuca, J. (2012). Altered effective connectivity during performance of an information processing speed task in multiple sclerosis. *Mult. Scler. J.* 18, 409–417. doi: 10.1177/1352458511423651

Lee, A. K., Babcock, S., and Shinn-Cunningham, B. G. (2008). Measuring the perceived content of auditory objects using a matching paradigm. *J. Assoc. Res. Otolaryngol.* 9, 388–397. doi: 10.1007/s10162-008-0124-0

Lefebvre, S., Demeulemeester, M., Leroy, A., Delmaire, C., Lopes, R., Pins, D., et al. (2016). Network dynamics during the different stages of hallucinations in schizophrenia. *Hum. Brain Mapp.* 37, 2571–2586. doi: 10.1002/hbm.23197

Li, L., Chao, T., Brant, J., O'Malley, B. Jr., Tsourkas, A., and Li, D. (2017). Advances in nano-based inner ear delivery systems for the treatment of sensorineural hearing loss. *Adv. Drug Deliv. Rev.* 108, 2–12. doi: 10.1016/j.addr.2016.01.004

Li, S., Qi, M., Yuan, W., and Chen, H. (2015). The impact of the depression and anxiety on prognosis of cervical total disc replacement. *Spine* 40, E266–E271. doi: 10.1097/BRS.0000000000000743

Lima, C. F., Krishnan, S., and Scott, S. K. (2016). Roles of supplementary motor areas in auditory processing and auditory imagery. *Trends Neurosci.* 39, 527–542. doi: 10.1016/j.tins.2016.06.003

Luo, Y., Qin, S., Fernandez, G., Zhang, Y., Klumpers, F., and Li, H. (2014). Emotion perception and executive control interact in the salience network during emotionally charged working memory processing. *Hum. Brain Mapp.* 35, 5606–5616. doi: 10.1002/hbm.22573

MacSweeney, M., Brammer, M. J., Waters, D., and Goswami, U. (2009). Enhanced activation of the left inferior frontal gyrus in deaf and dyslexic adults during rhyming. *Brain* 132(Pt 7), 1928–1940. doi: 10.1093/brain/awp129

Magni, E., Binetti, G., Bianchetti, A., Rozzini, R., and Trabucchi, M. (1996). Mini-mental state examination: a normative study in Italian elderly population. *Eur. J. Neurol.* 3, 198–202. doi: 10.1111/j.1468-1331.1996.tb00423.x

Manohar, S., Spoth, J., Radziwon, K., Auerbach, B. D., and Salvi, R. (2017). Noise-induced hearing loss induces loudness intolerance in a rat active sound avoidance paradigm (ASAP). *Hear. Res.* 353, 197–203. doi: 10.1016/j.heares.2017.07.001

Menon, V. (2011). Large-scale brain networks and psychopathology: a unifying triple network model. *Trends Cogn. Sci.* 15, 483–506. doi: 10.1016/j.tics.2011.08.003

Micarelli, A., Chiaravalloti, A., Viziano, A., Danieli, R., Schillaci, O., and Alessandrini, M. (2017). Early cortical metabolic rearrangement related to clinical data in idiopathic sudden sensorineural hearing loss. *Hear. Res.* 350, 91–99. doi: 10.1016/j.heares.2017.04.011

Moreno-Rius, J. (2018). The cerebellum in fear and anxiety-related disorders. *Prog. Neuropsychopharmacol. Biol. Psychiatry* 85, 23–32. doi: 10.1016/j.pnpbp.2018.04.002

Namkung, H., Kim, S. H., and Sawa, A. (2017). The insula: an underestimated brain area in clinical neuroscience, Psychiatry Neurol. *Trends Neurosci.* 40, 200–207. doi: 10.1016/j.tins.2017.02.002

Pascoe, M., Alamri, Y., Dalrymple-Alford, J., Anderson, T., and MacAskill, M. (2018). The symbol-digit modalities test in mild cognitive impairment: evidence from Parkinson's disease patients. *Eur. Neurol.* 79, 206–210. doi: 10.1159/000485669

Paul, B. T., Bruce, I. C., and Roberts, L. E. (2017). Evidence that hidden hearing loss underlies amplitude modulation encoding deficits in individuals with and without tinnitus. *Hear. Res.* 344, 170–182. doi: 10.1016/j.heares.2016.11.010

Petacchi, A., Laird, A. R., Fox, P. T., and Bower, J. M. (2005). Cerebellum and auditory function: an ALE meta-analysis of functional neuroimaging studies. *Hum. Brain Mapp.* 25, 118–128. doi: 10.1002/hbm.20137

Power, J. D., Barnes, K. A., Snyder, A. Z., Schlaggar, B. L., and Petersen, S. E. (2012). Spurious but systematic correlations in functional connectivity MRI networks arise from subject motion. *Neuroimage* 59, 2142–2154. doi: 10.1016/j.neuroimage.2011.10.018

Schmahmann, J. D., and Caplan, D. (2006). Cognition, emotion and the cerebellum. *Brain* 129(Pt 2), 290–292. doi: 10.1093/brain/awh729

Seeley, W. W., Menon, V., Schatzberg, A. F., Keller, J., Glover, G. H., Kenna, H., et al. (2007). Dissociable intrinsic connectivity networks for salience processing and executive control. *J. Neurosci.* 27, 2349–2356. doi: 10.1523/JNEUROSCI.5587-06.2007

Sepulcre, J. (2014). Functional streams and cortical integration in the human brain. *Neuroscientist* 20, 499–508. doi: 10.1177/1073858414531657

Seth, A. K., Barrett, A. B., and Barnett, L. (2015). Granger causality analysis in neuroscience and neuroimaging. *J. Neurosci.* 35, 3293–3297. doi: 10.1523/JNEUROSCI.4399-14.2015

Shirer, W. R., Ryali, S., Rykhlevskaia, E., Menon, V., and Greicius, M. D. (2012). Decoding subject-driven cognitive states with whole-brain connectivity patterns. *Cereb. Cortex* 22, 158–165. doi: 10.1093/cercor/bhr099

Sidlauskaite, J., Sonuga-Barke, E., Roeyers, H., and Wiersema, J. R. (2016). Altered intrinsic organisation of brain networks implicated in attentional processes in adult attention-deficit/hyperactivity disorder: a resting-state study of attention, default mode and salience network connectivity. *Eur. Arch. Psychiatry Clin. Neurosci.* 266, 349–357. doi: 10.1007/s00406-015-0630-0

Siedentopf, C. M., Ischebeck, A., Haala, I. A., Mottaghy, F. M., Schikora, D., Verius, M., et al. (2007). Neural correlates of transmeatal cochlear laser (TCL) stimulation in healthy human subjects. *Neurosci. Lett.* 411, 189–193. doi: 10.1016/j.neulet.2006.08.049

Sommer, I. E., Diederen, K. M., Blom, J. D., Willems, A., Kushan, L., Slotema, K., et al. (2008). Auditory verbal hallucinations predominantly activate the right inferior frontal area. *Brain* 131(Pt 12), 3169–3177. doi: 10.1093/brain/awn251

Song, J. J., De Ridder, D., Weisz, N., Schlee, W., Van de Heyning, P., and Vanneste, S. (2014). Hyperacusis-associated pathological resting-state brain oscillations in the tinnitus brain: a hyperresponsiveness network with paradoxically inactive auditory cortex. *Brain Struct. Funct.* 219, 1113–1128. doi: 10.1007/s00429-013-0555-1

Song, J. J., Vanneste, S., Lazard, D. S., Van de Heyning, P., Park, J. H., Oh, S. H., et al. (2015). The role of the salience network in processing lexical and nonlexical stimuli in cochlear implant users: an ALE meta-analysis of PET studies. *Hum. Brain Mapp.* 36, 1982–1994. doi: 10.1002/hbm.22750

Sridharan, D., Levitin, D. J., and Menon, V. (2008). A critical role for the right fronto-insular cortex in switching between central-executive and default-mode networks. *Proc. Natl. Acad. Sci. U.S.A.* 105, 12569–12574. doi: 10.1073/pnas.0800005105

Stokes, P. A., and Purdon, P. L. (2017). A study of problems encountered in granger causality analysis from a neuroscience perspective. *Proc. Natl. Acad. Sci. U.S.A.* 114, E7063–E7072. doi: 10.1073/pnas.1704663114

Stoodley, C. J., and Schmahmann, J. D. (2009). Functional topography in the human cerebellum: a meta-analysis of neuroimaging studies. *Neuroimage* 44, 489–501. doi: 10.1016/j.neuroimage.2008.08.039

Tombaugh, T. N., and McIntyre, N. J. (1992). The mini-mental state examination: a comprehensive review. *J. Am. Geriatr. Soc.* 40, 922–935. doi: 10.1111/j.1532-5415.1992.tb01992.x

Van Dijk, K. R., Sabuncu, M. R., and Buckner, R. L. (2012). The influence of head motion on intrinsic functional connectivity MRI. *Neuroimage* 59, 431–438. doi: 10.1016/j.neuroimage.2011.07.044

Vanneste, S., Song, J. J., and De Ridder, D. (2013). Tinnitus and musical hallucinosis: the same but more. *Neuroimage* 82, 373–383. doi: 10.1016/j.neuroimage.2013.05.107

White, T. P., Joseph, V., Francis, S. T., and Liddle, P. F. (2010). Aberrant salience network (bilateral insula and anterior cingulate cortex) connectivity during information processing in schizophrenia. *Schizophr. Res.* 123, 105–115. doi: 10.1016/j.schres.2010.07.020

Wu, X., Lin, P., Yang, J., Song, H., Yang, R., and Yang, J. (2016). Dysfunction of the cingulo-opercular network in first-episode medication-naive patients with major depressive disorder. *J. Affect. Disord.* 200, 275–283. doi: 10.1016/j.jad.2016.04.046

Yan, C. G., Cheung, B., Kelly, C., Colcombe, S., Craddock, R. C., Di Martino, A., et al. (2013). A comprehensive assessment of regional variation in the impact of head micromovements on functional connectomics. *Neuroimage* 76, 183–201. doi: 10.1016/j.neuroimage.2013.03.004

Yang, M., Chen, H. J., Liu, B., Huang, Z. C., Feng, Y., Li, J., et al. (2014). Brain structural and functional alterations in patients with unilateral hearing loss. *Hear. Res.* 316, 37–43. doi: 10.1016/j.heares.2014.07.006

Yang, X. H., Tian, K., Wang, D. F., Wang, Y., Cheung, E. F. C., Xie, G. R., et al. (2017). Anhedonia correlates with abnormal functional connectivity of the superior temporal gyrus and the caudate nucleus in patients with first-episode drug-naive major depressive disorder. *J. Affect. Disord.* 218, 284–290. doi: 10.1016/j.jad.2017.04.053

Yang, X. J., Jiang, H. M., Hou, X. H., and Song, J. (2015). Anxiety and depression in patients with gastroesophageal reflux disease and their effect on quality of life. *World J. Gastroenterol.* 21, 4302–4309. doi: 10.3748/wjg.v21.i14.4302

Zhang, J., Chen, Y. C., Feng, X., Yang, M., Liu, B., Qian, C., et al. (2015). Impairments of thalamic resting-state functional connectivity in patients with chronic tinnitus. *Eur. J. Radiol.* 84, 1277–1284. doi: 10.1016/j.ejrad.2015.04.006

Zhang, Y., Mao, Z., Feng, S., Liu, X., Lan, L., Zhang, J., et al. (2018). Altered functional networks in long-term unilateral hearing loss: a connectome analysis. *Brain Behav.* 8:e00912. doi: 10.1002/brb3.912

Changes in the Resting-State Cortical Oscillatory Activity 6 Months After Modified Tinnitus Retraining Therapy

*Sang-Yeon Lee[1], Jihye Rhee[2], Ye Ji Shim[3], Yoonjoong Kim[1], Ja-Won Koo[1], Dirk De Ridder[4], Sven Vanneste[5] and Jae-Jin Song[1]**

[1] Department of Otolaryngology-Head and Neck Surgery, Seoul National University Bundang Hospital, Seongnam, South Korea, [2] Department of Otolaryngology-Head and Neck Surgery, Seoul Veterans Hospital, Seoul, South Korea, [3] Department of Otolaryngology-Head & Neck Surgery, Seoul National University Hospital, Healthcare System Gangnam Center, Seoul, South Korea, [4] Unit of Neurosurgery, Department of Surgical Sciences, Dunedin School of Medicine, University of Otago, Dunedin, New Zealand, [5] Laboratory for Clinical and Integrative Neuroscience, School of Behavioral and Brain Sciences, The University of Texas at Dallas, Dallas, TX, United States

***Correspondence:**
Jae-Jin Song
jjsong96@snubh.org;
jjsong96@gmail.com

Although tinnitus retraining therapy (TRT) based on Jastreboff's classical neurophysiological model is efficacious in most patients, its effects on the cortical activity changes responsible for the improvement of tinnitus are still unclear. In this study, we compared pre- and post-TRT resting-state quantitative electroencephalography (rs-qEEG) findings to identify power changes that could explain TRT-induced improvements. Thirty-seven patients with severe tinnitus were enrolled in the study, and rs-qEEG data recorded before the initial TRT sessions and 6 months after TRT were compared. In addition, associations between the changes in qEEG and percentage improvements in Tinnitus Handicap Inventory (THI) scores and numeric rating scale (NRS) scores of tinnitus loudness and tinnitus perception were examined. The mean THI score decreased significantly 6 months after the initial TRT session. Also, significant improvements were observed 6 months after the initial TRT session compared with the pre-treatment scores in NRS loudness, distress, and perception. As compared with the pre-TRT status, post-TRT 6 months status showed significantly decreased powers in the left primary and secondary auditory cortices for the gamma frequency band. Changes in the alpha 1 frequency band power in the right insula and orbitofrontal cortex (OFC) appeared to be positively correlated with the percentage changes in NRS distress. These results suggested that TRT improved tinnitus-related distress by reducing the power of the top-down autonomic response modulator or peripheral physiological responses to emotional experiences. That is, TRT induced habituation via modulation of functional connections between the auditory system and the limbic and autonomic nervous systems. Our results confer additional basis for understanding the neurophysiological model and the newly suggested integrative model of tinnitus by De Ridder et al. (2014) in the context of the long-term efficacy of TRT.

Keywords: tinnitus retraining therapy, quantitative electroencephalography, neurophysiological model, cortical power, connectivity

INTRODUCTION

Subjective tinnitus is a common otological symptom characterized by the conscious auditory perception in the absence of an external stimulus, which is often called a "phantom sound" as there is no corresponding genuine physical source of the sound (Jastreboff, 1990). Although the precise mechanism remains unclear, the current consensus is that tinnitus may be a result of central maladaptive plastic changes reflecting a complex interplay of auditory and non-auditory brain regions responsible for tinnitus generation and tinnitus-related distress. That is, tinnitus is associated with functional changes not only in the auditory cortex but also in non-auditory regions such as the limbic, frontal, and parietal areas (De Ridder et al., 2011a; Adjamian et al., 2014; Lee et al., 2017).

Several management options, such as tinnitus retraining therapy (TRT), cognitive behavioral therapy, sound therapy, hearing rehabilitation using hearing aids or cochlear implants, pharmacotherapy, and brain stimulation, have been suggested for tinnitus (Langguth et al., 2013; Song et al., 2017). Of these modalities, TRT is a combination of directive counseling and sound therapy that seeks to manage tinnitus and reduce sound tolerance (Jastreboff, 1990). TRT is based on Jastreboff's classical neurophysiological model suggesting that the detection of tinnitus is made by neural network mechanisms, whereas the perception and evaluation involve the auditory cortical areas, limbic system, and sympathetic part of the autonomic nervous system (Jastreboff, 1999, 2007, 2015; Jastreboff and Jastreboff, 2000, 2003, 2006). TRT aims to suppress tinnitus by extinguishing functional connections between the auditory, limbic, and autonomic nervous systems, thus creating habituation to tinnitus-evoked reactions and ultimately the phantom perception itself (Jastreboff, 2015).

More than 100 studies have explored the effectiveness of TRT, and the majority of these studies indicated that TRT improved tinnitus significantly in approximately 80% of patients (Jastreboff, 2015). This implication has also been supported by the Cochrane review suggesting TRT as an effective treatment for patients with tinnitus, despite the conclusion based upon a single, low-quality randomized controlled trial (Phillips and McFerran, 2010). Although most studies have reported the effectiveness of TRT, changes in the cortical power responsible for the improvement of tinnitus are still unclear. A recent study demonstrated the neural substrates predicting short-term improvement of tinnitus loudness and distress by correlating resting-state source-localized quantitative electroencephalography (rs-qEEG) findings and the extent of tinnitus improvement 3 months after the first TRT session (Kim et al., 2016). In this study, pre-TRT activities in several cortical areas related to tinnitus generation, parasympathetic activity, and the descending noise-canceling system have been suggested as possible predictors of short-term improvement of tinnitus after TRT (Kim et al., 2016). However, the possible role of TRT in modulating abnormal cortical activities and thereby improving tinnitus remains unclear because there have been no studies comparing pre- and post-TRT cortical activities and correlating the cortical power changes with the degree of symptom improvement.

As a follow-up to our previous work (Kim et al., 2016), we compared rs-qEEGs measured before TRT and 6 months after the first TRT session in the present study. In addition, we correlated the extent of tinnitus improvement with the changes in rs-qEEG signals to determine the cortical activity changes responsible for the improvement of tinnitus using source localization complimented by connectivity analysis.

MATERIALS AND METHODS

Participants

The medical records of patients with subjective tinnitus who were enrolled in a modified TRT program at Seoul National University Bundang Hospital from May 2015 to April 2017 were retrospectively reviewed. Subjects with normal (<25 dB hearing level) or mild hearing loss (25–40 dB hearing level) calculated by averaging the pure tone thresholds at 0.5, 1, 2, and 3 kHz (Bae et al., 2017, 2018, 2019; Sunwoo et al., 2017; Song et al., 2018; Lee et al., 2019; Shim et al., 2019) on both ears were included in the present study. Subjects were excluded if they had the following conditions: (1) pulsatile tinnitus, Ménière's disease, otosclerosis, any psychiatric or neurological disorders, histories of drug or alcohol abuse, and chronic headache; (2) a history of head injury that caused loss of consciousness; (3) a history of seizures; and (4) subjects who were lost to follow-up were excluded from the study. Accordingly, the final study population consisted of 37 patients with subjective tinnitus. The study was approved by the Institutional Review Board of the Clinical Research Institute at Seoul National University Bundang Hospital, and was conducted in accordance with the Declaration of Helsinki (IRB-B-1708-412-128). The requirement for patient consent was waived. At the initial visit, we assessed the characteristics of tinnitus in a structured manner including the affected side, the nature of symptoms (pure-tone or narrow-band noise), and symptom duration. All participants underwent pure-tone audiometry, psychoacoustic tinnitus tests, such as tinnitus pitch matching, tinnitus loudness matching, and the minimum masking level test (Henry and Meikle, 2000), and an initial pre-TRT rs-qEEG. The perceived tinnitus handicap was measured by the Tinnitus Handicap Inventory (THI) (Newman et al., 1996). The THI consists of a total of 25 items, consisting of a functional subscale (11 items), an emotional subscale (9 items), and a catastrophic subscale (5 items). The total THI score (0–100 points) is used to determine a measure of the overall severity of the tinnitus annoyance or general tinnitus-related distress (Newman et al., 1996). The numeric rating scale (NRS) scores for tinnitus loudness (answering the question "how loud is your tinnitus?" on a scale from 0 to 10), tinnitus-related distress (answering the question "how bothered are you by your tinnitus?" on a scale from 0 to 10), and the percentage of the daytime during which the participant perceived tinnitus (NRS tinnitus perception, 0 to 100%) were used to evaluate the difficulties associated with tinnitus. All tests were conducted before and 6 months after the initial TRT session.

Modified TRT Program

After the initial evaluation, all subjects enrolled in the present study participated in our modified TRT program, which was based on the neurophysiological model of Jastreboff (Jastreboff, 1990, 1999, 2007, 2015; Jastreboff and Jastreboff, 2000, 2003, 2006). "The original TRT includes not only directive counseling and sound therapy but also stress management and facultative psychotherapeutic treatment. Meanwhile, the main point of modified TRT is the counseling, which based on the neurophysiological model of tinnitus (Mazurek et al., 2006)." During the initial session for 40 min, the subjects were educated regarding the background of tinnitus and TRT, such as the definition and incidence of tinnitus, simplified anatomy of the ear and auditory pathways, the subconscious processing and conscious perception of auditory stimuli, selective listening and the central noise-canceling mechanism (Song et al., 2015a), the neurophysiological model suggested by Jastreboff, tinnitus demystification, motivation and reassurance, explanation of habituation and ignoring tinnitus as the goal of TRT, the roles played by hearing aids and various sound therapies in treating tinnitus, and directed education on how to avoid silence and to add non-noxious sounds to the daily environment (i.e., ambient sound stimulation). All subjects were recommended to be exposed to ambient sound stimulation as much as possible and to avoid complete silence while they are awake. Hearing aids were not used in the present study population as only subjects with normal hearing or mild hearing loss were included to avoid bias with the cortical changes due to hearing loss and its improvement after hearing aid use. After the initial TRT session, all subjects were scheduled for monthly follow-up TRT sessions (30 min each). At each follow-up session, all subjects were reevaluated by follow-up THI and NRS score survey and counseled to determine subjective changes in their symptoms and to review the core content of the initial counseling session. In this way, a total of 7 TRT sessions were given to each subject.

EEG Recording

Rs-EEGs were obtained before and 6 months after the initial TRT session in all 37 subjects. Before measurement, the participants were asked not to drink alcohol for 24 h and to avoid caffeinated beverages on the day of recording to minimize alcohol-induced changes in EEG (Korucuoglu et al., 2016) or caffeine-induced alpha and beta power decreases (Siepmann and Kirch, 2002). EEGs were recorded with the patient in the sitting position with the eyes closed for 5 min using a tin-electrode cap (Electro-Cap, Eaton, OH, United States), a Mitsar amplifier (EEG-201; Mitsar, St. Petersburg, Russia), and WinEEG software version 2.84.44 (Mitsar) in a fully lit room shielded from sound and stray electric fields. The EEG was sampled with 19 electrodes in the standard 10–20 International placement, referenced to linked ears, and impedances were maintained below 5 kΩ at each electrode throughout the EEG measurements. We imported EEG as epoched data, and the data were collected for 100 2-second epochs eyes closed. The epochs remained after artifact removal differed from person to person according to the amount of removed data. The sampling rate was 1024 Hz, and the high- and low-pass frequencies used were 0.15 and 200 Hz, respectively. Initially recorded data were then resampled to 128 Hz and band-pass filtered using a fast Fourier transform filter and application of a Hanning window at 2–44 Hz. After importing the data into Eureka! Software (Sherlin and Congedo, 2005), plotting of the EEG stream and manual inspection for artifacts, such as eye movement, unconscious blinking, teeth clenching, and any form of body movements that can affect EEG stream, were performed to remove all episodic artifacts. As the vigilance level of participants may affect test results, we carefully monitored abnormal EEG patterns, such as slowing of the alpha rhythm or the emergence of sleep spindles (Moazami-Goudarzi et al., 2010). No participants included in the present study exhibited such abnormal EEG patterns throughout the measurements.

Source Localization Analysis

Low-resolution brain electromagnetic tomography (LORETA)-KEY software[1] designed for functional localization of standardized current densities based on certain electrophysiological and neuroanatomical constraints (Pascual-Marqui, 2002) was used to localize the cortical sources that generated the activities recorded from the scalp electrode in each of the following 8 frequency bands: delta (2–3.5 Hz), theta (4–7.5 Hz), alpha 1 (8–10 Hz), alpha 2 (10–12 Hz), beta 1 (13–18 Hz), beta 2 (18.5–21 Hz), beta 3 (21.5–30 Hz), and gamma (30.5–44 Hz) (Kim et al., 2015; Song et al., 2015a,b, 2017; Han et al., 2018; Vanneste et al., 2018).

Estimation of the position of the current sources from electrode potentials is known as the inverse problem or the neural source imaging problem (Grech et al., 2008; Lopez Rincon and Shimoda, 2016). In other words, the inverse problem involves the source reconstruction of images from electric neuronal activities based on extracranial measurements. Among various techniques available for EEG source localization, LORETA algorithm gives the best solution in terms of both localization error and ghost sources (Grech et al., 2008). The software makes assumptions with regard to orientations and strengths of the neighboring neuronal sources that are represented by adjacent voxels. This software implements revisited realistic electrode coordinates (Jurcak et al., 2007) and the lead field produced by Fuchs et al. (2002) resulting from standard electrode positions readjusted to a standard Montreal Neurological Institute (MNI)-152 head in combination with a boundary element method derived from the same standard anatomy (Jurcak et al., 2007). The LORETA-KEY anatomical template divides and labels the neocortical MNI-152 volume, including the hippocampus and anterior cingulate cortex, into 6239 voxels with dimensions of 5 × 5 × 5 mm, based on the Daemon Atlas (Lancaster et al., 2000). Anatomical labeling of significant clusters was performed automatically using a toolbox implemented in LORETA-KEY. The locations of significant clusters were initially investigated using the Anatomy toolbox (Eickhoff et al., 2005), and reconfirmed using the Talairach and Tournoux atlas (Talairach and Tournoux, 1988).

[1] http://www.uzh.ch/keyinst/NewLORETA/Software/Software.htm

Functional Connectivity Analysis

Phase synchronization over multiple frequency bands has been proposed to be the most plausible mechanism of large scale neuronal integration overcoming the distributed anatomical and functional organization of brain activity to enable coherent behavior and cognition (Varela et al., 2001). Therefore, phase synchronization and the amount of coherence between pre- and post-TRT qEEGs in different regions of interest (ROIs) were calculated to analyze functional connectivity by the built-in LORETA-KEY connectivity toolbox. The toolbox determines coherence and phase synchronization between multivariate time series; the measures are expressed as the sums of lagged/instantaneous dependencies. Of various methods, we analyzed lagged coherence as it excludes non-lagged parts of coherence that comprises effects of volume conduction (artificially increasing coherence), and effects of non-recorded sources that simultaneously drive recorded sources (Milz et al., 2014).

A total of 28 ROIs defined by Brodmann area were selected as possible nodes based on the previous literature on tinnitus: the bilateral primary and secondary auditory cortices (Rolls, 2004; Kringelbach, 2005; Smits et al., 2007), the bilateral parahippocampal (Landgrebe et al., 2009), the bilateral rostral/pregenual/subgenual anterior cingulate cortices (r/pg/sgACCs) (Vanneste et al., 2010; De Ridder et al., 2011b; Golm et al., 2013), the bilateral ventral medial prefrontal cortices (vmPFC) (Leaver et al., 2011, 2012), the bilateral insulae, bilateral precunei, and bilateral orbitofrontal cortices (OFC) (Vanneste et al., 2010; De Ridder et al., 2011b; Golm et al., 2016).

Statistical Analysis

Statistical non-parametric mapping (SnPM) was adapted for permutation tests for source localization and functional connectivity. SnPM yields results similar to those obtained with the statistical parametric mapping approach using a general linear model (GLM) with multiple comparison corrections derived from random field theory (Nichols and Holmes, 2002). That is, SnPM corrects for multiple tests performed for all voxels and all frequency bands. Due to its non-parametric nature, the validity of SnPM does not rely on any assumption of Gaussianity. In this regard, SnPM can be used to verify the validity of less computationally expensive parametric approaches and is suitable for functional neuroimaging studies involving multi-subjects or group analyses in small numbers of subjects (Nichols and Holmes, 2002). SnPM's permutation for correction for multiple comparisons (5,000 permutations in the current study) has previously been proven similar to those obtained using a standard GLM approach with multiple comparisons corrections (Holmes et al., 1996; Nichols and Holmes, 2002).

In this way, we compared pre- and post-TRT rs-qEEGs and correlated the extent of tinnitus improvement with the changes in rs-qEEG signals with regard to source-localized activity and functional connectivity. In addition, the paired t-test was used to evaluate the changes in perceived THI and NRS scores 6 months after TRT using SPSS (version 20.0; SPSS Inc., Chicago, IL, United States). In all analyses, $P < 0.05$ was taken to indicate statistical significance. The t-tests were based on one-tailed hypotheses.

RESULTS

Demographic and Clinical Characteristics of the Subjects

The clinical characteristics of the 37 subjects enrolled in this study are summarized in **Table 1**. The mean THI score of the subjects was 56.3 ± 16.8, and the enrolled subjects' tinnitus handicap ranged from "moderate" to "severe" as defined by Newman et al. (1998). The mean age of the subjects was 55.0 ± 11.9 years (range, 22–76 years), and 20 of the 37 subjects were male. Of the 37 subjects, 21 complained of unilateral tinnitus (15 with right tinnitus and 6 with left tinnitus), while the remaining 16 had bilateral tinnitus. Twenty-seven patients presented pure-tone tinnitus, while the other 10 presented narrow-band noise tinnitus. The mean symptom duration was 5.0 ± 4.1 years (range, 1–25 years).

Improvement in Questionnaire Scores 6 Months After the Initial TRT Session

As summarized in **Table 2**, the mean THI score improved significantly from 56.3 ± 16.8 to 37.5 ± 24.3 ($t = 5.83$, $P < 0.001$, Cohen's $d = 1.118$, paired t test) 6 months after the initial TRT session. In addition, significant improvements were observed 6 months after the initial TRT session compared with the pre-treatment scores in NRS loudness (from 6.9 ± 1.8 to 6.0 ± 2.0, $t = 3.525$, Cohen's $d = 0.484$, $P = 0.007$, paired t test), distress (from 7.0 ± 2.0 to 5.1 ± 2.6, $t = 3.096$, Cohen's $d = 0.916$, $P < 0.001$, paired t test), and perception (from 85.9 ± 22.2% to 64.2 ± 29.4%, $t = 3.451$, Cohen's $d = 0.981$, $P < 0.001$, paired t test).

TABLE 1 | Demographic and Clinical characteristics.

Parameters	Enrolled subjects (n = 37)
Sex	
Male	20 (54.1%)
Female	17 (45.9%)
Age (year)	
Mean [SD]	55.0 [11.9]
Range	22–76
Tinnitus laterality	
Unilateral	21 (56.8%)
Bilateral	16 (43.2%)
Tinnitus characteristics	
Pure tone	27 (73.0%)
Narrow band noise	10 (27.0%)
Duration (year)	
Mean	5.0 [4.1]
Range	1–25
Hearing level (dB)	
Normal	26 (70.2%)
Mild hearing loss	11 (29.8%)

TABLE 2 | Changes in the perceived tinnitus handicap scores 6 months after TRT.

Parameters	Pre-TRT	Post-TRT 6 months	*P*-value	Cohen's *d*
THI (0–100)	56.3 [SD:16.8]	37.5 [SD:24.3]	<0.001	1.118
NRS perception (%)	85.9 [SD:22.2]	64.2 [SD:29.4]	0.007	0.484
NRS loudness (0–10)	6.9 [SD:1.8]	6.0 [SD:2.0]	<0.001	0.916
NRS distress (0–10)	7.0 [SD:2.0]	5.1 [SD:2.6]	<0.001	0.981

TRT, tinnitus retraining therapy; NRS, numeric rating scale.

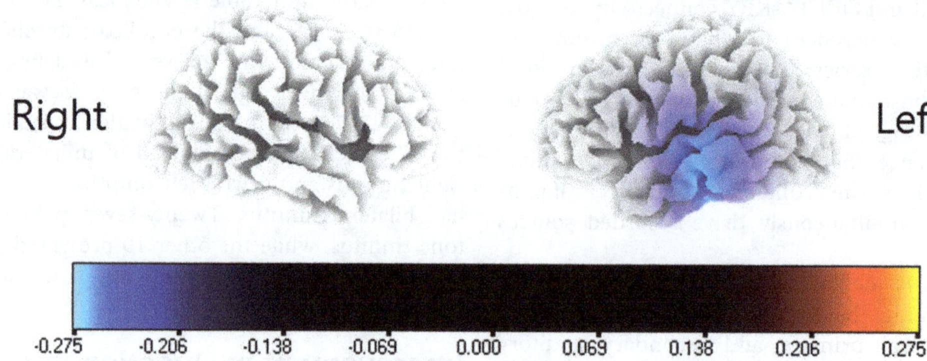

Weighted center	Anatomical area
(-65, -25, -15)	Secondary auditory cortex
(-59, -41, -15)	Primary auditory cortex

FIGURE 1 | Source-localized cortical power comparison between pre- and post-TRT conditions using repeatedly measured quantitative electroencephalography (qEEG) data. Post-TRT qEEG data showed decreased powers in the left primary and secondary auditory cortices (A1 and A2) for the gamma frequency band as compared with pre-TRT data.

Source-Localized Cortical Power and Connectivity Comparison Between Pre- and Post-TRT Conditions

The subjects enrolled in the present study showed significantly decreased powers in the left primary and secondary auditory cortices (A1 and A2) for the gamma frequency band 6 months after TRT in comparison with pre-TRT status ($P < 0.01$) (**Figure 1**). There were no other statistically significant differences between the pre- and post-TRT rs-qEEGs for the delta, theta, alpha 1 and 2, and beta 1–3 frequency bands.

No significant differences were found between pre- and post-TRT rs-qEEG data with regard to connectivity among the 28 ROIs.

Correlation Analyses Between NRS Changes and Source-Localized Cortical Power Changes

Changes in the source-localized cortical power in the right insula and OFC for the alpha 1 frequency band were positively correlated with the percentage improvements in NRS distress ($P = 0.04$) (**Figure 2**). Meanwhile, percentage improvements in NRS loudness or NRS perception showed no significant correlations with changes in source-localized cortical power after TRT.

Correlation Analyses Between Changes in NRS Parameters and Connectivity Changes

No significant correlations were observed in the percentage improvements in NRS loudness/distress/perception and connectivity among the 28 ROIs.

DISCUSSION

This study was performed to explore the role of modified TRT with regard to the modulation of abnormal cortical activities in subjects with debilitating tinnitus 6 months after the initial session by analyzing changes in resting-state cortical activities. By analyzing repetitively measured rs-qEEGs, we demonstrated that the cortical power of tinnitus subject changes after repeated modified TRT sessions and the improvement in symptoms is correlated with the changes in resting-state cortical oscillatory activities. To our knowledge, although the classical neurophysiological

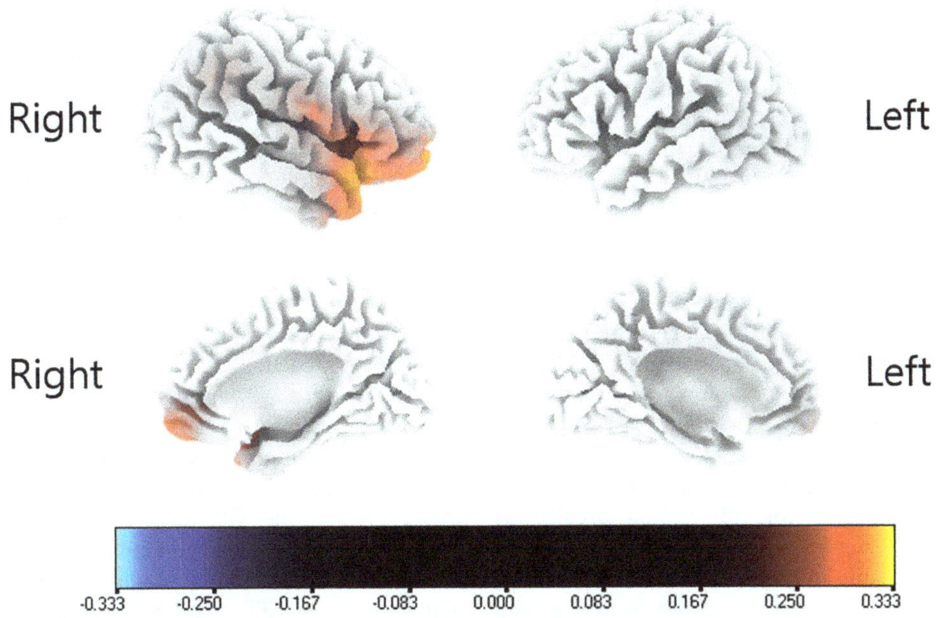

Weighted center	Anatomical area
(20, 65, -5)	Orbitofrontal cortex
(37, 15, -12)	Insula

FIGURE 2 | Source-localized correlation analysis between the percentage improvements in NRS of tinnitus distress and changes in TRT (pre- and post-TRT) resting-state qEEG data. EEG power changes in the right insula and orbitofrontal cortex (OFC) for the alpha 1 frequency band showed a positive correlation with the percentage changes in NRS distress ($P = 0.04$).

model of tinnitus suggested by Jastreboff postulated the involvement of cortical structures, such as the auditory cortex and limbic system, this is the first study to elucidate the cortical changes that may be relevant to the improvement of tinnitus after successful TRT sessions in subjects with severe tinnitus.

Sustained Improvement in Questionnaire Scores 6 Months After the Initial TRT Session

As a follow-up to our previous report (Kim et al., 2016), the present study was performed in a population of 37 patients enrolled in the TRT program of our institute and followed up for 6 months after the initial TRT session. As summarized in **Table 2**, the improvements in mean THI score (from 56.3 ± 16.8 to 37.5 ± 24.3), NRS loudness (from 6.9 ± 1.8 to 6.0 ± 2.0), distress (from 7.0 ± 2.0 to 5.1 ± 2.6), and perception (from 85.9 ± 22.2% to 64.2 ± 29.4%) indicated significant sustained improvements 6 months after the initial TRT session compared with the pre-treatment scores. The results were comparable to our previous preliminary report (Kim et al., 2016) as well as to other previous studies (Jastreboff and Jastreboff, 2006; Jastreboff, 2015).

Abnormal Auditory Cortical Power Is Suppressed 6 Months After Initial TRT Session

The perception of tinnitus has previously been suggested to be linked to increased neural activity in the auditory cortex, and A1 and A2 has been suggested to play important roles in tinnitus perception (De Ridder et al., 2015), and these areas have recently been suggested as a part of tinnitus core; i.e., the minimal brain area required to generate the phantom sound (De Ridder et al., 2014), along with the parahippocampus (PHC). Indeed, a recent meta-analysis of PET studies reported increased regional cerebral blood flow in A1 and A2 in tinnitus patients in comparison with normal controls, which supports the suggestion that A1 and A2 are important areas for tinnitus perception (Song et al., 2012). However, the included studies in this meta-analysis did not control for hearing loss, thereby might have been demonstrating correlates of hearing loss as well as, or instead of, tinnitus. Therefore, this awaits further confirmation.

Tinnitus was suggested to be caused by abnormal, spontaneous, and constant gamma-band activity generated as a consequence of hyperpolarization of the thalamic nuclei (Llinás et al., 1999). On the other hand, qEEG (Van Der Loo et al., 2009; Vanneste and De Ridder, 2012; Meyer et al., 2014) and MEG studies (Weisz et al., 2005, 2007) showed that tinnitus perception and its loudness are correlated with sustained high-frequency gamma-band activity in the auditory cortices. These results suggest that increased gamma-band activity in the auditory cortices is associated with the perception and loudness of tinnitus. The present study demonstrated significantly decreased gamma power at the left A1 and A2 at post-TRT 6 months as compared with pre-TRT baseline, showing decreased cortical power of the core tinnitus generator, i.e., the auditory cortices, after TRT. However, of note, reports on auditory cortical gamma power changes in patients with tinnitus appear to be controversial. For instance, other previous qEEG or MEG studies have failed to find gamma power changes between tinnitus- and control groups (Adjamian et al., 2012; Song et al., 2015b). Moreover, Sedley et al. revealed the differential patterns of gamma-band oscillations in the auditory cortex according to residual inhibition or excitation, suggesting a mutual inhibitory role of gamma oscillations on tinnitus symptoms (Sedley et al., 2012). These discrepant findings might be attributable to highly variable gamma-band frequency across studies (Weisz et al., 2007; Van Der Loo et al., 2009; Song et al., 2015b) and confounders such as laterality and hearing loss (Ortmann et al., 2011), and therefore further studies to elucidate the role of gamma power changes in the auditory cortex should be performed. Furthermore, reduced gamma power in the left A1 and A2 6 months after the initial session of modified TRT might also be biased by an effect of time, familiarity with EEG, or an indirect correlate of these such as attention. Future studies in a larger number of subjects should be performed to reconfirm our current findings.

Our preliminary study indicated that the percentage changes in improvement in tinnitus loudness were correlated with the gamma-band activities of A1 and A2 3 months after TRT (Kim et al., 2016). In this regard, decreased activities in the A1 and A2 in patients with tinnitus after TRT may be related to both short- and long-term TRT-mediated improvements in tinnitus. In addition, in a recent rs-qEEG study performed by Vanneste and De Ridder (2016), tinnitus was suggested to be more closely related to auditory cortical activity in patients with little or no hearing loss, but not to parahippocampal activity, whereas tinnitus appears to be related to parahippocampal mechanisms in those with more severe hearing loss. As the subjects enrolled in the present study had no or minimal hearing loss with thresholds better than 40 dB bilaterally, the deactivation of the auditory cortices in our subjects after TRT were consistent with that reported by Vanneste and De Ridder (2016).

TRT Attenuated Tinnitus-Related Distress via Modulation of the Interaction of the Limbic and Autonomic Nervous Systems

According to the classical neurophysiological model of tinnitus (Jastreboff, 1990, 2015), once an abnormal activity that causes tinnitus is classified as important, it spreads to the limbic system and autonomic nervous system. That is, tinnitus-related distress is attributable to changes in the limbic system and the autonomic nervous system as well as the interaction between these two systems. In an integrative model of tinnitus suggesting tinnitus as a unified percept of interacting separable subnetworks, the OFC has been suggested to be one of the cortical areas responsible for the emotional component of tinnitus (De Ridder et al., 2014). In addition, recent studies demonstrated that tinnitus-related distress is related to alpha oscillation over the network consisting of the amygdala-anterior cingulate cortex-insula-PHC (Vanneste et al., 2010; Golm et al., 2013). Moreover, another study demonstrated a correlation between tinnitus-related distress and sympathetic activation, mediated in part via the right anterior insula (van der Loo et al., 2011).

These previous studies were consistent with the present findings showing positive correlations between cortical power changes in the right insula/OFC and the percentage improvements in NRS distress 6 months after the initial TRT session. That is, greater normalization of OFC-mediated emotional components and right insula-mediated sympathetic activation by TRT showed an association with greater improvement in tinnitus-related distress. In addition, our preliminary study revealed a positive correlation between the pre-TRT activity of the insula and the percentage improvement in THI score, reflecting the improvement of psychological distress due to tinnitus, 3 months after the initial TRT session. Taken together with the results of our preliminary study, the findings presented here suggest that TRT may be more successful in subjects with severe distress due to abnormal autonomic nervous system activation.

Strengths and Limitations of the Current Study

To our knowledge, this is the first study to evaluate cortical power changes after TRT and to correlate these changes with improvements in subjective symptoms of tinnitus. Although this study not only replicated previous findings but also elucidated key changes responsible for the improvement of tinnitus and related distress, there are several potential limitations that warrant follow-up investigation.

First, we processed qEEG data by resampling to 128 Hz and band-pass filtering with the standard EEG wave range (2–44 Hz) in this study. A previous study, however, showed higher frequency (40–80 Hz) activities in the gamma range over auditory cortices in patients with intractable tinnitus (Ashton et al., 2007). The precise interpretation of the changes in gamma oscillation, which have been suggested to be neural correlates of perception and consciousness (Weisz et al., 2007), was not possible in the present study. Therefore, further studies using higher frequency band recording are required. Second, although we reported improvements in tinnitus-related symptoms 6 months after modified TRT, we cannot definitively conclude that these improvements were solely due to TRT. As tinnitus resolves spontaneously without any treatment during follow-up in some patients (Dobie and Snow, 2004) and as it is recommended for the TRT program to be continued for 18 months (Grewal et al., 2014), further studies comparing a TRT group with a "waiting list" control group with a longer follow-up duration are warranted. Third, tinnitus patients with relatively high levels of distress (mean THI score of 57.8) were enrolled in the present study. To explore the applicability of the present results to patients with different levels of distress, further studies in subjects with no or mild distress are required. Fourth, we enrolled tinnitus patients with normal hearing or only mild hearing loss and did not take combined hyperacusis into consideration. It has been reported that tinnitus patients show different cortical activity patterns according to the degree of hearing loss or combined hyperacusis (Vanneste and De Ridder, 2016). Therefore, further studies to explore the cortical power changes that occur after TRT in groups with different degrees of hearing loss and to evaluate the role of hyperacusis are required. Fifth, a recent study has suggested that there were no differences with regard to tinnitus improvement scores among TRT, partial TRT (counseling with placebo sound generator), and standard of care groups (Tinnitus Retraining Therapy Trial Research Group et al., 2019). Further research is warranted to reveal whether or not the effect of TRT is in a part of natural habituation. Sixth, our study subjects were heterogeneous with regard to tinnitus laterality (16 bilateral tinnitus, 15 right tinnitus, and 6 left tinnitus). In this regard, the findings in the current study are inconclusive as unilateral- and bilateral tinnitus subjects show different cortical oscillatory patterns according to previous literature (Vanneste et al., 2011). Future studies exploring different effects of TRT both in uni- and bilateral tinnitus groups should be performed to further explore the effect of tinnitus laterality.

CONCLUSION

Taken together, the results presented here indicated that TRT improves tinnitus by reducing the auditory cortical power and tinnitus-related distress by reducing the power of the top-down autonomic response modulator or peripheral physiological responses to emotional experiences. That is, TRT induces habituation via modulation of the functional connections between the auditory system and the limbic and autonomic nervous systems. The present study confers an additional basis for understanding the neurophysiological model and the newly suggested integrative model of tinnitus by De Ridder et al. (2014) in the context of the long-term efficacy of TRT. In addition, the present study suggested a mechanism by which TRT quiets tinnitus and relieves tinnitus-related distress in the context of psychological modulation of cortical power.

ETHICS STATEMENT

The study was approved by the Institutional Review Board of the Clinical Research Institute at Seoul National University Bundang Hospital and was conducted in accordance with the Declaration of Helsinki (IRB-B-1708-412-128). The requirement for patient consent was waived.

AUTHOR CONTRIBUTIONS

J-JS led the analysis and interpretation of the results, and drafted the first manuscript. S-YL, JR, and YS conceived the investigation, revised the manuscript for important intellectual content. All authors contributed to all aspects of the investigation, including methodological design, data collection and analysis, interpretation of the results, and revision of the manuscript for important intellectual content, and approved the final version of the manuscript and agreed to be accountable for all aspects of the work.

ACKNOWLEDGMENTS

The English in this document has been checked by at least two professional editors, both native speakers of English. For a certificate, please see: http://www.textcheck.com/certificate/G0JWRd.

REFERENCES

Adjamian, P., Hall, D. A., Palmer, A. R., Allan, T. W., and Langers, D. R. (2014). Neuroanatomical abnormalities in chronic tinnitus in the human brain. *Neurosci. Biobehav. Rev.* 45, 119–133. doi: 10.1016/j.neubiorev.2014.05.013

Adjamian, P., Sereda, M., Zobay, O., Hall, D. A., and Palmer, A. R. (2012). Neuromagnetic indicators of tinnitus and tinnitus masking in patients with and without hearing loss. *J. Assoc. Res. Otolaryngol.* 13, 715–731. doi: 10.1007/s10162-012-0340-5

Ashton, H., Reid, K., Marsh, R., Johnson, I., Alter, K., and Griffiths, T. (2007). High frequency localised "hot spots" in temporal lobes of patients with intractable tinnitus: a quantitative electroencephalographic (QEEG) study. *Neurosci. Lett.* 426, 23–28. doi: 10.1016/j.neulet.2007.08.034

Bae, Y. J., Jeon, Y. J., Choi, B. S., Koo, J. W., and Song, J. J. (2017). The role of MRI in diagnosing neurovascular compression of the cochlear nerve resulting in typewriter tinnitus. *AJNR Am. J. Neuroradiol.* 38, 1212–1217. doi: 10.3174/ajnr.A5156

Bae, Y. J., Shim, Y. J., Choi, B. S., Kim, J. H., Koo, J. W., and Song, J. J. (2019). Third window" and "single window" effects impede surgical success: analysis of retrofenestral otosclerosis involving the internal auditory canal or round window. *J. Clin. Med.* 8:E1182. doi: 10.3390/jcm8081182

Bae, Y. J., Song, J. J., Choi, B. S., Kang, Y., Kim, J. H., and Koo, J. W. (2018). Differentiation between intralabyrinthine schwannoma and contrast-enhancing labyrinthitis on MRI: quantitative analysis of signal intensity characteristics. *Otol. Neurotol.* 39, 1045–1052. doi: 10.1097/MAO.0000000000001901

De Ridder, D., Elgoyhen, A. B., Romo, R., and Langguth, B. (2011a). Phantom percepts: tinnitus and pain as persisting aversive memory networks. *Proc. Natl. Acad. Sci. U.S.A.* 108, 8075–8080. doi: 10.1073/pnas.1018466108

De Ridder, D., Vanneste, S., and Congedo, M. (2011b). The distressed brain: a group blind source separation analysis on tinnitus. *PLoS One* 6:e24273. doi: 10.1371/journal.pone.0024273

De Ridder, D., Vanneste, S., Langguth, B., and Llinas, R. (2015). Thalamocortical dysrhythmia: a theoretical update in tinnitus. *Front. Neurol.* 6:124. doi: 10.3389/fneur.2015.00124

De Ridder, D., Vanneste, S., Weisz, N., Londero, A., Schlee, W., Elgoyhen, A. B., et al. (2014). An integrative model of auditory phantom perception: tinnitus as a unified percept of interacting separable subnetworks. *Neurosci. Biobehav. Rev.* 44, 16–32. doi: 10.1016/j.neubiorev.2013.03.021

Dobie, R. A., and Snow, J. (2004). "Overview: suffering from tinnitus," in *Tinnitus: Theory and Management*, ed. J. B. Snow, (Lewiston, NY: BC Decker), 1–7.

Eickhoff, S. B., Stephan, K. E., Mohlberg, H., Grefkes, C., Fink, G. R., Amunts, K., et al. (2005). A new SPM toolbox for combining probabilistic cytoarchitectonic maps and functional imaging data. *Neuroimage* 25, 1325–1335. doi: 10.1016/j.neuroimage.2004.12.034

Fuchs, M., Kastner, J., Wagner, M., Hawes, S., and Ebersole, J. S. (2002). A standardized boundary element method volume conductor model. *Clin. Neurophysiol.* 113, 702–712. doi: 10.1016/s1388-2457(02)00030-5

Golm, D., Schmidt-Samoa, C., Dechent, P., and Kroner-Herwig, B. (2013). Neural correlates of tinnitus related distress: an fMRI-study. *Hear. Res.* 295, 87–99. doi: 10.1016/j.heares.2012.03.003

Golm, D., Schmidt-Samoa, C., Dechent, P., and Kroner-Herwig, B. (2016). Tinnitus- related distress: evidence from fMRI of an emotional stroop task. *BMC Ear Nose Throat Disord.* 16:10. doi: 10.1186/s12901-016-0029-1

Grech, R., Cassar, T., Muscat, J., Camilleri, K. P., Fabri, S. G., Zervakis, M., et al. (2008). Review on solving the inverse problem in EEG source analysis. *J. Neuroeng. Rehabil.* 5:25. doi: 10.1186/1743-0003-5-25

Grewal, R., Spielmann, P. M., Jones, S. E., and Hussain, S. S. (2014). Clinical efficacy of tinnitus retraining therapy and cognitive behavioural therapy in the treatment of subjective tinnitus: a systematic review. *J. Laryngol. Otol.* 128, 1028–1033. doi: 10.1017/S0022215114002849

Han, J. J., Jang, J. H., Ridder, D., Vanneste, S., Koo, J. W., and Song, J. J. (2018). Increased parietal circuit-breaker activity in delta frequency band and abnormal delta/theta band connectivity in salience network in hyperacusis subjects. *PLoS One* 13:e0191858. doi: 10.1371/journal.pone.0191858

Henry, J. A., and Meikle, M. B. (2000). Psychoacoustic measures of tinnitus. *J. Am. Acad. Audiol.* 11, 138–155.

Holmes, A. P., Blair, R. C., Watson, J. D., and Ford, I. (1996). Nonparametric analysis of statistic images from functional mapping experiments. *J. Cereb. Blood Flow Metab.* 16, 7–22. doi: 10.1097/00004647-199601000-2

Jastreboff, P. J. (1990). Phantom auditory perception (tinnitus): mechanisms of generation and perception. *Neurosci. Res.* 8, 221–254. doi: 10.1016/0168-0102(90)90031-9

Jastreboff, P. J. (1999). Tinnitus retraining therapy. *Br J Audiol.* 33, 68–70.

Jastreboff, P. J. (2007). Tinnitus retraining therapy. *Prog. Brain Res.* 166, 415–423. doi: 10.1016/S0079-6123(07)66040-3

Jastreboff, P. J. (2015). 25 years of tinnitus retraining therapy. *HNO* 63, 307–311. doi: 10.1007/s00106-014-2979-1

Jastreboff, P. J., and Jastreboff, M. M. (2000). Tinnitus retraining therapy (TRT) as a method for treatment of tinnitus and hyperacusis patients. *J. Am. Acad. Audiol.* 11, 162–177.

Jastreboff, P. J., and Jastreboff, M. M. (2003). Tinnitus retraining therapy for patients with tinnitus and decreased sound tolerance. *Otolaryngol. Clin. North Am.* 36, 321–336. doi: 10.1016/s0030-6665(02)00172-x

Jastreboff, P. J., and Jastreboff, M. M. (2006). Tinnitus retraining therapy: a different view on tinnitus. *ORL J. Otorhinolaryngol. Relat. Spec.* 68, 23–29. discussion 29-30. doi: 10.1159/000090487

Jurcak, V., Tsuzuki, D., and Dan, I. (2007). 10/20, 10/10, and 10/5 systems revisited: their validity as relative head-surface-based positioning systems. *Neuroimage* 34, 1600–1611. doi: 10.1016/j.neuroimage.2006.09.024

Kim, K., Punte, A. K., Mertens, G., Van de Heyning, P., Park, K. J., Choi, H., et al. (2015). A novel method for device-related electroencephalography artifact suppression to explore cochlear implant-related cortical changes in single-sided deafness. *J. Neurosci. Methods* 255, 22–28. doi: 10.1016/j.jneumeth.2015.07.020

Kim, S. H., Jang, J. H., Lee, S. Y., Han, J. J., Koo, J. W., Vanneste, S., et al. (2016). Neural substrates predicting short-term improvement of tinnitus loudness and distress after modified tinnitus retraining therapy. *Sci. Rep.* 6:29140. doi: 10.1038/srep29140

Korucuoglu, O., Gladwin, T. E., and Wiers, R. W. (2016). The effect of acute alcohol on motor-related EEG asymmetries during preparation of approach or avoid alcohol responses. *Biol. Psychol.* 114, 81–92. doi: 10.1016/j.biopsycho.2015.12.012

Kringelbach, M. L. (2005). The human orbitofrontal cortex: linking reward to hedonic experience. *Nat. Rev. Neurosci.* 6, 691–702. doi: 10.1038/nrn1747

Lancaster, J. L., Woldorff, M. G., Parsons, L. M., Liotti, M., Freitas, C. S., Rainey, L., et al. (2000). Automated talairach atlas labels for functional brain mapping. *Hum. Brain Mapp.* 10, 120–131. doi: 10.1002/1097-0193(200007)10:3<120::aid-hbm30>3.0.co;2-8

Landgrebe, M., Langguth, B., Rosengarth, K., Braun, S., Koch, A., Kleinjung, T., et al. (2009). Structural brain changes in tinnitus: grey matter decrease in auditory and non-auditory brain areas. *Neuroimage* 46, 213–218. doi: 10.1016/j.neuroimage.2009.01.069

Langguth, B., Kreuzer, P. M., Kleinjung, T., and De Ridder, D. (2013). Tinnitus: causes and clinical management. *Lancet Neurol.* 12, 920–930. doi: 10.1016/S1474-4422(13)70160-1

Leaver, A. M., Renier, L., Chevillet, M. A., Morgan, S., Kim, H. J., and Rauschecker, J. P. (2011). Dysregulation of limbic and auditory networks in tinnitus. *Neuron* 69, 33–43. doi: 10.1016/j.neuron.2010.12.002

Leaver, A. M., Seydell-Greenwald, A., Turesky, T. K., Morgan, S., Kim, H. J., and Rauschecker, J. P. (2012). Cortico-limbic morphology separates tinnitus from tinnitus distress. *Front. Syst. Neurosci.* 6:21. doi: 10.3389/fnsys.2012.00021

Lee, S. Y., Nam, D. W., Koo, J. W., De Ridder, D., Vanneste, S., and Song, J. J. (2017). No auditory experience, no tinnitus: lessons from subjects with congenital- and acquired single-sided deafness. *Hear. Res.* 354, 9–15. doi: 10.1016/j.heares.2017.08.002

Lee, S. Y., Song, S. K., Park, S. J., Park, H. G., Choi, B. Y., Koo, J. W., et al. (2019). Jugular bulb resurfacing with bone cement for patients with high dehiscent jugular bulb and ipsilateral pulsatile tinnitus. *Otol. Neurotol.* 40, 192–199. doi: 10.1097/MAO.0000000000002093

Llinás, R. R., Ribary, U., Jeanmonod, D., Kronberg, E., and Mitra, P. P. (1999). Thalamocortical dysrhythmia: a neurological and neuropsychiatric syndrome characterized by magnetoencephalography. *Proc. Natl. Acad. Sci. U.S.A.* 96, 15222–15227. doi: 10.1073/pnas.96.26.15222

Lopez Rincon, A., and Shimoda, S. (2016). The inverse problem in electroencephalography using the bidomain model of electrical activity. *J. Neurosci. Methods* 274, 94–105. doi: 10.1016/j.jneumeth.2016.09.011

Mazurek, B., Fischer, F., Haupt, H., Georgiewa, P., Reisshauer, A., and Klapp, B. F. (2006). A modified version of tinnitus retraining therapy: observing long-term outcome and predictors. *Audiol. Neurootol.* 11, 276–286. doi: 10.1159/000093526

Meyer, M., Luethi, M. S., Neff, P., Langer, N., and Buchi, S. (2014). Disentangling tinnitus distress and tinnitus presence by means of EEG power analysis. *Neural Plast.* 2014:468546. doi: 10.1155/2014/468546

Milz, P., Faber, P. L., Lehmann, D., Kochi, K., and Pascual-Marqui, R. D. (2014). sLORETA intracortical lagged coherence during breath counting in meditation-naive participants. *Front. Hum. Neurosci.* 8:303. doi: 10.3389/fnhum.2014.00303

Moazami-Goudarzi, M., Michels, L., Weisz, N., and Jeanmonod, D. (2010). Temporo-insular enhancement of EEG low and high frequencies in patients with chronic tinnitus. QEEG study of chronic tinnitus patients. *BMC Neurosci.* 11:40. doi: 10.1186/1471-2202-11-40

Newman, C. W., Jacobson, G. P., and Spitzer, J. B. (1996). Development of the Tinnitus Handicap Inventory. *Arch. Otolaryngol. Head Neck Surg.* 122, 143–148.

Newman, C. W., Sandridge, S. A., and Jacobson, G. P. (1998). Psychometric adequacy of the tinnitus handicap inventory (THI) for evaluating treatment outcome. *J. Am. Acad. Audiol.* 9, 153–160.

Nichols, T. E., and Holmes, A. P. (2002). Nonparametric permutation tests for functional neuroimaging: a primer with examples. *Hum. Brain Mapp.* 15, 1–25. doi: 10.1002/hbm.1058

Ortmann, M., Müller, N., Schlee, W., and Weisz, N. (2011). Rapid increases of gamma power in the auditory cortex following noise trauma in humans. *Eur. J. Neurosci.* 33, 568–575. doi: 10.1111/j.1460-9568.2010.07542.x

Pascual-Marqui, R. D. (2002). Standardized low-resolution brain electromagnetic tomography (sLORETA): technical details. *Methods Find. Exp. Clin. Pharmacol.* 24, 5–12.

Phillips, J. S., and McFerran, D. (2010). Tinnitus retraining therapy (TRT) for tinnitus. *Cochrane Database Syst. Rev.* 3:CD007330.

Rolls, E. T. (2004). The functions of the orbitofrontal cortex. *Brain Cogn.* 55, 11–29.

Sedley, W., Teki, S., Kumar, S., Barnes, G. R., Bamiou, D. E., and Griffiths, T. D. (2012). Single-subject oscillatory gamma responses in tinnitus. *Brain* 135(Pt 10), 3089–3100. doi: 10.1093/brain/aws220

Sherlin, L., and Congedo, M. (2005). Obsessive-compulsive dimension localized using low-resolution brain electromagnetic tomography (LORETA). *Neurosci. Lett.* 387, 72–74. doi: 10.1016/j.neulet.2005.06.069

Shim, Y. J., Bae, Y. J., An, G. S., Lee, K., Kim, Y., Lee, S. Y., et al. (2019). Involvement of the internal auditory canal in subjects with cochlear otosclerosis: a less acknowledged third window that affects surgical outcome. *Otol. Neurotol.* 40, e186–e190. doi: 10.1097/MAO.0000000000002144

Siepmann, M., and Kirch, W. (2002). Effects of caffeine on topographic quantitative EEG. *Neuropsychobiology* 45, 161–166. doi: 10.1159/000054958

Smits, M., Kovacs, S., De Ridder, D., Peeters, R. R., Van Hecke, P., and Sunaert, S. (2007). Lateralization of functional magnetic resonance imaging (fMRI) activation in the auditory pathway of patients with lateralized tinnitus. *Neuroradiology* 49, 669–679. doi: 10.1007/s00234-007-0231-3

Song, J. J., De Ridder, D., Van de Heyning, P., and Vanneste, S. (2012). Mapping tinnitus-related brain activation: an activation-likelihood estimation metaanalysis of PET studies. *J. Nucl. Med.* 53, 1550–1557. doi: 10.2967/jnumed.112.102939

Song, J. J., Hong, S. K., Lee, S. Y., Park, S. J., Kang, S. I., An, Y. H., et al. (2018). Vestibular manifestations in subjects with enlarged vestibular aqueduct. *Otol. Neurotol.* 39, e461–e467. doi: 10.1097/MAO.0000000000001817

Song, J. J., Kim, K., Sunwoo, W., Mertens, G., Van de Heyning, P., De Ridder, D., et al. (2017). A quantitative electroencephalography study on cochlear implant-induced cortical changes in single-sided deafness with Tinnitus. *Front. Hum. Neurosci.* 11:210. doi: 10.3389/fnhum.2017.00210

Song, J. J., Vanneste, S., and De Ridder, D. (2015a). Dysfunctional noise cancelling of the rostral anterior cingulate cortex in tinnitus patients. *PLoS One* 10:e0123538. doi: 10.1371/journal.pone.0123538

Song, J. J., Vanneste, S., Schlee, W., Van de Heyning, P., and De Ridder, D. (2015b). Onset-related differences in neural substrates of tinnitus-related distress: the anterior cingulate cortex in late-onset tinnitus, and the frontal cortex in early-onset tinnitus. *Brain Struct. Funct.* 220, 571–584. doi: 10.1007/s00429-013-0648-x

Sunwoo, W., Jeon, Y. J., Bae, Y. J., Jang, J. H., Koo, J. W., and Song, J. J. (2017). Typewriter tinnitus revisited: the typical symptoms and the initial response to carbamazepine are the most reliable diagnostic clues. *Sci. Rep.* 7:10615. doi: 10.1038/s41598-017-10798-w

Talairach, J., and Tournoux, P. (1988). *Co-Planar Stereotaxic Atlas of the Human Brain. 3-Dimensional Proportional System: an Approach to Cerebral Imaging.* New York, NY: G. Thieme.

Tinnitus Retraining Therapy Trial Research Group, Scherer, R. W., and Formby, C. (2019). Effect of tinnitus retraining therapy vs standard of care on tinnitus-related quality of life: a randomized clinical trial. *JAMA Otolaryngol. Head Neck Surg.* 145, 597–608. doi: 10.1001/jamaoto.2019.0821

van der Loo, E., Congedo, M., Vanneste, S., Van De Heyning, P., and De Ridder, D. (2011). Insular lateralization in tinnitus distress. *Auton. Neurosci.* 165, 191–194. doi: 10.1016/j.autneu.2011.06.007

Van Der Loo, E., Gais, S., Congedo, M., Vanneste, S., Plazier, M., Menovsky, T., et al. (2009). Tinnitus intensity dependent gamma oscillations of the contralateral auditory cortex. *PLoS One* 4:e7396. doi: 10.1371/journal.pone.0007396

Vanneste, S., and De Ridder, D. (2012). The auditory and non-auditory brain areas involved in tinnitus. An emergent property of multiple parallel overlapping subnetworks. *Front. Syst. Neurosci.* 6:31. doi: 10.3389/fnsys.2012.00031

Vanneste, S., and De Ridder, D. (2016). Deafferentation-based pathophysiological differences in phantom sound: tinnitus with and without hearing loss. *Neuroimage* 129, 80–94. doi: 10.1016/j.neuroimage.2015.12.002

Vanneste, S., Plazier, M., der Loo, E., de Heyning, P. V., Congedo, M., and De Ridder, D. (2010). The neural correlates of tinnitus-related distress. *Neuroimage* 52, 470–480. doi: 10.1016/j.neuroimage.2010.04.029

Vanneste, S., Plazier, M., van der Loo, E., Van de Heyning, P., and De Ridder, D. (2011). The difference between uni- and bilateral auditory phantom percept. *Clin. Neurophysiol.* 122, 578–587. doi: 10.1016/j.clinph.2010.07.022

Vanneste, S., Song, J. J., and De Ridder, D. (2018). Thalamocortical dysrhythmia detected by machine learning. *Nat. Commun.* 9:1103. doi: 10.1038/s41467-018-02820-0

Varela, F., Lachaux, J. P., Rodriguez, E., and Martinerie, J. (2001). The brainweb: phase synchronization and large-scale integration. *Nat. Rev. Neurosci.* 2, 229–239. doi: 10.1038/35067550

Weisz, N., Moratti, S., Meinzer, M., Dohrmann, K., and Elbert, T. (2005). Tinnitus perception and distress is related to abnormal spontaneous brain activity as measured by magnetoencephalography. *PLoS Med.* 2:e153. doi: 10.1371/journal.pmed.0020153

Weisz, N., Müller, S., Schlee, W., Dohrmann, K., Hartmann, T., and Elbert, T. (2007). The neural code of auditory phantom perception. *J. Neurosci.* 27, 1479–1484. doi: 10.1523/jneurosci.3711-06.2007

Permissions

All chapters in this book were first published by Frontiers; hereby published with permission under the Creative Commons Attribution License or equivalent. Every chapter published in this book has been scrutinized by our experts. Their significance has been extensively debated. The topics covered herein carry significant findings which will fuel the growth of the discipline. They may even be implemented as practical applications or may be referred to as a beginning point for another development.

The contributors of this book come from diverse backgrounds, making this book a truly international effort. This book will bring forth new frontiers with its revolutionizing research information and detailed analysis of the nascent developments around the world.

We would like to thank all the contributing authors for lending their expertise to make the book truly unique. They have played a crucial role in the development of this book. Without their invaluable contributions this book wouldn't have been possible. They have made vital efforts to compile up to date information on the varied aspects of this subject to make this book a valuable addition to the collection of many professionals and students.

This book was conceptualized with the vision of imparting up-to-date information and advanced data in this field. To ensure the same, a matchless editorial board was set up. Every individual on the board went through rigorous rounds of assessment to prove their worth. After which they invested a large part of their time researching and compiling the most relevant data for our readers.

The editorial board has been involved in producing this book since its inception. They have spent rigorous hours researching and exploring the diverse topics which have resulted in the successful publishing of this book. They have passed on their knowledge of decades through this book. To expedite this challenging task, the publisher supported the team at every step. A small team of assistant editors was also appointed to further simplify the editing procedure and attain best results for the readers.

Apart from the editorial board, the designing team has also invested a significant amount of their time in understanding the subject and creating the most relevant covers. They scrutinized every image to scout for the most suitable representation of the subject and create an appropriate cover for the book.

The publishing team has been an ardent support to the editorial, designing and production team. Their endless efforts to recruit the best for this project, has resulted in the accomplishment of this book. They are a veteran in the field of academics and their pool of knowledge is as vast as their experience in printing. Their expertise and guidance has proved useful at every step. Their uncompromising quality standards have made this book an exceptional effort. Their encouragement from time to time has been an inspiration for everyone.

The publisher and the editorial board hope that this book will prove to be a valuable piece of knowledge for researchers, students, practitioners and scholars across the globe.

List of Contributors

Jinghua Hu, Jin-Jing Xu, Yuanqing Wu and Jianwei Qi
Department of Otolaryngology, Nanjing First Hospital, Nanjing Medical University, Nanjing, China

Xuan Wei, Han Lv, Pengling Ren, Peng Zhang, Qian Chen, Yawen Liu, Pengfei Zhao, Zhenghan Yang and Zhenchang Wang
Department of Radiology, Beijing Friendship Hospital, Capital Medical University, Beijing, China

Songjian Wang, Meng Lin, Liwei Sun, Chunlin Li and Xu Zhang
School of Biomedical Engineering, Capital Medical University, Beijing, China
Beijing Key Laboratory of Fundamental Research on Biomechanics in Clinical Application, Capital Medical University, Beijing, China

Xueqing Chen, Xinxing Fu and LiLi Yan
Key Laboratory of Otolaryngology Head and Neck Surgery, Beijing Tongren Hospital, Beijing Institute of Otolaryngology, Ministry of Education, Beijing, China

Wenqing Xia, Yong Luo and Jianhua Ma
Department of Endocrinology, Nanjing First Hospital, Nanjing Medical University, Nanjing, China

Byung Yoon Choi
Department of Otorhinolaryngology-Head and Neck Surgery, Seoul National University Bundang Hospital, Seongnam, South Korea

Sang-Yeon Lee, Ja-Won Koo and Jae-Jin Song
Department of Otorhinolaryngology-Head and Neck Surgery, Seoul National University Bundang Hospital, Seongnam, South Korea
Department of Otolaryngology-Head and Neck Surgery, Seoul National University Bundang Hospital, Seongnam, South Korea

Yoonjoong Kim
Department of Otolaryngology-Head and Neck Surgery, Seoul National University Bundang Hospital, Seongnam, South Korea

Dirk De Ridder
Unit of Neurosurgery, Department of Surgical Sciences, Dunedin School of Medicine, University of Otago, Dunedin, New Zealand

Zhaodi Wang, Chunli Liu and Shusheng Gong
Department of Otolaryngology Head and Neck Surgery, Beijing Friendship Hospital, Capital Medical University, Beijing, China

Suijun Chen, Yanhong Chen, Maojin Liang, Yuexin Cai, Wenrui Li, Zhaopeng Tong, Wenchao Xu, Jiahong Li, Guisheng Chen, Liping Lan and Yiqing Zheng
Department of Otolaryngology, Sun Yat-sen Memorial Hospital, Sun Yat-sen University, Guangzhou, China
Institute of Hearing and Speech-Language Science, Sun Yat-sen University, Guangzhou, China

Mingwei Xie, Yun Su, Xiaoyan Wu and Jun Shen
Department of Radiology, Sun Yat-sen Memorial Hospital, Sun Yat-sen University, Guangzhou, China

Caiping Dang
Affiliated Brain Hospital of Guangzhou Medical University, Guangzhou, China
Department of Psychology, Guangzhou Medical University, Guangzhou, China

Xiaofeng Lin and Ningyi Jiang
Department of Nuclear Medicine, Sun Yat-sen Memorial Hospital, Sun Yat-sen University, Guangzhou, China
Department of Nuclear Medicine, The Seventh Affiliated Hospital, Sun Yat-sen University, Shenzhen, China

Yueyao Chen
Department of Radiology, Shenzhen Traditional Chinese Medicine Hospital, Shenzhen, China

Mingxia Wang
Department of Hearing and Speech Sciences, Xinhua College of Sun Yat-sen University, Guangzhou, China

Chao Song, Xiaoping Yuan and Qingyu Liu
Department of Radiology, Sun Yat-sen Memorial Hospital, Sun Yat-sen University, Guangzhou, China

Bingling Lin
Department of Radiology, Peking University Shen Zhen Hospital, Shenzhen, China

Haidi Yang
Department of Otolaryngology, Sun Yat-sen Memorial Hospital, Sun Yat-sen University, Guangzhou, China

Jae Joon Han
Department of Otorhinolaryngology-Head and Neck Surgery, Soonchunhyang University College of Medicine, Seoul Hospital, Seoul, South Korea

Sven Vanneste
Lab for Clinical and Integrative Neuroscience, Trinity College of Neuroscience, Trinity College Dublin, Dublin, Ireland
Laboratory for Clinical and Integrative Neuroscience, School of Behavioral and Brain Sciences, The University of Texas at Dallas, Dallas, TX, United States

Zihao Zhang, Xiuqin Jia, Yuelei Lyu and Tao Jiang
Department of Radiology, Beijing Chaoyang Hospital, Capital Medical University, Beijing, China

Xiaojiao Guan
Department of Radiology, Beijing Shijitan Hospital, Capital Medical University, Beijing, China

Yi Zhang and Jing Yang
Department of Hyperbaric Oxygen, Beijing Chaoyang Hospital, Capital Medical University, Beijing, China

Wan Chen
State Key Laboratory of Ophthalmology, Zhongshan Ophthalmic Center, Sun Yat-sen University, Guangzhou, China

Fei Zhao
Department of Speech Language Therapy and Hearing Science, Cardiff Metropolitan University, Cardiff, United Kingdom
Department of Hearing and Speech Science, Xinhua College, Sun Yat-sen University, Guangzhou, China

Yihsin Tai and Kelly Roth
Department of Speech and Hearing Science, University of Illinois at Urbana-Champaign, Champaign, IL, United States

Benjamin Zimmerman
Department of Speech and Hearing Science, University of Illinois at Urbana-Champaign, Champaign, IL, United States
Beckman Institute for Advanced Science and Technology, University of Illinois at Urbana-Champaign, Champaign, IL, United States

Megan Finnegan and Fatima T. Husain
Department of Speech and Hearing Science, University of Illinois at Urbana-Champaign, Champaign, IL, United States
Beckman Institute for Advanced Science and Technology, University of Illinois at Urbana-Champaign, Champaign, IL, United States
Neuroscience Program, University of Illinois at Urbana-Champaign, Champaign, IL, United States

Sara Schmidt
Beckman Institute for Advanced Science and Technology, University of Illinois at Urbana-Champaign, Champaign, IL, United States
Neuroscience Program, University of Illinois at Urbana-Champaign, Champaign, IL, United States

Subhadeep Paul
Department of Statistics, The Ohio State University, Columbus, OH, United States

Yuguo Chen
Department of Statistics, University of Illinois at Urbana-Champaign, Champaign, IL, United States

Lv Han, Zhao Pengfei, Wang Hao, Cheng Xu, Zhang Peng, Wang Zheng, Yang Zhenghan and Wang Zhenchang
Department of Radiology, Beijing Friendship Hospital, Capital Medical University, Beijing, China

Zeng Na
National Clinical Research Center for Digestive Diseases, Beijing Friendship Hospital, Capital Medical University, Beijing, China

Gong Shusheng
Department of Otolaryngology Head and Neck Surgery, Beijing Friendship Hospital, Capital Medical University, Beijing, China

Liu Chunli
Department of Otolaryngology Head and Neck Surgery, Beijing Friendship Hospital, Capital Medical University, Beijing, China
Department of Otolaryngology, Affiliated Hospital of Chengde Medical College, Chengde, China

Chen Yuchen
Department of Radiology, Nanjing First Hospital, Nanjing Medical University, Nanjing, China

Zhicheng Li
Department of Otolaryngology-Head and Neck Surgery, Third Affiliated Hospital of Sun Yat-sen University, Guangzhou, China
Department of Psychology and Center for Studies of Psychological Application, South China Normal University, Guangzhou, China

Min Qi, Jintian Cen, Shuqi Zhang, Jing Gu and Xiangli Zeng
Department of Otolaryngology-Head and Neck Surgery, Third Affiliated Hospital of Sun Yat-sen University, Guangzhou, China

Qi Chen
Department of Psychology and Center for Studies of Psychological Application, South China Normal University, Guangzhou, China

Ruolei Gu
Key Laboratory of Behavioral Science, Institute of Psychology, Chinese Academy of Sciences, Beijing, China

Chang-Dong Wang
School of Data and Computer Science, Sun Yat-sen University, Guangzhou, China

Cai-Ping Dang
Affiliated Brain Hospital of Guangzhou Medical University, Guangzhou, China
Department of Psychology, Guangzhou Medical University, Guangzhou, China

Jianheng Liang and Nannan He
College of Mathematics and Informatics, South China Agricultural University, Guangzhou, China

Xiao-Min Xu, Yun Jiao, Tian-Yu Tang, Chun-Qiang Lu, Sheng-Hong Ju, Jian Zhang and Gao-Jun Teng
Jiangsu Key Laboratory of Molecular and Functional Imaging, Department of Radiology, Zhongda Hospital, Medical School of Southeast University, Nanjing, China

Richard Salvi
Center for Hearing and Deafness, University at Buffalo, Buffalo, NY, United States

Ying Luan, Congxiao Wang and Tianyu Tang
Jiangsu Key Laboratory of Molecular and Functional Imaging, Department of Radiology, Zhongda Hospital, Medical School of Southeast University, Nanjing, China

Xiaoxiao Xie
Department of Radiology, The Second Affiliated Hospital and Yuying Children's Hospital of Wenzhou Medical University, Wenzhou, China

Yongbo Liu
Department of Radiology, Shanxi Lu'an General Hospital, Changzhi, China

Xiaowei Han
Graduate School, Chinese Academy of Medical Sciences, Peking Union Medical College, Beijing, China
Department of Radiology, Heping Hospital of Changzhi Medical College, Changzhi, China

Junfeng Li
Department of Radiology, Heping Hospital of Changzhi Medical College, Changzhi, China

Pei Liu
Graduate School, Beijing University of Chinese Medicine, Beijing, China

Hui Qiu
Graduate School, Changzhi Medical College, Changzhi, China

Huachen Yu
Department of Orthopedics, The Second Affiliated Hospital and Yuying Children's Hospital of Wenzhou Medical University, Wenzhou, China

Jihye Rhee
Department of Otolaryngology-Head and Neck Surgery, Seoul Veterans Hospital, Seoul, South Korea

Ye Ji Shim
Department of Otolaryngology-Head & Neck Surgery, Seoul National University Hospital, Healthcare System Gangnam Center, Seoul, South Korea

Jinluan Cui, Yuan Feng, Wei Yong, Huiyou Chen, Yu-Chen Chen and Xindao Yin
Department of Radiology, Nanjing First Hospital, Nanjing Medical University, Nanjing, China

Tao Zhang
Department of Otolaryngology–Head and Neck Surgery, The First Affiliated Hospital of Jinan University, Guangzhou, China

Wei-Wei Cai
Department of Otolaryngology–Head and Neck Surgery, The First Affiliated Hospital of Jinan University, Guangzhou, China
Department of Otolaryngology–Head and Neck Surgery, Panyu Central Hospital, Guangzhou, China

Zhi-cheng Li and Qin-tai Yang
Department of Otolaryngology–Head and Neck Surgery, The Third Affiliated Hospital, Sun Yat-sen University, Guangzhou, China

Index

www.ingramcontent.com/pod-product-compliance
Lightning Source LLC
LaVergne TN
LVHW082140200926
848484LV00008B/2084
9798887400815